Visit our website

to find out about other books from W.B. Saunders
and our sister companies in Harcourt Health S

Register free at
www.harcourt-international.com

and you will get

- **the latest information on new books, journals and electronic products in your chosen subject areas**

- **the choice of e-mail or post alerts or both, when there are any new books in your chosen areas**

- **news of special offers and promotions**

- **information about products from all Harcourt Health Sciences companies including W. B. Saunders, Churchill Livingstone and Mosby**

You will also find an easily searchable catalogue, online ordering, information on our extensive list of journals ... and much more!

Visit the Harcourt Health Sciences website today!

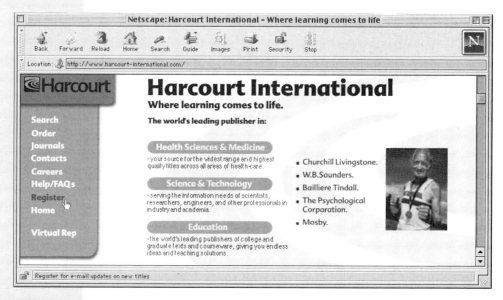

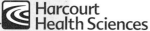

Commissioning Editor: Serena Bureau
Project Manager: Joanne Scott/Scott Millar
Production Manager: Mark Sanderson

Equine Locomotion

Edited by

Willem Back, DVM, PhD, Dipl. ECVS, Dipl. RNVA
Assistant Professor in Equine Surgery
Department of Equine Sciences
Faculty of Veterinary Medicine
Utrecht University
Utrecht
The Netherlands

and

Hilary M. Clayton, BVMS, PhD, MRCVS
McPhail Dressage Chair in Equine Sports Medicine
Department of Large Animal Clinical Sciences
College of Veterinary Medicine
Michigan State University
East Lansing
Michigan
USA

W.B. SAUNDERS

London • Edinburgh • New York • Philadelphia • St Louis • Sydney • Toronto 2001

WB SAUNDERS
An imprint of Harcourt Publishers Limited

© Harcourt Publishers Limited 2001

First published 2001

ISBN 0–7020–2483–X

British Library Cataloguing in Publication Data
A catalogue record for this book is available from the British Library

Library of Congress Cataloging in Publication Data
A catalog record for this book is available from the Library of Congress

Note
Medical knowledge is constantly changing. As new information becomes available,
changes in treatment, procedures, equipment and the use of drugs become
necessary. The editors and contributors and the publishers have taken care to ensure
that the information given in this text is accurate and up to date. However, readers are
strongly advised to confirm that the information, especially with regard to drug
usage, complies with the latest legislation and standards of practice.

The
Publisher's
policy is to use
paper manufactured
from sustainable forests

Printed in UK

Contents

Contributors

R. McNeill Alexander, FRS
Professor of Zoology
School of Biology
University of Leeds
Leeds
UK

Adam Arabian, BSC, MS
Department of Large Animal Clinical Sciences
College of Veterinary Medicine
Michigan State University
East Lansing, Michigan
USA

Fabrice Audigié, DVM, PHD
Assistant Professor in Equine Diagnostic Imaging
CIRALE-École Nationale Vétérinaire d'Alfort
Maisons-Alfort
France

Willem Back, DVM, PHD, DIPL. ECVS, DIPL. RNVA
Assistant Professor in Equine Surgery
Department of Equine Sciences
Faculty of Veterinary Medicine
Utrecht University
Utrecht
The Netherlands

Albert Barneveld, DVM, PHD, DIPL. RNVA
Professor in Equine and Bovine Surgery
Department of Equine Sciences
Faculty of Veterinary Medicine
Utrecht University
Utrecht
The Netherlands

Eric Barrey, DVM, PHD
INRA
Research Associate
Quantative Genetics Laboratory
Jouy-en-Josas
France

Helen L. Birch, BSC, PHD
Lecturer in Musculoskeletal Pathobiology
Royal Veterinary College and Institute of Orthopaedics UCL
Hatfield
Herts
UK

Anton J. van den Bogert, PHD
Department of Biomedical Engineering
Cleveland Clinic Foundation
Cleveland, OH
USA

H.H. Florian Buchner, DR. MED. VET., PHD
Associate Professor of Orthopedics in
    Large Animals
Clinic for Orthopedics in Ungulates
University of Veterinary Medicine Vienna
Vienna
Austria

Hilary M. Clayton, BVMS, PHD, MRCVS
McPhail Dressage Chair in Equine
    Sports Medicine
Department of Large Animal Clinical Sciences
College of Veterinary Medicine
Michigan State University
East Lansing, Michigan
USA

Jean Marie Denoix, DVM, PHD, AGRÉGATION
    IN ANATOMY
Professor in Equine Anatomy and Diagnostic
    Imaging
CIRALE-École Nationale Vétérinaire d'Alfort
Maisons-Alfort
France

Nancy R. Deuel, MS, PHD
Unit 16
St. Michaels
MA
USA

Mathew P. Gerard, BVSC, DIPL. ACVS
Department of Veterinary Clinical Sciences
Faculty of Veterinary Science
University of Sydney
Australia

Allen E. Goodship, BVSC, PHD
Professor of Orthopaedic Sciences
Royal Veterinary College and Institute of Orthopaedics UCL
Hatfield
Herts
UK

Albert Gramsbergen, PHD, MD
Professor of Developmental Neurosciences
Department of Medical Physiology
University of Groningen
Groningen
The Netherlands

David R. Hodgson, BVSC, PHD, FACSM, DIPL. ACVIM
Head, Department of Veterinary Clinical Sciences
Faculty of Veterinary Science
University of Sydney
Narellan Delivery Centre
Australia

At L. Hof, PHD
Associate Professor in Biomechanics
Department of Medical Physiology
University of Groningen
Groningen
The Netherlands

Mikael Holmström, DVM, PHD
Horse Interactive Sweden AB
Hollviken
Sweden

Liduin S. Meershoek, MSC
Department of Veterinary Anatomy and
    Physiology
Faculty of Veterinary Medicine
Utrecht University
Utrecht
The Netherlands

Henk C. Schamhardt, PHD
Associate Professor in Equine Biomechanics
Department of Veterinary Anatomy and
    Physiology
Faculty of Veterinary Medicine
Utrecht University
Utrecht
The Netherlands

P. René van Weeren, DVM, PHD, DIPL. ECVS, DIPL. RNVA
Associate Professor in Equine Surgery
Department of Equine Sciences
Faculty of Veterinary Medicine
Utrecht University
Utrecht
The Netherlands

Foreword

Horse locomotion has lost most of the practical importance it had in past centuries, but a great many people remain passionately interested in horses for leisure, racing or other purposes. This, and the high value of horses, sustain veterinary interest in the species.

Horses have also attracted the interest of many research scientists. Muybridge's (1899) sequences of photographs of horses in motion, taken with multiple cameras before the cine camera had been invented, have an honored place in the history of motion pictures. Camp and Smith's (1942) study of the digital ligaments of horses was an early recognition of the importance of tendon and ligament elasticity in running; horses, people, dogs, kangaroos and many other animals save energy by bouncing along, using their tendons like the spring of a child's pogo stick. Horses were particularly good material for this study because their adaptations for elastic energy savings are surpassed only by the camel (Dimery et al., 1986). Recent research provides many examples of research on horses that has wide significance for the understanding of animal and human movement. I will cite just a few of my favourites.

Most quadrupedal mammals walk, trot and gallop, but the significance of changing gaits became apparent only when Hoyt and Taylor (1981) trained ponies to change gait on command, so that they could be made (for example) to trot at speeds at which they would have preferred to walk, and vice versa. By measurements of oxygen consumption they showed that walking is the gait that needs least energy at low speeds, trotting at intermediate speeds, and galloping at high speeds, and that each gait is used in the range of speeds in which it is most economical. Bramble and Carrier (1983) depended largely on observations of horses for their demonstration that galloping mammals take one breath per stride, their breathing apparently driven by the movements of locomotion. They speculated that this might depend on the viscera functioning as an inertial piston, shifting forward and back in the trunk as the animal accelerated and decelerated in the course of each stride. Disappointingly, this seems not to be the case; the breathing of a galloping horse seems to be driven by the bending and extension of the back, functioning like a bellows (Young et al., 1992). Horses gave us valuable insight into the stresses that bones have to withstand when surgically implanted strain gauges were used to record strains in the lower leg bones of running and jumping horses (Biewener et al.,

1983). It was in a study of horses that Rome et al., (1990) showed us the remarkable range of properties that can be found within a single muscle. Some fibers in the soleus muscle of horses are capable of contracting ten times faster than others. And observations on horses were the first to show that tendons can be damaged by overheating, by heat liberated by the repeated stretching and recoil, that occurs in running (Wilson & Goodship, 1994).

Besides these studies that have wide significance, there have been others, equally fascinating, that concern horses alone. The reciprocal apparatus in the hindlimb makes movements of the stifle joint drive those of the hock (van Weeren et al., 1992). The hooves of horses have been shown to be designed in a remarkably sophisticated way, to withstand impact on the ground (Thomason et al., 1992). The hock joint of horses has bistable properties that make it click like an electric switch from one extreme position to the other, a property which, curiously, is much more marked in domestic horses than in zebra or Przewalski's horse (Alexander & Trestik, 1989).

These examples make it clear that horse locomotion has inspired a great deal of excellent and interesting science, much of which throws light on the biology of other animals, as well as of horses. That is one reason why this book will be so welcome. Another is that it has been written by a carefully chosen team of scientists whose research has added substantially to our knowledge of horse locomotion.

Sadly, the team has been depleted by the death of Henk Schamhardt, co-author of one of our chapters, who was pre-eminent among researchers in the field of equine biomechanics.

R. McNeill Alexander FRS
Professor of Zoology
University of Leeds

REFERENCES

Alexander, R. McN. and Trestik, C.L. (1989) Bistable properties of the hock joint of horses. *J. Zool.* **218**: 383–391.
Biewener, A.A., Thomason, J. and Lanyon, L.E. (1983) Mechanics of locomotion and jumping in the forelimb of the horse (*Equus*): *In vivo* stress developed in the radius and metacarpus. *J. Zool.* **201**: 67–82.

Bramble, D.M. and Carrier, D.R. (1983) Running and breathing in mammals. *Science* **219**: 251–256.

Camp, C.L. and Smith, N. (1942) Phylogeny and function of the digital ligaments of the horse. *University of California Memoirs in Zoology* **13**: 69–124.

Dimery, N.J., Alexander, R.McN. and Ker, R.F. (1986) Elastic extensions of leg tendons in the locomotion of horses (*Equus caballus*). *J. Zool.* **210**: 415–425.

Hoyt, D.F. and Taylor, C.R. (1981) Gait and the energetics of locomotion in horses. *Nature* **292**: 239–240.

Muybridge, E. (1899) *Animals in Motion.* London: Chapman and Hall.

Rome, L.C., Sosnicki, A.A. and Goble, D.O. (1990) Maximum velocity of shortening of three fibre types from horse soleus muscle: implications for scaling with body size. *J. Physiol.* **431**: 173–185.

Thomason, J.J., Biewener, A.A. and Bertram, J.E.A. (1992) Surface strain on the equine hoof wall *in vivo*: implications for the material design and functional morphology of the wall. *J. Exp. Biol.* **166**: 145–168.

van Weeren, P.R., Jansen, M.O., van den Bogert, A.J. and Barneveld, A. (1992) A kinematic and strain gauge study of the reciprocal apparatus in the equine hind limb. *J. Biomech.* **25**: 1291–1301.

Wilson, A.M. and Goodship, A.E. (1994) Exercise-induced hyperthermia as a possible mechanism for tendon degeneration. *J. Biomech.* **27**: 899–905.

Young, I.S., Alexander, R.McN., Woakes, A.J., Butler, P.J. and Anderson, L. (1992) The synchronisation of ventilation and locomotion in horses (*Equus caballus*). *J. Exp. Biol.* **166**: 19–31.

Preface

As a result of their diverse athletic abilities, horses have been used as beasts of burden, as vehicles of war and as partners in sports and recreation. The past century has seen an explosion in the popularity of equestrian sports with a concomitant increase in competition standards. The expectations for performance in today's competition horse require a high level of care and training, which can be achieved only through a comprehensive understanding of the anatomy and physiology of the elite equine athlete. The scientific community responded to this need for information by embracing the discipline of equine sports science, which has developed in parallel with the growth of equestrian sports. Gait analysis, which is the study of locomotion, is an area of equine sports science that has made great strides (quite literally) in the last 30 years.

By 1991, gait analysis was sufficiently established as a scientific discipline to warrant the establishment of an International Workshop on Animal Locomotion (IWAL). The idea of IWAL was conceived and brought to fruition by Henk Schamhardt and Ton van den Bogert at Utrecht University. Subsequent IWALs have been organized by Hilary Clayton in California in 1993 and by Eric Barrey in Saumur, France in 1996. By the time this book is published, Florian Buchner will have organized IWAL4 in Vienna and IWAL5 will be in the planning stages.

Each IWAL proceedings contains a collection of manuscripts that reflects the recent and on-going research projects in locomotion laboratories around the world. Although these proceedings have proven to be a valuable resource, the information they contain is not intended to cover the various aspects of the discipline completely. The need for a more comprehensive source of information on equine locomotion was recognized by Wim Back. W.B. Saunders supported the concept and Hilary Clayton was enlisted to assist in the editorial duties. Our goal in producing this book is to give the reader a complete picture of the horse in motion, as we now know it. The book begins with a history of man's association with the horse both in sports and in veterinary medicine, which sets the stage for a comprehensive description of the present state of knowledge beginning with the initiation of gait and ending with the more futuristic area of computer modeling. In areas where studies of horses are lacking, ideas from other species have been introduced. The list of authors comprises individuals who are acknowledged experts in their subject areas. We thank them for the enormous time and effort they have invested in producing this book.

Unfortunately, one of our most esteemed authors, Henk C. Schamhardt, PhD, died in an accident on June 26th 1999 during his sabbatical leave in Australia. As a leading member of the Utrecht Equine Biomechanics Research Group, Henk made an enormous contribution to the development of equine biomechanics across the world. Those who did not know Henk personally are familiar with his work through his excellent conference presentations, numerous publications, and his role as co-editor of the proceedings of the first two IWALs. As a result of his generosity in sharing his skills and knowledge, Henk acted as a mentor to a new generation of researchers in equine locomotion and biomechanics. It is a fitting tribute to dedicate this book to him.

It has been an honour and a pleasure to edit this millennium book about the locomotion of our mutual friend, the horse. As our Swedish colleagues would say while standing with one boot on a chair and the other one on the table "To the horse!"

Willem Back (Utrecht, The Netherlands)
Hilary Clayton (East Lansing, Michigan, USA)
2000

Acknowledgements

We thank the staff at W. B. Saunders, especially Catriona Byres, Deborah Russell, Rachel Robson, Joanne Scott, Samantha Tooby, Serena Bureau and Scott Millar for their help in completing this book.

We must also recognize the important role of our families, Wim's wife Tia and their children Niels, Floris and Milou, and Hilary's husband Richard. We appreciate their support and tolerance of the time we spent working on the book, which was usually during off duty hours.

Glossary

Nancy R. Deuel

Abduct, abductor, abduction: pertaining to the movement of a body part away from the midsagittal plane.

Acceleration: the time rate change of velocity.

Acceleration due to gravity: the acceleration of a body freely falling in a vacuum, the magnitude of which varies slightly with location. Standardized value at sea level is 9.807 m/s^2.

Accelerometer, accelerometry: pertaining to the measurement of accelerations.

Adduct, adductors, adduction: pertaining to the movement of a body part toward the midsagittal plane.

Advanced completion/lift-off: time elapsing between lift-off of two specified limbs.

Advanced placement: time elapsing between ground contact of two specified limbs.

Air resistance: drag on a body produced by the frictional effects of moving through air.

Airborne phase duration: the duration of a phase of a stride in which an animal is free from contact with the ground.

Allometry: the study of factors that change the shape and functionality of an animal with increasing size.

Angular acceleration: the time rate change of angular velocity.

Angular displacement: the change in orientation of a line segment, as the plane angle between initial and final orientation, regardless of the rotational path taken.

Angular velocity: the time rate change of angular displacement. A vector quantity.

Anterior, anteriorly: toward the head; cephalic or cranial; opposite of posterior or caudal.

Arthromere: one of the body segments of a jointed animal; somite.

Anthrometry: the study of joint movement range and mobility.

Articular, articulate, articulated, articulation: pertaining to a structure constructed of segments united by joints.

Axis: the intersection of two planes.

Biokinematics: kinematics applied to biological systems or entities.

Biokinetics: the study of the forces responsible for the movements of living organisms.

Biomechanics: the application of mechanical laws to living structures.

Biped, bipedal: having, utilizing, or supported by two feet.

Bipedal contact: a portion of the stride in which two limbs are in the stance phase simultaneously.

Biphasic: a movement or measurement with two distinct major amplitudes per cycle.

Canter, rotary: one of two footfall sequences of the canter gait in which the leading forelimb and leading hindlimb are on opposite sides of the body.

Canter, transverse: one of two footfall sequences of the canter gait in which the leading forelimb and leading hindlimb are on the same side of the body.

Caudal, caudad: toward the tail; posterior.

Center of mass: the point about which the total mass of a body is evenly balanced.

Central pattern generators: neural oscillators governing movement and other behaviors, located in the brainstem and/or spinal cord.

Contralateral: located on opposite (left or right) sides of the body.

Cost of transport: the energy expended by an animal in moving a given distance, which may be expressed in kcal/m.

Couplet: two limbs making ground contact relatively close together in time within a stride. A couplet may be diagonal/lateral/fore/hind.

Cranial, craniad: toward the head.

Damping:	a gradual reduction in the amplitude of an oscillating movement.
Density:	the concentration of matter, expressed as mass per unit volume.
Diagonal limb (pair):	a forelimb of one side and the hindlimb of the opposite side. Customarily, the 'right diagonal' is right fore and left hind; 'left diagonal' is left fore and right hind.
Diagonal stance, left/right:	a stride phase in which the diagonal fore and hindlimbs are in contact with the ground.
Diagonal step length, left/right:	the distance along the direction of motion between the diagonal fore and hindlimbs during diagonal stance.
Diagonal suspension, left/right:	a stride phase following left/right diagonal stance during which the animal is airborne, with no limbs in contact with the ground. Left diagonal suspension follows left diagonal stance.
Diagonal width:	the lateral distance between the placements of two diagonal limbs.
Digitize:	transform analog data, e.g. a photographic image, to digital form, e.g. an electronic file.
Direction of motion:	the course or projected course of a body in a straight line from the center of mass.
Displacement:	length measured along a straight line from starting point to finishing point. A vector quantity.
Distal:	away from the main mass of the body; opposite of proximal.
Distance:	a physical quantity of length with measurement units of meters.
Dorsal:	back or upper side, opposite of ventral.
Double support:	a portion of the stride in which exactly two limbs are in the stance phase simultaneously.
Drag:	resistance to motion within a fluid.
Duration:	the period of time during which a given state lasts.
Duty factor:	the duration of the stance phase of a specified limb as a proportion of the total limb cycle duration or stride duration.
Efficiency:	the ratio of useful energy delivered by a dynamic system to the energy supplied to it.
Elastic energy:	the potential energy stored by an object as a result of deformation.
Electrogoniometry, electrogoniometer, electrogoniometric:	pertaining to electrical signals generated by devices which monitor the change in angle of a joint.
Electromyography, electromyographer, electromyographic, EMG:	pertaining to electrical potentials generated by muscle cells during contractions.
Energetics:	the study of energy, force and efficiency.
Extend, extension, extensor (joint):	pertaining to factors which cause an increase in joint angle.
Extended suspension:	airborne phase of the stride that occurs with the vertebral column extended, between lift-off of the leading hindlimb and contact of the trailing forelimb.
Fatigue:	a reduction in power output, comfort, and/or efficiency associated with prolonged or excessive exertion.
Flex, flexion, flexor (joint):	pertaining to factors which cause a reduction in joint angle.
Force:	the mechanical action or effect of one body on another, which causes the bodies to accelerate relative to an inertial reference frame.
Force plate:	a device which measures ground reaction forces.
Frequency:	the number of repetitions of a periodic event which occur within a given time interval, usually expressed in Hz (cycles per second).
Gait:	cyclic pattern of limb movements. Each complete cycle is one stride.
Gallop, rotary:	one of two footfall sequences of the gallop gait in which the leading forelimb and leading hindlimb are on opposite sides of the body.
Gallop, transverse:	one of two footfall sequences of the gallop gait in which the leading forelimb and leading hindlimb are on the same side of the body.

Gathered suspension:	airborne phase of the stride that occurs with the vertebral column flexed, between lift-off of the leading forelimb and contact of the trailing hindlimb.
Ground reaction force:	force of the ground against the limb that acts in opposition to the force exerted by the limb against the ground.
Horsepower:	a quantity of power equal to 735.5 watts (or joules per second) metric system, or 745.7 watts (English system).
Hyperextension:	excessive or extreme extension of a joint, in a range which may cause injury.
Hyperflexion:	excessive or extreme flexion of a joint, in a range which may cause injury.
Impact interval:	the elapsed time between initial ground contacts of two specified limbs.
Ipsilateral limbs:	a forelimb and hindlimb of the same side, either the two left limbs or the two right limbs.
Jump suspension:	the phase during jumping when the horse has no contact with the ground.
Kinematics:	the branch of mechanics that is concerned with the description of movements.
Kinetic energy:	energy of a body associated with translational and rotational motion.
Kinetics:	the study of internal and external forces, energy, power and efficiency involved in the movement of a body.
Lateral:	pertaining to the sides, left and right.
Lateral limbs:	limbs on the same side of the body; ipsilateral fore and hindlimbs.
Lateral stance, left/right:	a stride phase in which two lateral limbs are in contact with the ground.
Lateral step length, left/right:	the distance along the direction of motion between the placements of two specified lateral limbs.
Lateral suspension, left/right:	a stride phase following left/right lateral stance during which the animal is airborne, with no limbs in contact with the ground. Left lateral suspension follows the left lateral stance phase.
Laterality:	asymmetry between the left and right sides of the body in motion or limb usage that occurs naturally and is not accounted for by pathology or injury, as in handedness in humans.
Levator, elevate, elevation:	pertaining to lifting a body part vertically.
Liftoff:	the moment at the end of stance in which the limb leaves the ground.
Liftoff interval:	the elapsed time between the moments when two specified limbs end their stance phases.
Limb, lead/leading:	the second of the two hindlimbs or two forelimbs to touch and leave the ground in each stride of an asymmetrical gait.
Limb, trail/trailing:	the first of the two hindlimbs or two forelimbs to touch and leave the ground in each stride of an asymmetrical gait.
Longitudinal axis:	a line in the median sagittal plane extending from head to tail; anteroposterior axis.
Mass:	characterization of a specific quantity of matter with units of kilograms.
Mass moment of inertia:	the measure of a body's resistance to accelerated angular motion about an axis.
Mechanical energy:	the capacity to do work, equal to the sum of potential energy and kinetic energy.
Modeling:	a theoretical, simplified mathematical construct of a physical phenomenon.
Moment of a couple:	the resultant moment of two equal but oppositely directed, non-collinear parallel forces (the couple).
Moment of a force:	the turning effect (torque) of a force about a point.
Morphometry, morphometric:	the study of the form and dimensions of a body.
Newtons:	the standard unit of force, equivalent to that which will cause a mass of 1 kg to accelerate 1 m/s^2
Normal:	perpendicular to a plane, usually the ground.
Normalize:	mathematically convert measurements to a common frame of reference, to facilitate comparisons between individuals or groups.
Ontogeny:	the sequential development of the individual organism.
Overlap:	one or more stride phases in which two limbs are simultaneously in stance.
Pedobarograph:	device for measuring the pressure distribution beneath the foot.
Phylogeny:	the complete developmental history through evolution of a group of animals.
Pitch:	a motion up and down of the forequarters and/or hindquarters about a lateral axis.

Placement interval:	elapsed time between the impacts of two specified limbs within a stride.
Placement, advanced:	elapsed time between the impacts of two specified limbs within a stride.
Potential energy:	energy of a body associated with position or configuration.
Power:	the rate at which work is done or energy is expended.
Pressure:	the force applied per unit area.
Pronate, pronator, pronation:	pertaining to movement toward a prone position; in locomotion, lateral rotation of the limb which brings the medial portion backward and downward.
Protract, protraction, protractor:	pertaining to moving a body part forward.
Quadriped, quadripedal:	having, utilizing or supported by exactly four feet.
Quadruple support:	a portion of the stride in which all four limbs are in the stance phase simultaneously
Retract, retraction, retractor:	pertaining to moving a body part backward (caudally).
Retrograde motion:	movement opposite to the accustomed direction, i.e. in the caudal direction.
Roll:	a turning motion about the cranial-caudal or longitudinal axis.
Rotation, endo-:	outward rotation of a limb or other body part.
Rotation, exo-:	inward rotation of a limb or other body part.
Rotator:	pertaining to twisting a body part.
Sagittal plane:	plane parallel to the median plane.
Scalar quantity:	a directionless variable expressed completely by its magnitude.
Single support:	a portion of the stride in which only one limb is in the stance phase.
Skin displacement:	movement of the skin relative to underlying skeletal landmarks.
Somit:	body segment
Speed:	the rate of change of distance. A scalar quantity.
Stance:	describes a limb in contact with the ground.
Stance phase:	the portion of the limb motion cycle when the limb is in contact with the ground.
Step:	the movement pattern involved in normal locomotion in transitioning from weight-bearing by one limb to another.
Step height:	the height to which a specified location on a limb is raised from the ground during locomotion.
Step length:	the horizontal distance in the plane of forward motion between two designated limbs at similar stages in their respective limb motion cycles.
Strain:	deformation resulting from the application of stress.
Strain rate:	the rate of strain generation.
Strength:	the maximal force produced by muscular contraction.
Stress:	an external force which acts on a body.
Stride:	a complete cycle of the repetitive series of limb movements that characterize a particular gait.
Stride contact duration:	the total time within the single normal cycle of locomotion in which one or more limbs are in the stance phase.
Stride duration:	the time required to complete one stride.
Stride frequency:	the number of repetitions of the stride per unit time.
Stride length:	the horizontal distance traveled in the plane of progression during a single stride, or between consecutive footprints of the same foot.
Supine, supinator, supination:	pertaining to movement toward a supine position; in locomotion, lateral rotation of the limb which brings the medial portion forward and upward.
Support, double:	ground contact and/or weight bearing by two limbs.
Support phase:	phase of the stride when one or more limbs are in contact with the ground.
Support, quadruple:	ground contact and/or weight bearing by four limbs.
Support, single:	ground contact and/or weight bearing by one limb.
Support, triple:	ground contact and/or weight bearing by three limbs.
Suspension:	a portion of the stride in which all four limbs are simultaneously in the swing phase and free from weight bearing.
Swing phase:	the portion of the limb motion cycle when the limb is free from contact with the ground.

Symmetrical:	a movement or morphology which is substantially similar as a mirror image on left and right sides of the body.
Symmetrical gaits:	those gaits in which the limb coordination pattern of one side repeats that of the other side, half a stride later.
Temporal:	concerning time, duration.
Tension:	the application of forces acting to stretch an object.
Tetrapod, tetrapodal:	having, utilizing, or supported by four feet.
Time:	measurable quantity in the temporal domain, with standardized international units of seconds.
Toe-off:	the instant at the end of stance phase in which the toe is no longer touching the ground.
Torque:	a turning or twisting force; also referred to as moment of force.
Triped, tripedal:	having, utilizing, or supported by three feet.
Tripedal contact:	a portion of the stride in which three limbs are in the stance phase simultaneously.
Ungulate:	hoofed mammal.
Uniped, unipedal:	having, utilizing, or supported by one foot.
Unipedal contact:	a portion of the stride in which one limb is in the stance phase alone.
Units, SI:	the units (or their standard multiples) accepted by the International Society of Biomechanics for scientific measurement, including length in meters; mass in kilograms; time in seconds; plane angle in radians.
Vector quantity:	a quantity that has both magnitude and direction.
Velocity:	the time rate change of displacement. A vector quantity.
Ventral:	toward the underside; opposite of dorsal.
Weight:	the force of gravity acting on a body, equal to the product of mass and the acceleration due to gravity.
Work:	the result of a force acting to displace a body in a given direction.
Yaw:	a turning motion about the dorso-ventral or vertical axis, deviating from a straight course.

Dedication

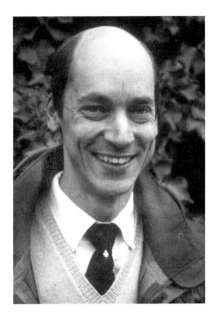

Dr. Henk C. Schamhardt
Respected Scientist, Colleague, Mentor and Friend.
1949–1999

1

History of Locomotor Research

P. René van Weeren

INTRODUCTION

Man has always been fascinated by the creatures that surrounded him. Rock paintings and engravings from prehistoric times show that, apart from man itself, it was the large mammalian species that were most often depicted. Among these, the horse played a prominent role in those latitudes where the species was abundant.

After the domestication of species interest in them naturally deepened as they changed their role from simple animals of prey to that of an important economic entity. The horse, unlike almost all other species, was domesticated for its locomotor capacities rather than as a supplier of food or clothing materials. It was this tremendous capacity to move that for millennia gave the horse its pivotal role in transport in many of the major civilizations on this planet and that also made it a most feared weapon in warfare from ancient times until very recently. As a result of this important role in transportation combined with its proximity to man, the horse became the primary focus when veterinary science developed in the ancient societies and later as it became a flourishing branch of science during the heyday of the Greek and Roman civilizations. It is therefore not surprising that it was during Antiquity that the first scientific comments were made on gait.

The decline of the Antique culture and the subsequent fall of the Roman Empire brought science to a virtual standstill in most of Europe during the dark Middle Ages and it is not until the Renaissance that we see a renewed scientific interest that also extends to veterinary medicine. First directed at the legacy of Antiquity, science took a step forward in the 18th century when the modern approach of making observations and drawing conclusions, later followed by the conjunction of hypotheses with subsequent experimental testing,

was adopted. Then we also see the founding of the first veterinary colleges. These focused almost exclusively on the horse which, throughout this entire period, had maintained its primary role in transport and warfare. It was France that took the lead and it was also French scientists that published the first scientific study completely dedicated to the locomotion of the horse. France retained the lead in veterinary medicine, and in equine gait analysis, for almost a century until the end of the 19th century. Then, with one notable exception in the United States, German scientists took over and explored the possibilities of novel techniques like cine film.

The outbreak of World War II brought this thriving research to a halt. There was no recovery after the end of the war because the mechanical revolution, which had already started during World War I, made horse power redundant and brought to a definitive end the traditional role the horse had played for millennia in transport and warfare. In fact, it looked as if the species would become entirely marginalised. However, interest in the species was revived at the end of the sixties and in the early seventies of the 20th century when equestrian sports enjoyed an immense popularity that still continues to increase today. This increase in popularity has again made the horse into an important economic factor, worthy of serious investment. At the same time, interest in locomotion analysis was revived. This time first in Sweden, but soon followed by other countries and regions where the horse has gained importance as a sports and leisure animal, e.g. North America and northwestern Europe. This renewed interest in equine locomotion coincided with the electronic revolution which made computer-aided analysis a reality, thus creating the possibility for much more advanced and profound studies of equine locomotion than ever before.

The science of equine locomotion is thriving. This book aims to present the state of the art in this branch of science. In the first chapter an attempt is made to give an overview of how this science developed over time against the background of evolving veterinary science, but more so against the background of the evolving relationship of mankind with what has been called our closest ally: the horse.

THE HORSE AND GAIT ANALYSIS IN HISTORY

Prehistoric times

The oldest known art to be produced by man is the rock art found in various caves in the Franco-Cantabrian region, covering what is nowadays south-western France and north-western Spain. Here, about 30 000 years ago the Cro-Magnon race of people began depicting their environment by means of large and impressive paintings on the walls of rock caves. Though at first still somewhat crude, artistic heights were reached about 15 000 years ago in the Magdalenian period, so called after the rock shelter of La Madeleine, near present-day Montauban. In those days of the last Ice Age, south-western Europe must have known abundant wildlife. In the paintings two

classes of animals prevail: ruminants such as cattle, bison, deer and ibex, and horses. The way horses were represented does not reveal a profound knowledge of equine locomotion. In most cases the animals were painted standing with all four legs on the ground, or in an unnatural jump-like action with the forelimbs extended forward and the hindlimbs backward, in much the same way as horses were still erroneously depicted in many 18th century and early 19th century paintings (Fig. 1.1). Species like rhinoceros, mammoth, bear and the felidae are present, but to a much lesser extent. Perhaps the plains which covered that part of Europe in this period looked much like the great plains of East Africa, such as the Serengeti, nowadays. Here too, ruminants like buffalo and wildebeest are abundant together with equids (zebras), while other species such as rhinoceros and the large cats occur in significantly smaller numbers.

Man was still a hunter–gatherer in those days and for this reason the wild animals comprised an essential part of his diet. Remains of large mammals eaten by man, including horses, have been found at many sites. It is interesting to note that the vast majority of rock paintings concerned animals, most of them large mammals, whereas man himself was depicted rarely and other parts of the environment such as the vegetation or topographical peculiarities were never shown. Also, non-mam-

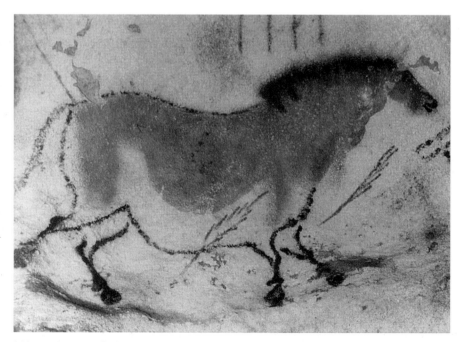

Fig. 1.1 Przewalski-type horse as depicted in the cave at Lascaux (about 15 000 BC). (From: Dunlop, R.H. & Williams, D.J. (eds) (1996) *Veterinary Medicine. An illustrated history*. St. Louis: Mosby.)

malian species such as birds, reptiles, fish or insects were virtually unrepresented. The rock art found in various parts of Zimbabwe and other parts of Southern Africa was somewhat different. These paintings were made by the Bushmen from 13 000–2000 years ago. Here again, the large mammalian species prevailed, with the zebra representating the equids, but man was depicted more often and there were some paintings of fish and reptiles (Adams & Handiseni, 1991). The Bushmen culture has survived until the present day, though in a very diminished and nowadays heavily endangered form, and it is known that these people, who were hunter–gatherers, lived in a very close relationship with their environment, forming an integral part of the entire ecosystem. It is easy to imagine that under such circumstances the large mammals, which were the most impressive fellow-creatures giving rise to mixed feelings of awe, admiration and a certain form of solidarity, inspired the creation of works of art.

The world changed dramatically when, at the beginning of the Neolithic period about 10 000–12 000 years ago, man changed from being a hunter–gatherer to practicing primitive forms of agriculture and pastoralism. The capacity of most natural savanna habitats to support fixed human nutritional requirements is estimated at only one or two persons per square mile (Dunlop & Williams, 1996). The advent of agriculture and pastoralism meant that the nutritional constraints on population growth were lifted and an unprecedented population growth followed. It also meant that man definitively and irreversibly placed himself apart from his fellow-creatures and outside the existing ecosystems where the numbers of species were determined by the unmanipulated carrying capacity of the environment.

These changes in human society were to a large extent possible thanks to a new phenomenon: the domestication of animal species. It is widely believed that the dog was the first animal to be domesticated about 12 000 years ago. Like most early domestications, this event took place in western Asia's Fertile Crescent (the area of fertile land from the Mediterranean coast around the Syrian desert to Iraq), which was the cradle of human civilization. There also the next domestication took place: small ruminants were domesticated approximately 10 000 years ago, sheep and goats in about the same period. Cattle were domesticated 2000 years later in Anatolia (western Turkey). Cats were domesticated (or they adopted man as some people state) as early as 9000 years ago. The first camelids to be domesticated were llamas in South America, perhaps as early as 7500 years ago. The horse arrived rather late on the scene. There is evidence that the first horses were domesticated in what is now southern Russia approximately 5000 years ago. However, the domestication of the horse dramatically influenced the history of mankind, mainly because of its enormous potency in warfare.

The horse was definitely the most revolutionary innovation in warfare before the invention of gunpowder. First, the animals were used to draw heavy war chariots which, used against traditional infantry, could provoke enormous massacres while being themselves rather invulnerable. Later, with the development of the skill of horse riding and increasing horsemanship, a real cavalry of mounted soldiers was developed which, with their greater agility, replaced the chariots. This development enabled rapid conquests of vast territories. The Hittites conquered Asia Minor (present-day Turkey) in 2000 BC with their horse-drawn chariots. A thousand years later the Scythians, originally a Eurasian nomadic tribe, settled in the area north of the Black Sea. The Scythians were excellent horse riders and they became masters in the tactics of cavalry-based steppe warfare, enslaving agricultural peoples and plundering what came in their way. Later other tribes that were mostly of Eastern origin succeeded. The Huns overran the Roman Empire from the 4th to the 6th century AD, and in the 13th century AD, Genghis Khan reached the gates of western Europe.

For those peoples the horse was more than just a domesticated animal; it was central in their culture, as a weapon, food, drink, a friend and a god. The warriors were capable of staying in the saddle for an entire day. They ate horsemeat, drank mare's milk and intoxicated themselves during their feasts with the fermented form of it. It is even said that soldiers, traveling without rations, opened the veins of their horses, drank the blood, closed the wounds, and remounted (Simpson, 1951).

The changes in attitude towards animals by man, including domestication and changes in the use of domestic animals that were partly dictated by changing environmental conditions, are magnificently demonstrated by the North African rock art found, for instance, in the Hoggar and Air mountain ranges in what is now the central Sahara Desert. Several thousands of years ago North Africa was not covered to such a large extent by the extremely arid and inhospitable Sahara Desert as it is now. The oldest art dates to about 7000 years ago and depicts wild animals such as buffalo, giraffe, elephant, ostriches, etc., suggesting that the area must have looked like large parts of eastern Africa do now. About 4000 BC cattle and fat-tailed sheep appeared as first representations of domestic species. Horses appeared around 1200 BC, first drawing chariots. These chariots are believed to have belonged to Cretan invaders because they are similar to pictures of chariots from this island (Lhote, 1988). In those days there was a Trans-Saharan route running from Tripoli and probably also Egypt to Gao on the Niger River, thus connecting the Mediterranean, Egyptian and Nubian cultures to the Bantu cultures of the Niger River valley. More recent rock art shows riders instead of chariots. With the increasing aridity of the Sahara, the horse became unsuitable for traveling large distances with ever-diminishing water resources, and was supplemented by camels around 100 BC.

The Ancient cultures

The first human civilizations, characterized by urbanization and the invention of a script, developed in Mesopotamia, the area around the Euphrates and Tigris rivers, about 3000 years BC. The first report on hippiatry dates from the 14th century BC from the Assyrian culture. In those days the city of Hethiter was famous for the procurement and training of horses. Also, donkeys were already crossbred with horses to produce the sturdier, but infertile mules. There is even evidence that horses were crossbred with the then abundant wild onagers.

After the decline of the Assyrian empire in the 8th century BC the Medean and Persian cultures took over. These were, to a large extent, horse-based societies where horsemanship was developed to great heights. In fact, the word 'Persia' is derived from the word for horseman. It was the forceful Persian cavalry that created the largest empire the world had ever seen until then, under Darius I – an empire that was only to be conquered by another horse-based army, that of Alexander the Great in 322 BC.

One of the other great ancient cultures, that of Egypt, lived its first periods of glory (the Old Kingdom from 2620–2170 BC and the Middle Kingdom from 2080–1760 BC) before the arrival of (horse-borne) invaders. During this period the horse was an unknown animal to the Egyptians who were surrounded by many domesticated species like dogs, cattle and cats, the last of which gradually obtained a divine status during the later periods of Egyptian culture. The horse was introduced in the New Kingdom when invaders from the Palestinian region, who used chariots drawn by swift Arabian horses, began to challenge Egyptian sovereignty. The only way to refute them was by using the same weapon: the horse. In the New Kingdom (1539–1078 BC) the Egyptians became masters in horsemanship and horse breeding, producing the finest Arabian horses. The horse even allowed them to expand their empire as far as the Euphrates River.

In China, where some think that a separate domestication of the horse had taken place, independent of the site in Southern Russia alluded to earlier (Simpson, 1951), the oldest reports of domesticated horses are

from the Shung dynasty (1766–1027 BC). Like everywhere else, the horse was used first to draw chariots, then for a mounted cavalry. From the latter period dates the famous 'army' of terracotta figures (including large numbers of horses) that was excavated at the burial site of Shih Hunagdi (259–210 BC). He is also called the first emperor as the formerly divided China was united by then. The horse gained great importance in China during the Han dynasty when Emperor Wu sent out a military expedition to capture 3000 horses of a heavier and sturdier breed, which he called the 'Horses of Heaven'. They were probably related to the Tarpan breed that still roamed the steppes of southern Russia; only 50 of them survived the 2000 mile journey home.

By the middle of the 7th century AD, during the Tang dynasty, horse breeding in China reached unprecedented heights when numbers increased from 5000 to over 700 000. The Chinese were excellent in designing saddlery and harnesses. They invented the trace harness, in which the power of the horse is transmitted by a belt around the chest, long before it was used in Europe where a collar-type of harness was common. This latter type of harness compresses the trachea and jugular veins when force is applied and therefore permits the exertion of a force only one-sixth that of using a trace harness. Also, stirrups are a Chinese invention, dating from the 3rd century AD.

A few reports on equine veterinary medicine have survived from these cultures, some of which are quite extensive and methodic, such as some Egyptian works. However, no specific studies on equine locomotion are known. Horses in general were depicted as they had been in prehistoric times and would remain until quite recently – either in a rather natural pose at a slow gait or in the characteristic unnatural pose that was used to indicate the gallop: forelimbs extended forward and hindlimbs backward.

The antique world

There is perhaps no revolution that has changed the course of human history more than the revolutionary change in thinking that originated in the Greek port towns of Asia Minor (western Turkey) and nearby islands around 600 BC. Leaving ordained preconceptions and supernatural speculations or dogmas behind as explanations for natural phenomena, nature was now studied in a rigorous, rational way. The proponents of this new way of thinking were called natural scientists or philosopher scientists (Dunlop & Williams, 1996). Here, the foundations were laid for the great Greek schools of philosophy, like the Athenian Academy. This institution became the intellectual center of the world a couple of centuries later, producing the great philosophers Socrates, Plato

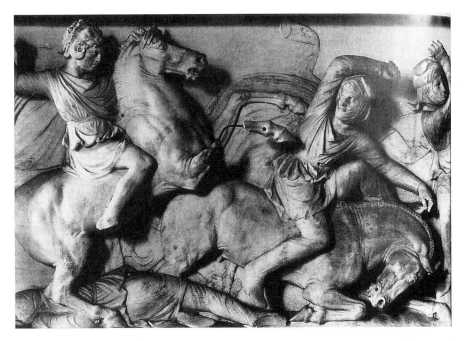

Fig. 1.2 Alexander the Great attacking Persian horsemen on Bucephalus. From the sarcophage of Alexander, Syria. (From: Dunlop, R.H. & Williams, D.J. (eds) (1996) *Veterinary Medicine. An illustrated history.* St. Louis: Mosby.)

and Aristotle. It can be stated without any hesitation that with the onset of the great Greek philosophical era science was born. Nature in all its aspects was studied for the first time by theoretical speculation (proposing hypotheses), followed by critical reappraisal and revision. What was still missing was the experimental testing of hypotheses which is essential to modern science. The Greek philosophical schools tried to resolve all problems by logical reasoning, so the balance was far to the intellectual side. Nowadays it is not uncommon to see a reversed tendency with strong emphasis on strictly controlled experimental testing, but with sometimes hardly any evidence of critical thinking.

Aristotle was a teacher of Alexander the Great who, seated on his black stallion Bucephalus, conquered most of the then known world. Alexander was a skilful rider who is said to have been the only one able to ride the horse. Bucephalus had been given to him by his father when Alexander was 12 years old and served him for 17 years (Fig. 1.2). Alexander greatly favored the development of science and created a center of learning in the city that was named after him: Alexandria. This city on the mouth of the Nile would remain the intellectual center of the world from 300 BC to 500 AD. In the vast library 700 000 scrolls were housed compiling all knowl-

edge that had been gained in the preceding millennium. The burning of the library on the orders of Caliph Omar in AD 642 was an act of barbarism, narrow-mindedness and, in its deepest meaning, fear for the unknown. It resembles the burning of books that took place in more recent history and is still taking place on the instigation of totalitarian regimes and intolerant sectarian cults.

The first extensive work on equine conformation was performed by Xenophon (430–354 BC). Apparently a man of great experience, he described in full detail the desirable and undesirable traits of horses. Many of his criteria were equal to those used today. Though his work was more of a hippiatric caliber than a scientific work, he already recognized the role of the hindquarters as the motor of locomotion.

It is not surprising that the first documented study on animal locomotion originated from one of the great Greek philosophers, Aristotle (384–322 BC). In his youth, Aristotle was intrigued by natural history, and he wrote various volumes on biological and medical matters. In his works *De motu animalium* and *De incessu animalium* ('On the movements of animals' and 'On the progression of animals') he accurately described quadrupedal locomotion, at least in the slower gaits. In *De incessu animalium* he states that:

Αἱ μὲν οὖν κάμψεις τῶν σκελῶν τοῦτόν τε τὸν τρόπον ἔχουσι καὶ διὰ τὰς αἰτίας τας εἰρμένας, κινεῖται δὲ τὰ ὀπίσθια πρὸς τὰ ἔμπροσθεν κατὰ διάμετρον· μετὰ γὰρ τὸ δεξιὸν τῶν ἔμπροσθεν τὸ ἀριστερὸν τῶν ὄπισθεν κινοῦσιν, εἶτα τὸ ἀριστερὸν τῶν ἔμπροσθεν, μετὰ δὲ

(The bendings, then, of the limbs take place in this manner and for the reasons stated. But the hindlimbs move diagonally in relation to the forelimbs; for after the right forelimb animals move the left hindlimb, then the left forelimb, and after it the right hindlimb)

The Romans were more doers than thinkers and lacked the intellectual drive that characterized the Greeks. Throughout the whole period of the Roman Empire, the intellectual center remained in Greece, Asia Minor and, of course, Alexandria. However, the Romans were excellent in organizing and implementing the scientific and technical advances of others. Consequently, they created one of the vastest empires the world has ever known and which still influences many aspects of daily life.

Horses played a pivotal role in the Roman army, which employed large numbers of veterinarians to care for them. These were first called *mulomedici*, but after an overhaul of the military regulations under Commodus (180–192 AD) the term *veterinarii* appears. Thanks to the enormous popularity of horse racing (chariots drawn by two or four horses), there was also employment for a category of veterinary specialists not unknown today: the racetrack veterinarian, of which Pelagonius in the 4th century was a famous example. However, these veterinarians were mainly engaged in the treatment of diseases and healing of the many wounds. Empiricists, they relied heavily on their Greek and Hellenistic counterparts for some theoretical basis. A noteworthy exception was the physician Galenus. Galenus was born in Pergamon, Asia Minor, in 130 AD, but he worked for decades in Rome. He conducted large numbers of experiments on animals to advance medical knowledge and can be seen as the founder of the experimental basis of comparative medicine. He produced vast numbers of treatises, of which about 20% have survived the ages. None of those is dedicated to the study of animal or human locomotion.

Emperor Diocletianus (284–306 AD) had divided the Roman Empire into an eastern and a western half. Constantine the Great reunited the empire in 324, but it was divided again in 395. The western part fell with the abdication of Romulus Augustus in 476; the eastern part was to survive for an additional 1000 years as the Byzantine Empire with Constantinople (Istanbul) as capital. The veterinary profession was at a high level as can be judged from the compilation of all that was known in

this field under the name *Corpus hippiatricorum Graecorum* or *Hippiatrika*. Though published in the 9th or 10th century, most of the contents date back to the 4th century. The contributions of Apsyrtos (300–360), the chief military veterinarian in the army of Constantine the Great, are of outstanding quality. Though the care and treatment of the locomotor system have a prominent position in this work, no specific comments on locomotion itself or gait analysis are made.

Through the Dark Ages to the Renaissance

After the fall of the western Roman Empire, the existing administrative structures collapsed and much of the knowledge that had been gained over the centuries was lost. For centuries most of Europe became an incoherent assembly of tribes and mini-states where insecurity and ignorance reigned. During this period the impressive Arab conquest started from Mecca in the Arabian peninsula where the prophet Muhammad had died in 632. Within a century, the Arabs conquered millions of square miles of land from northern India to Spain. This could be accomplished thanks to their aggressive light cavalry, which was based on the swift and enduring Arab horses, and their great horsemanship. They were halted by the troops of the Frankish king Charles Martel at Poitiers in 752. The Franks were only able to withstand them because they employed a heavily armored cavalry which was rather invulnerable to the light cavalry of the Arabs, a strategy not unlike the use of the first tanks in World War I.

While Europe was in cultural decline, the Arab culture flourished. It is thanks to many Arab scientists that at least a part of what had been written in Antiquity has survived to the present day. They translated the works into Arabic and in the later Middle Ages these Arabic versions were translated again into Latin to lay the foundation for the scientific revival in the Renaissance. The Arabs also contributed to veterinary medicine with original works. Akhi Hizam al-Furusiyah wa al-Khayl wrote the first book on the characteristics, behavior and diseases of horses in 860. Abu Bakr ibn el-bedr al Baytar (1309–1340) wrote an excellent work on veterinary medicine, the *Kamil as Sina'atayn*. This book features aspects of equine management and care including the tricks of horse dealers (!), together with remarks on appearance, conformation and gait (Dunlop & Williams, 1996). The horse had a very high standing in the Arab world. Abu Bakr held the opinion that the horse was so important to an Arab man that it would be reunited with him in paradise, together with his wives. There is also an Arab maxim stating that '*Every grain of barley given to a horse is entered by God in the register of Good Works*' (Simpson, 1951).

In the first part of the Middle Ages the medical and veterinary professions stood at a low level in most of Europe. The link with Antiquity had been broken and the Christian church, which saw diseases as a divine punishment to be cured with the help of supernatural power, had a hostile attitude towards the few rational natural scientists. In medieval matters mystics and superstition played an important role. It was not until the late Middle Ages that, mainly through the translation of Arab texts (originals and translations of classical works), the tide changed. The Emperor Frederick II was a man ahead of his time. He formed a bridge between the Christian Western world and the Islamic East. He was a great proponent of science and had a special interest in animals. It was his chief marshal, Jordanus Ruffus, who, supported by the emperor, published the first new work on equine medicine *De Medicina Equorum* in 1250. Frederick II was a great, but ruthless, innovator. At first supported by pope Innocent III, he fell into disgrace with his successors who deprived him of his kingdoms in 1245. This enlightened man can be seen as a very early protagonist of the wave of renewal that was to blow over Europe and which would mean an end to the Middle Ages: the Renaissance.

From the Renaissance to the 18th century

In Italy a shift in scientific attitude developed; this involved a change from the concept of life as the product of supernatural and mystical powers towards a more rational, naturalistic approach. Perhaps no one was so closely associated with this revolutionary process as the genial artist and scientist Leonardo da Vinci (1452–1519). Leonardo himself is known to have been interested in the movements of animals and he even projected to 'write a separate treatise describing the movement of animals with four feet, among which is man, who likewise in its infancy crawls on all fours' (Clayton, 1996). Da Vinci was intrigued by the flexibility of the equine spine and produced a series of fine drawings, now in the British Royal Collection at Windsor Castle, with horses in a number of exceptional, but not impossible poses. It has been stated that the renaissance in veterinary medicine started with the publication of the first great textbook on veterinary anatomy *Dell'Anatomia et dell'Infirmita del Cavallo* (*On the anatomy and diseases of the horse*) by Carlo Ruini in 1598. The anatomical part presented the first real new work since Antiquity. However, the part on diseases did not pass the standards of Jordanus Ruffus' *De Medicina Equorum* that had been published 350 years earlier.

It may not be surprising that this ambiance of emerging science fostered the first contribution to the science

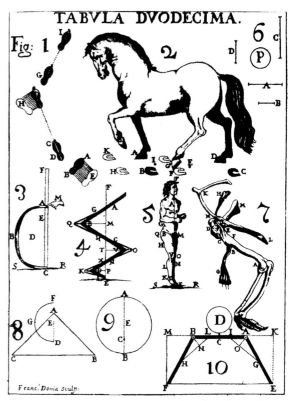

Fig. 1.3 Page from *De motu Animalium* by Giovanni Borelli, comparing equine and human locomotion. (From: Dunlop, R.H. & Williams, D.J. (eds) (1996) *Veterinary Medicine. An illustrated history.* St. Louis: Mosby.)

of equine locomotion since Aristotle. Giovanni Alphonso Borelli (1608–1679) was a professor of mathematics at Pisa University and applied physical theory to the study of animal locomotion. He calculated the force of muscle action and recognized that the muscles were under nervous control (Fig. 1.3). In his book *De motu Animalium* (*On the movement of animals*), he describes the center of gravity and also makes observations about limb placement in the various gaits (Borelli, 1681). He was obviously ahead of his time; this line of investigation would not be further pursued until the end of the 18th century.

The 17th century was the age of the great horse marshals. One of these was William Cavendysh, the first Duke of Newcastle (1592–1676). He was one of the most famous horse trainers of his days but was, as a royalist, forced to leave Britain when the army of Charles I was defeated by Cromwell's troops. In exile in Antwerp he wrote an extensive work on all aspects of the horse which first appeared in French. It includes a chapter on the gaits, which he studied with help of the sounds that the hooves make when they strike the ground (Cavendysh, 1674). Another great marshal of this era was Jacques de Solleysel from France. His great work *Le Parfait Maréchal qui enseigne a connoistre la beauté, la bonté et les défauts des chevaux* (*The perfect marshal who teaches how to know the beauty, the virtue and the defects of horses*) consists of two volumes. The first one is dedicated to horse management, the second to equine diseases. De Solleysel makes some remarks on limb placement in various gaits, but appears not to really have made a study of the subject (De Solleysel, 1733).

The start of veterinary education

Notwithstanding some progress in the preceding centuries, the veterinary profession was still far from any scientific status in the middle of the 18th century. George Leclerc, Comte de Buffon (1707–1778), who was the dominant personality in zoology during the second half of the 18th century, wrote at the end of his zoological description of the horse: 'I cannot end the story of the horse without writing with regret that the health of this useful and precious animal has been up to now surrendered to the care and practice, often blind, of people without knowledge and without qualification' (Dunlop & Williams, 1996).

However, the chances for the veterinary profession were to change for the better, mainly because of two reasons. On the one hand the need for better veterinary care became dramatically evident in this period by the huge losses of horses on the many battlefields of those days, and by the incredible losses of livestock caused by various waves of cattle plagues, mostly rinderpest, that swept over Europe. It has been estimated that more than 200 million cattle died in Europe in the years between 1711 and 1780 because of this disease which had a profound demoralizing effect on the rural areas. On the other hand, a new intellectual movement, which came to be known as the Enlightenment, was spreading through Europe from its origins in France. Philosophers such as Montesquieu, Rousseau and Voltaire rejected the idea of mere authority as the source of truth and emphasized the role of reason. These two concurrent circumstances created an optimal starting point for veterinary education. It was Claude Bourgelat, director of the Academy of Equitation in Lyon and himself one of the authors of the great work of the Enlightenment, a highly controversial and unorthodox encyclopedia that trampled the toes of many established authorities, who finally obtained royal permission to transform the riding school into the first veterinary school in 1761. A few years later he would establish a second one in the center of the French empire: Paris. Other European countries followed the French example with the Austro-Hungarian Empire as the first (1766).

The newly established veterinary center at Alfort near Paris did not fail to produce results. In 1779 the first modern work that focuses entirely on equine gait was published. The authors were the late M. Goiffon and his deputy Vincent, who was employed by the school and later became one of the first pupils of the Alfort School. The book of Goiffon and Vincent was primarily intended to help artists depict their horses in a more natural way, which had been a problem throughout the ages, but it was considered equally interesting for everybody dedicated to the art of horse riding. The work is of extreme importance in the history of equine gait analysis. Though not entirely correct with respect to limb placement in the faster gaits, the study is well done and enters into great detail. Gaits of horses are represented by a '*piste*' (a graphical representation of the footfall pattern), a kind of schematic stick diagram, an elaborate table, and by what we now call a gait diagram (Fig. 1.4). This latter representation of equine gait was invented by Goiffon and Vincent and has proved so useful that it is used in many present-day publications in an essentially unaltered form. Goiffon and Vincent called it an '*échelle odochronométrique*'. Regarding the origin of the word, they state: 'Cette denomination est composée de trois mots grecs, dont l'un signifie chemin, l'autre temps & le troisieme mesure. C'est la définition exacte de notre échelle; elle est la mesure du temps & du chemin fait pendant ce temps'. (This name is composed of three Greek words: one means distance, one means time and the third means measurement. This is the exact definition of our scale which in fact measures time and the distance covered in that time) (Goiffon & Vincent, 1779).

The 19th century

By the end of the first half of the 19th century veterinary schools had been founded in practically all countries that belonged to the then developed world, which did not yet include the United States. There, the first (private) veterinary school was the Veterinary College of Philadelphia, founded in 1852. However, progress was relatively slow and some of these institutions, an example being the Royal Veterinary College in London under Coleman, even had a questionable academic level. The profession still had a low status and the interest in the courses sometimes was marginal. In Holland, where veterinary education had started in 1821 with 24 first-year students, only 8 first-year students entered during the 7(!) years from 1848 until 1855 (Kroon *et al.*, 1921). In the second half of the century things would change dramatically thanks to decisive breakthroughs in microbiology, especially in bacteriology. Scientists such as Pasteur and Koch provided the clues for many diseases that so far had been of mysterious origin. The brilliant pathologist Virchow laid the basis for a cell-based pathology that broke with the old humoral theories. These discoveries had enormous implications, not only for human medicine but also for the veterinary sciences. It was the time that the great cattle plagues rinderpest and contagious pleuropneumonia came under control. In the horse the causative agent of glanders, then the greatest plague of this species and, as a zoonosis, a potential threat to man, was isolated by Schütz and Löffler in 1886. All these developments boosted the interest in veterinary medicine and stressed the importance of the profession.

Throughout the 19th century the horse retained its primary position in society. On the battlefields the cavalry remained as decisive as ever though heavier losses of horses were inflicted because of the increasing artillery firepower. Napoleon lost more than 30 000 horses (and over 300 000 men) during his Russian expedition. In the Boer war of 1899–1902, 326 073 horses perished. Over the entire century, millions more must have lost their lives in battle.

Horses remained equally important in the transport sector though in the second half of the century they were increasingly replaced by the rapidly expanding rail network for long distance transport. In Britain travel by mail coach peaked in the 1830s and then declined because of the increasing rail services. The extension of the rail network in Great Britain tripled between the years 1850 and 1875 from 5000 to 14 500 miles. However, horse-drawn transport remained important at a local level and in the rural areas until well into the 20th century.

In the field of locomotion analysis some progress was made in the first three-quarters of the 19th century. In Switzerland Conrad von Hochstätter published from 1821 to 1824 his *Theoretisch-praktisches Handbuch der äussern Pferdekenntniß, und der Wartung und Pflege der*

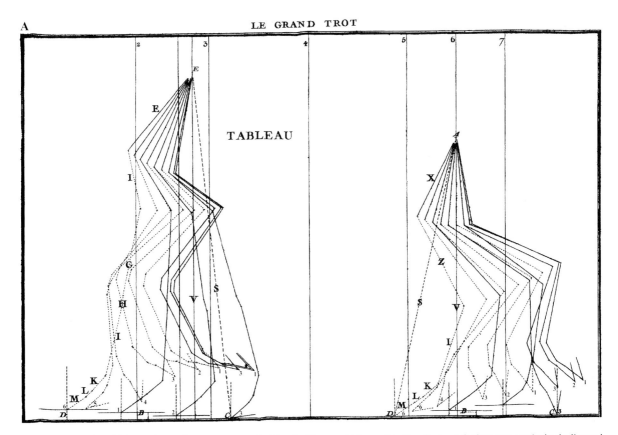

Fig. 1.4 Forms in which equine gait was represented by Goiffon and Vincent in the first work that was entirely dedicated to the subject. **A** Stick diagram. **B** Table. **C** Footfall pattern. **D** *'échelle odochronométrique,'* or the precursor of the present day gait diagram.

B

TABLE											

AVANT-MAIN.

Long.ᵈᵉˢ Sou tendan tes.	Appui			Vib.Rappel			Soutien					
	1	2	3	1	2	3	1	2	3	4	5	6
S	20.10.	20.4.	2010.	17.22.	17.20.	17.17.	17.10	17.11.	17.21.	19.13.	20.17.	21.6.
S V	12. 3/4	3. 1/2	6.	11. 1/2	11. 1/4	8. 3/4	5.	0. 3/4	3. 1/4	9. 1/4	18. 1/2	21. 3/4
V E	32.	23.	14.	10.	11.	14.	18. 1/2	23.	27. 1/2	32.	36. 1/2	41.
E F	116.	117.	117.	115.	114. 1/2	114.	113. 1/2	113. 3/4	114.	116. 1/2	120.	127.
F G	144. 1/2	147. 3/4	146. 3/4	90.	89. 1/2	89.	88. 1/2	88. 1/2	92.	104. 3/4	122.	155.
G H	175. 1/2	175. 1/2	175. 1/2	149.	148.	147. 3/4	146. 1/2	146.	148.	154. 1/2	160. 1/2	175. 1/2
H I	174. 3/4	174. 3/4	174. 3/4	149.	148.	147. 3/4	146. 1/2	146.	148.	154. 1/2	160. 1/2	174. 3/4
I K	134.	128. 3/4	148. 3/4	147.	147.	147.	147.	147. 1/2	149. 1/2	162.	159.	151. 3/4
K L	179.	173. 1/2	162. 1/2	158.	158.	158.	158.	158.	159.	168.	166.	173. 1/2
L M	175.	174.	165.	174.	174.	174.	174.	174.	173. 3/4	173. 1/2	164. 1/2	172. 1/2
M S	44. 1/2	53. 1/2	55. 1/2	64. 3/4	65. 1/2	66. 1/2	70. 3/4	67. 3/4	64. 1/2	39. 1/2	28. 1/2	35. 3/4
Élévation de la Pince sur le Sol.			3.2	3.3	2.19	2.13	2.16	2.11.	1.8.	0.22.	0.0.	

ARRIERE-MAIN.

Long.ᵈᵉˢ Sou tendan tes.	Appui			Vib.Rappel			Soutien					
	1	2	3	1	2	3	1	2	3	4	5	6
S	16.4.	16.5.	17.13.	16.11.	16.6.	16.1.	15.19.	15.13.	15.13.	15.23.	16.10.	16.22.
S V	2.	10.	20. 1/2	28. 1/2	26. 3/4	22. 3/4	17. 1/4	11.	5. 3/4	4. 1/2	9 3/4	13. 1/4
V X	16. 1/2	5. 3/4	5. 1/2	10. 1/2	9.	5. 1/2	0.	5. 1/2	11.	16. 1/2	22	27. 1/2
X Z	120. 3/4	118. 1/4	132.	124.	122.	120.	118.	116.	116.	116. 3/4	119. 1/2	124. 3/4
Z I	130 3/4	125. 1/2	119. 3/4	102.	98.	94.	90.	86.	86.	93.	112.	132. 3/4
I K	138.	164. 3/4	149. 3/4	138.	138.	138.	138	138.	138.	161. 1/2	175.	151. 3/4
K L	175. 3/4	164. 1/4	163. 3/4	152.	152.	152.	152.	152.	152.	167. 3/4	176. 1/2	176.
L M	178. 3/4	156. 1/2	164. 3/4	174.	174.	174.	174.	174.	174.	173.	172.	178. 1/4
M S	53.	65.	3. 3/4	24. 1/4	22. 1/2	20. 1/2	18. 3/4	16. 3/4	17. 3/4	12. 1/2	36. 3/4	41 3/4
Élévation de la Pince sur le Sol.			2.8.	2.6.	1.16.	1.5.	1.1.	1.0.	0.20.	0.14.	0.0.	

Fig. 1.4 *contd* **B** Table.

Pferde (Theoretical and practical handbook of the conformation of the horse and of horse grooming and care) which includes the first considerations of the mechanisms underlying equine gait, based on his own observations. He also discusses the consequences of a number of faulty conformations for performance. Unfortunately this work remained largely unnoticed by the veterinary profession (Schauder, 1923a).

In Germany there was an increasing interest in the explanation of locomotion by specific muscle action.

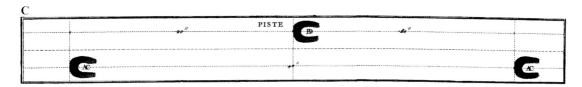

Fig. 1.4. *contd* **C** Footfall pattern

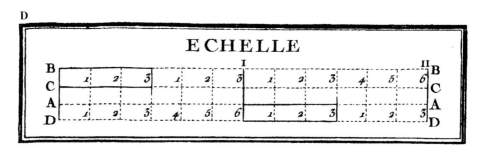

Fig. 1.4 *contd* **D** *'échelle odochronométrique,'* or the precursor of the present day gait diagram. (From: Goiffon & Vincent (1779) *Mémoire Artificielle des Principes Relatifs à la Fidelle Réprésentation des Animaux tant en Peinture, qu'en Sculpture. Alfort: Ecole Royale Vétérinaire.*)

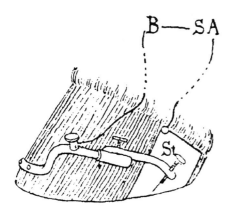

Fig. 1.5 Electrical device as developed by Bayer to measure the movement of the lateral hoof wall. St: needle; B: wire to battery; SA: wire to electric bell. (From: Bayer, J. (1882) Experimentelles über Hufmechanismus. *Oesterr. Monatsschr. Tierheilk.* 7: 72–74.)

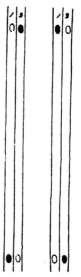

Fig. 1.6 Gait diagram as introduced by Lecoq (trot). Though later used by celebrities such as Muybridge, it did not find general acceptance because it provided information about the spatial position of the limbs only, but not on temporal aspects. This is in contrast to the original *'échelle odochronométrique'* invented by Goiffon and Vincent which, after modification by Marey, became the world standard. (From: Lecoq, F. (1843) *Traité de l'Extérieur du Cheval, et des Principaux Animaux Domestiques.* Lyon: Savy.)

This culminated in the classical work *Die topographische Myologie des Pferdes mit besonderer Berücksichtigung der lokomotorischen Wirkung der Muskeln* (*Topographical myology of the horse with special attention to the locomotor effect of muscles* by Karl Günther in 1866. In Austria Bayer (1882)) did some experimental work on the hoof mechanism using an electrical device (Fig. 1.5) while in Germany

Peters (1879) also dedicated himself to the hoof. In the meantime, in France attention remained focused on gait analysis as it was initiated by Goiffon and Vincent. In his book on the conformation of the horse, Lecoq (1843) introduced a different gait diagram from that of Goiffon and Vincent (Fig. 1.6). It did not find general acceptance because, although it was unequivocal regarding limb placement, it did not give temporal information.

In his book *Locomotion du cheval* (*Locomotion of the horse*, 1883), Captain Raabe presented an ingenious system consisting of two discs, a fixed one and a rotating one, with which the sequence of limb placement in all symmetrical gaits can be determined (Fig. 1.7). Raabe, who first published his work in 1857, divided the stride cycle of a limb into six periods. This was a simplification of the system used by Goiffon and Vincent who had used 12 time intervals. Raabe's division was also used by Lenoble du Teil (1873). In his 1893 publication, when he had a leading position

at the famous national stud Haras du Pin, Lenoble du Teil used his studies and similar works of others to take a strong stand against the classical Italian school of riding.

In the Anglo-Saxon world there was not much research on the topic. However, the problem of gait analysis was a point of discussion from time to time as exemplified by a scientific quarrel between Joseph Gamgee from Edinburgh and Neville Goodman from Cambridge in the *Journal of Anatomy and Physiology* in the early 1870s. Discussing the canter, Gamgee stated that 'The horse in the fast paces, as in the slowest movement, has never less than two of his feet acting on the ground.' This statement was (correctly) attacked by Goodman. However, there was, as yet, no means to prove this (Gamgee, 1869, 1870; Goodman, 1870, 1871). In 1873 Pettigrew published a book on animal locomotion in which he put forward some ideas that were later taken by Marey from France, who was to become much more famous.

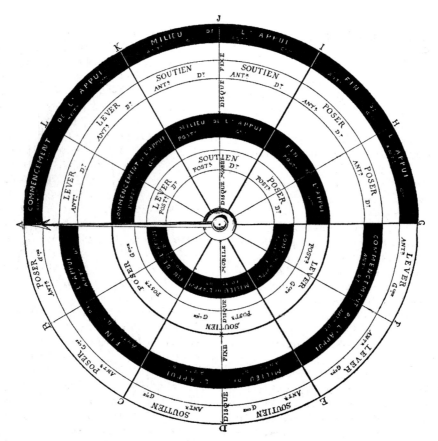

Fig. 1.7 System consisting of a fixed and a rotating disc to determine the sequence of limb placement in the symmetrical gaits. (From: Raabe (1883) *Locomotion du Cheval. Cadran Hippique des Allures Marchées*. Paris: T. Symonds.)

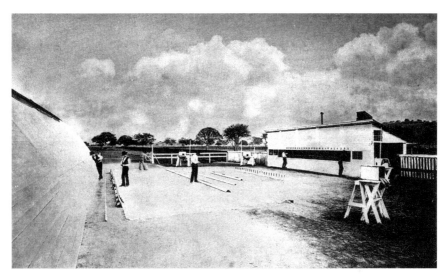

Fig. 1.8 The set-up at Palo Alto in California as used by Muybridge during his research on the locomotion of the horse for Leland Stanford, with 24 cameras in a linear array. (From: Stillman, J.D.B. (1882) *The Horse in Motion as shown by Instantaneous Photography with a Study on Animal Mechanics founded on Anatomy and the Revelations of the Camera in which is demonstrated the Theory of Quadrupedal Locomotion.* Boston: James R. Osgood & Co.)

MUYBRIDGE AND MAREY: REVOLUTION IN GAIT ANALYSIS

About a century after the French Revolution, which meant the end of an era and changed world politics forever, a revolution took place in the field of equine gait analysis. So far, treatises on gait analysis had largely consisted of theoretical considerations while conclusions based on experimental data were scarce. This was mainly due to the limitations of the human eye when observing the faster gaits. In the middle of the 19th century it was still contentious whether the faster gaits had moments when all limbs were in suspension or not, as illustrated by the dispute between Gamgee and Goodman alluded to above. It is thanks to the efforts of two men that decisive breakthroughs were made. The English-born American photographer Eadweard Muybridge and the French physiologist Etienne Jules Marey used the technology of their time to study equine gait.

It has been argued that 'the invention of motion pictures can be traced to an argument among the ancient Egyptians whether a trotting horse ever had all four feet off the ground at once' (Simpson, 1951). Though this certainly is a bit of an overstatement, it was this still unresolved question that led to Muybridge's first photographic experiments. The railroad magnate Leland Stanford, the founder of Stanford University, was intrigued by this question with respect to his trotter 'Occident' and it was at his farm in Palo Alto, California, that Muybridge commenced his experiments in 1872 (Fig. 1.8).

His first efforts were unsuccessful because his camera lacked a fast shutter. Then the project was interrupted because Muybridge was being tried for the murder of his wife's lover. Though acquitted, he found it expedient to travel for a number of years in Mexico and Central America taking publicity photographs for the Union Pacific railroad, owned by Stanford. In 1877 he returned to California and later pursued his work at the University of Pennsylvania (Fig. 1.9). Muybridge placed 24 single lens cameras in a row. The cameras were triggered in sequence by a series of thin threads that were stretched across the path of the animal. The thrust against each thread completed an electric circuit and effected a photographic exposure. He managed to get pictures of an excellent quality as, through an ingenious combination of clockworks and electromagnetic circuits, he had finally succeeded in bringing exposure time down to 1/6000 second (in a time when an exposure of 1/2 second was considered instantaneous!).

Muybridge did not only study equine locomotion, though it formed the major part of his work. He also focused on other domesticated species, wild animals and man. His book *Animal Locomotion*, first published in 1887, has been republished several times. Muybridge also invented the 'zoöpraxiscope,' a device that consisted of a large glass disc on which successive pictures were printed. By projecting these in rapid succession on a screen, it gave an impression of a moving picture. In fact, this was a forerunner of present-day cine film, the invention of which is usually credited to Thomas Edison,

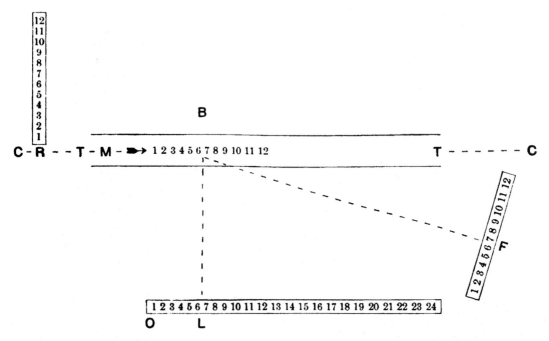

Fig. 1.9 Position of cameras and track as used in the studies conducted by Muybridge during his period at the University of Pennsylvania. B: lateral background; C: transverse backgrounds; F, R: batteries of 12 automatic photoelectric cameras; L: lateral battery of 24 automatic photoelectric cameras; O: position of operator; T: track. (From: Muybridge, E. *Animals in Motion*. Original edition 1899. Republished in 1957: Brown, L.S. (ed) New York: Dover Publications.)

though it is known that Edison derived some of his basic ideas from Muybridge. Early in 1888 Muybridge even discussed with Edison the possibility of producing talking pictures by synchronizing a zoöpraxiscope with a phonograph. As the phonograph at the time was not loud enough to be heard by an audience, the idea was abandoned (Muybridge, 1899). It would take another 40 years before the talking picture would conquer the world . . . .

Though originally a photographer, Muybridge was also something of a scientist. His book *Animals in motion* has a better scientific base than the book *The horse in motion as shown by instantaneous photography with a study on animal mechanisms founded on anatomy and the revelation of the camera in which is demonstrated the theory of quadrupedal locomotion* by the physician J.D.B. Stillman. Stanford provided many of Muybridge's photographs to Stillman without giving credit to the original photographer. Muybridge also suggested in a letter to *Nature* in 1883 that the photographic technique could be used to identify the winner of horse races when the finish was very close (Leach & Dagg, 1983). Indeed, in 1888 the world's first photo finish was made in New Jersey.

In the meantime, in France, the physiologist and university professor E.J. Marey investigated equine gait with

equally inventive, but somewhat different techniques. Marey was intrigued by the similarity of natural mechanisms and mechanical machinery and was convinced that a more profound study of the former, especially in the area of locomotion, would lead to substantial progress in mechanical engineering. In the preface of his book *La Machine Animale, Locomotion Terrestre et Aérienne* (1882a) he writes:

Quant à la locomotion aérienne, elle a toujours eu le privilège d'exciter vivement la curiosité chez l'homme. Que de fois ne s'est-il pas demandé s'il devrait toujours envier à l'oiseau et à l'insecte leurs ailes, et s'il ne pourrait aussi voyager à travers les airs, comme il voyage à travers les océans? A différentes époques, des hommes qui faisaient autorité dans la science ont proclamé, à la suite de longs calculs, que c'était là un rêve chimérique. Mais que d'inventions n'avons-nous pas vu réaliser qui avaient été pareillement déclarées impossibles?

(Aerial locomotion has always provoked a vivid curiosity in man. How many times did man wonder whether he would have to forever envy the birds and insects for their wings or whether it would be possible some day for him to travel through the skies as he travels the oceans? At various times scientific authorities have declared, after having made elaborate calculations, that this was an idle dream. But how many inventions did we

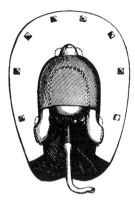

Fig. 1.10 A Devices developed by Marey to quantify equine locomotion. *'Chaussure exploratrice'* or exploratory shoe.

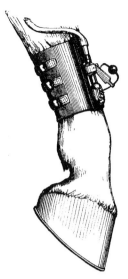

Fig. 1.10 *contd* **C** Air-filled bracelet for the discrimination between stance and swing phase on hard surfaces where the *'chaussure exploratrice'* could not be used. (From: Marey, E.J. (1882a) *La Machine Animale. Locomotion Terrestre et Aérienne*. Paris: Germer Baillière et Cie.)

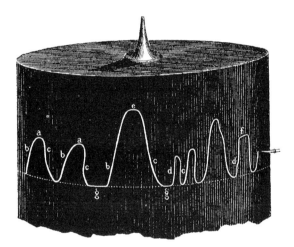

Fig. 1.10 *contd* **B** The recorder indicating limb placement of the horse.

not see that had been declared equally impossible beforehand?)

Twenty years later the Wright brothers would make their first flight and 80 years later long-distance maritime passenger transport would have been almost totally replaced by air travel.

In his book Marey studied both terrestrial and aerial locomotion. The studies on terrestrial gait focused on the horse. Three ingenious devices were used to study the equine gaits in a relatively accurate way. To discriminate between stance and swing phase Marey used a '*chaussure exploratrice*' or 'exploratory shoe' (Fig. 1.10A). This was essentially an India rubber ball filled with horse-hair that was attached to the horse's foot. At hoof placement the ball was compressed. The increase in pressure, transmitted by airtight rubber tubing, was registered by a

recorder in the rider's hand (Fig. 1.10B). The recorder consisted of a charcoal-blackened rotating cylinder on which traces were made by a needle that reacted to changes in air pressure. As this device wore rapidly on hard surfaces, a second instrument was made (Fig. 1.10C). It consisted of a kind of bracelet that was fastened to the distal limb just above the fetlock joint and that functioned according to the same principle. A third device consisted of two collapsible drums that were fastened to the withers and the croup, with levers attached to record vertical movements in the gaits.

Marey discussed various notations of gaits and concluded that the notation by Goiffon and Vincent was by far superior. He adapted this method somewhat and his notation, depicting limb placement by sequential open and filled bars, is still in common use today. Marey worked out the exact sequence of foot contacts, but his calculation of how long each foot remained on the ground was too short. Like Muybridge, he demonstrated the short suspension phase of the trot and he also correctly deduced that the hindquarters gave the main propulsion whereas the forequarters provided support (Leach & Dagg, 1983).

Though the techniques used in *La machine animale* are mainly of a mechanical nature and not photographic, Marey in fact is also one of the pioneers in photography (Marey, 1882b, 1883). At first he used multiple exposures on the same photographic plate, later he made a rotating plate not unlike Muybridge's 'zoöpraxiscope'. He also produced flight arcs of several segments of the body by repeated exposure of black objects with reflecting markers at anatomically defined points moving against a black background. Most of these techniques were applied to study human locomotion, but photographs of horses were also made. In the latter the superposition of hindlimb markers over forelimb markers using the repeated exposure technique made interpretation of the data a difficult job. He and his coworkers Pagès and Le Hello published a fine series of articles on the subject in the *Comptes Rendus Hebdomodaires des Séances de l'Academie des Sciences* (Le Hello, 1896, 1897, 1899; Marey & Pagès, 1886, 1887; Pagès, 1885, 1889).

Coincidentally, these two great men of equine gait analysis, Muybridge and Marey, were born one month apart in 1830 and died within one week from each other in 1904. They met in Marey's laboratory, in the presence of a large number of scientists from all over the world who attended the Electrical Congress in Paris in 1881. This was when Muybridge gave the first demonstration of his 'zoöpraxiscope' in Europe (Muybridge, 1899).

German supremacy until World War II

A nice synopsis of late 19th century state of the art in the field of equine gait analysis is given in the book by Goubaux and Barrier *De l'extérieur du cheval* (*On the conformation of the horse*, 1884). They describe both Marey's techniques and Muybridge's work. They cite Marey as saying that, if he had to do his experiments again, he would use an electric circuit instead of a pneumatic system. In fact, it appears that Barrier repeated his measurements in 1899 using an electrical device to improve accuracy (Schauder, 1923b). Goubaux and Barrier also described some other means to represent equine gait such as a kind of adjustable rattle that would reproduce the sounds made by the hoof beats in the various gaits, and a wooden table that was over 8 feet high through which limb placement in various gaits could be visualized (Fig. 1.11).

Following Goubaux and Barrier, the period of French supremacy in gait analysis ended. The French were very ingenious inventors, but it was the Germans who chose to follow the path indicated by Marey and Muybridge. It was only through sequential photography, soon followed by cine film which is essentially the same, that the faster equine gaits could be fully explored.

After laying the foundations in the late 19th century, German veterinary science had its golden age in the first half of the 20th century. Many disciplines flourished, but perhaps none so abundantly as the discipline of veterinary anatomy. Wilhelm Ellenberger (1848–1928) and Hermann Baum (1864–1932) published many editions of their *Handbuch der vergleichenden Anatomie der Haustiere*

(*Handbook of comparative anatomy of domestic animals*). This work was so complete that a facsimile version of the 1943 edition was still in print in the 1970s. Another excellent anatomist was Paul Martin who moved from Zürich to Gießen in the first years of the 20th century. Two of his pupils were to become famous anatomists themselves: Wilhelm Schauder at Gießen University and Reinhold Schmaltz in Berlin. In Germany, the study of muscle function and locomotion was in the hands of the anatomists. It is therefore not surprising that many of these individuals became involved in equine gait analysis and/or biomechanical studies. It has been reported that Ellenberger studied the gallop by attaching four different-sounding bells to the feet of the horses (Schauder, 1923b). Schmaltz was among the first to extensively use cine film for equine gait analysis, and Schauder published on equine gait and related topics throughout a long career that extended until after World War II.

Chief veterinary officer in the first Dragoon Regiment at Berlin, Werner Borcherdt used the pictures by Muybridge and the German photographer Otoman Anschütz for his largely theoretical treatise on the jumping horse (1912). In the proceedings of the *Kaiserlich-Königliche Botanische Gesellschaft* in Vienna in early 1917 Professor Keller showed the results of own kinematic experiments. Keller had constructed a turntable, that was moved by the horse itself, in the center of which was a camera. This system ensured a strictly lateral view although the horse was not walking along a straight line. Keller filmed at a rate of 32–50 frames per second (fps), and showed the film at the standard rate of 16 fps, thus creating a slow motion effect. Schmaltz (1922a,b) used essentially the same technique, but used the film mainly to produce a photographic series that shows the characteristics of each gait. It is Walter (1925) who, under the guidance of Schmaltz, extensively used the turntable in his study of limb placement sequence and changes in joint angles during walk, trot and gallop. Walter admits the disadvantage of the circular movement and indicates that the Clinical Department of the Berlin Veterinary High School made use of a linear rail over which a camera could be moved by mechanical power in order to keep up with a horse moving on a parallel path.

In a publication from 1923 A.O. Stoss from Munich used photographic methods to study the anatomy and kinematics of the equine limbs. In the section on the shoulder motion, he made a remark that it was a pity he could not use the pictures published by Muybridge to determine the exact location of the skeletal parts that make up the shoulder, because only skinny horses could be used for this purpose. Apparently, Muybridge's horses were too fat!

Studies using techniques other than photography were also being performed, again mainly by anatomists.

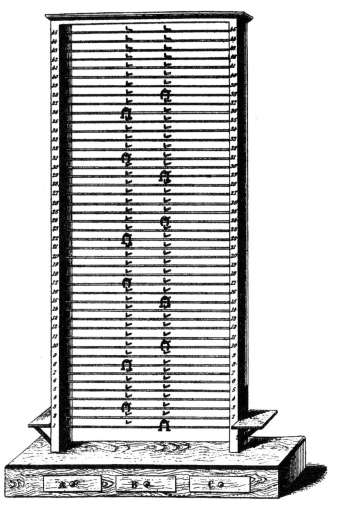

Fig. 1.11 Wooden table invented by Goubaux and Barrier to represent the footfall pattern in various gaits. Drawers A and B contain nickel-plated shoes for fore and hindlimbs; drawer C contains a series of cards on which the correct position of the feet in a certain gait are described (From: Goubaux, A. & Barrier, G. (1884) *'De l'extérieur du cheval.* Paris: Asselin et Cie.)

Dörrer (1911), working at the Königliche Tierärztliche Hochschule in Dresden, wrote a thesis on the tension in the flexor tendons and the suspensory ligament during various phases of the stride cycle. For his *in vitro* work he used a device that had originally been designed by Moser (Fig. 1.12). Strubelt (1928), who worked in Hanover, found that transecting either the lacertus fibrosus or the peroneus tertius muscle did not affect locomotion in the living animal, nor the anatomical relations in a specimen of the hindlimb that was brought under tension.

Bethcke (1930) focused on the relationship between morphometric data and performance in the trotter. Earlier studies on the subject had been performed by

Bantoiu (1922) in Berlin and Birger Rösiö (1927) who performed measurements on Standardbreds in Sweden, Germany and the United States. Bantoiu was one of a series of Rumanian vets who, under the guidance of Professor Schöttler in Berlin, studied the relationship between conformation and performance in various breeds. His colleagues Stratul (1922), Nicolescu (1923) and Radescu (1923) studied this relationship in Thoroughbreds and Hanoverian horses. Though Bethcke is able to give some data on anatomical differences between various breeds of horses, he has to conclude that he could not predict performance, stating that: '*Wenn uns so auch die Maße für die Beurteilung eines Trabers gewisse Anhaltspunkte geben, so*

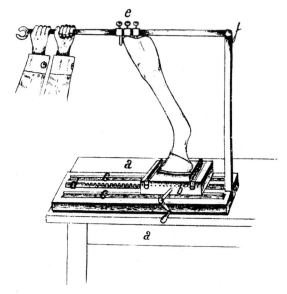

Fig. 1.12 Device to (semiquantitatively) determine the tension in the flexor tendons and the suspensory ligament in various positions of the limb as designed by Moser and used by Dörrer. (From: Dörrer, H. (1911) *Über die Anspannung der Beugesehnen des Pferdefußes während der verschiedenen Bewegungsstadien derselben.* Inaugural dissertation, Dresden.)

sind für seine Leistungsfähigkeit letzten Endes doch noch andere Faktoren wie Training, Temperament, Abstammung, Ausdauer, Beschaffenheit der inneren Organe usw. mit ausschlaggebend'

(Though the measurements may give us some clues for the judgement of a trotter, performance is in the end more determined by other factors such as training, character, descent, endurance and condition of the internal organs). This conclusion has not changed in the past 70 years.

The relationship of conformation and locomotion was heavily studied in pre-war Germany. Wiechert (1927) studied East Prussian cavalry horses to find morphometric criteria for performance potential. Though he finds some biometric differences between horses selected for specific purposes, the study lacks any statistical elaboration of the data. Buchmann (1929) focused mainly on stride length in various breeds. Kronacher and Ogrizek (1931) published a comprehensive study using 60 Brandenburger mares. A follow-up to this study was performed by Horst Franke (1935) who studied 186 mares from the famous stud in Trakehnen (East Prussia). A positive relationship between the length of some limb segments and stride length was found, but results on the influence of joint angulation were not consistent. While Kronacher and Ogrizek report a clear positive relation-

ship between stride length and shoulder and elbow angles, Franke is more cautious, stating that joint angles are much less important in determining stride length than the dimensions of limb segments. The study of Schmidt (1939) is even less conclusive. He studied 100 cavalry horses with the aim of determining conformational characteristics that were indicative of a long stride, which was a desirable trait of cavalry horses that often had to cover more than 30 miles a day, and concluded that no unequivocal conformational indications could be found. Therefore, it was better to accurately measure the actual stride length when buying cavalry horses! In 1934 Wagener published a comprehensive study on jumping horses and in 1944 Wehner wrote on the relation of bone axes and joint angles and stride length in the German coldblood.

In Munich research was more biomechanically oriented. Moskovits (1930) studied statical-mechanical aspects of the equine metacarpus. Max Kadletz studied the biomechanical behavior of the small tarsal joints in detail in relation to the pathogenesis of bone spavin (Kadletz, 1937). He also paid attention to the movements of front and hindlimbs, and addressed the age-old problem of how artists should depict horses, inventing some makeshifts for this purpose (Kadletz, 1926, 1932, 1933).

Possibly the most prolific of the pre-war German scientists was Wilhelm Krüger from Berlin. He published a very elaborate and authoritative study on the kinematics of both fore and hindlimbs (Krüger, 1937, 1938). Krüger did not use a turntable like his predecessors Schmaltz and Walter, but made use of a vehicle that moved alongside and at the same speed as the horse, probably the same installation that had already been described by Walter. He was well aware of the artifact introduced by the use of skin markers which had already been noted by Fick (1910) who had stated: '*Vor allem ist es schwierig, an den bewegten Gliedern bestimmte Punkte sicher zu markieren die ihre Lage auf der Körperoberfläche während der Bewegung nicht ändern, da sich ja auch die Haut in der Nähe der Gelenke beträchtlich verschiebt'*

(In the first place it is difficult on the moving limbs to mark sites that do not alter their positions on the body surface during movement, as the skin near the joints shifts considerably).

Krüger avoided the problem by oiling the skin and using oblique lighting, thus visualizing the position of the bones directly. Though the skin displacement artifact is taken into account in most pre-war research (in contrast to many much more recent studies), this was not always the case and Krüger does not hesitate to blame this artifact for the discrepancies of his findings with those by Aepli (1937) who, in his cinematographic measurements of joint angles during locomotion, failed

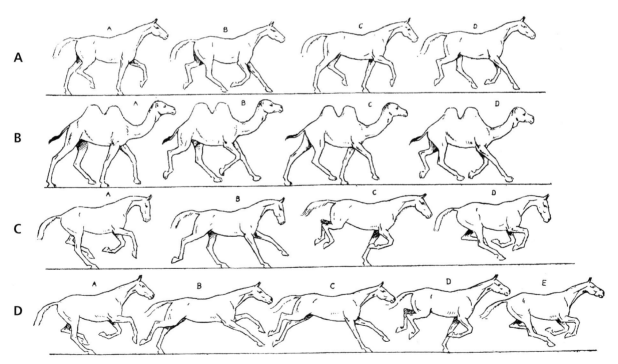

Abb. 1. Borelli'sche Schwerpunktswaage (Schema).
Erläuterungen im Text.

Fig. 1.13 The so-called *'Balance of Borelli'* as used by Krüger to determine the center of gravity of the horse. (From: Krüger, W. (1939) *Die Fortbewegung des Pferdes*. Berlin: Paul Parey.)

to correct for the artifact (Krüger, 1938). Krüger was a dedicated scientist and a prolific writer. Apart from his cinematographic work on gait analysis, which he summarized in a treatise on the movement of the horse

(1939a) (Fig. 1.13), he wrote on the oscillations of the vertebral column (1939b), specific limb placement during the gallop and while jumping (1939c,d), the position of the center of gravity during locomotion (1941a), and the effect of hauling heavy loads on the tendons in the forelimb (1941b).

Though German scientists were dominant in the era between the turn of the century and World War II, this was not the only site of activity. The work of Aepli (1937), which has been referred to already, was performed in Zürich. Before World War II, there were also scientists in South America who focused on equine gait analysis. When asked to write a series of articles for a sports magazine on the gaits of the horse, Magne de la Croix from Argentina started to study photographic material, including the series made by Muybridge, and became so interested in the subject that he wrote an article on the evolution of the gallop in which he stated that, in evolutionary terms, the rotatory gallop was more advanced than the transverse gallop (Magne de la Croix, 1928). He can be seen as a forerunner of the great American zoologist Milton Hildebrand, who four decades later stated that the various gaits are not that distinct as hitherto presumed but in fact form a continuum that

Fig. 1.14 Depiction of various gaits by Magne de la Croix. **A** Trotting horse; **B** pacing camel; **C** 3-beat gallop; **D** horse featuring 4-beat racing gallop. (From: Magne de la Croix, P. (1929) Filogenia de las locomociones cuadripedal y bipedal en los vertebrados y evolución de la forma consecutiva de la evolución de la locomoción. *Anal. Soc. Cient. Argent.* 108: 383–406.)

may gradually change into each other, when he writes: '*Un hecho en el cual nunca me había fijado, resaltó de repente a mis ojos, y es que el galope de carrera de los varios animales, en vez de presentarse sólo bajo dos formas: transverse gallop y rotatory gallop, como los llama Muybridge, ofrece, en realidad, una infinidad de variantes que constituyen una cadena insensible y continua*'

(A fact that so far had never occurred to me became suddenly clear. This is that the racing gallop of the various species, instead of presenting in only two forms: *transverse* and *rotatory gallop* as Muybridge calls them, in fact presents as an infinite number of variations that form a continuous, imperceptibly changing chain).

He developed the idea further and included all gaits and many different animals in his extensive paper on the phylogeny of quadrupedal and bipedal locomotion in vertebrates (Magne la Croix, 1929; Fig. 1.14). He continued publishing on the subject until the mid-1930s (Magne de la Croix, 1932, 1936).

Armando Chieffi in Brazil started his investigations of locomotion with a large study of the position of the center of gravity (Chieffi & de Mello, 1939). He continued with papers on the '*marcha*' (an artificial gait) in the Mangalarga Horse (Chieffi, 1943) and with studies comparing the stance phases of different gaits and the change of gallop (Chieffi, 1945, 1946). Finally he wrote a thesis (1949) on the subject of the transition of gaits, a subject on which little scientific work had been done as he concluded from his review of the literature: '*O exame de literatura a respeito . . . revelou que pouco ou nade existe sôbre transição de andamentos*'

(The literature search showed that there was very little if anything on the subject of changes of gait). It still is a relatively unexplored area.

In Belgium, Zwaenepoel published the same study on the impulse of gait in the horse twice in different journals (Zwaenepoel, 1910a,b, 1911a,b). In Holland, Kroon (1922, 1929) and van der Plank (1929) performed some detailed studies on the hoof mechanism using electric devices, not photography or cine film (Fig. 1.15). Captain Carnus from the military training school at Saumur was one of the few French authors of the era who wrote on the subject. His was a largely theoretical study on the role of the muscles of the neck in forelimb motion (Carnus, 1935). In Sweden the well-known veterinarian Forssell investigated the effect of the transection of various tendons and ligaments (Forssell, 1915) and Palmgren (1929) studied the angulation pattern of the elbow joint in relation to muscle use and muscle conformation ('feathering' of certain muscle groups) in Swedish Standardbreds using high-speed cine film. In Czechoslovakia Kolda (1937) published on the functional anatomy of the equine shoulder joint.

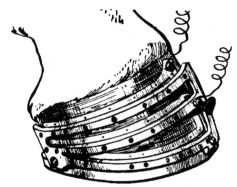

Fig. 1.15 Electric device to measure deformation of the hoof wall, adapted by Kroon (1922) from the original by Bayer (1882). (From: Kroon, H.M. (1922) Een bijdrage tot de studie van het hoefmechanisme. *Tijdschr. Dierg.* 49(11): 399–406.)

In the United States work in this area of research was scarce. In 1912 Gregory published a largely theoretical treatise on quadrupedal locomotion and Chubb of the American Museum of Natural History used photographs of horses as a help in the preparation of accurate specimens for the Museum (Berger, 1923). In 1934 Harry H. Laughlin, from the Carnegie Institution's Department of Genetics, published a study in which he developed a formula based on age, weight carried, distance run and time taken that quantified Thoroughbred performance in a given race. These figures were meant to serve as a 'mathematical yardstick' to be used in the search to find the natural laws governing the transmission of inborn racing capacity (Laughlin 1934 a,b). Less specific to the horse was the work of John T. Manter of South Dakota who wrote on the dynamics of quadrupedal walking (1938). The same applies to the book on speed of animals by A. Brazier Howell (1944). Also in 1944 J. Gray from Cambridge (UK) published a comprehensive study on the mechanics of the tetrapod skeleton. Even in Bolshevik Russia research was performed. Ivanov and Borissov (1935) continued the line set by Forssell (1915) and Strubelt (1928), studying the importance of the *lacertus fibrosus* in the standing and moving horse. Schtserbakow (1935) tried to use kinematic data for the determination of the optimal amount of work a horse should be given during training. Afanasieff (1930) claimed that he found correlations between some morphometric variables and maximal speed. He did not fail to mention that, whereas before the Russian Revolution there was a great interest in the American trotter and many crossings were made with the Russian Orlow trotter, the present breeding goal was to develop the pure Orlow trotter breed and to cut out any American influence . . . .

The horse in decline

World War II left large parts of Europe in ruins. Apart from the tragic loss of life for millions of people, the war had a devastating effect on many aspects of pre-war society. In Germany, where research on equine gait analysis and biomechanics had flourished as nowhere else, Bernhard Grzimek was still performing research on handedness in horses, parrots and monkeys in the Frankfurt Zoo in the summer of 1944 when the Allied Forces already were fighting their way to Paris through the heavily defended French province of Normandy. He submitted the paper on October 5, 1944, about at the time Montgomery's troops were defeated in the Battle of Arnhem which would prolong the war for about half a year. However, after the capitulation of the Third Reich in May 1945, science in Germany, like practically all aspects of public life, came to a grinding halt. Grzimek's paper finally was published in 1949.

Although public life regained its vitality earlier in the formerly occupied and now liberated parts of Europe, the situation was not essentially different. Attention was focused on repairing the enormous damage caused by the war, rather than on developing new scientific approaches. Apart from the direct consequences of the war, there were other developments that failed to stimulate new research in the field of equine locomotion. In World War I horses had been used extensively. The British Expeditionary Force in France in 1914 began with 53 000 horses, but it is estimated that in 1917 the army had more than 1 million horses in active service over all fronts (Dunlop & Williams, 1996). On the German side the number of horses was reported to be 1 236 000 in the same year, not counting those belonging to the army contingents employed at home or in the occupied territories (von den Driesch, 1989). In German East Africa (Tanzania) the commander of the relatively weak forces, First Lieutenant von Lettow-Vorbeck, developed a 'veterinary strategy' to combat an overwhelmingly more numerous army consisting of British, South African, Belgian and Portuguese forces. Using his superior knowledge of the local situation of tropical diseases, especially trypanosomiasis, and giving better prophylactic care to his own animals, he consistently retreated through the tsetse-infested areas, inflicting heavy losses in animals on the Imperial Forces. On Armistice Day in 1918 he still was at large with his last 1323 troops, pursued by an army of 120 000. At the start of World War II in September 1939 Polish Lancers tried to stop the invading German tanks. Not surprisingly, they suffered heavy losses and were not able to slacken the advance of the enemy. Though the German army still used horses extensively for transportation (a mean population of about 1 350 000 has been estimated, of which an average of 59% was lost), it became clear that the role of the horse in warfare finally had come to an end after 5000 years. There is no modern army in which the horse plays a prominent role, except perhaps for some ceremonial duties.

The increasing mechanization not only influenced the military role of the horse. Numbers of horses in the United States reached their peak in 1918 at 21 million. After that year, which is also the year that automobile production first passed the 1 million mark, the population more than halved to an estimated 8 million horses and 2 million mules in 1947 (Simpson, 1951). In Britain the agricultural horse population in 1913 was 1 324 400; in 1956 it was only 233 500 (Brayley Reynolds, 1957). It was to be expected that the day would not be far away that the last commercially used horse could be turned out to pasture after retirement. Of course, this trend affected the numbers of patients presented for treatment to the veterinary schools. In the pre-war period, the Utrecht Clinic of Large Animal Surgery received more equine than bovine patients. This ratio changed to 1:1 in the early post-war period and remained so through the early 1960s, followed by an increase in equine patients again from 1964 onwards, now in the form of sports and leisure animals (Offringa, 1981).

In view of the declining role of the horse in society, it is not surprising that research on equine locomotion received less priority than in the years before the war. Nevertheless, some activity remained. In Germany the old tradition had not completely been broken by the war, though the relative number of publications decreased considerably. Of the pre-war scientists Schauder, at Gießen University, continued publishing. He was principally interested in the functional development of the musculoskeletal system. In his pre-war publications he had focused on the development of various parts of the equine musculoskeletal system (Schauder, 1924a, 1924b, 1932). After the war he continued with this subject when quoting Goethe to express his basic presumption: '*Gestaltenlehre ist Verwandlungslehre*' (Morphology is the science of change) (Schauder, 1949). In the early 1950s he concentrated on shock-absorbing structures in the equine limbs and rump (Schauder, 1951, 1952, 1954), which he discussed on a theoretical basis.

The tradition at Gießen was continued by L. Krüger (not to be confused with Wilhelm Krüger from Berlin), who published on the hauling capacity of horses (and cattle) in order to determine performance capacity (Krüger, 1957). At the Institute of Animal Physiology of the University of Bonn (which had no veterinary faculty), Kaemmerer (1960) used photography to study the flight arcs of various parts of the equine limbs. He concluded that these flight arcs cannot be seen as parts of a circle, as had been stated before, but in fact are complicated cycloids which change their form when the horse is more heavily loaded. He stated, not without surprise, that the work by Walter (1925) had not received the recognition it merited. He had come across Walter's work only after finishing his own experiments, and concluded that both investigations, performed using different techniques, generally confirmed each other.

Equine gait analysis still formed a topic for a few of the many veterinary doctorate theses at the German universities. Richter (1953) in Berlin continued the tradition of the Rumanian veterinarians from the early 1920s when he studied the American-bred trotter in order to correlate morphometric data with performance. In Gießen, Maennicke (1961) and Genieser (1962) were among the first to work with (Shetland) ponies and not with horses. The Turkish veterinarian, Ihsan Aysan (1964), analyzed the gait of lame horses during his years in Gießen in which he prepared his thesis. He worked with a 3 m long track and with a fixed camera using a film speed of 132 fps. As the distance of the horse to the camera was not constant, complicated mathematical procedures were necessary to calculate the exact locations of certain anatomical sites. Though the principle of this mathematical data processing is the same in the modern video-based systems, one should be aware of the fact that this study was undertaken before the advent of the computer. As Aysan could not statistically process the data, his work basically consists of extended case reports of various types of lameness.

Though the interest in equine locomotion certainly was at a low in the period between the end of World War II and the early 1970s, some seeds were sown of what in later decades would become rich fruit-bearing trees. In Sweden Björck (1958) was the first to use a force-shoe to analyze the ground reaction forces exerted by the horse. In Vienna the opening of the reconstructed lecture hall of the Anatomy Department in 1950 was celebrated with a lecture by Schreiber on the old theme of the anatomically (in-)correct depiction of horses in art. The then young assistant Peter Knezevic used strain gauges and cinematography to study the hoof mechanism. With a 4-channel recorder he was able to make synchronous ungulographic recordings at walk, trot and gallop (Knezevic, 1962). In Holland, Slijper had already published an extensive study on the vertebral column and spinal musculature of mammals in 1946. However, the tradition of biomechanical research and gait analysis at Utrecht University, that is maintained to the present day, can be said to have started with the publication by Dick Badoux in *Nature* on the friction between feet and ground (1964). Many publications were to follow, all

focusing on the biomechanics of specific parts of the musculoskeletal system (Badoux 1966, 1970a, 1970b). There was also a start of the input of biomechanics in essentially clinical work, as shown by the thesis of Rathor (1968) on disorders of the equine and bovine femoropatellar articulation.

Elsewhere, activity was very limited in this field of research. In France a thesis was published by Marcel André (1949) on static, dynamic and cinematic aspects of equine locomotion. In Switzerland some work was performed on the biomechanics of the equine elbow joint in the late 1960s (Mosimann & Micheluzzi, 1969). In Eastern Europe there was some interest in the relation between conformation and performance. Fehér focused principally on biometric data concerning the horse with a normal configuration (Fehér, 1957, 1958). From the early 1960s Dušek from Czechoslovakia started a series of publications on the relation of a number of conformational parameters and performance like jumping ability and how to correctly evaluate these parameters. Unfortunately, some of this work was published in the Czech language which is not accessible to many scientists (Dušek & Dušek, 1963; Dušek *et al.*, 1970). In the German Democratic Republic some work was done on the conformation of trotters by von Lengerken and Werner (1969). However, the breed was not very important in socialist days as there was no more than one racetrack in the whole country. In the Soviet Union Sukhanov (1963) focused in a more general sense on the evolution of gait. In Japan Nomura published a series of reports on the mechanics of a number of equine joints in the early 1950s (Nomura, 1953 a,b,c)

In the Anglo-Saxon world the interest in equine gait analysis and biomechanics was still limited. In 1951 Grogan published a general descriptive article about gaits in horses which ominously opens with the words: '*With the drop in the number of working horses, the study of the horse has held less interest for most veterinarians and received less attention in the schools*'. In England H.W. Dawes (1957) published a paper on the relationship between conformation and soundness, giving detailed descriptions of some more or less desirable traits. The same topic is discussed by Pritchard in the US nearly a decade later (1965). Though interesting, both papers are based on clinical impressions rather than scientific research. This is different from the work of the great American zoologist Milton Hildebrand who studied, using film among other techniques, the gaits of tetrapods. Though he used the horse frequently as a study object, his interests were broader. The analysis and interpretation of the gaits of tetrapods, including the energetics of oscillating legs in relation to conformation and gait were his main targets, not the horse itself (Hildebrand, 1959, 1960, 1965, 1966). However, in the late 1960s some horse-specific research was published in the US (Taylor *et al.*, 1966; Rooney, 1968, 1969; Solá, 1969; Cheney *et al.*, 1970), indicating that we are in the wake of what may be called revolutionary changes in the science of equine biomechanical research and gait analysis.

THE REVIVAL IN EQUINE LOCOMOTION RESEARCH

In most countries in the world the era directly after World War II had been a period of hardship in which the damage caused by the war, either materially or economically, had to be repaired. In large parts of the world it was a period of lack of resources in which people were forced to work hard while leading a life deprived of any luxury. Gradually this picture changed as from the late 1950s or early 1960s economies began to boom. The mid 1960s onwards marked the start of a period of unprecedented economic growth and increasing prosperity in the developed world. While old sources of richness, such as the former colonial empires, disappeared new technological developments enabled manifold increases in human production capacity, leading to a large increase in cheap consumer goods. This development led to a period of wealth and prosperity in the industrial world.

The horse had lost its role in the military completely and in agriculture and transport to a large extent. However, it had, after 5000 years of close alliance, not lost its appeal to man. The horse had always been a very useful instrument for the satisfaction of one of the most fundamental drives of mankind, the need for competition. The official history of horse racing tells us that this sport started in 648 BC in Olympia in Greece (Simpson, 1951), but it is highly improbable that horse races were not common in the few thousand years between the domestication of the horse and that date. Apart from its role in competition, the horse, unlike any other animal with the possible exception of the dog, has always had man's affection. This special bond between man and the horse is already evident in the earliest human writings on the species in Antiquity and remains so, through the great horse marshals of the 17th century and many others in the course of time, to the present day.

With the booming economy in the 1960s, popular interest in the horse could be materialized. Equestrian sports had existed for thousands of years, but had always been restricted to the lucky few. Now they became within reach of the general public. From the end of the 1960s and beginning of the 1970s equestrian sports flourished as never before. This was evident in very old and well-known branches of the equestrian sports such as flat racing and harness racing all over the world, the Western-style activities in the US, and dressage and jumping in Europe. Popular interest also increased in other, less-known, areas such as three-day eventing, vaulting, four-in-hand driving and endurance competitions. New competitions were created in various of these disciplines and the time was ripe for the organization of large events like the World Equestrian Games, the first of which was held in Stockholm in 1990.

The increased interest in the horse was the trigger for the revival in equine locomotion research that started in the early 1970s. Though the economic role of the horse had disappeared (except for the increasing economic significance of the horse industry itself), the need for research into equine locomotion was now even greater than before. While in earlier times the horse had to be able to do its job properly, which required a functional, but not necessarily superior, locomotor system, the horse now had become an athlete upon which high demands were made. This prompted the need for a highly accurate analysis of normal and abnormal gait and of the ways in which equine locomotion could be influenced or improved. Rapid developments in computer technology enabled the production of both hardware and software that facilitated capture and analysis of the faster movements of the horse in intricate detail. These were the main factors that determined the explosion in equine locomotion research that started in the late 1970s and continues today.

It is beyond the scope of this chapter on history of equine locomotion research to give a comprehensive review of the recent literature on the topic. For such reviews, the reader is referred to the corresponding chapters further on in this book. In the following paragraphs a brief outline will be given of the development of the main centers of equine locomotion research in order to provide a link from the rich history of this area of research to the practice of today. References will be restricted to some key publications, but make no pretense of completeness.

Equine locomotion research centers and activities

Ingvar Fredricson and coworkers may be credited for the initiation of the revival of research on equine locomotion. In 1970 they published a report about the quantitative analysis of hoof motion patterns of harness horses using high-speed film in the proceedings of a congress on high-speed photography (Fredricson *et al.*, 1970). Shortly after that, the new method of investigating equine locomotion was published in the then recently founded *Equine Veterinary Journal* (Fredricson & Drevemo, 1971). Fredricson used high-speed film (with frame rates up to 500 fps) and analysis methods derived from the aviation industry to process his data. This approach enabled him to analyze in three dimensions the very fast movements of the distal limbs of Standardbreds trotting at high speed (Fig. 1.16). These investigations resulted in his thesis which may be seen as the starting point of the modern era of equine locomotion research (Fredricson, 1972).

The Swedish group, the nucleus of which was formed by Fredricson and Stig Drevemo, later joined by Gøran Dalín and Gunnar Hjertén, focused on kinematic analysis of the Swedish Standardbred. In Sweden, harness racing had always been a popular sport, but the industry boomed in the 1970s and 1980s with Sweden and France becoming the most important countries for harness racing in Europe. This increase in popularity of the sport

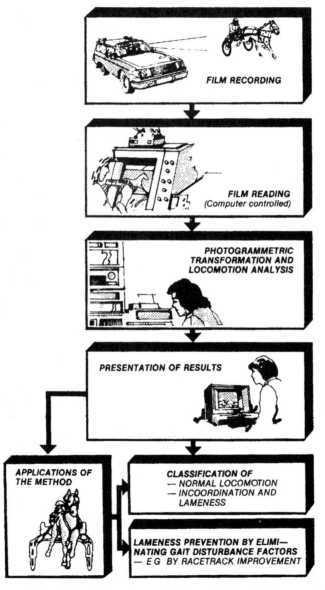

Fig. 1.16 Diagrammatic representation of the data capture and data analysis procedure as used by the Swedish group in the 1970s when they worked with high-speed film. (From: Fredricson, I., Drevemo, S., Dalín, G., Hjertén, G., Björne, K. (1980) The application of high-speed cinematography for the quantitative analysis of equine locomotion. *Equine Vet. J.* **12**(2): 54–59.)

was partly due to the very generous fiscal legislation for horse owners. The interest in harness racing was also evident in the extensive research this group has performed on the design of racetracks, signaling deleterious effects of poor racetrack design and giving possible solutions for improvement (Fredricson *et al.*, 1975a,b). Indeed, their work resulted in considerable improvements with respect to banking and curve geometry of many racetracks. The Swedish group may also be credited for being the first to use a treadmill for equine locomotion analysis (Fredricson *et al.*, 1983), an example that was soon to be followed by many research centers all over the world.

After Fredricson left the group to head the national stud at Flyinge, Stig Drevemo took the helm. He became a Professor of Anatomy at the Faculty of Veterinary Medicine of the Uppsala University of Agricultural Sciences into which the formerly independent Royal Veterinary College had been converted. His series of papers on equine locomotion that appeared in the *Equine Veterinary Journal* in 1980 can be considered as classic (Drevemo *et al.*, 1980a–c). Drevemo was a strong protagonist of international cooperation in the field of equine locomotion research. Together with Doug Leach from Saskatoon, Canada, he published the first (and unfortunately until now the last) edition of a *Bibliography of research in equine locomotion and biomechanics* in 1988. This reference list, though not complete and also not entirely free from errors, is still a great help for young researchers in this field as it also included the old literature that cannot be traced using modern electronic techniques.

The almost exclusive emphasis on kinematics of the Standardbred was broken by the arrival in Uppsala of the English-born globetrotter Leo Jeffcott. His broad interest in the field of equine orthopedics included problems related to the back. With the exception of the 1939 paper by Wilhem Krüger, little attention had been paid so far to the equine back. There is little doubt that this apparent lack in interest was partly caused by the inaccessibility of this structure. Jeffcott worked with Dalín and other members of the Swedish team on normal biomechanics of the back and on various back-related disorders (Jeffcott & Dalín, 1980; Jeffcott *et al.*, 1982, 1985).

After Jeffcott left for Australia, the Swedish group continued to perform equine locomotion research using high-speed cinematography. Though very reliable and accurate, the technique has a major drawback in that data analysis is extremely labor-intensive. The Swedes tried to overcome this problem by automizing as far as possible this analysis using advanced and expensive techniques such as the Trackeye® system (Drevemo *et al.*, 1993). In the 1990s they finally opted for the video-based Proreflex® system. Though older members of the group left or became absorbed in administrative functions, the Swedish group succeeded in maintaining momentum by attracting young researchers such as Holmström, Johnston and Roepstorff. Of these, Holmström focused on the kinematic analysis of top-level dressage horses (Holmström *et al.*, 1995), while Roepstorff and Johnston were engaged in the development of a force shoe suitable for use on the treadmill, in fact continuing the tradition begun by Björck in the late 1950s (Roepstorff & Drevemo, 1993). In this way the Swedish Equine Biomechanics Group continued in the 1990s as a key player in the field of equine locomotion research, which by then had taken global proportions.

Another center where research on equine locomotion was initiated in the 1970s was Vienna. Peter Knezevic had written a thesis on the biomechanics of the hoof using strain gauges when he was an assistant at the Veterinary High School. After he became head of the Department of Orthopedics of Even and Uneven-hoofed Animals of the Faculty of Veterinary Medicine of the University of Vienna, he strongly promoted further research in this field. From the late 1970s, the Vienna group started to publish regularly on both kinematic (using high-speed cinematography and later also the Selspot® system) and kinetic studies (using force plates) in the horse (Knezevic *et al.*, 1978; Knezevic & Floss, 1984). The historical interest of Knezevic is shown by his 1985 paper in the *Wiener Tierärztliche Monatsschrift* (where many of the papers from the first Golden Age of equine locomotion research had been published). However, this paper is principally a German copy of the *Equine Veterinary Journal* paper published on the same topic by Leach and Dagg in 1983. Knezevic's co-worker Girtler wrote an excellent and elaborate thesis on the temporal stride characteristics of lame horses at the walk and trot which, again, appeared in the *Wiener Tierärztliche Monatsschrift* (Girtler, 1988). Also after the retirement of Knezevic locomotion research remained a priority topic in Vienna. The research facilities greatly improved when the Faculty was moved to the vast new premises at the end of the 1990s. The group was substantially reinforced by the arrival of Florian Buchner in 1996 who had spent 4 years with the Utrecht Equine Biomechanics Research group working on his PhD thesis.

In Holland the foundation for the line on biomechanical research had been laid in the 1960s by Dick Badoux from the Department of Anatomy. One of the products of this line was the still authoritative study by Wentink on the biomechanics of the hindlimb of horse and dog (Wentink, 1978a,b). However, it was the strategic alliance between the Departments of Anatomy and of General and Large Animal Surgery that really boosted this kind of research from the end of the 1970s onwards. For this strategic alliance, the vision of the department heads,

Professors W. Hartman and A. W. Kersjes, respectively, should be given full credit. First, Schamhardt and Merkens focused on the analysis of the ground reaction forces in sound and lame horses using a force plate (Merkens *et al.*, 1986; Schamhardt & Merkens, 1987). Later, kinematic analysis was added. The Dutch group did not opt for high-speed film or the then recently introduced first video-based systems such as Selspot® or Vicon®, but chose a new invention from England: the CODA-3® system. This optoelectronic system used a concept that was basically different from any video-based system and thus avoided a number of disadvantages inherent to these systems. However, when the prototype with serial number 007 was delivered, it proved to be not exactly ready-to-use. In fact, it took about 4 years and a considerable amount of manpower before the machine was working well under the conditions encountered when performing gait analysis in the horse. It proved to have a high spatial and temporal (300 fps) resolution.

Van Weeren, who was intended to be the first user of the newly purchased system was forced to redirect his line of research. He started an investigation into a topic in equine kinematic gait analysis that had been correctly identified by most pre-war researchers, but which had been largely ignored so far in more recent research: the problem of skin displacement. Together with van den Bogert, Schamhardt and Barneveld he developed techniques using intra-osseous light-emitting diodes, which shone through the skin, and transcutaneous pins to produce correction factors for skin displacement (van Weeren & Barneveld, 1986; van Weeren *et al.*, 1992). In his study on the coupling between stifle and hock joint by the reciprocal apparatus, he was finally able to use the CODA-3® system for the first time (van Weeren *et al.*, 1990).

The first person to use the CODA-3® system extensively was Willem Back who, in a long-term project, studied the longitudinal development of gait from 4-month-old foal to adult horse (Back *et al.*, 1994a), concluding that the gait pattern of the individual horse does not essentially alter during this development. He also made comparisons between hard data from kinematic gait analysis and the subjective evaluation of horses as is done at horse shows and during sire selection procedures, identifying kinematic parameters that determine the judgment of quality of equine gait (Back *et al.*, 1994b). The Austrian veterinarian Florian Buchner used his time in Utrecht to study the kinematics of lame horses, and the symmetry of gait (Buchner *et al.*, 1996). Besides, he performed some important work on determining the centers of gravity of various body segments (Buchner *et al.*, 1997). Van den Bogert mathematically modeled equine gait (van den Bogert *et al.*, 1989). This excellent scientist included a floppy disc in his thesis

with an animation of equine gait, which was a novelty at the end of the 1980s.

Apart from the kinematic and kinetic studies, other lines of research were followed as well. Some work on bone strain in the tibia was performed (Hartman *et al.*, 1984; Schamhardt *et al.*, 1984). Riemersma started a line on tendon research using many techniques, including kinetic and kinematic analyses (Riemersma *et al.*, 1988a,b). This line was continued by Jansen, who made use of mercury in-silastic strain gauges (Jansen *et al.*, 1993) and Becker who focused on the inferior check ligament (Becker *et al.*, 1994).

In 1992 a specially constructed equine biomechanics research lab was opened in Utrecht, featuring a treadmill and a force plate track. This building greatly facilitated research. Recently, the CODA-3® system was complemented by a ProReflex® system (Fig. 1.17). By the early 1990s, the Utrecht Equine Biomechanics research group had become one of the world's leading centers for equine locomotion research. This had been possible in somewhat more than a decade because of the vision of the heads of department (after the retirement of Kersjes as head of the Department of General and Large Animal Surgery he had been succeeded by Ab Barneveld, who strongly supported this line of research), and the willingness to cooperate. This involved collaboration between departments, and between people with different scientific backgrounds. Henk Schamhardt, a driving force behind a large number of the research projects who unfortunately died as a consequence of a tragic accident in 1999, was a physicist, not a veterinarian, as is Ton van den Bogert, who later left for Canada, changing horses for humans.

In France, the cradle of modern equine locomotion research, work on the topic had been extremely limited after the turn of the century. However, here too interest in this kind of research regained momentum at the end of the 1970s which led to the resurfacing of France as one of the leading nations in equine locomotion research from the mid 1980s onwards. The new work originated in part from the veterinary faculties of the French universities, but also from institutions such as the '*Institut National de Recherches Agronomiques*' (INRA, National Institute for Agronomic Research) and the National Stud Services (*Service de Haras*), as is the case with the work by Langlois (1978) relating conformation with ability in trotting, galloping and jumping. In these institutions research work of a more applied than fundamental character has been carried out in various fields of equestrian sports, including jumping and harness racing, which is an important discipline in France.

Alfort took the lead among the veterinary schools. Eric Barrey studied the biomechanics of the equine foot extensively (Barrey, 1987), while Jean-Marie Denoix

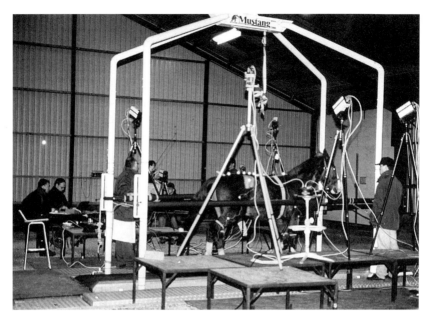

Fig. 1.17 Investigations on the kinematics of the equine spine at the Utrecht Biomechanics Research Lab at the end of the 1990s by a combined Dutch and Swedish team. A total of 7 Proreflex® cameras is used. (Photo: Utrecht Equine Biomechanics Research Group.)

started his very active career by studying contact areas in the fetlock joint (Denoix, 1987a) and the kinematics of the thoracolumbar spine (Denoix, 1987b). Originally an anatomist, Denoix' interest in clinical orthopedic disorders would later broaden considerably. His special interest in the biomechanics of the back, however, remained.

In the rest of Europe there were few developments. In Germany some isolated investigations were performed (Wilsdorf, 1971; Bayer, 1973; Preuschoft & Fritz, 1977), but no new centers of research emerged. In Switzerland the situation was similar (Koch, 1973; Hugelshofer, 1982). In Great Britain, where research in equine biomechanics and gait analysis had never been a strong area, a group interested in equine biomechanics emerged around Lance Lanyon and Allen Goodship. While Lanyon focused on biomechanics of bone (Lanyon, 1971; Lanyon & Rubin, 1980), Goodship dedicated himself and his group to the study of the equine tendon using force plate techniques (Goodship *et al.*, 1983). The latter technique was also used in the extensive evaluation of various treatments of tendon injury as documented in the first *Supplement* of the *Equine Veterinary Journal*, the famous Silver report (Silver *et al.*, 1983). Also from Britain, R. McNeill Alexander should be mentioned as the author of several studies on quadrupedal gait. Like the American zoologist Milton Hildebrand, Alexander regarded the horse as an example rather than a goal in itself (Alexander, 1980; Alexander & Jayes, 1983).

In North America work on equine biomechanics and gait analysis had been very limited after the great advances brought to this area of science by Eadweard Muybridge. Publications from the period that in Europe can be designated as the first Golden Age of equine locomotion research, the period between World Wars I and II, are virtually non-existent. After World War II this did not really change with only a few isolated publications on rather heterogenous topics. However, the scene changed dramatically after the revolution started by the Swedes. In just a few years a number of research groups were founded which would become very prolific. At the Western College of Veterinary Medicine in Saskatoon, Canada, Doug Leach founded a school of equine biomechanical research that was to foster a number of excellent scientists. Leach himself published on a variety of topics including the effects of fatigue (Leach & Sprigings, 1979) and temporal stride characteristics (Leach *et al.*, 1987). He was also interested in the history of equine locomotion research (Leach & Dagg, 1983) and was heavily involved in the definition of correct terminology (Leach *et al.*, 1984). Another researcher from Saskatoon was Hugh Townsend who dedicated his thesis to thoracolumbar kinematics and the relationships between vertebral morphology and pathologic changes which led to some important papers on this difficult subject (Townsend *et al.*, 1983, 1986; Townsend & Leach, 1984).

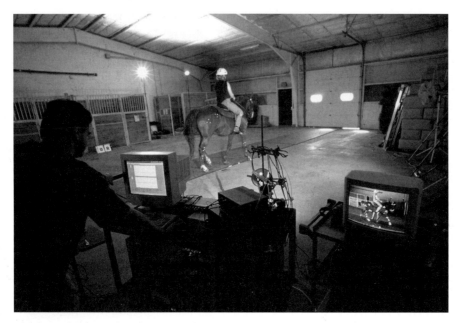

Fig. 1.18 Kinematic research conducted at the Equine Sports Medicine Center of Michigan State University, East Lansing. (Photo: Mary Anne McPhail Dressage Chair in Equine Sports Medicine.)

Leach's co-worker and later chair of the Department of Veterinary Anatomy, Hilary Clayton, was to become an even greater authority in the field. At first she focused on the kinematic analysis of various causes of lameness and on the performance of elite sport horses using high-speed film (Clayton, 1986, 1987). Later her research developed a more fundamental character when it was directed towards the kinematic analysis of elite sport horses (Clayton, 1993, 1994, 1997). Collaboration between Clayton and Bob Colborne, a human kinesiologist, and Joel Lanovaz, a mechanical engineer, broadened the scope of the work in Saskatoon to the calculation of net joint moments and joint powers at all joints of the equine limbs during both the stance and swing phases of the stride (Clayton *et al.*, 1998; Colborne *et al.*, 1998). In 1997 Clayton left Canada to become the first incumbent of the Mary Anne McPhail Dressage Chair in Equine Sports Medicine at Michigan State University in East Lansing (Fig. 1.18). The large research endowment that founded this unique chair and the construction of the new Mary Anne McPhail Equine Performance Center will ensure the continuance of equine locomotor research at Michigan State University for the foreseeable future.

In the United States, Jim Rooney, a pathologist in the Mecca of the American Thoroughbred industry, Kentucky, should be mentioned. In 1969 he published a book on the biomechanics of lameness in horses. After that, a long series of papers on a wide variety of biome-

chanical subjects followed. Rooney can to a certain extent be compared with the old scientists of the pre-World War II generation. The vast majority of his papers are single-authored and it sometimes is hard to tell which of his statements are personal opinions based on deductions from observations, and which are real facts based on hard, statistically sound, scientific data.

From the mid 1970s Marc Ratzlaff and his group at Washington State University in Pullman were one of the few who extensively used electrogoniometry for gait analysis in the horse, in addition to other techniques such as cinematography (Ratzlaff, 1974; Ratzlaff *et al.*, 1979). The gallop was the gait most intensively studied by this group (Ratzlaff *et al.*, 1995). The start of the work by George Pratt Jr. dates from about the same period. He used the force plate and concentrated on the Thoroughbred and the interaction with the race track (Pratt & O'Connor, 1976; Pratt, 1984).

Nancy Deuel, who spent most of her career at the University of Maryland in College Park, wrote her thesis on the kinematic analysis of the gallop in Quarter Horses (Deuel, 1985). She later became interested in top-level performance horses and obtained permission to make recordings during the World Equestrian Games in 1990 and the Olympic Games in 1988, 1992 and 1996 (Deuel & Park, 1990, 1991). Calvin Kobluk performed equine kinematic research, first using cinematography at Guelph

University, then the video-based Motion Analysis® system at the University of Minnesota (Kobluk *et al.*, 1989).

Apart from the fundamental research, more applied investigations were also being carried out. At Texas A&M University Gingerich *et al.* (1979) used the force plate to study the effect of pharmaceuticals on joint function. In the same university, Swiss-born Jörg Auer experimented with the so-called Kaegi-Straße, a 5 m long track of rubber matting consisting of a large number of tiny liquid-filled chambers which in fact were electrical circuits. The pressure of the hoof changed the electrical resistance and thus resulted in a change in the shape of the signal (Auer & Butler, 1985). This 'diagnostic street' was intended as an aid in diagnosing specific lameness causes. After the first enthusiastic reports, it died a silent death as things turned out not to be as simple as that. At Tufts University Howard Seeherman constructed his Equine Performance Lab which, among many other tests for equine performance, featured gait analysis techniques. Apart from the detection of gait irregularities, these were mainly used to correctly balance the hooves of the patients (Seeherman *et al.*, 1987, 1996).

Elsewhere in the world research remained limited. In Australia Leo Jeffcott began investigations into the non-invasive measurement of bone quality and the influence of exercise thereon (Jeffcott *et al.*, 1987), while Wilson *et al.* (1988a,b) did some work on the kinematics of trotters. However, no long-lasting research centers were founded. In Japan, Tokuriki and co-workers made advances in electromyography in the horse (Aoki *et al.*, 1984), while Niki and colleagues used the force plate for the study of equine biomechanics (Niki *et al.*, 1982).

By the beginning of the 1990s the second Golden Age of equine biomechanical and gait analysis research was well established with various centers where high-quality research was being performed in north-western Europe and North America. Besides these major research groups, smaller scale projects were undertaken in many other places underlining the importance given to this branch of research.

Concluding remarks

Since its domestication 5000 years ago, the horse has had a close relationship with man. There is no doubt that, from a historical viewpoint, the horse's most important role has been that of a machine of war, followed by its economic significance as a draft animal. However, from the very early days after domestication, the horse has had other roles also: as a sports and competition animal and as an animal with which man formed a bond of affection. It was the latter two aspects that ensured the horse's survival after mechanization relieved the horse of its former strongholds of military and economic

importance and, at the end of the 1940s, a total eclipse of the species threatened. Despite its retreat from many areas in society, the horse has remained within the public domain and is now more popular than ever.

The interest in the species from the veterinary perspective has kept pace with public appreciation of the horse. The same applies to equine locomotion research, though another factor should be mentioned too: the state of technology. The development of technology in general and photography in particular made possible the great breakthroughs accomplished by Muybridge and Marey at the end of the 19th century, which were the prelude to the first Golden Age of equine locomotion research. It was also the combination of the renewed interest in the horse and the rapidly developing computer technology which led to the second Golden Age of this branch of research.

What about the future? The bond between man and the horse has proved to be strong enough to survive the disappearance of what seemingly was the *raison d'être* of the alliance between the two species. There is no reason to suppose that interest in the horse will diminish as long as economic conditions do not become too harsh. As for technology, developments in this area seem to happen at ever increasing speed. It may be expected, therefore, that the present book will see many revised and updated editions, be it in a printed or electronic form.

REFERENCES

Adams, L. and Handiseni, T. (1991) *A Tourist Guide to Rock Art Sites in Northern Zimbabwe*. Harare: Queen Victoria Museum.

Aepli, A. (1937) Betrachtungen über die Messung der oberen Extremitätenwinkel sowie neue Meß-und Beobachtungsversuche durch die Filmaufnahme beim Pferd. *Inaugural dissertation, Zürich.*

Afanasieff, S. (1930) Die Untersuchung des Exterieurs, der Wachstumsintensität und der Korrelation zwischen Renngeschwindigkeit und Exterieur beim Traber. *Z. Tierz. Zücht. biol.* **18**: 171–209.

Alexander, R. McN. (1980) Optimum walking techniques for quadrupeds and bipeds. *J. Zool. Lond.* **192**: 97–117.

Alexander, R. McN. and Jayes, A.S. (1983) A dynamic similarity hypothesis for the gaits of quadrupedal mammals. *J. Zool. Lond.* **201**: 135–152.

André, M. (1949) Mécanique equestre. *Thèse, Lyon.*

Aoki, O., Tokuriki, M., Kurakawa, Y., Hataya, M. and Kita, T. (1984) Electromyographic studies on supraspinatus and infraspinatus muscles of the horse with or without a rider in walk, trot and canter. *Bull. Equine Res. Inst.* **21**: 100–104.

Aristotle (384–322 BC) Parts of animals; movements of animals; progression of animals. In: Peck, A.L. and Forster, E.S. (1961) (eds) *The Loeb Classical Library*. London: Heinemann.

Auer, J.A. and Butler, K.D. (1985) An introduction to the Kaegi equine gait analysis system in the horse. *Proc. 31st Annu. Conv. Am. Assoc. Equine Pract.*, pp. 209–226.

Aysan, I. (1964) Beitrag zur Analyse der Bewegungsanomalien beim Pferd mit Hilfe der kinematographischen Methode. *Inaugural dissertation, Gießen.*

Back, W., Barneveld, A., Schamhardt, H.C., Bruin, G. and Hartman, W. (1994a) Longitudinal development of the kinematics of 4-, 10-, 18- and 26-month-old Dutch Warmblood horse. *Equine Vet. J.* **17**(Suppl.): 3–6.

Back, W., Barneveld, A., Bruin, G., Schamhardt, H.C. and Hartman, W. (1994b) Kinematic detection of superior gait quality in young trotting warmbloods. *Vet. Quart.* **166** (S2): 91–96.

Badoux, D.M. (1964) Friction between feet and ground. *Nature* **202**: 266–267.

Badoux, D.M. (1966) Mechanics of the acropodium of the horse: a practical application of photoelastic research. *Tijdschr. Dierg.* **91**(19): 1207–1232.

Badoux, D.M. (1970a) Some biomechanical aspects of the elbow joint in the horse during normal gait. *Proc. K. Ned. Akad. Wetensch.* **73**(1): 35–47.

Badoux, D.M. (1970b) The statical function of some crural muscles in the horse. *Acta. Anat.* **75**: 396–407.

Bantoiu, C. (1922) Messungen an Trabern und die Beurteilung der Leistungsfähigkeit auf Grund der mechanischen Verhältnisse. *Inaugural dissertation, Berlin.*

Barrey, E. (1987) Biomécanique du pied du cheval: Étude experimental. *Thèse, École Nationale Vétérinaire d'Alfort.*

Bayer, A. (1973) Bewegungsanalysen an Trabrennpferden mit Hilfe der Ungulographie. *Zentbl. Vet. med. Reihe A* **20**: 209–221.

Bayer, J. (1882) Experimentelles über Hufmechanismus. *Oesterr. Monatsschr. Tierheilk.* **7**: 72–74.

Becker, C.K., Savelberg, H.H.C.M. and Barneveld, A. (1994) In vitro mechanical properties of the accessory ligament of the deep digital flexor tendon in horses in relation to age. *Equine Vet. J.* **26**: 454–459.

Berger, A.K. (1923/1980) In: *Natural History Magazine* (Nov/Dec) Mounting horse skeletons to exemplify different gaits and actions. A glimpse behind the scenes at the American Museum. Reprinted in: *Natural History* **89**(4): 100–102; 1980.

Bethcke (1930) Ist es möglich auf Grund der mechanischen Verhältnisse die Leistungsfähigkeit eines Trabers zu bestimmen? *Z. für Veterinärkunde* **42**(5): 161–170.

Björck, G. (1958) Studies on the draught forces of horses. Development of a method using strain gauges for measuring forces between hoof and ground. *Acta Agric. Scand.* **8**(Suppl. 4).

Borcherdt, W. (1912) Studien über die Sprungbewegung des Pferdes. *Inaugural dissertation, Bern.*

Borelli, G.A. (1681) *De motu animalium.* Roma.

Brayley Reynolds, E. (1957) In: Dawes, H.W. (ed): The relationship of soundness and conformation in the horse. *Vet. Rec.* **69**: 1367–1374.

Buchmann, J. (1929) Untersuchungen über Schritt-und Trabgang des Pferdes. *Dissertation, Breslau.*

Buchner, H.H.F., Schamhardt, H.C. and Barneveld, A. (1996) Limb movement adaptation in horses with experimentally induced fore or hind limb lameness. *Equine Vet. J.* **28**: 63–70.

Buchner, H.H.F., Savelberg, H.H.C.M., Schamhardt, H.C. and Barneveld, A. (1997) Inertial properties of Dutch Warmblood horses. *J. Biomech.* **30**: 653–658.

Carnus, (1935) Contribution à l'étude de la cinématique du cheval. L'action des muscles de l'encolure dans le jeu du membre antérieur. *Rev. Vét. Milit.* **19**: 563–570.

Cavendysh, G. (1674) *Méthode nouvelle et invention extraordinaire de dresser les chevaux et les travailler selon la nature.* Londres: Tho. Milbourne, pp. 119–126.

Cheney, J.A., Henwood, K. and Chen, C.K. (1970) Thoroughbred lameness, a report on research into its relationship to the composition of California racing surfaces. *The Thoroughbred of Calif.* (June): 906–924.

Chieffi, A. (1943) A marcha no cavalo mangalarga. *Rev. Fac. Med. Vet. S. Paulo.* **2**: 177–192.

Chieffi, A. (1945) Estudo comparativo de fases de apôio semelhantes, nos diversos andamentos do cavalo. *Rev. Fac. Med. Vet. S. Paulo.* **3**: 109–130.

Chieffi, A. (1946) Contribuição para o estudo da mudança do galope do cavalo pela cinematografia. *Rev. Fac. Med. Vet. S. Paulo* **3**(3): 61–69.

Chieffi, A. (1949) Contribuição para o estudo da transição dos andamantos, no cavalo, pela interpretação de filmes, em camara lenta. *Thesis, University of Sao Paulo.*

Chieffi, A. and de Mello, L.H. (1939) Contribuição para o estudo da localização do centro de gravidade no corpo dos animais domésticos e dos fatores que produzem seu deslocamento temporário ou permanente. *Rev. Fac. Med. Vet. S. Paulo* **1**: 97–154.

Clayton, H.M. (1986) Cinematographic analysis of the gait of lame horses. I: Fractured supraglenoid tubercle. *J. Equine Vet. Sci.* **6**(2): 70–78.

Clayton, H.M. (1987) Cinematographic analysis of the gait of lame horses. IV: Fracture of the third carpal bone. *J. Equine Vet. Sci.* **7**(3): 130–135.

Clayton, H.M. (1993) The extended canter: a comparison of some kinematic variables in horses trained for dressage and racing. *Acta Anat.* **146**: 183–187.

Clayton, H.M. (1994) Comparison of the stride kinematics of the collected, working, medium and extended trot in horses. *Equine Vet. J.* **26**(3): 230–234.

Clayton, H.M. (1997) Classification of collected trot, passage and piaffe based on temporal variables. *Equine Vet. J.* **23**(Suppl): 54–57.

Clayton, H.M., Lanovaz, J.L., Schamhardt, H.C., Willemen, M.A. and Colborne, G.R. (1998) Net joint moments and joint powers in the equine fore limb during the stance phase of the trot. *Equine Vet. J.* **30**(5): 384–389.

Clayton, M. (1996) *Leonardo da Vinci – a curious vision.* London: Merrell Holberton, pp. 158–159.

Colborne, G.R., Lanovaz, J.L., Sprigings, E.J., Schamhardt, H.C. and Clayton, H.M. (1998) Forelimb joint moments and power during the walking stance phase of horses. *Am. J. Vet. Res.* **59**(5): 609–614.

Dawes, H.W. (1957) The relationship of soundness and conformation in the horse. *Vet. Rec.* **69**: 1367–1374.

De Solleysel, J. (1733) *Le parfait maréchal, que enseigne a connoistre la beauté, la bonté et les défauts des chevaux,* 2ième partie. Paris: Pierre-Jean Mariette, p. 66.

Denoix, J.M. (1987a) Etude biomécanique de la main du cheval: extensometrie des rayons metacarpo-phalangiens et surfaces articulaires de contact (sur membre isolé soumis à compression). *Thèse, Université Claude-Bernard, Lyon.*

Denoix, J.M. (1987b) Kinematics of the thoracolumbar spine of the horse during dorsoventral movements: a preliminary report. *Proc. 2nd Int. Conf. Equine Exerc. Physiol.*, pp. 607–614.

Deuel, N.R. (1985) A kinematic analysis of the gallop of the horse. *Thesis, University of Illinois.*

Deuel, N.R. and Park, J.J. (1990) The gait patterns of Olympic dressage horses. *Int. J. Sport Biomech.* **6**: 198–226.

Deuel, N.R. and Park, J.J. (1991) Kinematic analysis of jumping sequences of Olympic show jumping horses. *Proc. 3rd Conf. Equine Exerc. Physiol.*, pp. 158–166.

Dörrer, H. (1911) Über die Anspannung der Beugesehnen des Pferdefußes während der verschiedenen Bewegungsstadien derselben. *Inaugural dissertation, Dresden.*

Drevemo, S., Dalín, G., Fredricson, I. and Hjertén, G. (1980a) Equine locomotion 1. The analysis of linear and temporal stride characteristics of trotting Standardbreds. *Equine Vet. J.* **12**(2): 60–65.

Drevemo, S., Fredricson, I., Dalín, G. and Björne, K. (1980b) Equine locomotion 2. The analysis of coordination between limbs of trotting Standardbreds. *Equine Vet. J.* **12**(2): 66–70.

Drevemo, S., Dalín, G., Fredricson, I. and Björne, K. (1980c) Equine locomotion 3. The reproducibility of gait in Standardbred trotters. *Equine Vet. J.* **12**(2): 71–73.

Drevemo, S., Roepstorff, L., Kallings, P. and Johnston, C. (1993) Application of TrackEye in equine locomotion research. *Acta Anat.* **146**: 137–140.

Dunlop, R.H. and Williams, D.J. (eds) (1996) *Veterinary Medicine. An illustrated history.* St. Louis: Mosby.

Dušek, J. and Dušek, J. (1963) Vyznam telesne stavby koni z hlediska pracovniho vykonu v zemedelstvi. *Sb. Zivoc. Výroba* **8**: 303–310.

Dušek, J., Ehrlein, H.J., von Engelhardt, W. and Hörnicke, H. (1970) Beziehungen zwischen Trittlänge, Trittfrequenz und Geschwindigkeit bei Pferden. *Z. Tierärztl. Zücht. biol.* **87**: 177–188.

Fehér, G. (1957) Beiträge zu den funktionellen Veränderungen der Form und Struktur des Schulterblatts beim Pferd. *Acta Vet. Acad. Sci. Hung.* **7**: 19–48.

Fehér, G. (1958) Beiträge zur Statik und Dynamik der vorderen Extremitäten des Pferdes. *Acta Vet. Acad. Sci. Hung.* **8**: 187–198.

Fick, R. (1910) Allgemeine Gelenk- und Muskelmechanik. In: von Bardeleben, K. (ed) *Handbuch der Anatomie des Menschen,* Bd. 2 Abt. 1. Jena: Fischer.

Forssell, G. (1915) Untersuchungen über die Wirkungsweise der Beugesehnen am Vorderfuß des Pferdes. *Z. Tiermed.* **18**: 184–188.

Franke, H. (1935) Untersuchungen über den Einfluß des Körperbaus auf die Schrittlänge des Pferdes. *Dissertation Landwirtschaftliche Hochschule, Berlin.*

Fredricson, I. (1972) Equine joint kinematics and co-ordination. *Thesis, Royal Veterinary College, Stockholm.* Published in: *Acta. Vet. Scand.* **37**(Suppl.): 1–136.

Fredricson, I. and Drevemo, S. (1971) A new method of investigating equine locomotion. *Equine Vet. J.* **3**(4): 137–140.

Fredricson, I., Andersson, S., Dandanell, R., Moen, K. and Andersson, B. (1970) Quantitative analysis of hoof motion patterns using high-speed films of harness horses. *Proc. 9th Int. Congr. High-Speed Photogr.*, pp. 347–350.

Fredricson, I., Dalín, G., Hjertén, G., Nilsson, G. and Alm, L.O. (1975a) Ergonomic aspects of poor racetrack design. *Equine Vet. J.* **7**(2): 63–65.

Fredricson, I., Dalín, G., Drevemo, S. and Hjertén, G. (1975b) A biotechnical approach to the geometric design of racetracks. *Equine Vet. J.* **7**(2): 91–96.

Fredricson, I., Drevemo, S., Dalín, G. et al. (1983) Treadmill for equine locomotion analysis. *Equine Vet. J.* **15**(2): 111–115.

Gamgee, J. (1869) On the action of the horse. *J. Anat. Physiol.* **3**: 370–376.

Gamgee, J. (1870) The action of the horse. *J. Anat. Physiol.* **4**: 235–236.

Genieser, D. (1962) Analyse der Bewegungswechsel beim Shetlandpony. *Dissertation, Gießen.*

Gingerich, D.A., Auer, J.A. and Fackelman, G.E. (1979) Force plate studies on the effect of exogenous hyaluronic acid on joint function in equine arthritis. *J. Vet. Pharmacol. Therap.* **2**: 291–298.

Girtler, D. (1988) Untersuchungen über die Dauer des

Bewegungszyklus – Stützbeinphase, Hangbeinphase, Phasenverschiebung – bei lahmen und bewegungsgestörten Pferden im Schritt und Trab sowie kinematische Beurteilungen zu deren Bewegungsmuster. *Wien. Tierärztl. Mon. schr.* **75**(5): 185–196; **75**(6): 217–231; **75**(7): 255–270; **75**(8): 310–324.

Goiffon and Vincent (1779) *Mémoire Artificielle des Principes Relatifs à la Fidelle Répresentation des Animaux Tant en Peinture, qu'en Sculpture.* I. Partie concernant le cheval. Alfort: Ecole Royale Vétérinaire.

Goodman, N. (1870) The action of the horse. *J. Anat. Physiol.* **4**: 8–11.

Goodman, N. (1871) The action of the horse. *J. Anat. Physiol.* **5**: 89–91.

Goodship, A.E., Brown, P.N., MacFie, H.J.H., Lanyon, L.E. and Silver, I.A. (1983) A quantitative force plate assessment of equine locomotor performance. *Proc. 1st Int. Conf. Equine Exerc. Physiol.*, pp. 263–270.

Goubaux, A. and Barrier, G. (1884) *De l'extérieur du cheval.* Paris: Asselin et Cie, pp. 547–582.

Gray, J. (1944) Studies in the mechanics of the tetrapod skeleton. *J. Exp. Biol.* **20**: 88–116.

Gregory, W.K. (1912) Notes on the principles of quadrupedal locomotion and on the mechanism of the limbs in hoofed animals. *Annals N Y Acad. Science* **22**: 267–294.

Grogan, J.W. (1951) The gaits of horses. *J. Am. Vet. Med. Assoc.* **119**: 112–117.

Grzimek, B. (1949) Rechts- und Linkshändigkeit bei Pferden, Papagaien und Affen. *Z. Tierpsychol.* **6**: 406–432.

Günther, K. (1866) *Die topographische Myologie des Pferdes mit besonderer Berücksichtigung der lokomotorischen Wirkung der Muskeln.* Hannover: Carl Rümpler.

Hartman, W., Schamhardt, H.C., Lammertink, J.L.M.A., Badoux, D.M. (1984) Bone strain in the equine tibia: An in vivo strain gauge analysis. *Am. J. Vet. Res.* **45**(5): 880–884.

Hildebrand, M. (1959) Motions of the running cheetah and horse. *J. Mamm.* **40**(4): 481–495.

Hildebrand, M. (1960) How animals run. *Scientific Am.* **202**(5): 148–157.

Hildebrand, M. (1965) Symmetrical gaits of horses. *Science* **150**: 701–708.

Hildebrand, M. (1966) Analysis of the symmetrical gaits of tetrapods. *Folia Biotheor.* **VI**: 9–22.

Holmström, M., Fredricson, I., Drevemo, S. (1995) Biokinematic effects of collection on the trotting gaits in the elite dressage horse. *Equine Vet. J.* **27**(4): 281–287.

Howell, A.B. (1944) *Speed in Animals.* New York: Hafner Publishing Co.

Hugelshofer, J. (1982) Vergleichende Kraft- und Belastungszeitmessungen an den Vorderhufen von gesunden und an Podotrochlose erkrankten Pferden. *Dissertation, Zürich.*

Ivanov, S. and Borissov, V.M. (1935) Importance of the lacertus fibrosus in standing and motion of the horse. *Archiv Anatomii, Gistologii i Embriologii* **14**: 51–55.

Jansen, M.O., van den Bogert, A.J., Riemersma, D.J. and Schamhardt, H.C. (1993) In vivo tendon forces in the forelimb of ponies at the walk validated by ground reaction force measurements. *Acta Anat.* **146**: 162–167.

Jeffcott, L.B. and Dalín, G. (1980) Natural rigidity of the horse's backbone. *Equine Vet. J.* **12**: 101–108.

Jeffcott, L.B., Dalín, G., Drevemo, S., Fredricson, I., Björne, K. and Bergqvist, A. (1982) Effect of induced back pain on gait and performance of trotting horses. *Equine Vet. J.* **14**(2): 129–133.

Jeffcott, L.B., Dalín, G., Ekman, S. and Olsson, S.E. (1985) Sacroiliac lesions as a cause of chronic poor performance in competitive horses. *Equine Vet. J.* **17**(2): 111–118.

Jeffcott, L.B., Buckingham, S.H.W. and McCartney, R.N. (1987) Noninvasive measurement of bone quality in horses and changes associated with exercise. *Proc. 2nd Int. Conf. Equine Exerc. Physiol.*, pp. 615–630.

Kadletz, M. (1926) Die Formenwechsel der Hinterhandmuskulatur des Pferdes während der Bewegung. *Wiener Tierärztl. Monatsschr.* **13**: 185–198.

Kadletz, M. (1932) Ueber die physiologischen Kreiselungen und über die Statik der Schultergliedmaße des Pferdes; gleichzeitig ein Erklärungsversuch der sog. Struppigkeit und des sog. Fuchtelns. *Münchn. Tierärztl. Wschr.* **83**(37): 433–436.

Kadletz, M. (1933) Ueber einige Behelfe zur Erkennung der Bewegungsarten des Pferdes. *Dtsch. Tierärztl. Wschr.* **41**(28): 433–438.

Kadletz, M. (1937) Über die Bewegungsweise des Tarsalgelenkes des Pferdes. 3. Beitrag zur Spatgenese. *Arch. wissensch. prakt. Tierheilk.* **71**(4): 279–296.

Kaemmerer, K. (1960) Deskriptives über einige Bahnkurven bei der Gliedmaßenbewegung des Pferdes. *Arch. Exp. Vet. Med.* **14**: 97–110.

Keller, K. (1917) Kinematographische Analyse der Bewegungen des Pferdes. *Verhandl. Zool. Botan. Ges. Wien* **67**: 93–94.

Knezevic, P. (1962) Klinik des Trachtenzwanghufes und Grundlagen der Ungulographie mit Dehnungsmeßstreifen beim Pferde. *Wien. Tierärztl. Mon. schr.* **49**(10): 777–824.

Knezevic, P.F. (1985) Zur Geschichte der Bewegungslehre des Pferdes – eine historische Betrachtung der Untersuchungstechniken. *Wien. Tierärztl. Mon. schr.* **72**(12): 399–405.

Knezevic, P.F. and Floss, F.N. (1984) Klinische Ergebnisse der rechnergestützten Bewegungsanalyse beim Pferd. *Arch. Tierärztl. Fortbild.* **8**:140–148.

Knezevic, P.F., Seebacher, M., Fischerleitner, F., Tauffkirchen, W. and Benedikter, G. (1978) Ermittlung des Zusammenhanges zwischen Bewegung und Belastung des Pferdehufes mit Hilfe von Hochfrequenzphotographie und Mehrkomponentenkraftmeßplatte. *Biomed. Tech.* **23**:154–155.

Kobluk, C.N., Schnurr, D., Horney, F.D., Summer-Smith, G., Willoughby, R.A. and DeKleer, V. (1989) Use of high-speed cinematography and computer generated gait diagrams for the study of equine hind limb kinematics. *Equine Vet. J.* **21**: 48–58.

Koch, A. (1973) Zeit- und Belastungsmessungen an den Vorderhufen des Pferdes mittels der Mehrkomponenten-Kraftmeßplatte 'Kistler'. *Dissertation, Zürich.*

Kolda, J. (1937) Srovnávací anatomie a mechanica pažního kloubo. *Zverolek Rozpr.* **11**: 265–276.

Kronacher, C. and Ogrizek, A. (1931) Exterieur und Leistungsfähigkeit des Pferdes mit besonderen Berücksichtigung der Gliedmaßenwinkelung und Schrittlängenverhältnisse. *Z. Zücht. Reihe B Tierz. u. Züchtungsbiol.* **32**(2): 183–228.

Kroon, H.M. (1922) Een bijdrage tot de studie van het hoefmechanisme. *Tijdschr. Dierg.* **49**(11): 399–406.

Kroon, H.M. (1929) Studie van het hoefmechanisme. *Tijdschr. Dierg.* **55**(19): 961–967.

Kroon, H.M., Paimans, W.J. and Ihle, J.E.W. (1921) *Een eeuw veeartsenijkundig onderwijs. 's Rijksveeartsenijschool – Veeartsenijkundige Hoogeschool 1821–1921.* Utrecht: Senaat der Veeartsenijkundige Hoogeschool.

Krüger, L. (1957) Die Bestimmung der Arbeitsfähigkeit bei Pferd und Rind durch Leistungsprüfungen, physiologische und psychologische Meßwerte und durch die Exterieurbeurteilung. *Z. Tierz. Zücht. Biol.* **69**: 289–320.

Krüger, W. (1937) Ueber den Bewegungsablauf an dem oberen Teil der Vordergliedmaße des Pferdes im Schritt, Trab und Galopp. *Tierärztl. Rundsch.* **43**(49/50): 809–816; 825–827.

Krüger, W. (1938) Ueber den Bewegungsablauf an dem oberen Teil der Hintergliedmaßedes Pferdes im Schritt, Trab und Galopp. *Tierärztl. Rundsch.* **44**(34): 549–557.

Krüger, W. (1939a) *Die Fortbewegung des Pferdes.* Berlin: Paul Parey.

Krüger, W. (1939b) Ueber die Schwingungen der Wirbelsäule – insbesondere der Wirbelbrücke – des Pferdes während der Bewegung. *Berl. Münchn. Tierärztl. Wschr.* **13**: 197–203.

Krüger, W. (1939c) Ueber die Arbeit der vier Gliedmaßen des Pferdes beim Galopp. *Tierärztl. Rundsch.* **45**(13): 250–265.

Krüger, W. (1939d) Bemerkungen zur Gliedmaßenfolge beim Renngalopp und beim Sprung des Pferdes. *Tierärztl. Rundsch.* **45**(15): 287–293.

Krüger, W. (1941a) Ueber das Verhalten des Schwerpunktes bei der normalen Fortbewegung des Pferdes. *Tierärztl. Rundsch.* **47**(12/13): 147–152; 162–166.

Krüger, W. (1941b) Die schwere Zugarbeit und ihre Auswirkungen auf die Sehnen der Vordergliedmaße des Pferdes. *Dtsch. Tierärztl. Wschr.* **49**(17): 203–208.

Langlois, P., Froidevaux, J., Lamarche, L. *et al.* (1978) Analyse des liaisons entre la morphologie et l'aptitude au galop, au trot et au saut d'obstacles chez le cheval. *Ann. Génét. Sél. Anim.* **10**: 443–474.

Lanyon, L.E. (1971) Use of an accelerometer to determine support and swing phases of a limb during locomotion. *Am. J. Vet. Res.* **32**(7): 1099–1101.

Lanyon, L.E. and Rubin, C.T. (1980) Loading of mammalian long bones during locomotion. *J. Physiol. Lond.* 303.

Laughlin, H.H. (1934a) Racing capacity in the Thoroughbred horse. Part 1. The measure of racing capacity. *The Sci. Monthly* **38**: 210–222.

Laughlin, H.H. (1934b) Racing capacity in the Thoroughbred horse. Part 2. The inheritance of racing capacity. *The Sci. Monthly* **38**: 310–321.

Leach, D.H. and Dagg A.I. (1983) Evolution of equine locomotion research. *Equine Vet. J.* **15**(2): 87–92.

Leach, D.H. and Sprigings, E. (1979) Gait fatigue in the racing Thoroughbred. *J. Equine Med. Surg.* **3**: 436–443.

Leach, D.H. and Ormrod, K., Clayton, H.M. (1984) Standardised terminology for the description and analysis of equine locomotion. *Equine Vet. J.* **16**(6): 522–528.

Leach, D.H., Sprigings, E.J. and Laverty, W.H. (1987) A multivariate statistical analysis of stride timing measurements of nonfatigued racing Thoroughbreds. *Am. J. Vet. Res.* **48**(5): 880–888.

Lecoq, F. (1843) *Traité de l'Extérieur du Cheval, et des Principaux Animaux Domestiques.* Lyon: Savy.

Le Hello, P. (1896) Du rôle des membres postérieurs dans la locomotion du cheval. *Cpt. Rend. Hebdom. des séances de l'acad. des sciences* **122**: 1356–1360.

Le Hello, P. (1897) Sur l'action locomotrice des membres antérieurs du cheval. *Cpt. Rend. Hebdom. des séances de l'acad. des sciences* **124**: 913–914.

Le Hello, P. (1899) Du rôle des organes locomoteurs du cheval. *Cpt. Rend. Hebdom. des séances de l'acad. des sciences* **129**: 179–181.

Lenoble du Teil, J. (1873) *Étude sur la Locomotion du Cheval et des Quadrupèdes en Général.* Paris: Librairie Militaire de J. Demaine.

Lenoble du Teil, J. (1893) *Les Allures de Cheval Dévoilées par la Méthode Expérimentale.* Paris: Berger-Levrault et Cie.

Lhote, H. (1988) La route des chars. In: Vaes, B., del Marmol, G. and d'Otreppe, A. (eds) *Guide du Sahara*. Paris: Hachette, pp. 464–466.

Maennicke, E.M. (1961) Untersuchungen über die Bewegungsvorgänge des Shetlandponys. *Dissertation, Gießen*.

Magne de la Croix, P. (1928) Sobre la evolución del galope de carrera y la consecutiva de la forma. Causa de la evolución en perisodáctiles y artiodáctiles. *Anal. Soc. Cient. Argent.* **106**(6): 317–331.

Magne de la Croix, P. (1929) Filogenia de las locomociones cuadripedal y bipedal en los vertebrados y evolución de la forma consecutiva de la evolución de la locomoción. *Anal. Soc. Cient. Argent.* **108**: 383–406.

Magne de la Croix, P. (1932) Evolución del galope transverso. *Anal. Soc. Cient. Argent.* **113**: 38–41.

Magne de la Croix, P. (1936) The evolution of locomotion in mammals. *J. Mamm.* **17**: 51–54.

Manter, J.T. (1938) The dynamics of quadrupedal walking. *J. Exp. Biol.* **15**: 522–540.

Marey, E.J. (1882a) *La Machine Animale. Locomotion Terrestre et Aérienne*, 3 ième ed. Paris: Germer Baillière et Cie., pp. 144–186.

Marey, E.J. (1882b) Emploi de la photographie instantanée pour l'analyse des mouvements chez les animaux. *Cpt. Rend. Hebdom. des séances de l'acad. des sciences* **94**: 1013–1020.

Marey, E.J. (1883) Emploi des photographies partielles pour étudier la locomotion de l'homme et des animaux. *Cpt. Rend. Hebdom. des séances de l'acad. des sciences* **94**: 1827–1831.

Marey, E.J. and Pagès C (1886) Analyse cinématique de la locomotion du cheval. *Cpt. Rend. Hebdom. des séances de l'acad. des sciences* **103**: 538–547.

Marey, E.J. and Pagès, C. (1887) Locomotion comparée. Mouvement du membre pelvien chez l'homme, l 'éléphant et le cheval. *Cpt. Rend. Hebdom. des séances de l'acad. des sciences* **105**: 149–156.

Merkens, H.W., Schamhardt H.C., Hartman, W. and Kersjes, A.W. (1986) Ground reaction force patterns of Dutch Warmblood horses at normal walk. *Equine Vet. J.* **18**(3): 207–214.

Mosimann, W. and Micheluzzi, P. (1969) Die Bewegung im Cubitus des Pferdes als gedämpfte, erzwungene Schwingung. *Zentbl. Vet. Med. Reihe A* **16**: 180–184.

Moskovits, S. (1930) Die statisch-mechanische Beurteilung der Arbeitstiere durchgeführt am Metacarpus der Pferde. *Wissensch. Arch. Landwirtsch. Abt. B Tiernähr. u. Tierz.* **2**(3): 372–421.

Muybridge, E. (1899/1957) *Animals in Motion*. Republished (1957): L. S. Brown (ed.). New York: Dover Publications.

Nicolescu, J. (1923) Messungen über die Mechanik des Hannoverschen Pferdes in Vergleich zum Vollblut und Traber. *Dissertation, Berlin*.

Niki, Y., Ueda, Y., Yoshida, K., Masumitsu, H. (1982) A force plate study in equine biomechanics. 2. The vertical and fore-aft components of floor reaction forces and motion of equine limbs at walk and trot. *Bull. Equine Res. Inst.* **19**: 1–17.

Nomura, S. (1953a) Mechanical studies on the elbow joint of the horse. *Jap. J. Vet. Sci.* **15**: 21–36.

Nomura, S. (1953b) On the so-called 'Fäderungsphänomen' of the elbow joint of the horse. *Jap. J. Vet. Sci.* **15**: 175–182.

Nomura, S. (1953c) A mechanical study on the tarsal joint of the horse. *Jap. J. Vet. Sci.* **15**: 281–293.

Offringa, C. (1981) *Van Gildestein naar Uithof*. D1. 2. Utrecht: Faculteit de Diergeneeskunde.

Pagès, C. (1885) Analyse cinématique de la locomotion du cheval. *Cpt. Rend. Hebdom. des séances de l'acad. des sciences* **101**: 702–705.

Pagès, C. (1889) De la marche chez les animaux quadrupèdes. *Cpt. Rend. Hebdom. des séances de l'acad. des sciences* **108**: 194–196.

Palmgren, A. (1929) Zur Kenntnis der sogenannten Schnappgelenke. II Die physiologische Bedeutung des Fäderungsphänomens. *Z. Ges. Anat. Abt. I Z. Anat Entwickl. ges.* **89**: 194–200.

Peters, F. (1879) *Mechanische Untersuchungen an den Gelenken und Hufe des Pferdes*. Berlin: August Hirschwald.

Pettigrew, J.B. (1873) *Animal Locomotion or Walking, Swimming and Flying with a Dissertation on Aeronautics*. London: Henry S. King & Co.

Pratt, Jr. G.W. (1984) Racing surfaces – A survey of mechanical behavior. *Proc. 30th Annu. Conv. Am. Assoc. Equine Pract.*, pp. 321–331.

Pratt, Jr. G.W. and O'Connor, Jr. J.T. (1976) Force plate studies of equine biomechanics. *Am. J. Vet. Res.* **37**: 1251–1255.

Preuschoft, H. and Fritz, M. (1977) Mechanische Beanspruchungen im Bewegungsapparat von Springpferde. *Fortschr. Zool.* **24**: 75–98.

Pritchard, C.C. (1965) Relationship between conformation and lameness in the foot. *Auburn Vet.* **22**: 11–26, 29.

Raabe (1883) *Locomotion du Cheval. Cadran Hippique des Allures Marchées*. Paris: T. Symonds.

Radescu, T. (1923) Biometrische Untersuchungen an Vollblutpferden in Vergleich mit Rennleistung. *Dissertation, Berlin*.

Rathor, S.S. (1968) Clinical aspects of the functional disorders of the equine and bovine femoro-patellar articulation with some remarks on its biomechanics. *Thesis, Utrecht*.

Ratzlaff, M. (1974) Locomotion of the horse. *Anat. Histol. Embryol.* **3**: 376–377.

Ratzlaff, M.H., Grant, B.D., Adrian, M. and Feeney-Dixon, C. (1979) Evaluation of equine locomotion using electrogoniometry and cinematography: research and clinical applications. *Proc. 25th Annu. Conv. Am. Assoc. Equine Pract.*, p. 381.

Ratzlaff, M.H., Shindell, R.M. and White, K.K. (1995) The interrelationships of stride length and stride times to velocities of galloping horses. *J. Equine Vet. Sci.* **15**: 279–283.

Richter, O. (1953) Korrelaten zwischen Körpermaßen und Leistungen bei dem auf amerikanischer Grundlage gezogenen deutschen Traber. *Inaugural dissertation, Berlin*.

Riemersma, D.J., Schamhardt, H.C., Hartman, W., Lammertink, J.L.M.A. (1988a) Kinetics and kinematics of the equine hindleg. In vivo tendon loads and force plate measurements in ponies. *Am. J. Vet. Res.* **49**(8): 1344–1352.

Riemersma, D.J., van den Bogert, A.J., Schamhardt, H.C. and Hartman, W. (1988b) Kinetics and kinematics of the equine hindleg. In vivo tendon strain and joint kinematics. *Am. J. Vet. Res.* **49**(8): 1353–1359.

Roepstorff, L. and Drevemo, S. (1993) Concept of a force-measuring horseshoe. *Acta Anat.* **146**: 114–119.

Rooney, J.R. (1968) Biomechanics of equine lameness. *Cornell Vet.* **58**(Suppl.): 49–58.

Rooney, J.R. (1969) *Biomechanics of Lameness in Horses*. Baltimore: Williams and Wilkins.

Rösiö, B. (1927) *Die Bedeutung des Exterieurs und der Konstitution des Pferdes für seine Leistungsfähigkeit*. Uppsala: Almqvist and Wiksells.

Schamhardt, H.C., and Merkens, H.W. (1987) Quantification of equine ground reaction force patterns. *J. Biomech.* **20**(4): 443–446.

Schamhardt, H.C. Hartman, W., Lammertink, J.L.M.A. and Badoux, D.M. (1984) Bone strain in the equine tibia: inertia as a cause of the presupport peak. *Am. J. Vet. Res.* **45**: 885–887.

Schauder, W. (1923a) Historisch-kritische Studie über die Bewegungslehre des Pferdes. (1. Teil) *Berl. Tierärztl. Wschr.* **39**(12): 123–126.

Schauder, W. (1923b) Historisch-kritische Studie über die Bewegungslehre des Pferdes. (2. Teil) *Berl. Tierärztl. Wschr.* **39**(13): 135–137.

Schauder, W. (1924a) Anatomische und metrische Untersuchungen über die Muskeln der Schultergliedmaße des Pferdes. *Z. f. d. ges. Anat. I. Abt.* **71**: 559–637.

Schauder, W. (1924b) Die fetale Entwicklung der 'Sehnenmuskeln' des Pferdes. *Arch. Mikrosk. Anat. u. Entwickl. mechanik.* **102**: 211–262.

Schauder, W. (1932) Ueber korrelative funktionelle Gestaltungen an den Gliedmaßen von Ungulaten besonders Equiden. *Münchn. Tierärztl. Wschr.* **83**(21): 241–244; (22): 257–261.

Schauder, W. (1949) 'Nur im Werden erfaßt, wird das Gewordene verständlich'. *Gießener Hochschulnachrichten*: 56–75.

Schauder, W. (1951) Allgemeine stoßbrechende Einrichtungen an den Gliedmaßen des Pferdes in funktionell-anatomische Hinsicht. *Dtsch. Tierärztl. Wschr.* **58**: 350–352.

Schauder, W. (1952) Die besonderen stoßbrechenden Einrichtungen an den Gliedmaßen des Pferdes, in angewandt-anatomische Hinsicht. *Dtsch. Tierärztl. Wschr.* **59**: 35–38.

Schauder, W. (1954) Stoßabfangende Einrichtungen in Rumpfe des Pferdes. *Dtsch. Tierärztl. Wschr.* **61**: 7–9.

Schmaltz, R. (1922a) Analyse der Gangarten des Pferdes durch den Film. *Berl. Tierärztl. Wschr.* **38**(46): 523–527.

Schmaltz, R. (1922b) Die Analyse der Gangarten des Pferdes durch den Film. Bemerkung dazu. *Berl. Tierärztl. Wochenschr.* **38**: 551.

Schmidt, H. (1939) Beziehungen zwischen Schrittlänge und Bau der Gliedmaßen des Pferdes. *Dtsch. Tierärztl Wschr.* **47**(46): 689–692.

Schreiber, J. (1950) Gestalt und Bewegung. Eine anatomische Betrachtung des Pferdes in der darstellenden Kunst. *Wien. Tierärztl. Monatsschr.* **37**(2): 73–105.

Schtscherbakow, N.M. (1935) The determination of the work for which a horse is suitable by means of measurement of its gait. *Bull. Moscow Vet. Inst.* **2**: 113–146.

Seeherman, H.J., Morris, E.A. and Fackelman, G. (1987) Computerized force plate determination of equine weight-bearing profiles. *Proc. 2nd Int. Conf. Equine Exerc. Physiol.*, pp. 536–552.

Seeherman, H.J., Morris, E. and O'Callaghan, M.W. (1996) Comprehensive clinical evaluation of performance. In: Auer, J.A. (ed) *Equine Surgery*. Philadelphia: Saunders, pp. 1133–1173.

Silver, I.A., Brown, P.N., Goodship, A.E. *et al.* (1983) A clinical and experimental study of tendon injury, healing and treatment in the horse. *Equine Vet. J.* (Suppl. 1): 23–35.

Simpson, G.G. (1951) *Horses*. New York: Oxford University Press.

Slijper, E.J. (1946) Comparative biologic-anatomical investigations on the vertebral column and spinal musculature of mammals. *Proc. K. Ned. Acad. Wetensch.* **42**(5): 1–128.

Solá, G.A. (1969) Environmental factors affecting the speed of pacing horses. *MS Thesis, Ohio State University.*

Stillman, J.D.B. (1882) *The Horse in Motion as shown by Instantaneous Photography with a Study on Animal Mechanics founded on Anatomy and the Revelations of the Camera in which is demonstrated the Theory of Quadrupedal Locomotion.* Boston: James R. Osgood & Co.

Stoss, A.O. (1923) Anatomie und Kinematik der Gelenke der Pferdeextremitäten. *Z. Anat. Entwickl. ges.* **69**: 5–31.

Stratul, J. (1922) Biometrische Untersuchungen an Vollblutpferden mit Rückschlüssen auf Rennleistung. *Inaugural dissertation, Berlin.*

Strubelt (1928) Über die Bedeutung des Lacertus fibrosus und des Tendo femorotarseus für das Stehen und die Bewegung des Pferdes. *Arch. Tierheilk.* **57**: 575–585.

Sukhanov, V.B. (1963) Forms of movement (gaits) of land vertebrates (a theory of locomotion and of the evolution of its forms). *Byull. Mosk. Obshch. Ispyt. Prirody Otd. Biol.* **67**(5): 136–137.

Taylor, B.M., Tipton, C.M., Adrian, M. and Karpovich, P.V. (1966) Action of certain joints in the legs of the horse recorded electrogoniometrically. *Am. J. Vet. Res.* **38**(10): 1675–1677.

Townsend, H.G.G. and Leach, D.H. (1984) The relationship between intervertebral jont morphology and mobility in the equine thoracolumbar spine. *Equine Vet. J.* **16**(5): 461–465.

Townsend, H.G.G., Leach, D.H. and Fretz, P.B. (1983) Kinematics of the equine thoracolumbar spine. *Equine Vet. J.* **15**(2): 117–122.

Townsend, H.G.G., Leach, D.H., Doige, C.E. and Kirkaldy-Willis, W.H. (1986) The relationship between spinal biomechanics and pathological changes in the equine thoracolumbar spine. *Equine Vet. J.* **18**(2): 107–112.

van den Bogert, A.J., Schamhardt, H.C. and Crowe, A. (1989) Simulation of quadrupedal locomotion using a dynamic rigid body model. *J. Biomech.* **22**(1): 33–41.

van der Plank, G.M. (1929) De verdeeling der lichaamslast over de draagvlakte van den voorhoef, bij verhooging der verzenen. *Tijdschr. Dierg.* **55**(10): 498–500.

van Weeren, P.R. and Barneveld, A. (1986) A technique to quantify skin displacement in the walking horse. *J. Biomech.* **19**(10): 879–883.

van Weeren, P.R., van den Bogert, A.J. and Barneveld, A. (1992) Correction models for skin displacement in equine kinematic gait analysis. *J. Equine Vet. Sci.* **12**(3): 178–192.

van Weeren, P.R., van den Bogert, A.J., Barneveld, A., Hartman, W. and Kersjes, A.W. (1990) The role of the reciprocal apparatus in the hind limb of the horse investigated by a modified CODA-3 opto-electronic gait analysis system. *Equine Vet. J.* **9**(Suppl.): 95–100.

von den Driesch, A. (1989) *Geschichte der Tiermedizin. 5000 Jahre Tierheilkunde.* München: Callwey.

von Hochstätter, C (1821–24) *Theoretisch-praktisches Handbuch der äussern Pferdekenntniß, und der Wartung und Pflege der Pferde.* Bern: Haller.

von Lengerken and Werner K (1969) Das Exterieur der Zucht- und Renntraber in der DDR. *Wiss. Z. Univ. Halle* **18**(5): 505–534.

Wagener, H. (1934) Untersuchungen an Spitzenpferden des Spring- und Schulstalles der Kavallerie-Schule Hannover. *Arbeiten der Deutschen Gesellsch. für Züchtungsbiol.* **65**: 1–117.

Walter, K. (1925) Der Bewegungsablauf an den freien Gliedmaßen des Pferdes im Schritt, Trab und Galopp. *Arch. wissensch. prakt. Tierheilk.* **53**: 316–352.

Wehner, R. (1944) Lassen sich Beziehungen der Knochenachsen und Gliedmaßenwinkel und Schrittlänge beim Rheinisch-Deutschen Kaltblut nachweisen? *Z. Tierz. Zücht. biol.* **56**: 321–353.

Wentink, G.H. (1978a) An experimental study on the role of the reciprocal tendinous apparatus of the horse at walk. *Anat. Embryol.* **154**: 143–151.

Wentink, G.H. (1978b) Biokinetical analysis of the movements of the pelvic limb of the horse and the role of the muscles in the walk and trot. *Anat. Embryol.* **154**: 261–272.

Wiechert, F. (1927) Messungen an ostpreußischen Kavalleriepferden und solchen mit besonderen Leistungen und die Beurteilung der Leistungsfähigkeit auf Grund der mechanischen Verhältnisse. *Arbeiten der Deutschen Gesellsch. Für Züchtungskunde* **34**: 1–67.

Wilsdorf, G. (1971) Beitrag zur Biomechanik der Vorderextremität des Galopprennpferdes und deren Beziehung zur sogenannten Schienbeinerkrankung. *Mon. hefte Vet. med.* **26**(24): 939–944.

Wilson, B.D., Neal, R.J., Howard, A. and Groenendyk, S. (1988a) The gait of pacers. I. Kinematics. *Equine Vet. J.* **20**(5): 341–346.

Wilson, B.D., Neal, R.J., Howard, A. and Groenendyk, S. (1988b) The gait of pacers. II. Factors influencing racing speed. *Equine Vet. J.* **20**(5): 347–351.

Xenophon (430–354 BC) Über die Reitkunst. In: Widdra, K. (ed.) (1965) *Xenophon. Reitkunst.* Berlin: Schriften und Quellen der Alten Welt 16.

Zwaenepoel, M. (1910a) Démonstration expérimentale du mécanisme de l'impulsion et du recul chez le cheval. *Ann. de méd. Vétérin.* **59**: 322–334.

Zwaenepoel, M. (1910b) Démonstration expérimentale du mécanisme de l'impulsion et du recul chez le cheval. *Ann. et Bull. De la Soc. Roy. des Sciences Méd. et Natur. de Bruxelles* **68**: 83–91.

Zwaenepoel, M. (1911a) Démonstration expérimentale du mécanisme de l'impulsion chez le cheval. *Ann. de méd. Vétérin.* **60**: 461–478.

Zwaenepoel, M. (1911b) Démonstration expérimentale du mécanisme de l'impulsion chez le cheval. *Bull. de l'Acad. Roy. de Méd. IVe Série,* Tôme XXV: 527–558.

2

The Neurobiology of Locomotor Development

Albert Gramsbergen

INTRODUCTION

Kinematic aspects of locomotion have been studied extensively in the horse (e.g. Muybridge 1887/1957; Hildebrand 1962). This is in contrast to the lack of data on morphological and neurophysiological aspects of the equine central nervous system (CNS). Older textbooks on comparative neuroanatomy are limited to comparing primitive vertebrates such as teleosts, reptiles, amphibians and birds with smaller mammals and man. Larger mammals are seldom included in these comparisons (e.g. Ariens Kappers *et al.*, 1967). Very little is known about neural projections in horses. Verhaart and Sopers-Jurgens (1957) studied Bagley's bundle in horses, which runs from the cerebral cortex to the mesencephalic and pontine tegmentum and is considered to be the phylogenetic predecessor of the corticospinal tract in higher mammals. However, the CNS of horses has not been studied systematically.

Recent studies on neuroanatomy are based upon tract tracing methods and neurotransmitter biochemistry, and are generally limited to the neural systems in cats, rats and primates (Nieuwenhuys *et al.*, 1997). In the 1940s and 1950s degenerating fiber projections were stained after creation of experimental lesions. More recently a variety of retrogradely and anterogradely injected tracing techniques have been developed, but these require surgical interference and imply the death of the animal after a short survival period. Such studies have not been performed in larger mammals partly due to their economical value, but also because of the long distances that must be traveled by the intravital stains and the large quantities of stains that are needed. For similar reasons, the implantation of depth electrodes for recording or for stimulation in central nervous structures have not been performed systematically in larger mammals.

Description of the neurobiological basis of movements in horses is, therefore, based upon extrapolation from knowledge obtained in laboratory animals such as rats and cats. In humans, ethical considerations prohibit invasive experiments, so modern imaging techniques are combined with extrapolation from animal research to unravel the relationships between the brain and behavior. A similar approach in larger mammals might open promising possibilities.

Comparative studies in neuroanatomy, neurophysiology and ethology have shown the need for caution in making intraspecies extrapolations. Differences in the ecological biotope and behavioral competence of the animal are mutually interconnected with neural organization. The relation between the degree of manipulative skills and the nature of the terminal projections of the corticospinal tract, e.g. in rabbits and in higher primates, is a case in point. Rabbits are unable to manipulate objects by means of independent movements of the toes of their forepaws and have no direct corticospinal connections to motoneurons of the toe muscles. In higher primates, however, such monosynaptic connections exist and enable apes and the human to move their fingers independently (Lawrence & Hopkins, 1976). Differences in size affect locomotor behavior and the neuromuscular system, and these are addressed in chapter 15.

This chapter reviews current knowledge of locomotion and its neurobiological substrate. The information on the neuroanatomy and neurophysiology of motor systems is largely based on studies in the rat, which can be used as a basis for extrapolation to the horse. Also included are data on the segmental circuitry in the spinal cord and the neuronal circuitry involved in locomotion obtained from research in cats. Since limb movements are intimately connected to postural control, data on postural control will also be presented.

The neuro-ontogenetic approach, in which the function of neural structures is analyzed during early development, has made an important contribution to our understanding of the neurobiological background of walking and postural maintenance. For this reason, locomotion and postural maintenance will be discussed from a developmental perspective. The rat is the animal of choice for such studies; it is born at an early stage of brain development, so investigation of the early stages can be performed postnatally, which has important experimental advantages.

THE ONSET OF MOVEMENTS

Movements indicate life and the onset of movements has intrigued scientists for a long time. In antiquity, the onset of motility of chick embryos and mammalian fetuses was investigated, including horse fetuses (see, e.g. Adelmann's foreword in Fabricius' *De Formatu Foetu* 1604/1967). Motion as the expression of the soul, the relation between form and function as well as the animation of form, were key notions in Aristotle's thinking and his authority was appreciated until the 16th century.

Modern research into the development of the nervous system only emerged at the end of the 19th century (see Hamburger, 1988). This 'experimental neuroembryology' was directed towards aspects of the developmental process, and research into brain and behavior relationships during development is a special field within this research. During development the relatively simple organization of the nervous system becomes increasingly complex and its functional repertoire expands simultaneously. A major aim is to unravel these mutual relationships (Hamburger, 1988). It is noteworthy that this neuro-ontogenetical research led to the conceptualization of the neuron theory.

Fetal movements in mammals such as cats, rats and sheep can be observed when the uterine horns are exposed by surgical intervention. In rats, which are born after a gestational period of 23 days, the first movements occur from the 15th or 16th embryonic day (E15–E16). Angulo y Gonzalez (1932) described these movements as gradually changing from patterns involving the whole body into movements of certain segments of the extremities at later stages. Narayanan *et al.* (1971), however, first observed movements in the extremities and these later included larger parts of the body. Similar studies in cat fetuses (Windle, 1940) and sheep fetuses (Barcroft & Barron, 1939) reported that the first movements occurred in single extremity segments with single movements becoming part of the movement patterns at later

stages. Coghill (1929), however, observed movement patterns from the onset in amphibiae while later on movements of single extremities developed. These data, which are highly confusing, resulted in a vivid debate from the 1920s and over the 20 years thereafter on the nature of the first movements. The question was whether the first movements are mass patterns that developed by a process of individuation, or reflexes which later by integration became organized into movement patterns. For retrospections on the individuation–integration controversy and discussions on the roots of this debate see Kuo (1963), Oppenheim (1978) and Hamburger (1988).

Recent investigations into the development of movements in human fetuses with real-time ultrasound scanning have made an important contribution to our knowledge regarding the nature of motor development (de Vries *et al.*, 1982, 1985; Prechtl, 1984). Initially, at the 6th–7th week of gestation, there are minor head and neck movements but a few days later trunk and extremity movements also occur. Soon after, a rich repertoire of arm and limb movements develops, with trunk flexion and extension as well as sucking and breathing movements. These longitudinal observations on human fetuses revealed that both 'mass patterns' and 'local movements' develop in parallel soon after the onset of spontaneous motility.

In fetal rats, the first movements can be observed at E15–E16. Motoneuronal axons from the lumbar segments form contacts with the muscles of the hindlimbs shortly before this age, but afferent fibers from neurons in the dorsal ganglia at the lumbar levels do not reach their motoneuronal pools until E18.5 (Kudo & Yamada, 1987). Electrophysiological research demonstrated that, from this age onwards, muscle contractions can be elicited by electrical stimulation of the dorsal roots. This sequence of development indicates that reflexes in rats develop a few days after the first occurrence of spontaneous movements. As supraspinal descending projections are not yet present, the movement patterns involving trunk and extremities are autonomously generated by spinal circuits. Given the complexity of the movements and the number of body segments involved, this indicates that motoneurones are already coupled via

Summary

The first movements of the fetus occur spontaneously. Their onset coincides with the arrival of motor axons at the (primitive) muscles at the stage when proprioceptive feedback from the muscles and supraspinal projections are not yet established.

segmental and propriospinal interneurons. In the opossum, it was demonstrated that these propriospinal interneurons are indeed among the first long range projections to develop (Cassidy & Cabana, 1993).

DEVELOPMENT OF LOCOMOTION

In fetal rats the first movements occur from E15–E16 and consist of dorso-ventral and lateral trunk movements as well as isolated movements of extremities (Angulo y Gonzalez, 1932; Narayanan *et al.*, 1971). From E20, coordinated movements in single limbs occur (Bekoff & Lau, 1980) and soon after birth the first signs of interlimb coordination may be observed. Bekoff & Trainer (1979) demonstrated that rhythmic swimming movements in all four paws could be evoked by immersing the neonatal rats in water. Rhythmic stepping movements of the four paws can also be elicited a few days after birth, when supporting the body with one paw in contact with the floor. Moving the rat slowly ahead or aside leads to the so-called hopping reflex (Gramsbergen & Mulder, 1998). However, neonatal rats left alone and unstimulated in an overground situation lie with their ventral body surface on the floor of the cage and crawling movements occur only intermittently when they are awake (Gramsbergen *et al.*, 1970). The interpretation of Bekoff and Trainer's observations is that when posture is adequately supported (in their case by the upward pressure of water) it permits alternating walking movements. Interestingly, Jamon and Clarac (1998) recently demonstrated that stimulating neonatal pups with odorous material from their maternal litter induced vigorous walking movements and even lifting of the ventral body surface from the floor. Olfactory stimulation, which is obviously a potent factor in eliciting trunk and extremity muscles even in the first days of life, probably increases the activation level of the limbic motor system which, in turn, activates spinal motoneurons (see below).

The development of movements and reflexes during further postnatal development has been studied extensively (e.g. Small, 1899; Bolles & Woods 1964; Blanck *et al.*, 1967; Smart & Dobbing, 1971; Altman & Sudarshan, 1975; Almli & Fisher, 1977; Geisler *et al.*, 1993). Crawling movements in neonatal rats mostly occur during so-called pivoting, a behavior in which a circular field is explored with the hindlimb at its center (Gramsbergen *et al.*, 1970). From the 8th day after birth (P8) rats are able to stand with their ventral body surface off the floor and from that age, stepping movements gradually develop. However, these bouts of 'free walking' only involve a few steps and the movements remain staggering in the week to follow. The environment is scanned by head

movements in ventro-dorsal and in lateral directions but before doing so, they have to stand still.

At P15–P16 the immature pattern of locomotion is replaced by a smooth walking pattern. From that age onwards rats can walk swiftly and vary their speed abruptly. Head movements may occur during walking. Before P16 the hindlimbs are abducted during walking but afterwards they remain adducted. Meticulous behavioral observations by Clarke and Williams (1994) revealed that hind paw movements and foot placing are not yet fully adult-like at this age and that the adult pattern only develops between P22 and P30.

Obviously, adequate postural control is an important factor in the development of standing and locomotion. Posture may be defined as the relative positions of the head, trunk and the extremities as well as the orientation of the body in space. In adults both feedback ('static') and feed-forward ('dynamic') control mechanisms play a role (see, e.g. Massion, 1992). Although it is impossible to distinguish them from a behavioral point of view, it should be remembered that the neural systems governing posture and movement are organized differently and have a different evolutionary descent. Specific central motor areas, specialized sensory systems and medially descending spinal projections are involved in postural control. Other neural systems with laterally descending fiber projections are involved in single movements of the extremities. Obviously, intimate connections exist between these systems.

Recent experiments by Geisler *et al.* (1996a) indicated that vestibular deprivation by plugging the semicircular canals from P5 induces a retardation in postural development. The development of grooming (self-cleaning behavior) was retarded by one to two days but the emergence of rearing (standing on the hindlimbs without support from the wall) was delayed by as much as 5 days. Development of the adult-like walking pattern was retarded by 3–4 days, indicating that postural development is the limiting factor for development of this walking pattern. It has been suggested that feedback control of posture prevails during the slow and staggering walking pattern before P15, while after the transition into the smooth adult-like walking pattern feed-forward control gradually adds to postural maintenance (Gramsbergen, 1998).

Rats open their eyes around P14 (Smart & Dobbing, 1971; Gramsbergen & Mulder, 1998) and an obvious question is whether the development of the smooth walking pattern around that age is related to opening of the eyes. Suturing the eyelids from P9 and rearing in a dark environment did not change the time course of walking or postural development, although it influenced the organization of motor behavior (Gramsbergen, unpublished results).

Summary

Rhythmic limb movements in the rat may be elicited from birth. Around the end of the second week after birth the immature walking pattern is replaced by a smooth adult-like walking pattern. The development of postural control seems to be the limiting factor for this transition.

Summary

Research has mainly concentrated upon walking at slower speeds. When speed increases the swing phase duration remains relatively unchanged but the stance phase duration decreases. The hindlimbs are used for acceleration and the forelimbs for deceleration.

Walking in adult rats

During walking, adult rats extend and flex their limbs in a vertical plane. Limbs are in contact with the ground during the stance phase and are moved forward during the swing phase. During both stance and swing the limbs show relative extension and flexion phases.

The foot placement sequence during walking at moderate speeds is typically LH–LF–RH–RF, with the body always being supported by three limbs. The extension phases of the two hindlimbs are phase shifted by 0.5, which implies that when one limb is starting its cycle of movement the other limb is halfway through its cycle. When walking along irregular trajectories, these phase shifts change. This alternating gait pattern (Grillner, 1981) applies not only for rats but to many quadrupeds, including horses, during walking at lower speeds.

When walking speed increases there is an increase in stride length and a decrease in stance duration, but swing duration remains more or less constant (Westerga & Gramsbergen, 1990). During further increases in speed, walking changes into a trot and then to a gallop, which are characterized by different footfall patterns. Transitions between gaits during acceleration or deceleration occur at variable speeds (Grillner, 1975, 1981). The kinematic and neurophysiological aspects of these patterns have not been studied in detail. In the few studies that have been performed, the goal was to investigate energy expenditure and force production by muscles during such patterns (e.g. in mice: James *et al.*, 1995; in rats: Sullivan & Armstrong, 1978; Taylor *et al.*, 1982; Perry *et al.*, 1988).

An important difference between smaller and larger animals during faster types of locomotion is that in species such as rats, cats and dogs the hindlimbs are used for acceleration and maintenance of speed and the forelimbs for braking, while in larger animals such as horses the hind and forelimbs subserve similar functions during acceleration and braking (Heglund *et al.*, 1982). These differences could well be reflected in neural circuitries as well as muscular and skeletal specializations of the hind and forelimbs.

EMG RECORDINGS DURING WALKING

Most of the investigations into correlations between electromyographic (EMG) patterns and limb movements during walking have been restricted to the hindlimb in rats and cats (for reviews, Grillner, 1975, 1981; Grillner *et al.*, 1991). Globally, the extensors of the hip, knee, ankle and digits are activated during the stance phase and the flexors are active during the swing phase (Fig. 2.1). EMG patterns in the forelimb have been studied less frequently. In the newt, extensors and flexors of the forelimb are activated rhythmically and reciprocally but the EMG patterns are more complex and co-contractions are often observed (Szekely *et al.*, 1969).

In the literature on kinematic and electromyographic aspects of the step cycle in cats, the 'extension phase' generally is subdivided into an E1 phase indicating the onset of limb extension before contacting the ground, the E2 phase during the midphase of ground contact and the E3 phase with the foot still in contact with the ground but shortly before toe off. The swing phase thus consists of the F (flexion) and E1 phase, and the stance phase consists of the E2 and E3 phases.

In the hindlimbs of freely moving rats, the tibialis anterior (ankle flexor) and the semitendinosus muscles (knee flexor) are activated shortly before the onset of the swing phase. Bursts in these muscles are characterized by a short 'attack' phase and the bursts generally only last during the first part of the swing phase (the F phase). Between the bursts EMG activity generally is absent. Remarkably, the onsets of the bursts in these muscles coincide, despite the fact that they move different limb segments and that slight phase shifts in joint angle trajectories occur (Westerga & Gramsbergen, 1990). During increases in speed, the burst durations in these flexor muscles remain unchanged, but the EMG amplitudes increase (Westerga & Gramsbergen, 1993a; Gramsbergen *et al.*, 1999). In cats, EMG recordings in the iliopsoas and the extensor digitorum longus muscles as well as in the tibialis anterior muscle showed similar results (e.g. Engberg & Lundberg, 1962, 1969).

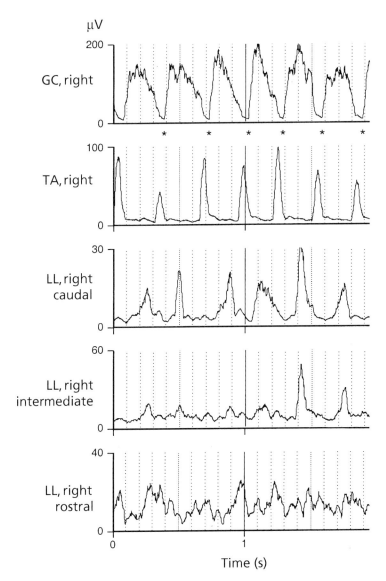

Fig. 2.1 Averaged EMG records of a rat aged 32 days. Recordings from the gastrocnemius (GC) muscle at the right side, the tibialis (TA) muscles at the right side, and the longissimus (LL) muscles at caudal, intermediate and rostral levels. Asterisks indicate the onsets of the stance phase in the hindlimb at the right side. (Gramsbergen *et al.*, 1999. Reproduced with permission from Elsevier Science.)

The gastrocnemius, the soleus (ankle extensors) and the quadriceps femoris (knee extensor) muscles are activated shortly before the onset of the stance phase (during the E2 phase) and EMG activity lasts until shortly before the onset of the next swing phase (Westerga & Gramsbergen, 1993a, 1994; Gramsbergen *et al.*, 1999). Remarkably, the bursts in these extensors start simultaneously (as occurs in the flexors) and their profiles are more or less identical. During increases in speed, the burst amplitudes in these muscles remain the same but the burst durations decrease (Fig.

2.2), which agrees with the data from cats (Grillner, 1981).

EMG activity in the postural muscles in the back is related in a complex way to the activity in the hindlimb extensors and flexors. In adult rats EMG patterns were recorded in the medially located multifidus muscles and the laterally located longissimus muscles (Geisler *et al.*, 1996b; Gramsbergen *et al.*, 1999). The multifidus muscle is tonically active during all movements that require stabilization of the trunk, and during locomotion the activity in this muscle modulates slightly with the frequency of

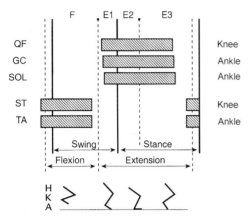

Fig. 2.2 Schematic representation of EMG activity in a few hindlimb muscles in relation to extension and flexion phases and swing and stance phases. QF: quadriceps femoris muscle, GC: gastrocnemius muscle, SOL: soleus muscle, ST: semitendinosus muscle, TA: tibialis anterior muscles (extensors and flexors of the knee and ankle, respectively). Blocks indicate burst activity. E1: extension of hindlimb before stance phase, E2: mid-stance phase, E3: extension shortly before toe off, F: flexion. Stick diagrams are derived from video recordings; H: hip, K: knee, A: ankle.

Summary

Flexors in the hindlimb are activated simultaneously, shortly before the swing phase of the hindlimb and extensors are activated shortly before the stance phase. The longissimus muscles in the back are activated during extension of the hindlimbs and EMG activity in this muscle is strongest during the stance phase of the ipsilateral hindlimb.

Development of EMG patterns during walking

Before P15, EMG activity in the gastrocnemius and the soleus muscles, as well as the tibialis anterior muscle, is irregular and spiky, with coactivation of flexors and extensors being observed during all phases of the step cycle (Westerga & Gramsbergen, 1993a, 1994). From P15–P16 an interference pattern develops and from then onwards, EMG recordings show regular bursts with increased amplitudes. These bursts become increasingly accurate in their phase relation with the step cycle.

The transition from irregular into smooth interference patterns in the EMG coincides with the development of the adult-like smooth walking patterns. These changes in the EMG could be induced by increased activation of motoneurons due to developmental changes in supraspinal fiber projections, which have been shown to have a facilitating effect on motoneurons during adult locomotion (Zomlefer et al., 1984), and the emergence of an interference pattern in the EMG from P15–P16 may indicate that these projections are inducing increased activation of motoneurons.

EMG recordings in the longissimus muscles show complicated trends during development. This muscle is tonically but irregularly active at early ages but from P12 clear-cut EMG bursts develop which are in phase with the step cycle. Interestingly, until P22 the strongest activity accompanies the stance phase in the contralateral hindlimb but after this age the bursts with the highest amplitudes are coupled to the stance phase in the ipsilateral hindlimb. Ipsilateral coupling is probably the most effective mode of propulsion and is possibly more efficient metabolically (Gramsbergen, 1998). In rats that were vestibularly deprived from P5, Geisler and Gramsbergen (1998) demonstrated that the coupling of activities in the longissimus and hindlimb extensors remained highly variable at least until P28, and sometimes persisted until older ages. This suggests that the shift in coordination depends on developmental changes in central motor areas.

the left and right hindlimb. The EMG in the longissimus muscle, on the other hand, is more phasic in character. EMG bursts in these muscles are phase-linked to bursts in the gastrocnemius muscle during the stance phase (Gramsbergen et al., 1999). This is remarkable because intuitively, it seems that a swing phase in one of the hindlimbs induces a relative instability of the trunk which should be counteracted by activity in the trunk muscles. During one step cycle of both hindlimbs two bursts in the longissimus muscles occur. The burst with the higher amplitude accompanies extension of the ipsilateral hindlimb. EMG activity at more rostral levels in the longissimus muscle is variable in amplitude, duration and phasing of the bursts. During rapid acceleration and fast walking, simultaneous contractions may occur over the entire length of the muscle but at slower speeds the rostral portions of the longissimus muscles show only tonic activity without modulations in amplitude (Fig. 2.2).

These data on adult rats are in agreement with results from adult cats. Carlson et al. (1979) reported a similar coupling in the activation of back muscles with the vastus lateralis muscle in the hindlimb during treadmill walking. Their data, however, indicate that the two bursts per step cycle in both hindlimbs and in the longissimus muscles are more or less identical in amplitude, which might be a peculiarity of treadmill walking.

Summary

In hindlimb muscles EMG bursts alternating with silent periods that are phase linked to the swing and stance phases develop around the time when the adult-like walking pattern emerges. An interference pattern in the EMG develops around the age when the adult-like walking pattern emerges. Activity in the longissimus muscles is initially linked to the contralateral hindlimb and later to the ipsilateral hindlimb. Vestibular deprivation from early ages leads to a retardation in this development.

MUSCLES AND MOTONEURONES

Histological and neurophysiological aspects of muscles at adult age have been reviewed repeatedly (Burke, 1981; Partridge & Benton, 1981; Kernell, 1998) and will be repeated only briefly here. Histologically, different fiber types can be distinguished in muscles that are classified into three or more types depending on the method. In a classical method, the histological material is preincubated at different pHs and ATPase staining enables differentiation between type I, IIa and IIb muscle fibers (Dubowitz & Brooke, 1973). More recent methods apply myosin-related antibodies to identify several subtypes of muscle fibers (Schiaffino *et al.*, 1986).

The metabolism of the type I muscle fibers is based upon glucose oxidation which is also used to a certain degree by type IIa muscle fibers. The contractile properties of these muscle fibers depends upon a continuous supply of glucose from the blood vessels. The type IIb fibers on the other hand (and this holds to a certain degree also for the type IIa muscle fibers, which have a mixed metabolism) obtain their energy supply from the anaerobic metabolism of glycogen which is stored within the muscle fibers. Obviously, after long periods of activity, these stores are exhausted.

Physiologically, groups of muscle fibers are innervated by one motoneuron (together with a motor unit) and the muscle fibers of a motor unit tend to have the same properties. Four types of units can be discerned on the basis of isometric twitch speed, maximum tetanic force and fatigue resistance: S-type, slow-twitch and fatigue resistant units; FR, fast-twitch, fatigue resistant units; Fint, fast twitch and intermediate fatigue resistant units; and FF, fast-twitch and fatigable units (Burke, 1981). Muscle fibers of S-type units are identical to the type I muscle fibers and fibers of the F-type units to the type IIa and IIb muscle fibers.

The properties of the a-motoneurons are matched to the properties of the motor units. Electrophysiologically it has been demonstrated that the smallest a-motoneurons innervate the S-type units and the largest innervate the FF-type units. Due to differences in their membrane properties, the smaller motoneurons are recruited first and progressively larger motoneurons are recruited in an orderly fashion with increasing stimulation intensities (Henneman & Mendell, 1981). Interestingly, the relative force of additional motor units over a wide range of forces is more or less the same (Milner-Brown *et al.*, 1973).

Most of the muscles in the rat contain a majority of type IIa and IIb fibers and a minority of type I muscle fibers but a few muscles are characterized by high proportions of fatigue resistant type I muscles fibers. Most notable in this respect are the multifidus and the longissimus muscles in the back, the soleus muscle in the hindlimb as well as an important portion of the flexor carpi ulnaris muscle in the forelimb (Gramsbergen *et al.*, 1996). These particular muscles are fatigue resistant and highly efficient in their energy metabolism, which makes them ideally suited for postural functions, such as keeping the trunk straight and carrying the body weight (for a review on muscle regionalization, see, Kernell, 1998).

Apart from their sizes, motoneurons also differ in other morphological characteristics. Motoneurones of muscles with important postural tasks have their dendrites running in dendrite bundles (Gramsbergen *et al.*, 1996), which have also been described in the spinal cord of the cat (Scheibel & Scheibel, 1970) and in the human (Schoenen, 1982).

Investigations into the development of the dendritic tree of motoneurons revealed that until P14, dendrites of motoneurons in lumbar segments innervating the tibialis anterior muscle (a flexor) and the soleus muscle (an extensor) are seemingly disorganized. From that age the dendrites of the motoneurones to the soleus muscle become organized into bundles but the motoneurons innervating the tibialis anterior muscle remain essentially unchanged (Westerga & Gramsbergen, 1992). This reorganization depends on the ingrowth of descending projections. In rats, spinal cord transection at P10 prevents these bundles from developing (Gramsbergen *et al.*, 1995) and in cats such interference at later ages leads to their hypotrophy or even atrophy (Reback *et al.*, 1982).

Dendrite bundles consist of up to 15 dendrites in close vicinity for several hundreds of millimeters, running in longitudinal and transverse directions (Fig. 2.3), and connected via long-stretched gap-junctions (Matthews *et al.*, 1971; van der Want *et al.*, 1998). Recently we demonstrated that dendrite bundles specifically occur in pools of axial muscles in the trunk and neck as well as in extremity muscles with an important postural task, such

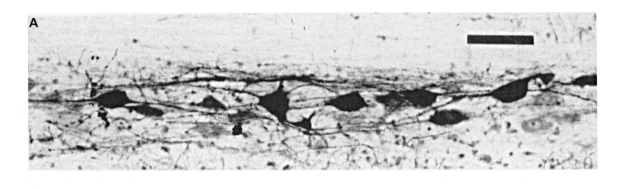

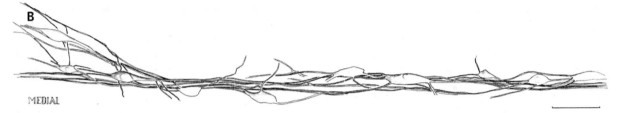

Fig. 2.3 Motoneuronal pools of the longus capitis muscle: microphotograph (**A**) and reconstruction of another pool (**B**). Bars: 100 µm. (From Gramsbergen *et al.*, 1996, with permission from Academic Press.)

as the soleus and the gastrocnemius muscle in the hindlimb and the flexor carpi ulnaris muscle in the forelimb. These are the same muscles that contain high percentages of type I muscle fibers (see above). The physiological significance of dendrite bundles is not known but one possibility is that they serve to electrotonically couple motoneurones in pools stretching over several spinal cord segments which innervate long muscles, for example in the back or abdomen.

Myogenic development

Histologically, the trunk muscles arise from the segmentally arranged myotomes while the extremity muscles develop from the limb buds. Cytologically, myocytes develop from a longitudinal array of mesenchymal cells that fuse around P13, possibly under the influence of ingrowing motoneuronal axons. The first generation of multinuclear muscle fibers, the primary myotubes, are soon innervated at the future endplate region by a multitude of motoneuronal axons. At a later stage, a second generation of secondary myotubes develops and these are innervated initially by several motoneuronal axons (Ontell & Dunn, 1978; Goldspink & Ward, 1979; Bennett, 1983). Wilson *et al.* (1988) studied the effects of severe undernutrition of rats from early gestation and through the lactation period on muscular development. The number of primary myotubes remained unaffected but they detected a dramatic decrease in the number of secondary myotubes. These results led them to hypothesize that development of primary myotubes is genetically determined while that of the secondary myotubes is susceptible to environmental factors, such as undernutrition, but possibly also hormonal factors. As they (and others) suggested that the primary myotubes are the precursors of type I muscle fibers and the secondary myotubes of the type II muscle fibers, this implies that the relative proportions of type II fibers in muscles could be influenced during early development.

During further development, the contractile proteins actin and myosin increase such that the nuclei in the myocytes are pushed aside in the cell. The motor end-

Summary

Most muscles in the rat contain a majority of fast-twitch type II muscle fibers. Muscles involved in postural tasks are characterized by relatively high percentages of slow twitch fatigue resistant type I muscle fibers. Motoneuronal properties are matched to those of the muscle units. The dendrites of motoneurones that innervate muscles with important postural tasks are organized in bundles.

Summary

Trunk and extremity muscles descend from myotomes and limb buds, respectively. Cytologically they develop from primary and secondary myotubes. Muscle fibers are polyneurally innervated at early stages and the regression into mononeural innervation is related to neural and muscular activity.

plate develops its folded appearance and from a certain stage of development these cells have acquired the characteristics of the mature myocyte.

A puzzling phenomenon is the polyneural innervation of the muscle fibers at early stages and subsequently a regression towards mononeural innervation (for reviews, Bennett, 1983; Jansen & Fladby, 1990). Obviously a relation exists between activity in muscle fibers and the regression of polyneural innervation. Respiratory muscles in the rat are mononeurally innervated already from around birth but the regression of polyneural innervation in the soleus muscle is completed only around P16 and in the psoas muscle by P20 (IJkema-Paasen & Gramsbergen, 1997). In experimental research it has been demonstrated that the blockade of neuromuscular transmission by α-bungarotoxin stops this regression (Greensmith & Vrbova, 1991) while electrical stimulation accelerates it (O'Brien *et al.*, 1978).

It has been considered that a great excess of axons randomly innervate the primitive muscle fibers at early stages and that selective regression of supernumerary axon endings matches the properties of muscle fibers with their motoneurones. More recent research has indicated, however, that even at the earliest stages ingrowing axons follow a specific trajectory towards certain muscular regions with a preponderance of one or other muscle fiber type. Therefore, the development of innervation patterns should be regarded as a fine-tuning of this matching. The problem remains, however, why this requires such massive over-innervation during the early stages.

Central pattern generators

Graham Brown (1914) was the first to convincingly demonstrate that rhythmic and alternating movements of the extremities can occur after several dorsal roots of the lumbar spinal cord had been severed. A few years earlier, Sherrington (1910) had demonstrated rhythmic limb movements after transection of the thoracic spinal cord at lower levels. Brown hypothesized that so-called half-centers in the spinal cord generate these rhythmic patterns autonomously although a certain amount of

sensory input appeared necessary for the automatic movements to occur. Somewhat later, von Holst (1935) described rhythmic swimming movements of the trunk after differentiation and transection of the spinal cord in teleosts and Weiss reported similar results in salamanders after deafferentation of the limbs (Weiss, 1936). The relevance of these observations has to be understood in the perspective of investigations of other neuroscientists, who at that time theorized that a chain of reflexes should be considered as the neural substrate for rhythmic limb movements. The experiments referred to above, however, demonstrate that the spinal cord is capable of autonomously generating rhythmic activities necessary to activate trunk and extremity muscles, provided some afferent input remains intact. Such rhythmic neural activity has also been implicated in wing movements of birds as well as in breathing movements. The neural substrate for this clock-like activation is known as the central pattern generator (CPG).

Most of the studies on CPGs for extremity movements have concentrated on the hindlimb. Grillner and Zangger (1975) demonstrated that adult cats with a low thoracic spinal cord transection maintained a delicate pattern of orderly starting and stopping of EMG activities in the hindlimb flexors and extensors during walking on a treadmill. Forssberg *et al.* (1980) demonstrated that the coordination patterns of the limbs follows the increasing speed of the treadmill, provided that the limb afferents were left intact. At higher speeds they even observed a gallop-like coordination. Shik and Orlovsky (1976) studied cats after spinal cord transection when walking on a treadmill with two belts, driven at different speeds. When the speed differences became too large the frequencies of the CPG shifted to a 1:2 relationship and on the basis of this and other evidence it is considered that each limb has its own CPG.

The neural principles involved in CPGs have been studied in the lamprey which has a less complex spinal cord. In an impressive series of experiments the neural elements constituting the CPGs in the spinal cord segments were identified. Basically, the spinal cord segments on the left and right side have two networks consisting of a few types of excitatory and inhibitory interneurons and with the motoneurons as output elements. The networks on both sides are connected via inhibitory connections and these connected networks function as coupled oscillators. Networks in adjacent spinal cord segments are connected via propriospinal interneurons.

Based on the neuroanatomical and neurochemical studies in the lamprey, the network was modeled and computer simulations indicated that increased excitability of the neurons in the segmental circuitry induced decreases in cycle times. Increases in frequency of the most rostral segment (or oscillator) are spread along the spinal cord by a process of entrainment and this leads to higher swimming speeds (Grillner *et al.*, 1991). Such increases in natural life are induced by supraspinal influences and possibly also by afferent input.

The CPG for extremity movements in tetrapods might also consist of a series of coupled oscillators for the different muscle groups, but it should be realized that the interactions between these oscillators and, consequently, the neural structure might be more complex. Recently, experiments have been performed in the isolated spinal cord of newborn rats by Cazalets *et al.* (1995) in which so-called fictive locomotion was recorded from electrical activity in the ventral roots. In other experiments, the isolated spinal cord remained connected to one of the hindlimbs (Kjaerulff & Kiehn, 1996). Such preparations allow study of the CPGs for limb movements in tetrapods and in the future such experiments may reveal the neural circuitry involved. Cazalets and co-workers showed that the CPG for hindlimb movements in the rat is located in the first lumbar segment. Although indications have been gathered by both these groups on the neural transmitters that are involved, such as excitatory amino acids (EAA) – (probably L-glutamate and aspartate), 5-HT, dopamine and GABA, the neural elements and the circuitry of these CPGs for rhythmic alternating limb movements in higher vertebrates are still unknown. Several models have been devised, most of which are based upon reciprocal inhibition of groups of neurons and computer modeling has shown that these models faithfully mimic rhythmic activity. Such reciprocal inhibitory circuitries do exist in the CNS of mammals as has been demonstrated by neuroanatomical and neurophysiological techniques. Due to the immense complexity of the segmental circuitry in the spinal cord combined with methodological difficulties, it has not yet been possible to unravel the structure of CPGs for hindlimb movements by neuroanatomical or neurophysiological methods.

Obviously, locomotion in intact animals is adapted to environmental constraints. Avoiding an object in the trajectory, walking on a slope or anticipating an unevenness in the path lead to adjustments of the limb excursions or their rhythmicity. Exteroceptive and proprioceptive information influences the extension and flexion phases of the step cycle via segmentally arranged circuitry. Stumbling over unexpected objects on the trajectory leads to adjustments of the step cycle (Rossignol *et al.*, 1988) and other experiments have demonstrated that increasing the load on the extended limb and input from Golgi-tendon organs via group II afferents also leads to adjustments of the step cycle (Duysens & Pearson, 1980). On the other hand, the CPG itself influences the input from proprioceptive afferents. This

Summary

CPGs in the spinal cord are able to autonomously generate rhythmical locomotor patterns in the trunk muscles in fish and amphibiae and in the extremities in quadrupeds and bipeds. Afferent feedback and CPGs mutually influence each other. In rats the CPG for hindlimb movements is localized in the first lumbar segment.

probably is effected by activating the inhibitory interneurons mediating the reciprocal Ia inhibition (Hultborn, 1972). Input from the visual and the vestibular system is relayed along descending projections and cerebellar circuitry probably plays an important role in adjustments (see below).

Developmental aspects of CPGs

The output pattern and, therefore, the circuitry of CPGs is specified already in the neurula stage during early neuro-ontogeny. Straznicky (1963) has demonstrated that interchanging brachial and lumbar segments of the spinal cord in the chick embryo at the third day of incubation results in movement patterns which are related to the origin of these spinal cord segments; after these operations the wings produced alternating movements and the limbs moved simultaneously. This demonstrates that the global coordination pattern is determined by the neural circuitry independent of the neuromuscular connections.

In rats, rhythmic activity can already be evoked at E15.5 by adding EAAs or 5-HT to the isolated spinal cord kept *in vitro*, with clear signs of coordination between the left and right side (Iizuka *et al.*, 1998). This suggests that the CPGs in the spinal cord develop at a very early stage. Rhythmic and alternating limb movements in human fetuses occur already from the 12th–14th week of gestation (de Vries *et al.*, 1982). In newborn babies during the first weeks of life a stepping response can be elicited, consisting of alternating limb movements (Forssberg, 1985). After a silent period of several months walking movements reappear around one year of age. Strong arguments exist indicating that the CPG for the alternating limb movements in the human fetus is identical to the CPG operating at later and at adult ages.

Although the circuitry and the output pattern of the CPG probably remains largely unchanged through an animal's lifetime, experimental interference during early development may induce slight changes in the tuning of CPGs. In young rats restriction of the movements of one hindlimb during the first 3 weeks after birth leads to subtle but consistent changes in the phasing of EMG activation of muscles in the previously restricted hindlimb that persist long after the termination of the restriction (Westerga & Gramsbergen, 1993b). These results suggest that some reorganization of the CPG might occur but the overall rhythmicity remains undisturbed.

Investigations into CPGs in quadrupeds have largely been restricted to extremity movements. An intriguing problem is how the fluent postural adjustments during locomotion at various speeds are effected. It is well known from kinematic studies in horses that the activation and coordination of trunk muscles differs importantly between walking, trotting and galloping. Theoretical possibilities are that the trunk muscles are activated via the CPG for limb movements, that the rhythmic activity in the trunk muscles is produced by a separate CPG (perhaps similar to those in fish) which is entrained to the CPG for limb movements, or that the trunk muscles are activated and adjusted via supraspinal influences. Our own experiments involving EMG recordings of limb muscles and dorsal trunk muscles in adult rats indicated that at low walking speeds the back muscles are activated variably and only tonic activation appeared. At higher speeds, and particularly during accelerations, stronger and more uniform activation patterns were observed (Fig. 2.2; Gramsbergen et al., 1999).

Experiments in which we attempted to selectively sever the spinal afferents from the longissimus muscles and other trunk muscles have been unsuccessful, so the nature of the neural circuitry involved in the rhythmic trunk muscle activity has not been determined. However, given that vestibular deprivation from P5 leads to longlasting abnormalities in the coordination between extremity movements and trunk control (Geisler & Gramsbergen, 1998) it seems that in adult rats supraspinal influences take an important part in the control of axial muscles (Gramsbergen, 1998). On the other hand, before P22 rats showed a coupling between activation of the stance phase in one limb and activation of the contralateral longissimus muscle, much like the pattern

observed in salamanders (Weiss, 1936). This might indicate that in young rats a CPG for rhythmic trunk movements is effective, which later becomes dominated by other neural influences.

Descending motor projections and their development

The architecture of the components of the descending projections of the somatic motor system reflect their phylogenetical descent. Axial muscles in the trunk descend from the segmentally arranged myotomes and the ventromedially located motoneurons of these muscles are innervated by medially descending motor projections. The extremity muscles, developing from the limb buds and the motoneurones of these muscles, which are located laterally in the ventral horn, are innervated by the laterally descending tracts. In quadrupeds the rubrospinal tract (RST) is particularly important for activation of the latter motoneurones but in primates the corticospinal tract (CST) has largely taken over this function (Kuypers, 1982).

The medially descending projections, such as the vestibulospinal, reticulospinal and tectospinal projections, are particularly important for innervation of the muscles in the neck and trunk and also muscles in the proximal segments of the extremities. Anatomical investigations in rats demonstrated that these projections descended before birth and electrical stimulation of the medial structures during the first day of life demonstrated that they are functional, although not in an adultlike fashion (Thoman & Korner, 1971; L. Vinay 1998, personal communication).

The RST arises from the red nucleus and descends laterally. This tract arises mainly from the most caudally located magnocellular part but also from the rostral parvocellular part. It crosses in the ventral tegmental decussation and descends via the lateral funiculus. The axons terminate upon excitatory and inhibitory interneurons in the spinal cord. The red nucleus receives its major input from the deep cerebellar nuclei and also from the motor cortex both via direct connections and via collaterals from the CST. The cerebellum and the vestibular complex play an important role in the regulation of locomotor movements and the regulation of postural maintenance (see below). With regard to the development of its circuitry, efferent projections from the deep cerebellar nuclei develop even before the cerebellar cortex starts to form. The first cerebello-rubral connections have been demonstrated from E16 (Cholley et al., 1989) and the first RST fibers in the spinal cord have been demonstrated from E17 (Lakke et al., 1991). The cerebellar cortex, however, develops largely after birth (Altman & Bayer, 1985). No data are available on the

Summary

CPGs probably are amongst the first neural circuitries to develop in neuro-ontogeny. CPGs essentially remain unaltered during an animal's lifetime although slight adjustments might take place. Postural adjustments during walking might be governed largely by supraspinal influences.

further development of terminal patterns in relation to segmental circuitry. Functionally, however, the cerebellum and the RST seem to mature relatively late. Cerebellar hemispherectomy in rats at P5 or at P10 leads to motor handicaps after P14 (Gramsbergen, 1982) and this might indicate that the fibers in the RST after having descended, wait for some time until definite and functional synaptic connections are established. Similar evidence was obtained with regard to other descending projections in the opossum (Cassidy & Cabana, 1993) and to the CST in monkeys (Lemon et al., 1997).

The crossed CST arises from the somatosensory areas of the cerebral cortex. As the axons of this projection terminate mainly in the dorsal quadrants of the spinal cord it has been suggested that in rats the CST is important for adjusting and gating afferent proprioceptive and exteroceptive feedback. The main portion of the CST in rodents descends through the contralateral dorsal funiculus onto lumbar levels and the uncrossed part descends in the ventral funiculus. In carnivores, such as the cat, this tract courses through the dorsolateral funiculus. In man four tracts can be distinguished: crossed and uncrossed dorsolateral and crossed and uncrossed ventral tracts. In other species such as rabbits (Hobbelen et al., 1992) and probably also in horses (Verhaart & Sopers-Jurgens, 1957) the CST is less well expressed compared to rats and cats. For example, in rabbits the unmyelinated fibers of this tract end at the 2nd cervical segment (for review see Nudo & Masterton, 1988). The large degree of variation of the CST may be attributed to the fact that the corticospinal tract is phylogenetically young (Armand, 1982).

Most of the fibers of the crossed CST, which courses through the dorsal funiculus, have reached cervical levels by E20 and reach lumbar levels only during the second postnatal week (Gribnau et al., 1986; Joosten et al., 1987). After the corticospinal fibers have made definite synaptic contacts, myelination starts, first in the largest fibers as indicated from research in rats (Gribnau et al., 1986).

Parallel to the projections of the so-called somatic motor system referred to above, another system of diffusely projecting monoaminergic fibers has been distinguished which plays an important role in motor steering. This system was termed the limbic motor system (LMS) by Kuypers (1982) and the emotional motor system by Holstege (1991, 1995). In this chapter I will refer to this system as the LMS. The LMS originates in the medial portions of the hypothalamus and the mesencephalon. Its medial components influence the excitatory state of interneurons and motoneurons via diffusely projecting monoaminergic fibers. This motor system probably is the most advanced in its development at birth having descended already to lumbar levels and established 5-HT

Summary

Medially descending projections impinge upon axial muscles and laterally descending projections impinge upon extremity muscles. The phylogenetically oldest systems, the vestibulospinal and the reticulospinal tracts, are functional at early stages but the crossed rubrospinal tract matures later around the end of the second week of life. The corticospinal tract reaches lumbar levels in the second week.

containing synapses in rats (Rajaofetra et al., 1989). As the terminals initially are widespread but later are restricted to the dorsal and ventral horns, Rajofetra hypothesized that these 5-HT containing fibers might play a role in the stabilization of the innervation patterns of other projections in the spinal cord.

INITIATION OF LOCOMOTION AND SUPRASPINAL MODULATION OF WALKING PATTERN AND POSTURE

Strong evidence has been collected from research in cats that locomotion is initiated by activity in a group of cells in the mesencephalic brain stem. Electrical stimulation of this area in intact cats on a moving treadmill induced locomotion (Shik et al., 1966) and since then this area has been termed the mesencephalic locomotor region (MLR). Anatomically, these cells are localized around the pedunculopontine tegmental nucleus (Spann & Grofova, 1989). Descending fibers from this cell group probably course via the reticulospinal tract and impinge upon the CPG where they might induce rhythmical activity.

When the stimulus intensity was increased the walking speed increased and eventually the animals made a transition to trot or gallop (Shik et al., 1966). The increases in speed and the transitions into other coordination patterns probably are mediated by indirect activation of noradrenergic projections arising from the locus coeruleus and adjacent cell groups which are located close by the MLR and are part of the LMS (see above). On the other hand, the gait transitions probably are induced by alternative coordination patterns produced by the CPGs.

Cerebellar lesions (e.g. Brooks, 1975; Gramsbergen, 1982) or cooling of the cerebellum (Udo et al., 1979) lead to atactic gait and irregularities in foot placing, and for this reason it is generally considered that the cerebellum plays a key role in the fine adjustments of limb movements during the step cycle and also in postural control.

The cerebellum receives information from spinal sources via several inputs. Most important are the ventral spinocerebellar tract (VSCT) and the spinoreticulo-cerebellar pathway (SRCP). The VSCT transmits information from the interneurons near to the motoneurones, the premotor neurons, to the cerebellar cortex via the parallel (or mossy) fiber system and phasic activity in this tract has been recorded during walking (Arshavsky *et al.*, 1972). This phasic activity has also been recorded in the SRCP, which transports information via the lateral reticular nucleus to the cerebellar parallel fiber system. Both systems also send collaterals to the deep cerebellar nuclei, the anterior interposed nuclei (AIN) and the lateral vestibular nuclei (LVN). This information might be processed in the B and the C zones of the cerebellar cortex and then fed back to the AIN and the LVN via the Purkinje cell axons (Voogd, 1995).

The other important input to the cerebellum is via the inferior olivary nucleus (ION), which receives indirect information from the spinal cord and several areas in the CNS. Axons from ION neurons reach the cerebellum as climbing fibers, each of which has thousands of synaptic contacts with one Purkinje cell (Ruigrok & Cella, 1995). The physiological significance of the input from the ION to the cerebellum remains unclear. In one theory, the climbing fiber system, together with the parallel fiber system, is ascribed a decisive role in motor learning (Marr, 1969). A more recent theory suggests that the ION plays an important role in regulating a distributed processing of afferent information in the cerebellar cortex (Llinas & Muhletaler, 1988).

Information from the AIN in the cerebellum is transported via the red nucleus and along the RST to the spinal cord. Information from the LVN is relayed via the lateral vestibulospinal tract (the LVST) to the spinal cord. Activity in both these tracts is modulated in phase with the step cycle (Arshavsky *et al.*, 1972, 1986). The LVST is particularly active during the stance phase, while the RST is active during the swing phase. Input from these descending tracts reaches motoneurons of extrem-ity muscles via interneurons and this input probably is crucial for postural adjustments and differential postural control during walking and running.

A synthesis

Rhythmic and alternating limb movements may be elicited in newborn rats (Jamon & Clarac, 1998). Strong olfactory stimulation induces this behavior, swimming induces alternating limb movements (Bekoff & Trainer, 1979) and electrophysiological experiments in the isolated spinal cord have indicated that the CPG is already producing rhythmic and alternating bursts of activity (Cazalets *et al.*, 1995). These results indicate that around birth the descending projections from the MLR and probably from the LMS are already functional. Around P8, rats are able to stand on their four limbs, with the ventral body surface elevated from the ground, and to make a few steps. Investigations demonstrated that the force produced by the muscles at earlier ages cannot be the limiting factor for standing to occur (Gramsbergen, 1998), so maturational processes in the CNS are probably responsible. At this age the staggering type of walking and its slow speed suggest that feedback regulation of standing and walking prevails. From the end of the second week after birth the smooth, adult-like walking pattern develops and evidence from several sources indicates that from this age a feed-forward type of postural control becomes effective. Ablating the cerebellar hemispheres interferes with this development and we hypothesize that from then onwards the cerebellar and vestibular processing becomes functional.

From this time until the end of the third week of life the coordination of trunk muscles still shows signs of an evolutionary older pattern of coordination (Geisler *et al.*, 1996b) and also extremity movements and footfall patterns are not yet mature (Clarke & Williams, 1994). Possibly it is only after P22 that the CPG for limb movements along with cerebellar and vestibular circuitry assume full control (Gramsbergen, 1998).

The development of postural control is the limiting factor for the adult walking pattern to emerge. Vestibular deprivation from P5 has demonstrated that smooth walking and other behavior patterns that require elaborate control are not influenced until P15 but from then onwards retardations in walking, rearing and other motor patterns occur (Geisler *et al.*, 1996b, Geisler & Gramsbergen, 1998). In addition, long-lasting or even permanent deficits are observed in the coordination of the trunk muscles during walking.

Particular muscles and regions of other muscles are specialized to subserve postural tasks. They contain large

Summary

Locomotion is initiated by activity in the MLR, which in turn might be activated by higher centers. The LMS plays a role in the acceleration or deceleration of walking speed. Cerebellar circuitry plays a role in adjustments and fine tuning of walking.

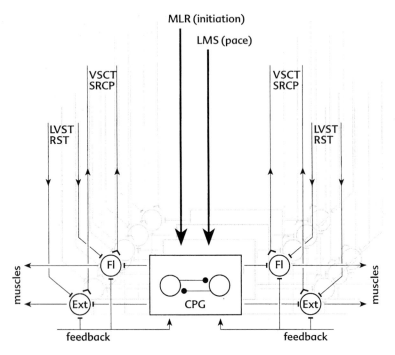

Fig. 2.4 Diagram representing CPG in relation to motoneurons (Fl: flexors, Ext: extensors) and ascending and descending tracts. CPG: central pattern generator; Feedback: proprioceptive feedback from muscles, tendons and joint receptors; RST: rubrospinal tract; LVST: lateral vestibulospinal tract; VSCT: ventral spinocerebellar tract; SRCP: spinoreticulocerebellar tract; MLR: mesencephalic locomotor region; LMS: limbic motor system.

proportions of type I muscle fibers. These muscles are innervated by motoneurons which are characterized by dendrite bundles (Gramsbergen *et al.*, 1996). Muscles composed mainly of type I muscle fibers are innervated by motoneuronal pools with conspicuous bundles (as in the soleus muscle and the trunk muscles), whereas those with limited regions with a high proportion of type I muscle fibers, such as the gastrocnemius and vastus medius, have a few regions with dendrite bundles. The bundles in the pools for the hindlimb muscles develop around P14–P16 (Westerga & Gramsbergen, 1992) and they probably develop by virtue of ingrowing descending fiber projections around P15 (Gramsbergen *et al.*, 1995).

At adult age, the basic rhythmicity in alternating limb movements during walking is produced by a CPG, which in the rat is located in the first lumbar segment (Fig. 2.4). Walking starts by activation from the MLR in the mesencephalic brain stem. This cell group, in turn, is activated by other brain areas, possibly by the sensory-motor cortex. The speed of walking is adjusted by the LMS. In situations of fear, strong activation by the LMS may lead the CPG to switch to other coordination patterns. Information from the premotor neurons in the

spinal cord is relayed via the VSCT and the SRCP and via other ascending tracts to the cerebellum and the vestibular complex. The information, which is processed and output via the RST and LVST, leads to fine-tuning of activations of the hindlimb and trunk muscles during each step. This activity together with afferent feedback ensures the smooth walking pattern and postural adjustments.

Future research into the neurobiology of locomotion should concentrate upon elucidating the circuitry and the properties of the CPG. *In vitro* preparations of the spinal cord offer promising perspectives for this enterprise. In addition, neuroanatomical and neurophysiological aspects of the cerebellar processing of afferent input and the nature of efferent influences on limb movements and postural control during locomotion should be studied. Solving these problems is not only necessary for understanding the neurobiology of locomotion but this also would be of great help in alleviating clinical problems in the human, such as cerebral palsy. Obviously, a sound description of kinematic aspects of locomotion as well as kinesiological research as given by the dynamical systems approach is of the greatest value to these investigations.

A

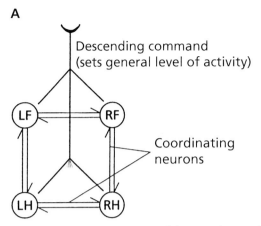

Fig. 2.5 Schematic representation of the neural control of locomotion in the horse.

A Dorsal view. Interlimb coordination is achieved by interaction of the central pattern generators (CPGs) of each of the four limbs. The general level of activity in the different generators that are capable of rythmic activity is set by a supraspinal descending command, whereas actual coordination is due to interaction between the four different generators via coordinating neurons. (Adapted from Grillner, S. (1975) Locomotion in vertebrates: central mechanisms and reflex interaction. *Physiological Reviews* **55**(2): 247–304).

B

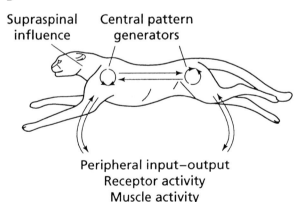

B Lateral view. The CPG of each limb is influenced by peripheral input from a variety of somatosensory receptors as well as descending influence from supraspinal centers. Through peripheral output pathways, appropriate muscles are contracted to perform their task and result in intralimb coordination.
(Adapted from Goslow, G.E. (1985) Neural control of locomotion. In: Hildebrand, M., Bramble, D.M., Liem, K.F. and Wake, D.B. (eds) *Functional Vertebrate Morphology*. Harvard University Press, Fig. 17.1, p. 339).

EPILOGUE AND INTERSPECIES COMPARISONS

In this chapter, I concentrated upon the neurobiological aspects of walking in the rat and data from research in cats were included. Extrapolations to research in horses should take into account size differences and also differences in neural circuitary between these small mammals and horses. Kinematic and kinesiological research in rats and in cats is in its infancy but such data are urgently needed to make extrapolations from rats and cats to problems in equine research. Inverse and forward dynamics from kinematic research should lead to basic principles which then could be applicable in problems of locomotion in horses. On the other hand, neuroanatomical and neurophysiological data are needed in horses. In the future, the use of modern and non-invasive imaging techniques may lead to such insight (Fig. 2.5).

REFERENCES

Almli, C.R. and Fisher, R.S. (1977) Infant rats: sensorimotor ontogeny and effects of substantia nigra destruction. *Brain Res. Bull.* **2**: 425–459.

Altman, J. and Bayer, S.A. (1985) Embryonic development of the rat cerebellum III. Regional differences in the time of origin, migration, and settling of Purkinje cells. *J. Comp. Neurol.* **231**: 42–65.

Altman, J. and Sudarshan, K. (1975) Postnatal development of locomotion in the laboratory rat. *Anim. Behav.* **23**: 896–920.

Angulo y Gonzalez, A.W. (1932) The prenatal development of behavior in the albino rat. *J. Comp. Neurol.* **55**: 395–442.

Ariens Kappers, C.U., Huber, G.C. and Crosby, E.C. (1967) *The Comparative Anatomy of the Nervous System of Vertebrates including Man*. New York: Hafner.

Armand, J. (1982) The origin, course and terminations of corticospinal fibers in various mammals. In: Kuypers, H.G.J.M. and Martin, G.F. (eds) *Descending pathways to the spinal cord. Progress in Brain Research*, vol. 57, pp. 327–360. Amsterdam: Elsevier.

Arshavsky Yu. I., Berkinblit, M.B., Fukson, O.I., Gelfand, I.M. and Orlovsky, G.N. (1972) Origin of modulation in neurones of the ventral spinocerebellar tract during locomotion. *Brain Res.* **43**: 276–279.

Arshavsky Yu. I., Gelfand, I.M. and Orlovsky, G.N. (1986) *Cerebellum and Rhythmical Movements*. Berlin, Heidelberg: Springer.

Baldissera, F., Hultborn, H. and Illert, M. (1981) Integration in spinal neuronal systems. In: Brooks, V.B. (ed) *Handbook of Physiology*. Bethesda, Md.: American Physiological Society, pp. 509–597.

Barcroft, J. and Barron, D.H. (1939) The development of behaviour in foetal sheep. *J. Comp. Neurol.* **70**: 447–502.

Bekoff, A. and Lau, B. (1980) Interlimb coordination in 20-day-old rat fetuses. *J. Exp. Zool.* **214**: 173–175.

Bekoff, A. and Trainer, W. (1979) The development of interlimb co-ordination during swimming in postnatal rats. *J. Exp. Biol.* **83**: 1–11.

Bennett, M.R. (1983) Development of neuromuscular synapses. *Physiol. Rev.* **63**: 915–1048.

Blanck, A., Hard, E. and Larsson, K. (1967) Ontogenetic development of orienting behavior in the rat. *J. Comp. Physiol. Psychol.* **63**: 427–441.

Bolles, R.C. and Woods, P.J. (1964) The ontogeny of behaviour in the albino rat. *Anim. Behav.* **12**: 427–441.

Brooks, V.B. (1975) Roles of the cerebellum and basal ganglia in initiation and control of movements. *Can. J. Neurol. Sci.* **2**: 265–277.

Brown, T.G. (1914) On the nature of the fundamental activity of the nervous centers; together with an analysis of the conditioning of rhythmic activity in progression, and a theory of the evolution of function in the nervous system. *J. Physiol. (Lond.)* **48**: 18–46.

Burke, R.E. (1981) Motor units: anatomy, physiology, and functional organization. In: Brooks, V.B. (ed) *Handbook of Physiology*. Bethesda, Md.: American Physiological Society, pp. 345–423.

Carlson, H., Halbertsma, J. and Zomlefer, M. (1979) Control of the trunk during walking in the cat. *Acta. Physiol. Scand.* **105**: 251–253.

Cassidy, G. and Cabana, T. (1993) The development of the long descending projections in the opossum, Monodelphis domestica. *Dev. Brain Res.* **72**: 291–299.

Cazalets, J.R., Borde, M. and Clarac, F. (1995) Localization and organization of the central pattern generator for hind limb locomotion in newborn rat. *J. Neurosci.* **15**: 4943–4951.

Cholley, B., Wassef, M., Arsénio-Nunes, L., Bréhier, A. and Sotelo, C. (1989) Proximal trajectory of the brachium conjunctivum in rat fetuses and its early association with the parabrachial nucleus. A study combining in vitro HRP anterograde axonal tracing and immunohistochemistry. *Dev. Brain Res.* **45**: 185–202.

Clarke, K.A. and Williams, E. (1994) Development of locomotion in the rat, spatiotemporal footfall patterns. *Physiol. Behav.* **55**: 151–155.

Coghill, G.E. (1929) *Anatomy and the Problem of Behavior.* Cambridge: Cambridge University Press.

Dubowitz, V. and Brooke, M.H. (1973) Muscle biopsy: A modern approach. In: Walton, J.N. (ed) *Major Problems in Neurology*, vol. 2, London: W.B. Saunders, pp. 10–100.

Duysens, J. and Pearson, K.G. (1980) Inhibition of flexor burst generation by loading ankle extensor muscles in walking cats. *Brain. Res.* **187**: 321–332.

Engberg, I. and Lundberg, A. (1962) An electromyographic analysis of stepping in the cat. *Experientia* **18**: 174.

Engberg, I. and Lundberg, A. (1969) An electromyographic analysis of muscular activity in the hind limb of the cat during unrestrained locomotion. *Acta. Physiol. Scand.* **75**: 614–630.

Fabricius ab Aquapendente, H. (1967) De formatione ovi et pulli and de formatio foetu, a facsimile edition by Adelman, H.B. Ithaca, NY: Cornell University Press.

Forssberg, H., Grillner, S., Halbertsma, J. and Rossignol, S. (1980) The locomotion of the low spinal cat. 2: Interlimb coordination. *Acta. Physiol. Scand.* **108**: 283–295.

Forssberg, H. (1985) Ontogeny of human locomotor control: I. Infant stepping, supported locomotion, and transition to independent locomotion. *Exp. Brain Res.* **57**: 480–493.

Geisler, H.C. and Gramsbergen, A. (1998) The EMG development of the longissimus and multifidus muscles after plugging the horizontal semicircular canals. *J. Vestib. Res.* **8**: 1–11.

Geisler, H.C., Westerga, J. and Gramsbergen, A. (1993) Development of posture in the rat. *Acta. Neurobiol. Exp.* **53**: 517–523.

Geisler, H.C., van der Fits, I.B.M. and Gramsbergen, A. (1996a) The effect of vestibular deprivation on motor development in the rat. *Behav. Brain Res.* **86**: 89–96.

Geisler, H.C., Westerga, J. and Gramsbergen, A. (1996b) The function of the long back muscles; and EMG study in the rat. *Behav. Brain Res.* **80**: 211–215.

Goldspink, G. and Ward (1979) Changes in rodent muscle fiber types during postnatal growth, undernutrition and exercise. *J. Physiol. (Lond.).* **296**: 453–469.

Gramsbergen, A. (1982) The effects of cerebellar hemispherectomy in the young rat. I Behavioural sequelae. *Behav. Brain Res.* **6**: 85–92.

Gramsbergen, A. (1998) Posture and locomotion in the rat: independent or interdependent development. *Neurosci. Bio. Behav. Rev.* **22**: 547–554.

Gramsbergen, A. and Mulder, E.J.H. (1998) The influence of betamethasone and dexamethasone on motor development in the developing rat. *Pediatr. Res.* **44**: 1–6.

Gramsbergen, A., Schwartze, P. and Prechtl, H.F.R. (1970) The postnatal development of behavioural states in the rat. *Develop. Psychobiol.* **3**: 267–280.

Gramsbergen, A., IJkema-Paassen, J. and Klok, F. (1995) Factors influencing the development of dendrite bundles in the rat spinal cord. *Soc. Neurosci. Abstr.* **21**: 1790.

Gramsbergen, A., IJkema-Paassen, J., Westerga, J. and Geisler, H.C. (1996) Dendrite bundles in motoneuronal pools of trunk and extremity muscles in the rat. *Exp. Neurol.* **137**: 34–42.

Gramsbergen, A., van Eykern, L.A., Taekema, H. and Geisler, H.C. (1999) The activation of back muscles during locomotion in the developing rat. *Dev. Brain Res.* **112**: 217–228.

Greensmith, L. and Vrbova, G. (1991) Neuromuscular contacts in the developing rat soleus depend on muscle activity. *Dev. Brain. Res.* **62**: 121–129.

Gribnau, A.A.M., De Kort, E.J.M., Dederen, P.J.W.W.C. and Nieuwenhuys, R. (1986) On the development of the corticospinal tract in the rat II. An anterograde tracer study of the outgrowth of the corticospinal fibers. *Anat. Embryol.* **175**: 101–110.

Grillner, S. (1975) Locomotion in vertebrates: central mechanisms and reflex interaction. *Physiol. Rev.* **55**: 247–304.

Grillner, S. (1981) Control of locomotion in bipeds, tetrapods, and fish In: Brooks, V.B. (ed) *Handbook of Physiology.* Bethesda, Md.: American Physiological Society, pp. 1179–1236.

Grillner, S. and Zangger, P. (1975) How detailed is the central pattern generator for locomotion? *Brain. Res.* **88**: 367–371.

Grillner, S., Wallén, P., Brodin, L. and Lansner, A. (1991) Neuronal network generating locomotor behaviour in lamprey: circuitry, transmitters, membrane properties, and simulation. *Ann. Rev. Neurosci.* **14**: 169–199.

Hamburger, V. (1988) Ontogeny of neuroembryology. *J. Neuroscience* **8**: 3535–3540.

Heglund, N.C., Cavagna, G.A. and Taylor, C.R. (1982) Energetics and mechanics of terrestrial locomotion. III Energy changes of the center of mass as a function of speed and body size in birds and mammals. *J. Exp. Biol.* **97**: 41–56.

Heimer, L. and Zaborszky, L. (1989) *Neuroanatomical Tract-tracing Methods* 2. New York, London: Plenum Press.

Henneman, E. and Mendell, L.M. (1981) Functional organization of motoneuronal pool and its inputs. In: Brooks, V.B. (ed) *Handbook of Physiology.* Bethesda, Md.: American Physiological Society, pp. 43–106.

Hildebrand, M. (1962) Walking running and jumping. *Am. Zool.* **2**: 151–155.

Hobbelen, J.F., Gramsbergen, A. and van Hof, M.W. (1992) Descending motor pathways and the hopping response in the rabbit. *Brain. Behav. Res.* **51**: 217–221.

Holst, E. von (1935) Über den Prozess der zentralnervösen Koordination. *Pflugers Arch.* **236**: 149–158.

Holstege, G. (1991) Descending motor pathways and the spinal motor system: limbic and non-limbic components. *Prog. Brain Res.* **87**: 307–421.

Holstege, G. (1995) The basic, somatic, and emotional components of the motor system in mammals. In: Paxinos, G. (ed) *The Rat Nervous System*, 2nd edn. San Diego: Academic Press, pp. 137–154.

Hultborn, H. (1972) Convergence on interneurons in the reciprocal Ia inhibitory pathway to motoneurones. *Acta. Physiol. Scand.* **375** (Suppl.): 1–42.

Iizuka, M., Nishimaru, H. and Kudo, N. (1998) Development of the spatial pattern of 5-HT-induced locomotor rhythm in the lumbar spinal cord of rat fetuses *in vitro. Neurosci. Res.* **31**: 107–111.

IJkema-Paassen, J. and Gramsbergen, A. (1998) Regression of polyneural innervation in the psoas muscle of the developing rat. *Muscle and Nerve.* **21**: 1058–1063.

James, R.S., Altringham, J.D. and Goldspink, D.F. (1995) The mechanical properties of fast and slow skeletal muscles of the mouse in relation to their locomotory function. *J. Exp. Biol.* **198**: 491–502.

Jamon, M. and Clarac, F. (1998) Early walking in the neonatal rat: a kinematic study. *Behav. Neurosci.* **112**: 1218–1228.

Jansen, J.K.S. and Fladby, T. (1990) The perinatal reorganization of the innervation of skeletal muscle in mammals. *Prog. Neurobiol.* **34**: 39–90.

Joosten, E.A.J., Gribnau, A.A.M. and Dederen, P.W.J.C. (1987) An anterograde tracer study of the developing corticospinal tract in the rat: Three components. *Dev. Brain Res.* **36**: 121–130.

Kernell, D. (1998) Muscle regionalization. *Can. J. Appl. Physiol.* **23**: 1–22.

Kjaerulff, O. and Kiehn, O. (1996) Distribution of networks generating and coordinating locomotor activity in the neonatal spinal cord *in vitro*: a lesion study. *J. Neurosci.* **16**: 5777–5794.

Kudo, N. and Yamada, T. (1987) Morphological and physiological studies of development of the monosynaptic pathway in the rat lumbar spinal cord. *J. Physiol. (Lond).* **389**: 441–459.

Kuo, Z.-T. (1963) Total patterns, local reflexes or gradients of response? *Proc. 16th Int. Congr. Zool.* **4**: 371–374.

Kuypers, H.G.J.M. (1982) A new look at the organization of the motor system. In: Kuypers, H.G.J.M. and Martin, G.F. (eds) *Descending pathways to the spinal cord. Progress in Brain Research.* Amsterdam: Elsevier, vol. 57, pp. 381–403.

Lakke, E.A.J.F. and Marani, E. (1991) The prenatal descent of rubro-spinal fibers through the spinal cord of the rat: a study using retrograde transport of (WGA-)HRP. *J. Comp. Neurol.* **314**: 67–78.

Lawrence, D.G. and Hopkins, D.A. (1976) The development of motor control in the rhesus monkey: evidence concerning the role of corticomotoneuronal connections. *Brain.* **99**: 235–254.

Lemon, R.N., Armand, J., Olivier, E. and Edgley, S.A. (1997) Skilled action and the development of the corticospinal tract in primates. In: Connolly, K.J. and Forssberg, H. (eds) *Neurophysiology and Neuropsychology of Motor Development.* London: MacKeith Press.

Llinas, R. and Muhletaler, M. (1988) Electrophysiology of guinea pig cerebellar nuclear cells in the in vitro brainstem-cerebellar preparation. *J. Physiol. (Lond).* **404**: 241–258.

Marr, D. (1969) A theory of cerebellar cortex. *J. Physiol. (Lond.)* **202**: 437–470.

Massion, J. (1992) Movements, posture and equilibrium: interaction and coordination. *Prog. Neurobiol.* **38**: 35–56.

Matthews, M.A., Willis, W.D. and Williams, V. (1971) Dendrite bundles in lamina IX of cat spinal cord. A possible source for electrical interaction between motoneurons? *Anat. Rec.* **171**: 313–328.

Milner-Brown, H.S., Stein, R.B., and Yemm, R. (1973) The orderly recruitment of human motor units during voluntary isometric contractions. *J. Physiol. (Lond.)* **230**: 359–370.

Muybridge, E. (1957) *Animals in Motion.* New York: Dover.

Narayanan, C.H., Fox, M.W. and Hamburger, V. (1971) Prenatal development of spontaneous and evoked activity in the rat. *Behaviour* **40**: 100–134.

Nieuwenhuys, R., Ten Donkelaar, H.J. and Nicholson, C. (1997) *The Central Nervous System of Vertebrates.* Berlin: Springer.

Nicolopoulos-Stournaras, S. and Iles, J.F. (1983) Motor neurons columns in the lumbar spinal cord of the rat. *J. Comp. Neurol.* **217**: 74–85.

Nudo, R.J. and Masterton, R.B. (1988) Descending pathways to the spinal cord: a comparative study of 22 mammals. *J. Comp. Neurol.* **277**: 53–79.

O'Brien, R.A.D., Ostberg, A.J.C. and Vrbova, G. (1978) Observations on the elimination of polyneural innervation in developing mammalian skeletal muscle. *J. Physiol. (Lond.)* **282**: 571–582.

Ontell, M. and Dunn, R.F. (1978) Neonatal muscle growth: a quantitative study. *Am. J. Anat.* **152**: 539–556.

Oppenheim, R.W. (1978) Coghill, G.E. (1872–1941) pioneer, neuroembryologist and development psychobiologist. *Persp. Biol. Med.* **22**: 45–64.

Partrdge, L.D. and Benton, L.A. (1981) Muscle, the motor. In: Brooks, V.B. (ed) *Handbook of Physiology.*Bethesda, Md.: American Physiological Society, pp. 43–106.

Perry, A.K., Blickhan, R., Biewener, A.A., Heglund, N.C. and Taylor, C.R. (1988) Preferred speeds in terrestrial vertebrates: are they equivalent? *J. Exp. Biol.* **137**: 207–219.

Prechtl, H.F.R. (1984) Continuity and change in early neural development. In: Prechtl, H.F.R. (ed) Continuity of Neural Functions from Prenatal to Postnatal Life. Oxford: Spastics International Medical Publications, pp. 1–15.

Rajaofetra, N., Sandillon, F., Geffard, M. and Orivat, A. (1989). Pre- and post-natal ontogeny of serotonergic projections to the rat spinal cord. *J. Neurosc. Res.* **22**: 305–321.

Reback, P.A., Scheibel, A.B. and Smith, J.L. (1982) Development and maintenance of dendrite bundles after cordotomy in exercised and nonexercised cats. *Exp. Neurol.* **76**: 428–440.

Rossignol, S., Lund, J.P. and Drew, T. (1988) The role of sensory inputs in regulating patterns of rhythmical movements in higher vertebrates. In: Cohen, A.H., Rossignol, S., Grillner, S. (eds) *Neural Control of Rhythmic Movements in Vertebrates.* New York: Wiley, pp. 201–283.

Ruigrok, T.J.H. and Cella, F. (1995) Precerebellar nuclei and red nucleus. In: Paxinos, G. (ed.) *The Rat Nervous System.* 2nd edn. San Diego: Academic Press, pp. 277–300.

Scheibel, M.E. and Scheibel, A.B. (1970) Developmental relationship between spinal motoneuron dendrite bundles and patterned activity in the hind limb of cats. *Exp. Neurol.* **29**: 328–335.

Sherrington, C.S. (1910) Flexion reflex of the limb, crossed extension reflex and reflex stepping and standing. *J. Physiol. (Lond.)* **40**: 28–121.

Schiaffino, S., Saggin, L., Viel, A., Ausoni, S., Sartore, S. and Gorza, L. (1986) Muscle fiber types identified by monoclonal antibodies to myosin heavy chains. In: Benzi, G., Packer, L., Siliprandi, N. (eds) *Biochemical Aspects of Physical Exercise.* Amsterdam: Elsevier, pp. 27–34.

Schoenen, J. (1982) Dendritic organization of the human spinal cord: The motoneurons. *J. Comp. Neurol.* **21**: 226–247.

Shik, M.L. and Orlovsky, G.N. (1976) Neurophysiology of locomotor automatism. *Physiol. Rev.* **56**: 465–501.

Shik, M.L., Severin, F.V. and Orlovsky, G.N. (1966) Control of walking and running by means of electrical stimulation of the midbrain. *Biophysics* **11**: 756–765.

Small, W.S. (1899) Notes on the psychic development of the young white rat. *Am. J. Psychol.* **11**: 80–100.

Smart, J.L. and Dobbing, J. (1971) Vulnerability of developing brain. II. Effects of early nutritional deprivation on reflex ontogeny and development of behaviour in the rat. *Brain Res.* **28**: 85–95.

Spann, B.M. and Grofova, I. (1989) Origin of ascending and spinal pathways from the nucleus tegmenti pedunculopontinus in the rat. *J. Comp. Neurol.* **283**: 13–27.

Straznicky, K. (1963) Function of heterotopic spinal cord segments investigated in the chick. *Acta. Biol. Hung.* **14**: 145–155.

Sullivan, T.E. and Armstrong, R.B. (1978) Rat locomotory muscle fiber activity during trotting and galloping. *J. Appl. Physiol.* **44**: 358–363.

Szekely, G., Czeh, G. and Vörös, G. (1969) The activity pattern of limb muscles in freely moving and deafferented newts. *Exp. Brain Res.* **9**: 53–62.

Taylor, C.R., Heglund, N.C. and Maloiy, G.M. (1982) Energetics and mechanics of terrestrial locomotion. I. Metabolic energy consumption as a function of speed and body size in birds and mammals. *J. Exp. Biol.* **97**: 1–21.

Thoman, E.B. and Korner, A.F. (1971) Effects of vestibular stimulation on the behavior and development of infant rats. *Develop. Psychobiol.* **5**: 92–98.

Tracey, D.J. (1995) Ascending and descending pathways in the spinal cord In: Paxions, G. (ed.) *The Rat Nervous System,* 2nd edn. San Diego: Academic Press, pp. 67–80.

Udo, M., Matsukawa, K. and Kamei, H. (1979) Effects of partial cooling of cerebellar cortex at lobules V and IV of the intermediate part in decerebrate walking cats under monitoring vertical floor reaction forces. *Brain Res.* **160**: 559–564.

Verhaart, W.J.C. and Sopers-Jurgens, M.R. (1957) Aspects of comparative anatomy of the mammalian brain stem. *Acta. Morph. Neerl-Scand.* **1**: 246–255.

Voogd, J. (1995) Cerebellum. In: Paxinos, G. (ed) *The Rat Nervous System,* 2nd edn. San Diego Academic Press, pp. 309–350.

Vries, J.I.P., de, Visser, G.H.A. and Prechtl, H.F.R. (1982) The emergence of fetal behaviour. I. Qualitative aspects. *Early Human Develop.* **7**: 301–322.

Vries, J.I.P., de, Visser, G.H.A. and Prechtl, H.F.R. (1985) The emergence of fetal behaviour. II. Quantitative aspects. *Early Human Develop.* **12**: 99–120.

Want, J.J.L., van der, Gramsbergen, A., IJkema-Paassen, J., Weerd, H. de and Liem, R.S.B. (1998) Dendro-dendritic connections between motoneurons in the rat spinal cord. An electronmicroscopic investigation. *Brain Res.* **779**: 342–345.

Weiss, P.A. (1936) A study of motor coordination and tonus in deafferented limbs of amphibia. *Am. J. Physiol.* **115**: 461–475.

Westerga, J. and Gramsbergen, A. (1990) The development of locomotion in the rat. *Develop. Brain Res.* **57**: 163–174.

Westerga, J. and Gramsbergen, A. (1992) Structural changes of the soleus and the tibialis anterior motoneuron pool during development in the rat. *J. Comp. Neurol.* **319**: 406–416.

Westerga, J. and Gramsbergen, A. (1993a) Changes in the EMG of two major hind limb muscles during locomotor development in the rat. *Exp. Brain Res.* **92**: 479–488.

Westerga, J. and Gramsbergen, A. (1993b) The effect of early movement restriction in the rat: an EMG study. *Brain Behav. Res.* **59**: 205–209.

Westerga, J. and Gramsbergen, A. (1994) Development of the EMG of the soleus muscle in the rat. *Dev. Brain Res.* **80**: 233–243.

Wilson, S.J., Ross, J.J. and Harris, A.J. (1988) A critical period for formation of secondary myotubes defined by prenatal undernourishment in rats. *Development* **102**: 815–821.

Windle, W.F. (1940) *Physiology of the Fetus.* Philadelphia: Saunders.

Zomlefer, M.R., Provencher, J., Blanchette, G. and Rossignol, S. (1984) Electromyographic study of lumbar back muscles during locomotion in acute high decerebrate and in low spinal cats. *Brain Res.* **290**: 249–260.

3
Measurement Techniques for Gait Analysis

Hilary M. Clayton and Henk C. Schamhardt

INTRODUCTION

In daily life, almost everybody is using gait analysis, often without realizing it. While walking in the street, it usually takes only a fraction of a second to determine whether an approaching person is male or female, and whether that person is familiar or a complete stranger. The human eye, which captures the image, and the human brain, which processes it, are a surprisingly powerful system for recognition and identification. After a little training, the human observer is also able to judge the quality of gait: one can determine whether a particular walking pattern is supple and graceful or clumsy and incoordinated. This statement holds true not only for observations of people moving in various activities (walking or running, dancing or sport), but also for judging the performance of animals.

The eye of the experienced judge determines the outcome of equestrian sports such as dressage, reining, cutting and show hunters. Selection of horses for inclusion in breed registries and for approval as breeding stock is also based, to a certain extent, on the opinion of a committee of judges. However, this kind of 'gait analysis,' based on the judgment of an observer carries all the risks that are inherent in subjectivity.

Qualitative gait analysis is also applied successfully in the diagnosis of equine lameness. Clinicians use a semi-quantitative method of evaluation when assigning a lameness grade. While repeatability of lameness scores by an experienced clinician may be good (Back *et al.*, 1993), there is considerable variation between clinicians (Keegan *et al.*, 1998).

However, there are applications for which a qualitative evaluation of locomotion is inadequate, necessitating the use of a quantitative method of analysis that offers greater accuracy without the biases that are inherent in a subjective analysis. Chapter 1 provided an eloquent description of the evolution of different methods of gait analysis, and the explosion of research studies that have exploited the new capabilities for data storage and data processing in the computer age. This chapter describes the current and emerging techniques for equine gait evaluation in the areas of kinematic analysis, kinetic analysis, electromyography (EMG) and computer modeling. The value of the treadmill for data collection is also considered.

Kinematic analysis measures the geometry of movement without considering the forces that cause the movement. At the present time, the majority of kinematic evaluations are performed using videographic or optoelectronic systems consisting of integrated hardware and software components. Kinetics is the study of the forces that are responsible for the movements. A variety of transducers, including strain gauges, piezoelectric and piezoresistive transducers and accelerometers, are used in kinetic studies. Several transducers can be combined to develop force plates and force shoes for measuring ground reaction forces (GRFs). EMG detects the electrical activity associated with muscular contraction as a means of determining muscular activation patterns during different activities. The variables that are measured during gait analysis can be used to compute other quantities that are not or cannot be measured directly through computer modeling. The development of appropriate models facilitates a deeper understanding of the behavior of the musculoskeletal system and allows predictions to be made regarding its response to various perturbations without the need for live animal experiments.

INTERPRETING THE EFFECTS OF BIOLOGICAL VARIABILITY

It is widely recognized that a certain variability is inherent to data obtained from repeated measurements on biological material, and it is necessary to give consideration as to how to treat these data correctly. As an example, consider the measurement of GRFs using a force plate. When the horse is guided over the force plate, the chance for a correct hit by one fore hoof is about 50%, with the number of hits being approximately evenly distributed between the right and left limbs. After several runs, it is likely that a different number of correct hits will have been recorded from the right and left limbs. When calculating the mean and the standard error of the mean (SEM) for a force variable (e.g. peak vertical force) by averaging the data of these runs, the mean of the data obtained from the limb with the higher number of correct hits usually has a lower SEM. Are data from that limb more 'correct' than those from the other limb? Obviously not, but it is not easy to define a universal, statistically correct recipe to deal with this problem. In practice, most laboratories collect data until a certain minimum number of correct hits have been recorded from each limb. In sound horses, both the kinematic and force variables are quite stable, and analysis of a relatively small number of strides is representative of the gait pattern. It has been suggested that 3–5 strides are sufficient for kinematic (Drevemo et al., 1980a) or GRF (Schamhardt, 1996) analysis. The data describing an equal number of strides for each limb are averaged and considered to be 'representative' for that limb. The mean value is then used in further stages of the analysis as being representative of that variable for a particular limb in one horse. Most of the stride variables show good repeatability over the short and long term (Drevemo et al., 1980b; van Weeren et al., 1993), and the stride kinematics of a young horse have already assumed the characteristics that they will have at maturity by the time the foal is 4 months of age (Back et al., 1994).

Variability between individual horses affects the response to certain interferences, such as drug treatment and shoeing, which differ qualitatively and quantitatively in different animals. Impressive libraries of statistical routines have been developed to extract trends in the data, to detect differences between groups, or to identify a 'statistically significant' response to a certain treatment. Unfortunately, the prerequisites for these statistical tests may invalidate their use in a particular study. For example, data may not be normally distributed, or data describing different variables may be correlated with each other. Therefore, it is very important to plan the experiment and treat the data in a statistically appropriate manner. Before any experiment is carried out, a

Summary

Summary statistical analysis of biological data is important, but rather difficult to perform correctly and the literature contains many examples of incorrect applications. Furthermore, it is not only the statistical significance or lack thereof that is important in interpreting the results of a study; the findings should also be interpreted in terms of trends that are indicative of the biological relevance of the outcome.

thorough evaluation of the problem should be conducted. An hypothesis is formulated, and an appropriate experimental design and statistical model are determined to test that hypothesis. After collection of data, it is not unusual to find dependency within series of data, which disqualifies a particular statistical test. A detailed discussion of the pitfalls and problems associated with statistical testing is beyond the scope this text. Readers are advised to consult a suitable statistical text or a statistician to avoid using incorrect analyses, which have appeared frequently in the literature.

A statistical test determines the likelihood that a certain hypothesis can be accepted, or has to be rejected. However, the answer is not absolute: for example, having selected an uncertainty level of $p < 0.05$, the correct decision to accept or reject the hypothesis will be made in 95% of cases. Conversely, there is a 5% chance of being wrong, and one observation out of 20 will differ significantly due to chance. Therefore, statistical tests are not proof that a certain hypothesis is true or false. The majority of equine locomotion studies are based on a rather small number of subjects, which may be insufficient to give the required power for a statistical analysis. In these cases, trends in the data may suggest a biologically significant effect that cannot be proven statistically but is, nevertheless, important.

KINEMATIC ANALYSIS

Kinematic analysis quantifies the features of gait that are assessed qualitatively during a visual examination. The output is in the form of temporal (timing), linear (distance) and angular measurements that describe the movements of the body segments and joint angles. The data may be transferred to a spreadsheet for further analysis, e.g. detection of asymmetries between lame and sound limbs, or it may be displayed graphically or as stick

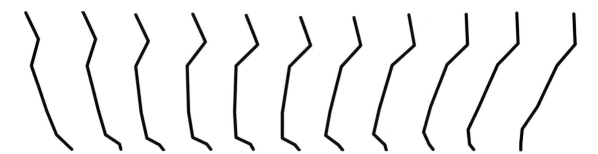

Fig. 3.1   Stick figure of the forelimb of a horse trotting overground. The figures are shown at intervals of 10% of stance duration.

figures (Fig. 3.1). In the past high-speed cinematography was the most commonly used technique for kinematic analysis, but it was an expensive and tedious method. TrackEye (Innovativ Vision AB, Linköping, Sweden) is an image digitizing system that processes high-speed film to provide accurate two-dimensional data with software for three-dimensional reconstruction. Today, the most popular techniques for studying kinematics are videographic analysis combined with a commercial software package, or optoelectronic systems that are based on the emission and detection of infrared or visible light. Analyses may be two-dimensional or three-dimensional. Two-dimensional studies are relatively simple to perform but the results are adversely affected by image distortion due to out-of-plane image movements of the body segments. Three-dimensional analysis overcomes these problems, but is a more complex procedure, particularly with regard to calibration of the movement space.

Videographic systems

Videography is a popular method of kinematic analysis in horses. Turnkey systems are available that produce useful data within a reasonable period of time by autodigitizing reflective markers on the subject either on-line or during post-processing. However, the user must check the accuracy of the digitization before accepting the data for further analysis. Problems arise when different markers cross each other in the field of view or when a marker is temporarily obscured. Errors in the raw data will give rise to problems throughout the subsequent analysis. Some video systems also offer a manual digitizing option that can be used when there are no markers on the subject, for example when videos are recorded during a competition. Manual digitizing is also a useful option when the autodigitizing system has difficulty differentiating between markers that are placed close together or that cross each other during locomotion.

The sequence of events for video analysis involves marker application to the subject, setting up and calibrating the recording space, video recording, digitization, transformation, smoothing and normalization. Analyses may be performed in two or three dimensions. Since the limbs of the horse have evolved to move primarily in a sagittal plane, most of the useful information is captured by the two-dimensional lateral view, and in many situations the extra effort involved in extracting three-dimensional data is not warranted. However, there are times when a knowledge of the abduction and adduction or internal and external rotations would be useful, especially during sporting activities and in relation to lameness. Most video systems are capable of three-dimensional analysis, but there are some additional requirements beyond those for two-dimensional analysis. These include using a minimum of two camera views and ensuring that each marker is visible to at least two cameras throughout the movement.

Video-based kinematic analysis systems used in horses include the Ariel Performance Analysis System (Ariel Dynamics Inc., Trabuco Canyon, CA), ExpertVision (Motion Analysis Corp., Santa Rosa, CA) and Peak Performance System (Peak Performance Technologies Inc., Englewood, CO).

Skin markers

Most video systems offer automated digitization if appropriate markers are placed on the skin and the lighting is controlled to provide sufficient contrast between the edge of the markers and the surroundings. Black acrylic paint, available from artist's supply stores, can be used to draw a bullseye target around a marker to improve its contrast against white hairs. For two-dimensional analysis, circular markers, 2–3 cm in diameter are used, with the bigger markers giving better accuracy when the resolution of the system is poor (Schamhardt *et al.*, 1993a). Retro reflective material can be purchased in sheets

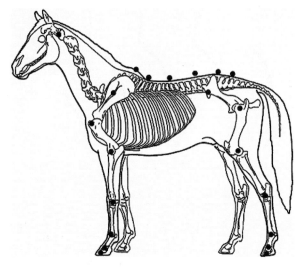

Fig. 3.2 The black dots represent locations that are commonly used for skin marker placement for kinematic analysis.

(Scotchlite, 3M Corp., St Paul, MN) and cut into markers of a suitable size or precut circles can be purchased at a higher price. The self-adhesive backing may not be adequate to hold the markers in place, especially when the horse sweats. Cyanoacrylate glue (super glue) is effective for securing the markers, but some brands are difficult to remove completely at the end of the study, which may pose a problem in client-owned horses. A little experimentation may be needed to find appropriate products for use under a variety of circumstances. Retro reflective paint (Scotchlite 7210 Silver, 3M Corp., St Paul, MN) is also available, but the reflective beads tend to clump, making it a less satisfactory method of marking. For three-dimensional studies spherical or hemispherical markers are used because they retain their circular shape when viewed from different angles. Spherical markers can be purchased ready-made or they can be made from polystyrene balls, about 3 cm in diameter, which are purchased from hobby stores. If necessary, the balls are cut in half before covering them with strips of reflective tape or reflective paint.

Marker locations are chosen in accordance with the purposes of the analysis. Calculation of the angle between two limb segments in two dimensions requires a minimum of three markers. Figure 3.2 shows the approximate centers of joint rotation on the fore and hindlimbs, which can be used for marker placement during two-dimensional analyses in the sagittal plane, using software packages that require the markers to be placed over the joint centers. Other software allows the use of two markers per segment that are aligned along the long

axis of the segment, without necessarily being placed over the joint centers. Markers on the dorsal midline of the back are used to evaluate trunk motion (Licka & Peham, 1998). Markers on the neck, withers and croup are useful for evaluating left–right asymmetries in the vertical excursions of these reference points.

On the limbs, skin movements relative to specific underlying bony landmarks have been quantified and correction algorithms have been developed for walking and trotting Dutch warmblood horses (van Weeren et al., 1990a, 1990b, 1992). However, these algorithms are only valid for horses of similar conformation, moving at the same gaits and at similar speeds. Figure 3.3 illustrates the effect of skin displacement on the angular motions of the stifle and tarsal joints during walking. It shows that the effects of skin movement are much greater at the stifle joint than at the tarsal joint. Distal to the elbow of the forelimb and the stifle of the hindlimb, skin movement artifact is small enough to be neglected. In the more proximal parts of the limb, however, skin movements as large as 12 cm have been measured, which is sufficient to change the entire shape of the angle–time diagrams at the proximal joints. In these locations, uncorrected data cannot be used for absolute angular computations or for measuring muscle or tendon lengths based on limb kinematics.

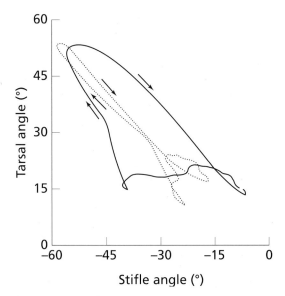

Fig. 3.3 Angle–angle diagrams of the stifle and tarsal joints of a horse at walk. The movements of the skin markers are shown before (continuous line) and after (broken line) correction for skin displacement. (Reprinted with permission from Schamhardt, H.C. (1996) In: *Measuring movement and locomotion: from invertebrates to humans* © R.G. Landes Company.)

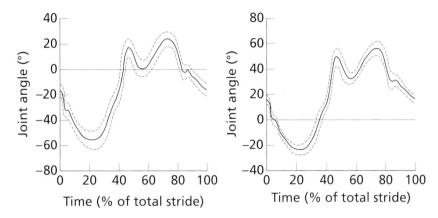

Fig. 3.4 Angle–angle diagrams of the fetlock joint of the forelimb of a horse trotting on a treadmill at 4 m/s. The diagram on the left shows the joint angles measured relative to the position in which the proximal and distal segments are aligned. The diagram on the right shows the angles relative to those recorded with the horse standing squarely. For both diagrams flexion is positive and extension is negative. (Reprinted with permission from Schamhardt, H.C. (1996) In: *Measuring movement and locomotion: from invertebrates to humans* © *R.G. Landes Company*.)

The repeatability in positioning the skin markers must also be considered. Usually, markers are applied in the standing horse and care should be taken that the horse is standing squarely with weight on all four limbs. When the limb is unloaded or when the horse is not standing still, it is difficult to fix the markers with an accuracy better than about 0.5 cm. Inevitably, this has consequences for repeated measurements in one horse, when the markers have to be removed between sessions, unless remnants of glue remain or paint is used to mark the spot. Another possibility for avoiding this problem is to standardize joint angular measurements to those obtained in the square standing horse (Back *et al.*, 1994), so that the angles are reported as deviations from this square standing position, with relative flexion being assigned a positive value and relative extension being assigned a negative value. Repeated measurements of horses positioned in a square standing position, however, have indicated poor reliability (Sloet, personal communication). Other methods of displaying joint angles include reporting the absolute joint angle, which is usually measured on the anatomical flexor aspect of the joint, or measuring the flexion (positive) and extension (negative) angles relative to the position at which the proximal and distal segments are aligned. Although the patterns are the same regardless of the method of measurement (Fig. 3.4), the values differ considerably, which impairs comparisons between data from different studies.

The requirements for three-dimensional analysis are similar to those for two-dimensional analysis in that the chosen marker locations show minimal skin displacement or have correction algorithms to compensate for skin displacement. In addition, each marker must be vis-ible to at least two cameras throughout the movement. This combination of requirements is difficult to fulfil during some movements. One way to overcome these problems is to use a virtual targeting system (Nicodemus *et al.*, 1999). This method relies on the fact that, for rigid body motion, the location of any point on a body does not change with respect to that body. Therefore, if the location of a point on a segment is known with respect to the segment, and the orientation of the segment is known in a global coordinate system, then the location of that point on that segment can be calculated in the global coordinate system. The virtual targeting method employs two sets of markers: tracking markers and virtual markers. Three virtual markers are attached to each segment to define the segmental coordinate system: two are oriented along the long axis of the segment and the third is perpendicular to that axis. Three non-colinear tracking markers are placed on the segment in appropriate positions to track the motion of the segment in the global coordinate system, i.e. at locations that are readily visible to the cameras during locomotion and at locations for which the skin displacement is known. The coordinates of the tracking markers are used in a transformation that converts the global coordinate system to a segmental coordinate system. A standing file is recorded with both the virtual and tracking markers in place, after which the virtual markers are removed. Recordings are made with the tracking markers in place. During the subsequent data processing, algorithms are used to calculate the locations of the virtual markers with respect to a segmental coordinate system and to track that target in the global coordinate system.

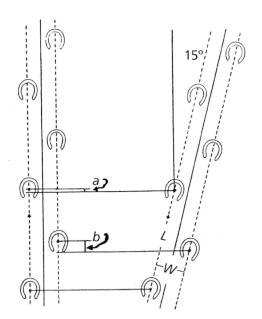

Fig. 3.5 Influence of the horse moving obliquely across the force plate, at an angle of 15° to the long axis of the plate. The erroneously calculated stride length (L * cos α = L * 0.9) differs from the actual length L by the distance a, which is fairly small. The calculated placement of the right limb in front of the left limb is much more affected (distance b), because b is proportional to w * sin α = w * 0.26. (Reprinted with permission from Schamhardt, H.C. (1996) In: *Measuring movement and locomotion: from invertebrates to humans* © *R.G. Landes Company*.)

Video recording

For two-dimensional studies, the camera is precisely oriented so that its axis is perpendicular to the plane of interest. For three-dimensional studies, precise camera positioning is not important, so long as each marker is visible to at least two cameras at all times. However, if the angle between the cameras is small, it reduces the accuracy along the axis running toward the cameras. The field of view should always be somewhat larger than the movement space to avoid errors due to distortion at the periphery of the lens, especially with a wide-angled lens.

An important decision relates to the type of video camera to be purchased and whether it is worth investing in a high-speed camera. A standard camcorder records 30 frames/s in the NTSC format and 25 frames/s in the PAL format. Each frame is made up of two video fields recorded 1/60 s (NTSC) or 1/50 s (PAL) apart. The gait analysis software may be able to display successive fields sequentially giving an effective sampling rate of 60 fields/s (NTSC) or 50 fields/s (PAL). High-speed video cameras are available and are

useful for studies of short-duration events or rapid movements but the lighting conditions become more critical at faster recording speeds. Comparisons of joint displacement data from horses cantering on a treadmill showed minimal loss of information in terms of angular data when the sampling rate was reduced from 200 Hz to 50 Hz (Lanovaz, unpublished). Linford (1994) compared the temporal stride variables in horses trotting on a treadmill by analysing the same ten strides with two cameras sampling at 60 Hz and at 1000 Hz, respectively. Mean values for stride duration, stance duration, swing duration, and breakover did not differ by more than 3.3 ms. A camcorder that records at 60 Hz is adequate for kinematic analysis of some aspects of equine locomotion, but a large number of strides must be analyzed to produce a representative mean value for temporal events of short duration. At gaits faster than a walk, a faster camera is preferable, especially if the displacement data will be processed further.

During a recording session the markers on the horse are illuminated by a lamp (usually 300–500 W) directed along the axis of the lens. If there is too much ambient light, it may not be possible to autodigitize the markers, so controlled lighting conditions are an advantage. When the exposure time is very short, as when using high-speed cameras, more illumination is needed to maintain decent quality of the video image.

Calibration

A calibration frame is recorded in the field of view to scale the coordinate data. For two-dimensional analysis, a rectangular frame or a linear ruler is positioned along the horse's line of progression. If the horse deviates from the plane of calibration but continues to move parallel to the intended plane of motion, errors are introduced in the linear data, though the timing data are not affected. Correction algorithms can be used to adjust the linear data if the horse moves along a line parallel to the intended plane of motion. However, if the horse moves at an oblique angle to the camera, it causes image distortion. Length measurements along a line in the longitudinal direction (e.g. stride length) are proportional to the cosine of the angle at which the horse moves relative to the desired direction (Fig. 3.5). As long as the oblique movement angle is less than about 15°, this error is smaller than 5%. If a transverse distance is involved, such as step length between the left and right limbs, the distances show a larger error that is proportional to the sine of the oblique movement angle. Again, assuming the horse moves at an angle of 15°, the error in the transverse direction can be as large as 26% (Fig. 3.5).

For three-dimensional studies a calibration frame with non-coplanar control points is used. A larger number of control points gives a more accurate reconstruction. The accuracy of the data is markedly reduced outside the area of volume of the calibration frame, so a large, custom-designed frame is required for equine studies. The accuracy of the calibration completely determines the accuracy of the final three-dimensional data (DeLuzio *et al.*, 1993), which emphasizes the importance of investing the necessary effort into calibration of the volume space in which the measurements are made.

Digitization

Through the process of digitization the coordinates of the body markers are determined in two-dimensional or three-dimensional space. Digitization may be performed manually, or it may be performed automatically with the system locating each marker by edge detection then calculating the position of its center. If the software allows, it is preferable for the operator to check each digitized field and make adjustments for digitizing errors or invisible markers before accepting the data into memory. In some situations, for example when there is too much ambient light or when markers cannot be applied as in a competition, manual digitization is necessary. In addition to the time required, this tedious process creates more digitizing noise than automated digitization.

Transformation

The transformation process integrates the calibration information with the digitized coordinates to scale the data. For three-dimensional studies direct linear transformation (DLT) is the standard procedure for combining two or more two-dimensional views into a single three-dimensional view. This method has the advantage of not needing any information about camera locations; the transformation is based on knowledge of the coordinates of the control points on the calibration frame, which are determined for each camera view.

Smoothing

During digitization small errors are introduced that constitute 'noise' in the signal. The effect of noise is not too great in the displacement data, but it becomes increasingly apparent in the time derivatives, i.e. the velocity and acceleration data (Fioretti & Jetto, 1989) as shown in Fig. 3.6. Smoothing removes high-frequency noise introduced during the digitization process using one of two general approaches: a digital filter followed by finite difference technique or a curve-fitting technique (e.g. polynomial or spline curve fitting). Selection of an appropriate smoothing algorithm and smoothing parameter for a specific purpose requires some expertise. As a guideline, a low-pass digital filter with a cut-off frequency of 10–15 Hz is adequate for most videographic studies of equine gait. However, the movement of a marker may have an oscillatory component, especially when loose connective tissue is interposed between the skin and the underlying bones. Since these oscillations are essentially tied to the movements themselves, they cannot be removed by smoothing (Schamhardt, 1996).

Normalization

Normalization or standardization of data facilitates comparisons between different horses by standardizing certain parameters. Normalization to the stride duration expresses the values of the temporal variables as a percentage of stride duration. This facilitates comparisons between strides that have slightly different durations, and allows the construction of mean curves from a number of strides. In other studies, normalization to stance duration or swing duration may be more appropriate depending on the objectives of the study. The most common method of performing the normalization is to use cubic spline interpolation, which resamples the curve at a set number of intervals (usually 100 or 101).

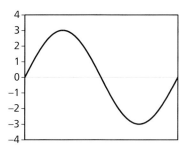 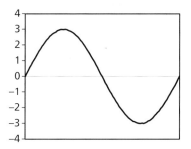 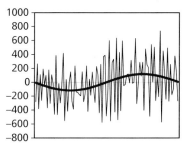

Fig. 3.6 Effect of noise on derived functions. The graphs show a smooth curve (left) to which a small amount of noise has been added (center) and the second derivative from the smooth (——) and noisy (——) data (right).

Optoelectronic systems

Many aspects of data collection and data processing using an optoelectronic system are similar to those described above for videographic systems. Procedures such as marker attachment, smoothing and normalization of data that have been described for videographic analysis will not be repeated here.

Several systems are available that use either active markers (markers that emit a signal) or passive markers (markers that detect or reflect a signal). Use of these systems is usually confined to the laboratory, because of the need for a hard-wired connection to the subject and/or controlled lighting conditions. Optoelectronic systems are suitable for equine research include MacReflex and ProReflex (Qualisys Inc., Glastonbury, CT), Optotrack and Watsmart (Northern Digital Inc., Waterloo, ON), Selspot Motion Measurement System (Innovision Systems, Warren, MI), Vicon (Oxford Metrics, Oxford, England) and CODA (Charnwood Dynamics Ltd, Barrow-upon-Soar, England). These systems perform the digitizing on-line, so data are usually available quite quickly. Many of the systems have a built-in method for distinguishing between individual markers, for example by sequencing the temporal output of different markers or by using markers of different shapes or colors. The loss of direct control of digitizing sometimes leads to errors in the data, especially in the systems that do not distinguish between markers.

The CODA system used for many of the studies at Utrecht University is one of a kind, having been modified from the original CODA-3 system (Schamhardt *et al.*, 1992). It tracks up to 12 markers simultaneously in three-dimensional space with a sampling frequency of 300 samples/s. The markers are connected by a long umbilical cord to the portable scanner unit that consists of three light sources fixed to a steel frame. An advantage of the CODA system is that it does not need to be calibrated prior to each use because the coordinates are calculated relative to the frame of the scanner. At a measuring distance of 8 m, the accuracy in the transverse plane is about 0.3 mm.

MacReflex and ProReflex are used in a number of equine gait analysis labs. They are relatively easy to use and provide data rapidly without the need for digitization. However, they do require a controlled lighting environment.

Electrogoniometry

An electrogoniometer or elgon is a device for measuring joint angle changes. It consists of a potentiometer attached to two rotating metal arms. These arms are fixed to the limb with tape or straps, so that the center of the elgon lies over the center of rotation of the joint (Fig. 3.7). Joint angle changes alter the electrical resistance of the potentiometer, which is calibrated with a protractor to produce a proportional displacement of known magnitude. Permanent records, or goniograms, can be recorded on an oscilloscope. The data can be stored in a computer for later analysis.

In horses, electrogoniometry has been used to record joint movements at different gaits in normal and lame horses (Adrian *et al.*, 1977), to diagnose obscure lameness, and to evaluate the changes in joint motion after medical or surgical treatment (Taylor *et al.*, 1966; Ratzlaff *et al.*, 1979).

Kinematic data

Kinematic data consist of temporal, linear and angular variables. Temporal data, which describe the stride duration and the limb coordination patterns, are calculated from the frame numbers and the sampling frequency. Distance data, computed from the coordinates of the markers combined with the calibration information, describe the stride length, the distances between limb placements, and the flight paths of the body parts. Angular data describe the displacements, velocities and accelerations of the body segments and joints.

In two-dimensional studies the angular data are usually reported as flexion and extension in the sagittal plane. This is a reasonable simplification because the horse's joints have evolved to swing primarily in this plane as an energy-saving mechanism. The centers of joint rotation in the sagittal plane have been described (Leach & Dyson, 1988), and these locations are often used as land-

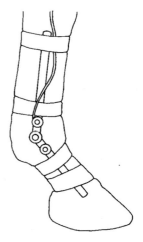

Fig. 3.7 Electrogoniometer placed over the equine fetlock joint.

marks for placement of skin markers for kinematic analysis (Fig. 3.2).

In three-dimensional analysis the problems of standardization become much more complicated. First, each length measurement has three components in space and a segment requires three angle measurements to define its orientation. One approach that has been used in equine studies is to define the joint angles with the same landmarks used in the two-dimensional studies and project the joint angles onto three mutually perpendicular planes that are tied to the global coordinate system (Fredricson & Drevemo 1972). Providing that the horse is moving in a direction parallel to a global coordinate axis, the planes become the sagittal, frontal and transverse planes. In effect, this method degrades the three-dimensional analysis into a quasi-two-dimensional analysis. This type of analysis is limited by the fact that joint motion that is not parallel to one of the projection planes cannot be accurately measured. Additionally, since this method usually defines segments as simple lines between landmarks, rotations along the long axis of a segment are impossible to measure.

An alternative is to establish a three-dimensional joint coordinate system for the equine joints that is based on the axes of the limb segments, which are independent of the joint centers of rotation. This allows the true measurement of three types of joint motion; flexion/extension, adduction/abduction, and internal/external rotation.

Establishment of a three-dimensional joint coordinate system requires that an axis system be defined for each limb segment that corresponds to an anatomically meaningful direction, such as the long axis of the bone. The segments themselves are defined by a minimum of three landmarks each. With one method of calculating joint angles (Grood & Suntay, 1983), an appropriate axis on the proximal segment of a joint is used as the flexion/extension axis and an axis on the distal segment becomes the internal/external rotation axis. The adduction/abduction axis is then defined as perpendicular to both the flexion/extension axis and the internal/external rotation axis. This is sometimes called the floating axis since it is not necessarily aligned with the planes of either limb segment. The three joint angles are usually expressed as motions of the distal segment relative to the proximal segment (Fig. 3.8) and the angles can be expressed independently of each other. This allows for examination of complex coupled motion in a joint.

KINETIC ANALYSIS

Kinetic analysis measures locomotor forces, both external and internal to the body. Forces developed by

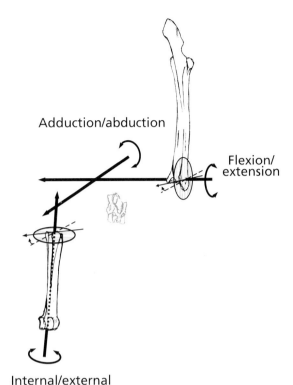

Adduction/abduction

Flexion/extension

Internal/external

Fig. 3.8 Three-dimensional joint coordinate system for kinematic analysis. Flexion/extension and external/internal rotation are expressed in terms of the distal segment rotating relative to the proximal segment. Abduction and adduction are relative to the floating axis.

muscles are transformed into rotations of the limb segments that ultimately produce movement. The GRFs during locomotion can be recorded using a force plate (Pratt & O'Connor, 1976) or a force shoe (Frederick & Henderson, 1970; Ratzlaff et al., 1990; Roepstorff & Drevemo, 1993). Transmission of forces and accelerations through the body are recorded by strain gauges and accelerometers attached directly to the tissues. Intrinsic forces in other parts of the locomotor system are calculated from a knowledge of the GRFs.

Force shoes

A force shoe is attached directly to the hoof and allows the GRF to be recorded during a large number of successive stance phases, which overcomes one of the limitations of the force plate. Force shoes also have the advantages of being amenable to use on different surface types, and being able to collect data from more than one limb at a time. Several researchers have used force shoes experimentally, but none is currently marketed commercially.

Frederick and Henderson (1970) described a device with three force sensors sandwiched between a base plate that was nailed to the hoof wall and a ground plate that was attached to the base plate, thus preloading the force sensors. Some years later, a force shoe designed at Washington State University was based on a piezoelectric transducer located in a housing over the frog. A later version with three transducers located at the medial heel, the lateral heel and the toe, gave a better correlation with simultaneous force plate recordings. It was used primarily in studies of galloping Thoroughbreds (e.g. Ratzlaff et al., 1990), and provided unique data when a horse wearing the shoe sustained a rupture of the distal sesamoidean ligaments while galloping on a training track (Ratzlaff et al., 1994).

A Swedish force shoe based on three strain gauge measuring units, one at the toe and one at each quarter, measures vertical, longitudinal and transverse forces (Roepstorff & Drevemo, 1993). The output has been shown to correlate well with that of a force plate, provided all three measuring units are in contact with the ground. When one or more sensors lose contact with the ground, for example during breakover, the force shoe and force plate signals do not compare well with each other. This shoe has been used to compare GRFs during exercise on treadmill belts with different compositions (Roepstorff et al., 1994). Yet another type of force shoe, this time with four transducers, one on each side of the toe and quarters, was integrated into the bottom of an easy boot (Barrey, 1990).

Although a force shoe would be an ideal method of measuring GRFs, the technical difficulties in con-structing an accurate and reliable device have restricted their use to the laboratories in which the various models have been developed. To date, the majority of published GRF data have been derived from force plate studies.

Force plate

A force plate is a steel plate, recessed into the ground then covered with a non-slip material (Fig. 3.9). When a horse steps on the plate, the force is detected by transducers at its corners, and is converted to an electrical signal that is amplified and recorded. Variables measured by the force plate include the stance duration, the magnitude of the vertical, longitudinal (horizontal craniocaudal) and transverse (horizontal mediolateral) forces, the time when the peak forces occur, the impulses (area under the force–time curves), and the point of application of the force (center of pressure).

Selection and installation

In selecting a force plate for equine use, it is important to choose one that has a linear response over an appropriate range of forces, taking into account the weight of the horses and the gaits and speeds to be studied. The dimensions of the plate should maximize the chance of getting a good strike from one fore hoof followed by the hind hoof on the same side at a walk or trot. If two hooves strike the plate simultaneously, it is not possible to separate their effects, and the trial must be discarded. Shorter force plates (60–90 cm) are preferred for collecting data at the walk, but a length of 90–120 cm is preferable for use at the faster gaits. Width of the plate is

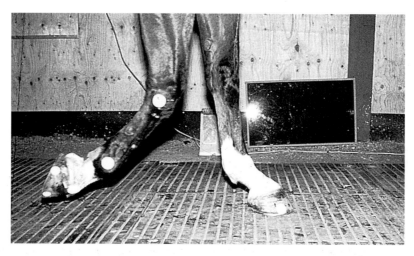

Fig. 3.9 Horse stepping on a force plate during data collection.

not generally a limiting factor: 50–60 cm is adequate. A good strike has been recorded for every 2–6 passes at the walk, trot and canter (Niki *et al.*, 1982; Merkens *et al.*, 1986, 1993a, 1993b). During jumping the obstacle is moved to increase the likelihood of getting a good strike with a particular limb at take off or landing (Schamhardt *et al.*, 1993b). The horse should move parallel with the long axis of the force plate to avoid cross talk between the horizontal transducers (Fig. 3.10). Companies that manufacture force plates suitable for equine use include Advanced Medical Technology (AMTI, Watertown, MA), Bertec Corporation (Columbus, OH) and Kistler Instruments Corp. (Amherst, NY).

Installation and calibration of the force plate are critically important to the quality of the data collected. The plate is embedded in a concrete pit to isolate it from surrounding vibrations. The supporting surface must be absolutely level to avoid cross talk between the vertical and horizontal channels. Before recording data, the calibration should be checked by placing a known weight, that is similar in magnitude to the loads that will be applied during normal use, at different locations on the force plate. The same vertical force should be recorded independent of the location, and the position indicated by the force plate should match the actual location of the load.

Data collection

GRFs vary with speed (McLaughlin *et al.*, 1996). Provided the horse's velocity over the force plate is maintained within a narrow range, the GRFs are consistent and repeatable between strides, with analysis of five strides being sufficient to provide representative data (Merkens *et al.*, 1986). The horse's average velocity over the plate can be checked using timing lights to record the time taken to cover a known distance as the horse moves over the force plate; data from runs that fall outside the required time range are discarded. Sensors for a simple infrared timing device can be purchased inexpensively. Alternatively, the average horizontal velocity of a marker on the horse during the stride can be determined when the data are analyzed, with strides that fall outside a certain range being discarded. It is sometimes

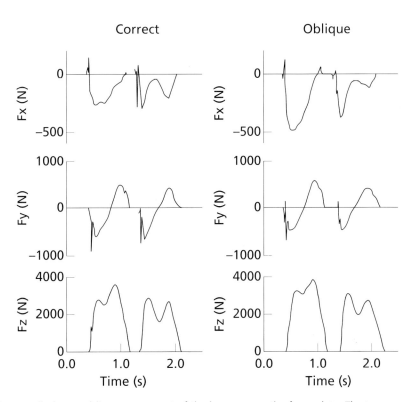

Fig. 3.10 Effect of cross talk due to oblique movement of the horse across the force plate. The transverse (F*x*), longitudinal (F*y*) and vertical (F*z*) ground reaction forces were obtained from the hindlimb of a horse as it walked across the force plate perpendicular to its long axis (graphs on left) or obliquely (graphs on right). (Reprinted with permission from Schamhardt, H.C. (1996) In: *Measuring movement and locomotion: from invertebrates to humans* © R.G. Landes Company.)

useful to screen strides in this manner before performing a more detailed analysis.

Bad runs occur when the horse fails to strike the force plate, when the hoof contacts the edge of the plate, or when more than one hoof is on the plate simultaneously. These problems are recognized by the force traces having an unusual shape or magnitude, or failing to return to the baseline between individual limb contacts. It may be helpful to have a video camera focussed on the surface of the force plate to verify the limb placements on its surface.

Normalization

GRFs vary with the body mass of the horse (Barr *et al.*, 1995). Comparisons between horses are facilitated by normalizing the force traces to the horse's weight, so they are expressed in newtons/kilogram body weight (N/kg). GRFs may also be normalized to the duration of the stance phase, which allows the timing of specific events to be expressed as a percentage of the stance duration.

Standard GRF patterns have been developed for Dutch warmbloods at a walk (Merkens *et al.*, 1988), trot (Merkens *et al.*, 1993a) and canter (Merkens *et al.*, 1993b). Adaptation to other breeds could be accomplished by incorporating appropriate parameters and weighting factors into the formulae used to develop the standard patterns.

Data

Figure 3.11 shows the force patterns of the three force components (vertical, longitudinal, transverse) during the stance phase of a forelimb at a walk and trot. The vertical force, which represents the support function of the limb, has a magnitude of the order of 60% of body weight at the walk and 90% of body weight at a moderate speed trot. In the walk the vertical force trace may be biphasic. If this is the case, the second peak is higher in the forelimbs, the first peak is higher in the hindlimbs. In the trot sharp spikes usually occur immediately after initial ground contact during the period of impulsive loading (impact phase). The trace then rises smoothly to peak when the limb is at its midstance position, which is marked by the cannon segment being vertical, after which it decreases to lift off. For both the walk and trot, in the early part of the stance phase the longitudinal force brakes (decelerates) the horse's forward movement as a result of friction that prevents the hoof slipping forward. Later in the stance phase, it changes to a propulsive (accelerating) force (Fig. 3.11). The direction of the horse's motion across the force plate determines whether acceleration or deceleration is recorded as positive. Software correction is applied to standardize the sign

convention. The peak value of the longitudinal force is 10–15% of the horse's body weight at the walk and trot, with marked spiking occurring during the impact phase at the trot. The transverse force is much smaller in magnitude, of the order of 2% body weight at the trot. The left to right values recorded by the force plate are converted to represent medial and lateral values for each limb. The center of pressure is located under the middle of the hoof during most of the stance phase, moving rapidly toward the toe at the start of breakover.

Values representing the peak forces and their times of occurrence are extracted from the force tracings. The impulses are determined by time integration of the force curves. A procedure that combined over 90 numbers describing the peak amplitudes, their times of occurrence, and the impulses has been described as the H(orse) INDEX (Schamhardt & Merkens, 1987). This method is valid but has some drawbacks in that the variables used to calculate the index are selected by the user and are essentially dependent on the shape of the signal. Moreover, it does not take account of the real pattern of the curve, which can be accomplished by different techniques that are more suitable for comparing curve patterns.

The stance durations, GRF amplitudes and impulses are symmetrical in sound horses at the walk (Merkens *et al.*, 1986, 1988) and trot (Seeherman *et al.*, 1987; Merkens *et al.*, 1993a). Evaluations of a variety of lamenesses have shown a similar pattern of changes in the GRF, consisting of a reduction in the horizontal decelerating force and reductions in the vertical force amplitude and impulse in a lame forelimb, with compensatory changes in the compensating forelimb. Lameness models that produce these changes include pressure on the hoof sole (Merkens & Schamhardt, 1988); collagenase-induced tendinitis in the flexor tendons or desmitis of the suspensory ligament (Keg *et al.*, 1992); and surgical creation of a full thickness cartilage defect on the radial carpal bone (Morris & Seeherman, 1987). In addition to its value for detecting lameness, the force plate is a sensitive tool for measuring the response of lame horses to diagnostic anesthesia (Keg *et al.*, 1992) or to therapeutic intervention (Gingerich *et al.*, 1979), and for detecting abnormalities in postural sway in horses with neurological diseases (Clayton *et al.*, 1999).

Strain gauges

Body tissues deform in response to an applied load. When a tensile force is applied to a solid material, it causes the length to increase, whereas a compressive force causes the length to decrease. A bending force causes both increases and decreases in length in different parts of the tissue. In ideally elastic materials, the deformation is proportional to the applied force and the

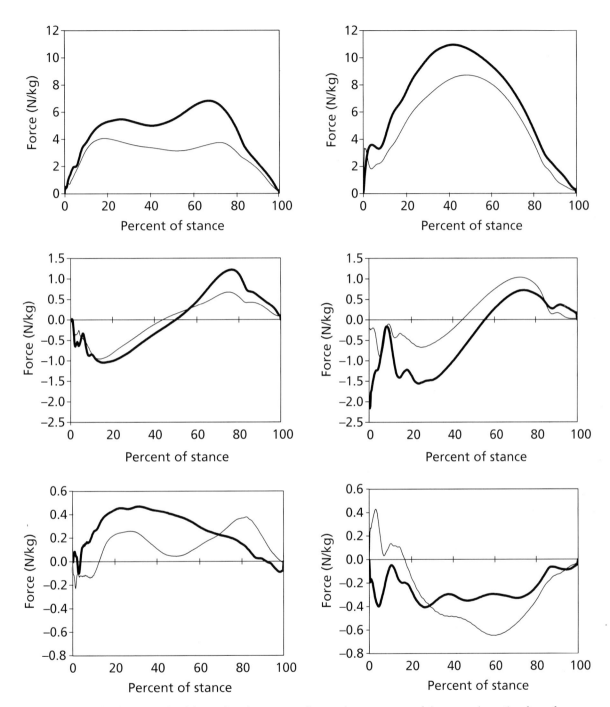

Fig. 3.11 Vertical (top), longitudinal (center) and transverse (bottom) components of the ground reaction force for a horse at the walk (left) and at the trot (right). For the longitudinal force the cranial direction is positive and for the transverse force the medial direction is positive. Forelimb (━━); hindlimb (───).

material restores its original shape as soon as the deforming force is removed. The deformation of the material, usually expressed in terms of *strain* (ε), is defined as:

$$\varepsilon = \frac{l_1 - l_0}{l_0}$$

where l_0 is the original (or resting) length, l_1 is the length after deformation, and $l_1 - l_0$ represents the change in length. Usually, the resting length is defined as the length at zero loading force. Because strain is a relative measure, it has no units. It is expressed as a fraction or as a percentage strain.

A strain gauge changes its electrical resistance in response to deformation in a certain direction; the change in resistance is converted to a voltage output that is proportional to the strain and is stored for later processing by a computer. A combination of three strain gauges stacked at 45° angles to each other forms a rosette gauge capable of measuring three-dimensional strains. Strain gauges, which are a component of force plates and force shoes, can also be used independently to provide direct strain measurements for body tissues.

Measuring strains in hard tissues

Hard tissues, such as bones, deform slightly in multiple directions as a result of the combined effects of weight bearing, tension in the muscles and tendons, and inertial effects due to acceleration and deceleration of the limb. Rosette (three-dimensional) gauges, bonded to a bone surface using a thin layer of cyanoacrylate glue, deform with the surface to provide information about the compressive and tensile forces (Lanyon, 1976). The best sites for attachment of strain gauges to bones are in areas where the bone lies subcutaneously, so soft tissue trauma during surgery is minimized. Attachment of strain gauges requires meticulous preparation of the bone surface. The periosteum is removed and the underlying bone is dried before bonding the strain gauges to the bone using cyanoacrylate adhesive. The wires exit the skin through a separate incision. It is important to shield the wires from movement and trauma, since damage to or loosening of the wires is the most frequent reason for failure of the gauges. During data collection, the gauges deform as if they were part of the bone surface. The resulting electrical signal is amplified and transmitted to a data recorder or computer for storage. Strain gauges have been bonded to equine long bones to investigate bone loading under various conditions (e.g. Hartman *et al.*, 1984; Schamhardt *et al.*, 1985; Davies *et al.*, 1993)

A practical problem in quantifying bone strain is that the resting length of bone is difficult to identify. When the horse is standing quietly with the limb lifted from the ground, the loading may be assumed to be small. However, the effects of muscular contraction cannot be excluded completely, and the influence of gravity may also affect the zero-strain determination. Software has been developed to calculate a 'zero-strain compensation' for *in vivo* strain gauge data of horses at the walk, using the assumption that strain is minimal in the middle of the swing phase, when the limb is moving forward with an almost constant velocity (Schamhardt & Hartman, 1982).

Surface strain is a consequence of the forces loading the bone. However, the relationship between surface strain and load is very complicated, especially in non-homogeneous, nonlinear, viscoelastic structures such as bones (Rybicki *et al.*, 1974). Roszek *et al.* (1993) presented an elegant technique to quantify the loading forces from a post-mortem calibration using multiple strain gauges and known bending and torsional loading forces. Without this kind of calibration, however, bone strain recordings are a valuable, but qualitative, estimate of bone loading.

By using three or four strain rosettes around the perimeter of a long bone shaft, and combining their output with a knowledge of the bone's geometry, the distribution of principal strains can be determined. It has been shown that the loading pattern of each bone is fairly consistent in different activities, though the peak strain and the strain rate vary with gait and speed (Rybicki *et al.*, 1974). This information has been applied in locating the tension surface of various long bones, which is the surface of choice for the application of bone plates. Strain gauges are easily bonded to the hoof wall to study the functional anatomy of the hoof capsule under a variety of loading conditions (Thomason *et al.*, 1992).

Measuring strains in tendons and ligaments

The long tendons in the lower limb of the horse can be considered as elastic, more or less homogeneous cables. When loaded, their length increases. However, strain in tendons is not as well defined as in bones. An unloaded tendon shrinks in length and the tendon fibers become wrinkled. When elongated, the crimp in the fibers is first straightened out, then the fibers are stretched elastically up to a point, beyond which permanent elongation occurs.

In tendons and ligaments, unidirectional strain gauges are adequate to record tensile strains during loading. The load–elongation curve for a tendon has a 'toe' region, which is characterized by having a large elongation for a small load. This region represents straightening of the crimp in the collagen fibers. As loading increases beyond the 'toe' region, there is a linear relationship between load and elongation in the elastic region until the yield point, which occurs around 10–12% strain. Beyond the yield point permanent elongation results as the tendon fibers begin to rupture. A problem in measuring tendon strain lies in defining the initial length of the tendon and the position of zero load, which affects the magnitude of the strains recorded throughout the physiological range. It appears that the resting length, or the length at zero force, can only be approximated. Studies that rely on different criteria for defining zero load give very different strain values during similar activities and at the yield point. An objective method of determining the transition between the toe and the elastic region has been described (Riemersma & Bogert, 1993). Figure 3.12 shows the strain pattern in the suspensory ligament during walking.

Several types of strain gauges have been used to study tendon strains in horses. In a buckle transducer, the tendon is wound over a buckle and preloaded it as it passes over the middle support bar. Tensile loading straightens the tendon and loads the buckle, and this loading is detected by a strain gauge. Calibration of a buckle strain gauge requires transection of the tendon and application of known weights, which limits the use of this type of transducer to a research setting. Another problem with the buckle transducer is that, by forcing the tendon to follow a curved course, its initial strain and tension are altered.

Liquid metal (e.g. mercury in silastic) strain gauges have the advantage of being calibrated *in vivo*, but they have to be custom made, which is a tricky process. Micro damage in the area of implantation alters the tensile properties of the tendon within a few days after implantation, so readings must be taken as soon as possible after surgery (Jansen *et al.*, 1998). Liquid metal strain gauges have been used to investigate the load distribution between the flexor tendons and suspensory ligament (Jansen *et al.*, 1993), and to detect changes in the loading pattern in response to changes in surface type or shoeing adaptations (Riemersma *et al.*, 1996a, 1996b).

A transducer based on the Hall effect, in which the voltage output of a semiconductor is proportional to the strength of a magnetic field, was used to measure strain in the superficial digital flexor tendon. Although the strains recorded were higher than would be expected, this may have been due to the definition of initial length as the length at heel strike (Stephens *et al.*, 1989).

A novel type of force transducer that detects the strain from a very small part of the tendon has been applied in horses (Platt *et al.*, 1994). A drawback to this type of transducer is that it samples a very small area that is not necessarily representative of strain in the entire tendon.

Accelerometers

Accelerometers measure acceleration of the surface to which they are attached. In equine studies they have most often been applied to the hoof wall, where they are used to detect initial ground contact and to measure the associated acceleration. A hoof-mounted accelerometer is probably the most effective means of measuring certain characteristics of the footing (Barrey *et al.*, 1991) and the efficiency of shock absorbing shoes and pads (Benoit *et al.*, 1991). By mounting accelerometers to the hoof wall and to the bones of the digit, Lanovaz *et al.* (1998) studied the attenuation of impact shock in the distal digit *in vitro*; Willemen *et al.* (1997) performed similar measurements both *in vitro* and *in vivo*.

In another application, two accelerometers were secured beneath the horse's sternum to measure longitudinal and dorsoventral accelerations of the trunk segment (Barrey *et al.*, 1994). The data were transmitted telemetrically to a receiver connected to a portable computer. Analysis of the left/right symmetry of the trunk acceleration patterns during trotting detected subtle asymmetries in lame horses (Barrey & Desbrosse, 1996). The same device has been used to study the accelerations of the trunk during jumping (Barrey & Galloux, 1997).

Accelerometers attached to the saddle have been used to measure the acceleration at different gaits and the findings have been applied in the development of a mechanical horse that simulates the motions during walking, trotting, cantering and jumping (Galloux *et al.*, 1994).

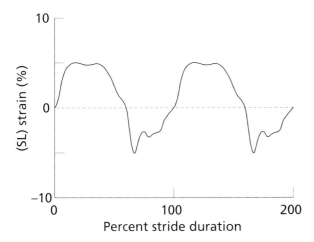

Fig. 3.12 Strain pattern in the suspensory ligament (SL) of a walking horse measured using a liquid metal filled strain gauge implanted into the ligament. The stride starts and ends at ground contact of the instrumented limb, which occurs at times 0%, 100% and 200%. (Reprinted with permission from Schamhardt, H.C. (1996) In: *Measuring movement and locomotion: from invertebrates to humans* © *R.G. Landes Company.*)

TREADMILL EVALUATION

The treadmill is extremely useful for equine gait analysis because the speed of movement is controlled, allowing the horse's gait to be evaluated at the same speed under different circumstances. Theoretically, treadmill locomotion does not differ from overground locomotion (Ingen Schenau, 1980), but differences in kinematic stride variables have been reported (Fredricson et al., 1983; Barrey et al., 1993; Buchner et al., 1994b).

A period of habituation is required before horses move consistently on the treadmill, with habituation occurring more rapidly at faster gaits. Rapid adaptation is seen during the first few training sessions, and by the end of the third 5-min session, the kinematics of the trot have stabilized (Fig. 3.13), whereas the walk kinematics are not fully adapted even at the tenth session (Buchner et al., 1994a). During the first session and, to a lesser extent at the start of subsequent sessions, the initial steps are short and quick, with the withers and hind quarters lowered, and the feet splayed to the side to give the horse a larger base of support. Even horses that are experienced on the treadmill take at least one minute for their gait pattern to stabilize each time the belt starts moving (Buchner et al., 1994a).

Comparisons between overground and treadmill locomotion in horses trotting at the same speed under both conditions have shown that speed on the treadmill is achieved with a higher stride frequency and a longer stride length (Barrey et al., 1993). On the treadmill there is an increase in stance duration, earlier placement of the forelimbs, greater retraction of both fore and hindlimbs and reduced vertical excursions of the hooves and the withers (Buchner et al., 1994b).

Horses moving on a treadmill use less energy than horses moving overground at the same speed, which may be partly due to a power transfer from the treadmill to the horse. Although the speed of the treadmill belt is assumed to be constant, in fact it is reduced by about 9% during the first part of the stance phase due to the frictional effect of the vertical force component and the decelerating effect of the longitudinal force component exerted by the horse's limb. In the later part of the stance phase the frictional effect of the vertical force declines while the propulsive longitudinal force tends to accelerate the belt (Schamhardt et al., 1994).

Although the kinematics and energetics of treadmill locomotion are not exactly equivalent to overground locomotion, this does not diminish its value for clinical and research studies involving comparisons between treadmill locomotion under different conditions. Videographic analysis of a horse moving on a treadmill is particularly useful for evaluating hoof balance and the flight arc of the hoof: even without a gait analysis system the tapes can be viewed at normal speed and in slow motion to visualize events that happen too rapidly to be perceived by the human eye.

Kinematic analysis of horses moving on a treadmill has been used to study the movements of the limbs (Back et al., 1995a, 1995b), ontogeny of the trot (Back et al., 1994), the response to training (van Weeren et al., 1993; Corley & Goodship, 1994), the development of gait

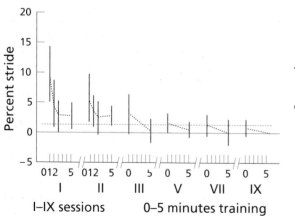
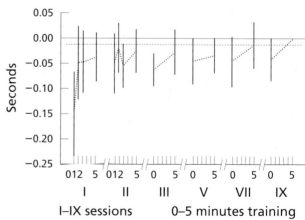

Fig. 3.13 Habituation to treadmill locomotion in 10 horses determined by changes in hindlimb stance duration, expressed as a percentage of stride duration (left) and in seconds (right). The horizontal axis shows the number of training sessions, each of 5 min duration. The vertical axis shows the relative stance duration. Reductions in stance duration are regarded as a sign of habituation. The horizontal line indicates the 'habituation limit' based on data of the final recording session. Vertical bars indicate standard deviations within 10 horses. (Reprinted with permission from Buchner et al. (1994b) *Equine Vet. J.* **17**(Suppl.): 13–15.)

asymmetries (Drevemo *et al.*, 1987) and adaptations used by the horse to manage lameness (Peloso *et al.*, 1993; Buchner *et al.*, 1995, 1996b, 1996c).

At the University of Zurich, a force plate suitable for equine use has been embedded in a treadmill to measure the vertical forces of all four limbs over an unlimited number of steps at any gait (Weishaupt *et al.*, 1996). The force measuring system consists of 16 piezoelectric force transducers mounted between the treadmill frame and the supporting steel plate over which the belt moves. Each transducer measures the vertical force at the corresponding bearing of the supporting plate. Transfer coefficients have been determined for each of the 16 transducers for each square centimeter of the treadmill surface by the application of a test force. These values are shown as a table that is used in the calculation procedures. The coordinates of each hoof on the treadmill surface are calculated by triangulation based on angle values derived from two electrogoniometers. For each sampling instant, a set of 16 linear equations can be formulated containing the four unknown hoof forces, the four $x–y$ coordinates of the hoof force application, their corresponding transfer coefficients and the 16 forces from the sensors, from which the individual hoof forces are extracted.

ELECTROMYOGRAPHY

Muscular contraction generates forces that stabilize and move the limbs. Muscle contraction is preceded by electrical activation, which can be detected and recorded as the electromyogram. Electromyography (EMG) gives information on the state of activity of the motor neurones at rest, during reflex contraction and during voluntary contraction. Since it is relatively non-invasive, EMG can be performed on the conscious horse, and can be used during locomotion (Korsgaard, 1982; Tokuriki *et al.*, 1989; Jansen *et al.*, 1992; Tokuriki & Aoki, 1995). The recognition of new neurologic disorders, such as equine motor neurone disease (EMND), hyperkalemic periodic paralysis, myotonia congenita and equine myotonic dystrophy, has resulted in EMG becoming a useful diagnostic tool. However, the characteristic features of neuromuscular disease may be difficult to detect and evaluate without sedation or anesthesia.

The nerve impulse

EMG studies the functional unit of the muscle, the motor unit, which consists of the motor neurone and the muscle fibers it innervates. A resting muscle fiber has a 90 mV potential difference across its surface membrane, with the outer side being positive. During excitation the resting potential is temporarily reversed to 40 mV, with the outside being negative. As the action potential travels along the muscle fiber, the small electrical potential generated across the surface membrane is dissipated in the surrounding interstitial fluid, which is a good electrical conductor. The summation of the electrical changes in the interstitial fluid is recorded as the EMG.

The number of muscle fibers per motor unit is inversely related to the precision of movements. Muscles that direct very precise movements have motor units composed of a small number of muscle fibers, whereas muscles that are primarily concerned with force production can have thousands of muscle fibers innervated by a single motor neurone. The force of muscular contraction is regulated by adjusting the number of motor units that are activated and/or the firing rate of the motor neurones. These factors interact to produce smooth and graded muscle contraction.

EMG equipment

The essential components of an EMG system are electrodes for recording potentials, an amplifier to enlarge the small electric potentials, a filter to reduce unwanted noise, and a data recording device. Data are transferred from the electrodes to the amplifier through wires (Denoix, 1989; Jansen *et al.*, 1992) or via telemetry (Aoki *et al.*, 1984; Tokuriki *et al.*, 1989).

The electrodes function as the antenna to pick up the electrical signal. They may be placed on the skin surface, inserted percutaneously into the muscle or implanted surgically. Surface electrodes have the advantage of being non-invasive but they provide only a gross estimation of muscle activity in the large superficial muscle groups. Jansen *et al.* (1992) found surface EMG to be a reliable and reproducible technique. However, many locomotor muscles of the horse are deeply placed or lie beneath the thick cutaneous muscles, making them unsuitable for study by surface electrodes. The percutaneous technique involves using a hypodermic needle to introduce fine wires into the muscle belly. Barbed ends usually hold the wires in place. This simple technique does not damage the muscle tissue, but has the disadvantage that the position of the electrodes cannot be visualized directly. Surgical implantation is a more complex, time-consuming and potentially damaging procedure, but it provides the best results in terms of electrical and mechanical reliability, since the operator has direct visual control of the position of the electrodes.

Several electrode configurations are used. A unipolar electrode usually has a single strand of wire coated with an insulating material except for a small length at its distal end. The wire is inserted percutaneously through a small hypodermic needle and the end of the wire is bent back on itself to act as a barb. The potential is measured between the uninsulated tip of the wire and a reference electrode on the skin. Unipolar electrodes detect the time of activation of the muscle, rather than the amplitude of the contraction. Bipolar electrodes measure the voltage difference between two electrical contacts. A simple bipolar design has two hooked wires inserted through a hypodermic needle. Another type is the concentric bipolar electrode, which measures the potential difference between a point-like recording contact and an average of all the potentials in a ring surrounding it at some fixed distance. The advantages of this configuration are that the recording electrode is shielded by the outer needle from electromagnetic noise and the reference is kept as close to the electrode as possible.

The muscle potentials may be displayed on a cathode ray oscilloscope using the convention that a positive potentials is indicated by a downward deflection. A chart recorder may be used to produce a hard copy of the output. The data are usually converted from analog to digital format and stored in a computer. Special software is used to process the information, to measure variables such as the amplitude and frequency of the spikes, to rectify the output, to construct an envelope that touches the peaks of the spikes and to measure the areas under the resulting curves.

The electromyogram

During EMG examination there are three phases of electrical activity: insertional activity, resting activity and activity during muscle contraction. The mechanical stimulation associated with insertion or movement of the EMG needle precipitates a discharge of potentials that last only a few milliseconds, end abruptly, and are followed by electrical silence (Fig. 3.14). Increased electrical activity lasting more than 10 ms after insertion or moving the needle is abnormal and thought to be due to hyperirritability and instability of the muscle fiber membrane, which is usually a sign of early denervation atrophy, but it is also seen in myotonic disorders and myositis (Kimura, 1984) and in EMND (Podell et al., 1995). Changes in insertional activity and action potentials may be difficult to detect objectively in standing horses.

Positive sharp waves (PSWs) are monophasic, with a short positive phase followed by a longer, very large negative phase (Fig. 3.14). PSWs occur in muscular diseases such as myositis, exertional rhabdomyolysis and EMND.

Fibrillation potentials are the most commonly observed abnormal electromyographic findings. They have a bi- or triphasic waveform with an initial positive potential that is represented by a downward deflection. They are thought to be spontaneous discharges from

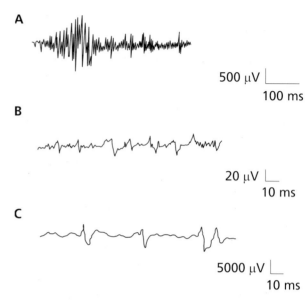

Fig. 3.14 Normal electromyographic findings. **A:** Insertional activity; **B:** endplate noise; **C:** motor unit action potential (MUAP). (Reprinted with permission from van Wessum, R. Sloet, M.M. and Clayton, H.M. (1999) *Vet. Quart.* **21:** 3–7.)

acetylcholine-hypersensitive denervated muscle fibers. Fibrillation potentials strongly suggest denervation and may be present as early as 4 to 10 days after denervation, though in horses they may not be seen until 2 weeks or longer after denervation. When denervation persists and atrophy commences, the fibrillation potentials decrease in number and amplitude, finally ceasing when the muscle is completely atrophied. Fibrillations were found in 45% of horses with EMND (Podell et al., 1995), and have been reported in draft horses affected by shivers (Cox, 1992). Fasciculations, which are spontaneously contracting motor units that may be visible at gross inspection, often occur in association with fibrillation potentials in EMND (Podell et al., 1995) and in shivers (Cox, 1992).

Relaxed skeletal muscle is electrically silent, and the resulting fairly flat trace is the baseline electromyogram. When the electrode is positioned near an endplate or nerve twig it gives rise to endplate noise (Fig. 3.14) and endplate spikes, which are usually eliminated by repositioning the needle.

Motor unit action potentials (MUAPs) are the summation of muscle action potentials from the voluntary or reflex contraction of myofibers in a motor unit. Approximately 50 muscle fibers around a needle electrode contribute to the observed potential. Dedicated software is used to measure the amplitude and frequency of the MUAPs, rectify the curves, construct envelopes and calculate the area under the curves.

Polyphasic MUAPs are potentials during submaximal muscle contraction that have more than four phases and a decreased amplitude and duration. These are indicative of a diffuse loss of muscle fibers resulting in the need for extra motor unit stimulation in order to perform the work normally done by fewer motor units, as in primary myopathies (Andrews & Fenner, 1987).

Myotonic discharges are the result of repeated spontaneous electrical discharges of individual myofibers or groups of myofibers, not followed by a muscle contraction. Myotonic discharges have a long duration of 4–5 s, and their amplitude waxes and wanes during the discharge. In the horse myotonic discharges occur in myotonic dystrophy (Hegreberg *et al.*, 1990), hyperkalemic periodic paralysis (Naylor *et al.*, 1992) and Australian stringhalt (Huntington *et al.*, 1989).

Studies of athletic horses have described the activation pattern of various muscles during normal locomotion (Wentink, 1978; Korsgaard, 1982; Tokuriki *et al.*, 1989). On the basis of EMG activity, muscles were shown to be active at times that were different from expectations based on their topography (Wentink, 1978). This work led to an appreciation of the importance of muscles for stabilizing the joints rather than simply acting as prime movers. Recent studies describing the net joint moments at different joints and the work done across these joints is shedding new light on the interpretation of EMG findings (Colborne *et al.*, 1998; Clayton *et al.*, 1999; Lanovaz *et al.*, 1999).

The amplitude of the EMG signal depends on the dimensions of the electrodes, their electrical contact with the muscle, and the kind of electrodes: signals from indwelling wire electrodes usually are much lower than those obtained from surface electrodes. However, the major influence on the EMG signal amplitude is caused by the degree of activation of the muscle. When the muscle is completely activated, the EMG signal will reach a maximum. This relationship allows the EMG signal amplitude to be used as a measure of the degree of activation, and thus indirectly, of the muscle force development (Hof, 1984). However, it is not possible to determine a reliable estimate of muscle force development on the basis of EMG signal analysis alone. This requires the development of a sophisticated muscle model that incorporates the muscle architecture, the force–length and force–velocity relationships of the muscle fibers, and the activation of the muscle (possibly from EMG signal analysis).

ARTIFICIAL NEURAL NETWORKS

Artificial neural networks (ANN) are computer programs consisting of cells that are organized in analogy with the architecture of the human brain. They can be used for qualitative and quantitative pattern recognition. ANNs are trained using a set of input data that are provided together with a target output. Training sessions are repeated until the ANN 'learns' to interpret the input data to produce an appropriate output. For example, in training an ANN for lameness diagnosis, input might be in the form of kinematic data, while the target output is the clinical diagnosis.

Preliminary studies have indicated that the GRF may be estimated from hoof wall strain using as few as two gauges, one at the toe and one on the lateral hoof wall. Since the relationship between hoof wall strain and GRF is nonlinear, common analytical tools are not applicable. ANNs, however, excel in performing this type of complex pattern recognition task (Savelberg *et al.*, 1997). They have also shown the ability to detect the lame limb and to assess the lameness degree with reasonable accuracy if adequate data were used to train the ANN (Schlobesberger, 1996; Savelberg *et al.*, 1997).

REFERENCES

Adrian, M., Grant, B., Ratzlaff, M., Ray, J. and Boulton, C. (1977) Electrogoniometric analysis of equine metacarpophalangeal joint lameness. *Am. J. Vet. Res.* **38**: 431.

Andrews, F.M. and Fenner, W.R. (1987) Indications and use of electrodiagnostic aids in neurologic disease. *Vet. Clin. North Am.: Equine Pract.* **3**: 293–322.

Aoki, O., Tokuriki, M., Kurakawa, Y., Masaaki, M. and Kita, T. (1984) Electromyographic studies on supraspinatus and infraspinatus muscles of the horse with or without a rider in walk, trot and canter. *Bull. Equine Res. Inst.* **21**: 100–104.

Back, W., Barneveld, A., Weeren, P.R. van and Bogert, A.J. van den (1993) Kinematic gait analysis in equine carpal lameness. *Acta Anat.* **146**: 86–89.

Back, W., Barneveld, A., Schamhardt, H.C., Bruin, G. and Hartman, W. (1994) Longitudinal development of the kinematics of 4-, 10-, 18- and 26-month-old Dutch Warmblood horses. *Equine Vet. J.* **17**(Suppl.): 3–6.

Back, W., Schamhardt, H.C., Savelberg, H.C.C.M., Bogert, A.J van den, Bruin, G., Hartman, W. and Barneveld, A. (1995a) How the horse moves. 1. Significance of graphical representations of equine forelimb kinematics. *Equine Vet. J.* **27**: 31–38.

Back, W., Schamhardt, H.C., Savelberg, H.C.C.M., Bogert, A.J. van den, Bruin, G., Hartman, W. and Barneveld, A. (1995b) How the horse moves. 2. Significance of graphical representations of equine hindlimb kinematics. *Equine Vet. J.* **27**: 39–45.

Barr, A.R.S., Dow, S.M. and Goodship, A.E. (1995) Parameters of forelimb ground reaction forces in 48 normal ponies. *Vet. Rec.* **136**: 283–286.

Barrey, E. (1990) Investigation of the vertical hoof force distribution in the equine forelimb with an instrumented horseboot. *Equine Vet. J.* **9**(Suppl.): 35–38.

Barrey, E. and Desbrosse, F. (1996) Lameness detection using an accelerometric device. *Pferdeheilkunde* **12**: 617–622.

Barrey, E. and Galloux, P. (1997) Analysis of the equine jumping technique by accelerometry. *Equine Vet. J.* **23**(Suppl.): 45–49.

Barrey, E., Landjerit, B and Wolter, R. (1991) Shock and vibration during hoof impact on different track surfaces. *Equine Exerc. Physiol.* **3**: 97–106.

Barrey, E., Galloux, P., Valette, J.P., Auvinet, B. and Wolter, R. (1993) Stride characteristics of overground versus treadmill locomotion. *Acta Anat.* **146**: 90–94.

Barrey, E., Hermelin, M., Vaudelin, J.L., Poirel, D. and Valette, P. (1994) Utilisation of an accelerometric device in equine gait analysis. *Equine Vet. J.* **17**(Suppl.): 7–12.

Benoit, P., Barrey, E., Regnault, J.C. and Brochet, J.L. (1991) Comparison of the damping effect of different shoeing by the measurement of hoof acceleration. *Acta Anat.* **146**: 109–113.

Buchner, H.H.F., Savelberg, H.H.C.M., Schamhardt, H.C. *et al.* (1994a) Habituation of horses to treadmill locomotion. *Equine Vet. J.* **17**(Suppl.): 13–15.

Buchner, H.H.F., Savelberg, H.H.C.M., Schamhardt, H.C. *et al.* (1994b) Kinematics of treadmill versus overground locomotion in horses. *Vet. Quart.* **16**(Suppl. 2): S87–90.

Buchner, H.H.F., Savelberg, H.H.C.M., Schamhardt, H.C. *et al.* (1995) Temporal stride patterns in horses with experimentally induced fore or hind limb lameness. *Equine Vet. J.* **18**(Suppl.): 161–165.

Buchner, H.H.F., Savelberg, H.H.C.M. and Becker, C.K. (1996a) Load redistribution after desmotomy of the accessory ligament of the deep digital flexor tendon in adult horses. *Vet. Quart.* **18**(Suppl. 2): S70–74.

Buchner, H.H.F., Savelberg, H.H.C.M., Schamhardt, H.C. *et al.* (1996b) Limb movement adaptations in horses with experimentally induced fore or hind limb lameness. *Equine Vet. J.* **28**: 63–70.

Buchner, H.H.F., Savelberg, H.H.C.M., Schamhardt, H.C. *et al.* (1996c) Head and trunk movement adaptations in horses with experimentally induced fore or hind limb lameness. *Equine Vet. J.* **28**: 71–76.

Clayton, H.M., Schamhardt, H.C., Lanovaz, J.L., Colborne, G.R. and Willemen, M.A. Superficial digital flexor tendinitis: 2. Net joint moments and joint powers. *Am. J. Vet. Res.* (in press).

Clayton, H.M., Schott, H.C., Littlefield L and Lanovaz, J.L. (1999) Center of pressure analysis in horses. *Am. Coll. Vet. Int. Med.* **13**; 241.

Colborne, G.R., Lanovaz, J.L., Sprigings, E.J., Schamhardt, H.C. and Clayton, H.M. (1998) Forelimb joint moments and power during the walking stance phase of horses. *Am. J. Vet. Res.* **59**: 609–614.

Corley, J.M. and Goodship, A.E. (1994) Treadmill training induced changes to some kinematic variables measured at the canter in Thoroughbred fillies. *Equine Vet. J.* **17**(Suppl.): 20–24.

Cox, J. (1992) Neuromuscular disorders. In: Mills, L. (ed.) *Current Therapy in Equine Medicine.* Philadelphia: W.B. Saunders, pp. 571–573.

Davies, H.M.S., McCarthy, R.N. and Jeffcott, L.B. (1993) Strain in the equine metacarpus during locomotion. *Acta Anat.* **146**: 148–153.

DeLuzio, K.J., Wyss, U.P., Li, J. and Costigan, P.A. (1993) A procedure to validate three-dimensional motion assessment systems. *J. Biomech.* **26**: 753–759.

Denoix, J.M. (1989) Biomechanical studies in the athletic horse. Present methods and objectives. *Rec. Med. Vet.* **165**: 107–115.

Drevemo, S., Dalin, G., Fredricson, I. and Hjertén, G. (1980a) Equine locomotion 1: The analysis of linear and temporal stride characteristics of trotting Standardbreds. *Equine Vet. J.* **12**: 60–65.

Drevemo, S., Dalin, G., Fredricson, I. and Björne, K. (1980b) Equine locomotion 3: The reproducibility of gait in Standardbred trotters. *Equine Vet. J.* **12**: 71–73.

Drevemo, S., Fredricson, I. and Hjertén, G. (1987) Early development of gait asymmetries in trotting Standardbred colts. *Equine Vet. J.* **19**: 189–191.

Fioretti, S. and Jetto, L. (1989) Accurate derivative estimation from noisy data: a state-space approach. *Int. J. Systems Sci.* **20**: 33–53.

Frederick, F.H. Jr and Henderson, J.M. (1970) Impact force measurement using preloaded transducers. *Am. J. Vet. Res.* **31**: 2279–2283.

Fredricson, I. and Drevemo, S. (1972) Methodological aspects of kinematics of the joints in the forelimbs of fast moving horses. *Acta Vet. Scand.* **37**: 93–136.

Fredricson, I., Drevemo, S., Dalin, G., *et al.* (1983) Treadmill for equine locomotion analysis. *Equine Vet. J.* **15**: 111–115.

Galloux, P., Richard, N., Dronka, T. *et al.* (1994) Analysis of equine gait using three-dimensional accelerometers fixed on the saddle. *Equine Vet. J.* **17**(Suppl.): 44–47.

Gingerich, D.A., Auer, J.A. and Fackelman, G.E. (1979) Force plate studies on the effect of exogenous hyaluronic acid on joint function in equine arthritis. *J. Vet. Pharmacol. Therap.* **2**: 291–298.

Grood, E.S. and Suntay, W.J. (1983) A joint coordinate system for the clinical description of three-dimensional motions: applications to the knee. *J. Biomech. Eng.* **105**: 136–144.

Hartman, W., Schamhardt, H.C., Lammertink, J.L.M.A. and Badoux, D.M. (1984) Bone strain in the equine tibia: An in vivo strain gauge analysis. *Am. J. Vet. Res.* **45**: 880–884.

Hegreberg, G.A. and Reed, S.M. (1990) Skeletal muscle changes associated with equine myotonic dystrophy. *Acta Neuropathol.* **80**: 426–431.

Hjertén, G. and Drevemo, S. (1987) A method to analyze forces and moments in the extremities of the horse during the stance phase at the trot. *Equine Exerc. Physiol.* **2**: 587–598.

Hof, A.L. (1984) EMG and muscle force: an introduction. *Human Movement Sci.* **3**: 119–153.

Huntington, P.J., Jeffcott, L.B., Friend, S.C.E., Luff, A.R., Finkelstein, D.I. and Flynn, R.J. (1989) Australian stringhalt – epidemiological, clinical and neurological investigations. *Equine Vet. J.* **21**: 266–273.

Ingen Schenau, G.J. van (1980) Some fundamental aspects of the biomechanics of overground versus treadmill locomotion. *Med. Sci. Sports Exerc.* **12**: 257–261.

Jansen, M.O., Raaij, J.A.G.M. van, Bogert, A.J., van den, Schamhardt, H.C. and Hartman, W. (1992) Quantitative analysis of computer-averaged electromyographic profiles of intrinsic limb muscles in ponies at the walk. *Am. J. Vet. Res.* **53**: 2343–2349.

Jansen, M.O., Bogert, A.J. van den and Schamhardt, H.C. (1993) In vivo tendon forces in the forelimb of ponies at the walk, validated by ground reaction force measurements. *Acta Anat.* **146**: 162–167.

Jansen, M.O., Schamhardt, H.C., Bogert, A.J. van den and Hartman, W. (1998) Mechanical properties of the tendinous equine interosseus muscle affected by *in vivo* transducer implantation. *J. Biomech.* **31**: 485–490.

Keegan, K.G., Wilson, D.A., Wilson, D.J. *et al.* (1998) Evaluation of mild lameness in horse trotting on a treadmill by clinicians and interns or residents and correlation of their assessments with kinematic gait analysis. *Am. J. Vet. Res.* **59**: 1370–1377.

Keg, P.R., Belt, A.J.M. van den, Merkens, H.W., Barneveld, A. and Dik, K.J. (1992) The effect of regional nerve blocks on the lameness caused by collagenase induced tendonitis in the midmetacarpal region of the horse: a study using gait analysis, and ultrasonography to determine tendon healing. *J. Vet. Med.* **A39**: 349–364.

Kimura, J. (1984) *Electrodiagnosis in Disease of Nerve and Muscle: Principles and Practice.* Philadelphia: F.A. Davis.

Korsgaard, E. (1982) Muscle function in the forelimb of the horse. An electromyographical and kinesiological study. *PhD thesis, Kopenhagen.*

Lanovaz, J.L., Clayton, H.M. and Watson, L.G. (1998) In vitro attenuation of impact shock in equine digits. *Equine Vet. J.* **26**(Suppl.): 96–102.

Lanovaz, J.L., Clayton, H.M., Colborne, G.R. and Schamhardt, H.C. (1999) Forelimb kinematics and joint moments during the swing phase of the trot. *Equine Vet. J.* **30** (suppl.); 235–239.

Lanyon, L.E. (1976) The measurement of bone strain *in vivo. Acta Orthop. Belg.* **42**(Suppl. 1): 98–108.

Leach, D.H. and Dyson, S. (1988) Instant centres of rotation of equine limb joints and their relationship to standard skin marker locations. *Equine Vet. J.* **6**(Suppl.): 113–119.

Licka, T. and Peham, C. (1998) An objective method for evaluating the flexibility of the back of standing horses. *Equine Vet. J.* **30**: 412–415.

Linford, R.L. (1994) Camera speeds for optoelectronic assessment of stride-timing characteristics in horses at the trot. *Am. J. Vet. Res.* **55**: 1189–1195.

McLaughlin, R.M., Gaughan, E.M., Roush, K. and Skaggs, C. (1996) Effects of subject velocity on ground reaction force measurements and stance times in clinically normal horses at the walk and trot. *Am. J. Vet. Res.* **57**: 7–11.

Merkens, H.W. and Schamhardt, H.C.C. (1988) Evaluation of equine locomotion during different degrees of experimentally induced lameness 1: Lameness model and quantification of ground reaction force patterns of the limbs. *Equine Vet. J.* **6**(Suppl.): 99–106.

Merkens, H.W., Schamhardt, H.C., Hartman, W. and Kersjes, A.W. (1986) Ground reaction force patterns of Dutch Warmblood horses at normal walk. *Equine Vet. J.* **18**: 207–214.

Merkens, H.W., Schamhardt, H.C., Hartman, W. and Kersjes, A.W. (1988) The use of Horse(INDEX), a method of analysing the ground reaction force patterns of lame and normal gaited horses at the walk. *Equine Vet. J.* **20**: 29–36.

Merkens, H.W., Schamhardt, H.C., Osch, G.J.V.M. and Bogert, A.J. (1993a) Ground reaction force patterns of Dutch Warmblood horses at normal trot. *Equine Vet. J.* **25**: 134–137.

Merkens, H.W., Schamhardt, H.C., Osch, G.J.V.M. van and Hartman, W. (1993b) Ground reaction force patterns of Dutch Warmbloods at canter. *Am. J. Vet. Res.* **54**: 670–674.

Morris, E.A. and Seeherman, H.J. (1987) Redistribution of ground reaction forces in experimentally induced carpal lameness. *Equine Exerc. Physiol.* **2**: 553–563.

Naylor, J.M., Robinson, J.A., Crichlow, E.C. and Steiss, J.E. (1992) Inheritance of myotonic discharges in American quarter horses and the relationship to hyperkalemic periodic paralysis. *Can. J. Vet. Res.* **56**: 62–66.

Nicodemus, M.C., Lanovaz, J.L., Corn, C. and Clayton, H.M. (1999) The application of virtual markers to a joint coordinate system for equine three-dimensional motions. *Proc. Equine Nutr. Physiol. Soc.* **16**: 24–25.

Niki, Y., Ueda, Y., Yoshida, K. and Masumitsu, H. (1982) A force plate study in equine biomechanics. 2. The vertical and fore-aft components of floor reaction forces and motion of equine limbs at walk and trot. *Bull. Equine Res. Inst.* **19**: 1–17.

Peloso, J.G., Stick, J.A., Caron, J.P., Peloso, P.M. and Soutas-Little, R.W. (1993) Computer-assisted three-dimensional gait analysis of amphotericin-induced carpal lameness in horses. *Am. J. Vet. Res.* **54**: 1535–1543.

Platt, D., Wilson, A.M., Timbs, A., Wright, I.M. and Goodship, A.E. (1994) Novel force transducer for the measurement of tendon forces *in vivo. J. Biomech.* **27**: 1489–1493.

Podell, M., Valentine, B.A., Cummings, J.F. *et al.* (1995) Electromyography in acquired equine motor neuron disease. *Prog. Vet. Neurol.* **6**: 128–134.

Pratt, G.W. Jr and O'Connor, J.T. Jr (1976) Force plate studies of equine biomechanics. *Am. J. Vet. Res.* **37**: 1251–1255.

Ratzlaff, M.H., Grant, B.D., Adrian, M. and Feeney-Dixon, C. (1979) Evaluation of equine locomotion using electrogoniometry and cinematography: research and clinical applications. *Proc. Am. Assoc. Equine Practnrs.* **25**: 381.

Ratzlaff, M.H., Hyde, M.L., Grant, B.D., Balch, O. and Wilson, P.D. (1990) Measurement of vertical forces and temporal components of the strides of galloping horses using instrumented shoes. *J. Equine Vet. Sci.* **10**: 23–25.

Ratzlaff, M.H., Grant, B.D., Hyde, M.L. and Balch, O.K. (1994) Rupture of the distal sesamoidean ligaments of a horse: vertical forces and temporal components of the strides before, during and after injury. *J. Equine Vet. Sci.* **14**: 45–52.

Riemersma, D.J. and Bogert, A.J. van den (1993) A method to estimate the initial length of equine tendons. *Acta Anat.* **146**: 120–122.

Riemersma, D.J., Bogert, A.J. van den, Jansen, M.O. and Schamhardt, H.C. (1996a) Tendon strain in the forelimbs as a function of gait and ground characteristics, and in vitro limb loading in ponies. *Equine Vet. J.* **28**: 133–138.

Riemersma, D.J., Bogert, A.J. van den, Jansen, M.O. and Schamhardt, H.C. (1996b) Influence of shoeing on ground reaction forces and tendon strains in the forelimbs of ponies. *Equine Vet. J.* **28**: 126–132.

Roepstorff, L. and Drevemo, S. (1993) Concept of a force-measuring horseshoe. *Acta Anat.* **146**: 114–119.

Roepstorff, L., Johnston, C. and Drevemo, S. (1994) The influences of different treadmill constructions on ground reaction forces as determined by the use of a force-measuring shoe. *Equine Vet. J.* **17**(Suppl.): 71–74.

Roszek, B., Loon, P. van, Weinans, H. and Huiskes, R. (1993) In vivo measurements of the loading conditions on the tibia of the goat. *Acta Anat.* **146**: 188–192.

Rubin, C.T. and Lanyon, L.E. (1982) Limb mechanics as a function of speed and gait: A study of functional strains in the radius and tibia of horse and dog. *J. Exp. Biol.* **101**: 187–211.

Rybicki, E.F., Simonen, F.A., Mills, E.J. *et al.* (1974) Mathematical and experimental studies on the mechanics of plated transverse fractures. *J. Biomech.* **7**: 377–384.

Savelberg, H.H.C.M., Loon, J.P. van and Schamhardt, H.C. (1997) Ground reaction forces in horses assessed from hoof wall deformation using artificial neural networks. *Equine Vet. J.* **23**(Suppl.): 6–8.

Schamhardt, H.C. (1996) Quantitative analyses of equine locomotion. In: Ossenkopp, K.-P., Kavakiers, M. and Sanberg, P.R. (eds) *Measuring Movement and Locomotion: from Invertebrates to Humans,* Springer-Verlag, Heidlberg, pp. 189–211.

Schamhardt, H.C. and Hartman, W. (1982) Automatic zero strain compensation of in vivo bone strain recordings. *J. Biomech.* **15**: 621–624.

Schamhardt, H.C. and Merkens, H.W. (1987) Quantification of equine ground reaction force patterns. *J. Biomech.* **20**: 443–446.

Schamhardt, H.C., Hartman, W. and Lammertink, J.L.M.A. (1985) In vivo bone strain in the equine tibia before and after transection of the peroneus tertius muscle. *Res. Vet. Sci.* **39**: 139–144.

Schamhardt, H.C., Bogert, A.J. van den, Lammertink, J.L.M.A. and Markies, H. (1992) Measurement and analysis of equine locomotion using a modified CODA-3 kinematic analysis system. *Proc. 8th Mtg. Eur. Soc. Biomech.*, p. 270.

Schamhardt, H.C., Bogert, A.J. van den and Hartman, W. (1993a) Measurement techniques in animal locomotion analysis. *Acta Anat.* **146**: 123–129.

Schamhardt, H.C., Merkens, H.W., Vogel, V. and Willekens, C. (1993b) External loads on the limbs of the jumping horse at take-off and landing. *Am. J. Vet. Res.* **54**: 675–680.

Schamhardt, H.C.C., Bogert, A.J. van den and Lammertink, J.L.M.A. (1994) Power transfer from treadmill engine to athlete. *Proc. Can. Soc. Biomech.* pp. 306–307.

Schlosberger, H. (1996) Einsatz eines neuronalen Netzes bei der Lahmheitsuntersuchung von Pferden im Trab. *Dissertation, Wien.*

Schryver, H.F., Bartel, D.L., Langrana, N. and Lowe, J.E. (1978) Locomotion in the horse: Kinematics and external and internal forces in the normal equine digit in the walk and trot. *Am. J. Vet. Res.* **39**: 1728–1733.

Seeherman, H.J., Morris, E.A. and Fackelman, G.E. (1987) Computerized force plate determination of equine weightbearing profiles. *Equine Exerc. Physiol.* **2**: 537–552.

Stephens, P.R., Nunamaker, D.M. and Butterweck, D.M. (1989) Application of a Hall-effect transducer for measurement of tendon strain in horses. *Am. J. Vet. Res.* **50**: 1089–1095.

Sustronck, B. (1994) Electromyographic examination in the horse. *Vet. Annual* **34**: 97–106.

Taylor, B.M., Tipton, C.M., Adrian, M. and Karpovich, P.V. (1966) Action of certain joints in the legs of the horse recorded electrogoniometrically. *Am. J. Vet. Res.* **27**: 85–89.

Thomason, J.J., Biewener, A.A. and Bertram, J.E.A. (1992) Surface strains on the equine hoof wall *in vivo*: implications for the material design and functional morphology of the wall. *J. Exp. Biol.* **166**: 145–168.

Tokuriki, M., Aoki, O., Niki, Y., Kurakawa, Y., Hataya, M. and Kita, T. (1989) Electromyographic activity of cubital joint muscles in horses during locomotion. *Am. J. Vet. Res.* **50**: 950–957.

Tokuriki, M. and Aoki, O. (1995) Electromyographic activity of the hindlimb muscles during the walk, trot and canter. *Equine Vet. J.* (Suppl.): 152–155.

Weeren, P.R. van, Bogert, A.J. van den and Barneveld, A. (1990a) A quantitative analysis of skin displacement in the trotting horse. *Equine Vet. J.* **9**(Suppl.): 101–109.

Weeren, P.R. van, Bogert, A.J. van den and Barneveld, A. (1990b) Quantification of skin displacement in the proximal parts of the limbs of the walking horse. *Equine Vet. J.* **9**(Suppl.): 110–118.

Weeren, P.R. van, Bogert, A.J. van den and Barneveld, A. (1992) Correction models for skin displacement in equine kinematic gait analysis. *J. Equine Vet. Sci.* **12**: 178–192.

Weeren, P.R. van, Bogert, A.J. van den, Back, W., Bruin, G. and Barneveld, A. (1993) Kinematics of the Standardbred trotter measured at 6, 7, 8 and 9 m/s on a treadmill, before and after 5 months prerace training. *Acta Anat.* **146**: 154–161.

Weishaupt, M.A., Hogg, H.P., Wiestner, T., Demuth, D.C. and Auer, J.A. (1996) Development of a technique for measuring ground reaction force in the equine on a treadmill. *Abstr. 3rd Int. Conf. Equine Locomotion*, Saumur, France.

Wentink, G.H. (1978) Biokinetical analysis of the movements of the pelvic limb of the horse and the role of the muscles in the walk and trot. *Anat. Embryol.* **152**: 261–272.

Willemen, M.A., Jacobs, M.W.H. and Schamhardt, H.C. (1997) In vitro transmission and attenuation of impact vibrations in the lower forelimb of the horse. In: Willemen, M.A. (ed.) Horseshoeing: a biomechanical analysis. *PhD thesis, Utrecht University.*

4

Inter-limb Coordination

Eric Barrey

INTRODUCTION

The locomotor apparatus is a complex set of systems including muscle, bone segments and joints, that are controlled by the central nervous system to produce well-coordinated locomotion. Biomechanically, locomotion involves moving all the body and limb segments in rhythmic and automatic patterns which define the various gaits. A great diversity exists in equine gait patterns because quadrupedal locomotion allows many combinations of inter-limb coordination. Furthermore, horse breeds have been genetically selected for different occupations: draft, riding, driving and meat production. Sport horses compete in a variety of sports, including pacing, trotting and

Table 4.1 Classification and main characteristics of equine gaits.

Classification	Gait	Gait variations	Footfall sequence	Rythm (beat/ stride)	Type of symmetry	Speed (m/s)	Stride length (m)	Stride frequency (stride/s)	Limb stance phase (s or % stride)	Suspension Phase (s or % stride)
Walking gaits	Walk	collected, medium, extended	RH,RF,LH,LF	4	Right/left bipedal	1.2–1.8	1.5–1.9	0.8–1.1	65–75 %	0
	Toelt = Paso = Rack = Fox-trot	medium	RH,RF,LH,LF	4	Right/left lateral	3.4–5.3	1.7–2.3	2.23–2.36	40–55%	0
Running gaits	Trot	piaffe, passage, collected, medium, extended, flying-trot	RH-LF, Susp., LH-RF, Susp.	2	Right/left diagonal	2.8–14.2	1.8–5.9	0.9–2.52	26–53%	0–09%
	Pace	medium, extended	RH-RF, Susp., LH-LF, Susp.	2	Right/left lateral	9.1–16.0	4.5–6.3	1.8–2.4	0.130–0.138 s	0.081–0.094 s
	Canter	collected, medium, extended, desunited	Trail. H, Lead. H, Trail .F, Lead.F, Susp.	3	Asymmetry with a phase lag between limb pair	2.9–9	1.9–4.6	1.6–2.0	0.28–0.30 s	0–0.013 s
	Gallop	transverse, rotary	Transverse: Trail. H, Lead. H, Trail. F, Lead. F, Susp.	4	Asymmetry with a phase lag between limb pair	9–20	4.5–7.2	2.27–2.92	0.085–0.09 s	0.063–0.114 s 16–28 %

galloping races, eventing, show jumping, dressage, endurance and Western disciplines. Consequently, a large range of gaits and gait variations can be observed in horses, including the walk and its many variations, trot, pace, canter and gallop. These gaits can be analyzed and classified according to their linear, temporal and dynamic characteristics using the measuring techniques that have been described in Chapter 2. The variety and complexity of gaits have always created difficulties in defining a terminology that is, at the same time, broad enough and also sufficiently specific to describe the locomotor phenomenon. Some efforts have been made to define a standard terminology for describing equine locomotion (Leach *et al.*, 1984a; Clayton, 1989; Leach, 1993). The gait terminology used in this book is defined in the Glossary (pp. xii).

CLASSIFICATION AND DESCRIPTION OF GAITS

A *gait* can be defined as a complex and strictly coordinated, rhythmic and automatic movement of the limbs and the entire body of the animal, which results in the production of progressive movements. In horses, a 2, 3 or 4 beat gait corresponds to the number of footfalls that can be heard during each stride of trot, canter and gallop, respectively. The sounds are related to the footfall pattern of the gait but when the interval between footfalls is very short, the human ear is not able to perceive the separation.

One method of classifying gaits depends on the symmetry between the left and right sides. In a symmetric gait the left and right footfalls of the fore and hindlimbs are evenly spaced in time. In an asymmetric gait, the footfalls of the fore and/or hindlimbs occur as couplets. The first limb of a couplet to contact the ground is the trailing limb, the second is the leading limb.

- *Symmetric gaits*: walk, trot, running walk, rack, toelt, fox trot, paso, stepping pace
- *Asymmetric gaits*: canter, transverse and rotary gallop, half bound.

Another type of gait classification distinguishes between stepping or walking gaits that have no period of suspension (there is always a contact with the ground) and running gaits that have one or more suspension phases in each stride (no foot in contact with the ground). The main characteristics of the equine gaits are described in Table 4.1. Within each gait there exist continuous variations from a collected type of gait with a slow speed to an extended type of gait with a higher speed.

Many types of illustrations have been proposed to describe the limb movements more precisely in time and space: drawings, chronophotographs, bar diagrams,

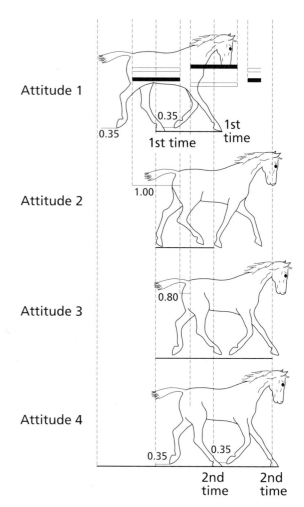

Fig. 4.1 Methods for representing the footfall sequences and temporal characteristics of the gaits. **Fig. 4.1A** (above) Drawings of the footfall sequence observed at the trot (Barroil, 1887).

phase diagrams and pie diagrams (Fig. 4.1). Some of the methods are only descriptive and show either temporal or linear characteristics of gaits:

- Drawings of the footfall sequence (Barroil, 1887) (Fig. 4.1A)
- Stick diagrams and hoof imprints which shows tracks and linear distances (Lenoble du Teil, 1893) (Fig. 4.1B). Stick diagrams can also describe temporal footfall sequence (Marey, 1873) (Fig. 4.5B)
- Pie gait diagram showing the footfall sequence and relative durations of the suspension phase, stance phases and overlaps (Deuel & Lawrence, 1987) (Fig. 4.1C).

Two other methods represent and classify the gaits in a more functional way using phase lag or advance between the footfalls:

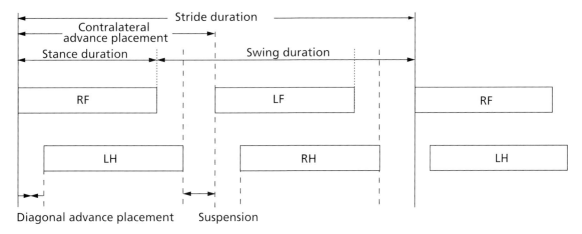

Fig. 4.1B Stick diagram of the trot. The sticks represent the stance phase duration of each limb.

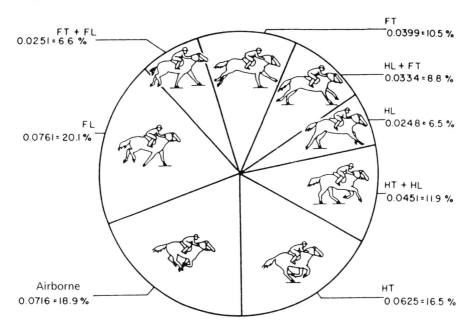

Fig. 4.1C Pie gait diagram of the gallop in Quarter Horses showing the footfall sequence and the durations of the suspension phase, stance phases and overlaps expressed in seconds and as a percentage of stride duration. The sequence rotates counterclockwise (Deuel & Lawrence, 1987). F: fore; H: hind; L: leading; T: trailing.

1. The continuum of symmetric gaits was described by a diagram proposed by Hildebrand (1965) (Fig. 4.2). The stance duration of the hindlimb was plotted against the lateral advanced placement. On the x-axis, the stance duration of the hindlimb indicates if the gait is classified as walking (no suspension phase) or running (two suspension phases per stride in the symmetric gaits). On the y-axis, the lateral advanced placement quantifies the phase lag of the lateral fore and hindlimbs. The 2 beat gaits are at the top and bottom of the diagram, with the 4 beat gaits between them. A similar diagram has been proposed

   for illustrating and comparing the diagonal gaits by plotting the hind stance phase duration against the diagonal advanced placement (Clayton, 1997).

2. A group of methods describe the type of coupling between the four limbs. All the running gaits can be modeled using the relative phases of the limb cycle (Alexander, 1984) (Fig. 4.1D). However this diagram describes only the footfalls sequence but does not give any linear of duration characteristics of the stride. A more sophisticated method based on a series of coupled oscillators has been proposed to describe and simulate both symmetric and asymmetric gaits (Collins

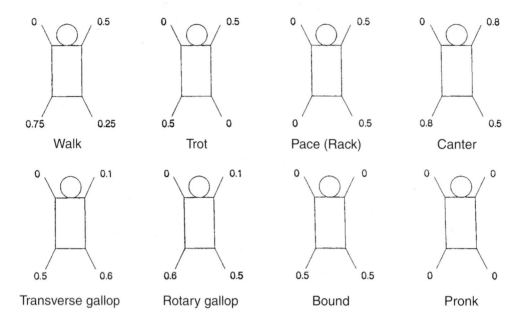

Fig. 4.1D Drawings of the relative phases between the limbs in various quadrupedal gaits (Alexander, 1984, © The Massachussetts Institute of Technology).

& Stewart, 1993). This model has the advantage of being able to describe gait transitions and abnormal gaits like the aubin, in which the hindlimbs trot while the forelimbs gallop, and traquenard, in which the hindlimbs gallop while the forelimbs trot. The model consists of four coupled oscillators that simulate the cyclical patterns of the four limb movements. It is possible to generate all types of equine gaits using five ways of coupling the oscillators. This type of functional model can be useful for understanding locomotor control by the central nervous system. Experimental results in neurophysiology demonstrated that the rhythmic activity of the skeletal muscles of each limb comes from the central nervous system (Barebeau & Rossignol, 1987). There are four distinct rhythm generators for the two hindlimbs and two forelimbs (Forssberg *et al.*, 1980a,b). Such a generator has been identified in lumbar spinal cord of the newborn rat (Cazalets *et al.*, 1996). In horses, the characteristics of these rhythm generators should determine the stride frequency and its variability. A great stability is required in dressage while rapid changes are necessary for jumping or racing horses.

Walk

The walk is a 4 beat gait with large overlap times between stance phases of the limbs and no period of suspension (Fig. 4.3). It is the slowest equine gait but probably one of the more complex gaits because of the variability in the overlap and lag time between limbs. In a lameness examination, the variability in the regularity and symmetry of the stride measured at the walk was higher than at the trot (Barrey & Desbrosse, 1996). In dressage horses, the speed of the walk increases from the collected walk (1.37 m/s) to the extended walk (1.82 m/s) with only a small increase in stride frequency (Clayton, 1995). The speed change was mainly the result of lengthening the stride by increasing the over-tracking distance. Even in highly trained dressage horses, a regular 4 beat rhythm of the footfalls was observed in only one of the six horses.

Other walking gaits

Icelandic horses, Paso Finos, and certain other gaited breeds exhibit a 4 beat symmetric gait in which the footfalls of the lateral pair of limbs occur as couplets (Fig. 4.4). Gaits with these characteristics are called toelt, paso, running walk, rack, stepping pace or slow gait. These gaits are comfortable for the rider because the amplitude of the dorsoventral displacement is lower than at the trot, which is a consequence of not having a period of suspension. The speed ranges between 1.7 and 2.3 m/s for the toelt and the natural gait transition sequence is walk–toelt–canter (Graselli *et al.*, 1991).

Hind limb stancephase (% of stride duration)

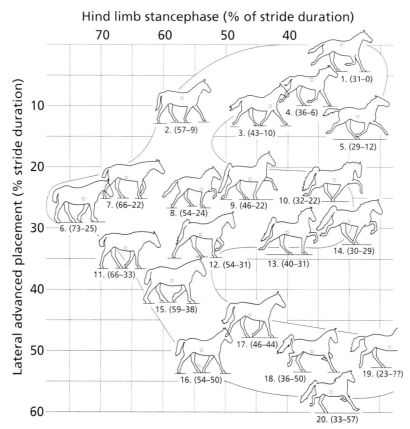

Fig. 4.2 Classification of symmetrical gaits according to the temporal characteristics of the gait (Hildebrand, 1965). In the background is shown the area of the basic graph within which fall nearly all gait formulas for symmetrical gaits of horses. Twenty specific formulas are located (small circles) and around each is drawn a silhouette of a horse moving as represented by the formula. In every sketch the left hind foot has just touched the ground.

Trot

The trot is a 2 beat, symmetric, diagonal gait (Fig. 4.5). The variations of the trot of saddle horses are the collected, working, medium and extended trots, with the speed of the gait increasing from collected to extended trot. A positive diagonal advanced placement has been measured at the collected trot in elite dressage horses (Holmström *et al.*, 1994; Clayton, 1997), with the hindlimb contacting the ground about 20–30 ms before the diagonal forelimb. Passage and piaffe are diagonal exercises derived from collected trot. From trot in hand to passage, the speed (–2.18 m/s) and stride length (–1.18 m) are reduced while the stride duration (+ 0.279 s) and diagonal advanced placement (+ 9.7 ms) increase (Holmström *et al.*, 1995). The dressage finalists at the Olympic Games in Barcelona showed differences between the temporal variables of the collected trot, passage and piaffe (Clayton, 1997). The stride duration is longer for piaffe (1.08 s) and passage (1.09 s) than for collected trot (0.84 s), which means that passage and piaffe have a lower

stride frequency. For most of the other temporal variables, collected trot and passage were very similar to each other except that the suspension phase was shorter in passage.

In harness trotters, the trot is so extended that it can reach a maximum speed of 14.2 m/s with a maximum stride frequency of 2.52 strides/s and a maximum stride length of 5.92 m (Barrey *et al.*, 1995). The diagonal sequence is usually affected with a 4 beat rhythm due to asynchrony of the impact (and lift-off) of the diagonal limb pairs (Drevemo *et al.*, 1980). This particular gait is named the flying trot (Fig. 4.6). The hindlimb touches the ground first (positive advanced placement), and the dissociation at lift-off is greater than at impact.

Various irregularities in the rhythm of the trot can occur during a harness race, which may result in the horse being disqualified by the gait judges. Irregular gait patterns that occur relatively frequently are called the aubin and the traquenard in French. At the *aubin*, the forelimbs gallop and the hindlimbs trot, while at the *traquenard*, the hindlimbs trot and the forelimbs gallop.

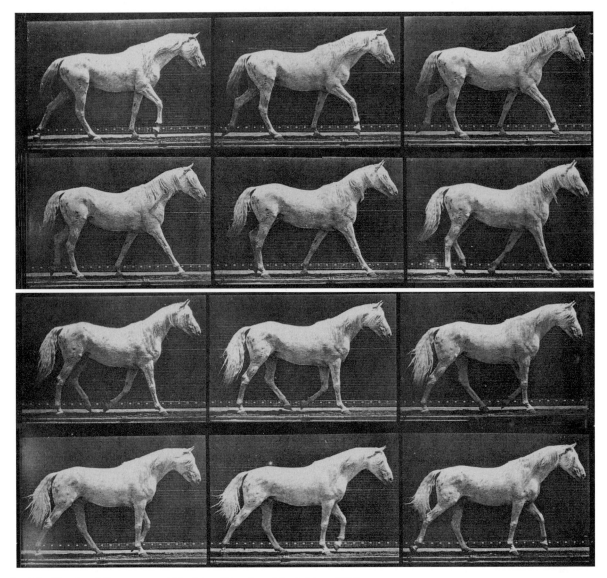

Fig. 4.3 The footfall sequence of 'Eagle' walking free (Muybridge, 1887).

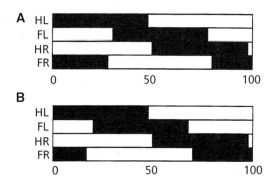

A trotter is also disqualified for pacing or galloping. With increasing speed the stride length increases linearly but interference between the hindlimb and the lateral forelimb becomes a limiting factor. A large amount of over-reaching by the hindlimbs is possible only if the hindlimbs move outside (lateral to) the forelimbs during the swing phase.

Fig. 4.4 Stick diagrams illustrating two types of footfall sequences of the toelt in Icelandic horses: diagonal couplets (**A**) and lateral couplets (**B**) (Graselli *et al.*, 1991). HL: left hindlimb; HR: right hindlimb; FL: left forelimb; FR: right forelimb.

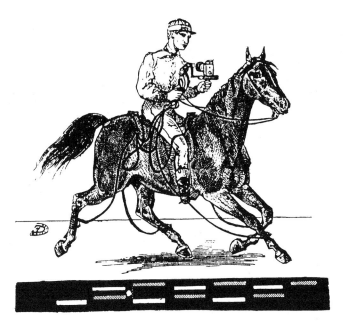

Fig. 4.5 Footfalls sequence recorded at the trot using a pneumatic gait recorder (Marey, 1873). **Fig 4.5A** (above) Horse equipped with pneumatic accelerometers attached to the limbs, saddle and tuber sacrale for measuring temporal gait parameters. The white spot indicates the suspension phase as shown on the figure.

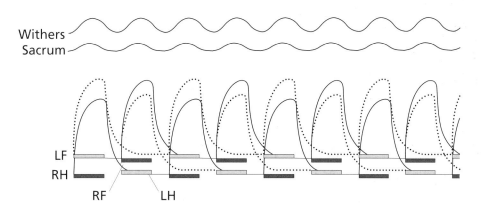

Fig. 4.5B Time-related changes in the pressure obtained from the pneumatic accelerometers at the trot (LF: left forelimb; RF: right forelimb; RH: right hindlimb; LH: left hindlimb). The shaded bars indicate the stance phase duration of each limb. The gaps between the shaded bars are the suspension phase between the diagonal supports.

The foxtrot is a 4 beat symmetric gait in which the footfalls of the diagonal limbs occur as couplets. The interval between footfalls of the fore hoof and the diagonal hind hoof is 15% of stride, compared with 35% of stride between footfalls of the hind hoof and the lateral fore hoof. During a complete stride the overlap periods were tripedal with two hindlimbs and one forelimb (8.9%), diagonal bipedal (60.6%), tripedal with one hindlimb and two forelimbs (8.9%) and lateral bipedal (21.7%) (Clayton & Bradbury, 1995).

Pace

This lateral symmetric gait is used in harness racing mainly in North America and Australia (Fig. 4.7). The maximum speed is higher than at the flying trot. At racing speed, the pace, like the trot, becomes a 4 beat

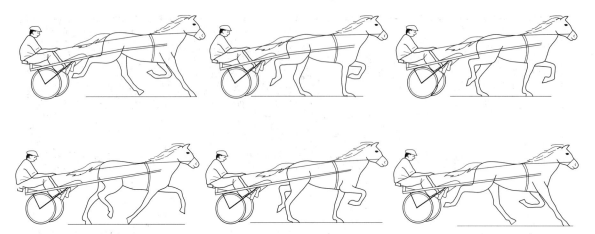

Fig. 4.6 Flying trot of a Standardbred (Drevemo *et al.*, 1980).

gait, with dissociation of the lateral limb pairs at impact and lift-off. The hindlimb contacts the ground about 26–30 ms before the lateral forelimb (Wilson *et al.*, 1988a). In comparison with the flying trot, there is less problem of limb interference at the pace because the lateral sequence avoids any contact between the ipsilateral limbs. Consequently, there are fewer coordination problems and it is easier for the horse to increase stride length. These differences may explain the higher speed records obtained by pacers: 9.4–16.0 m/s (Wilson *et al.*, 1988b) than by trotters: 11.8–14.2 m/s (Barrey *et al.*, 1995).

Canter and gallop

Canter and gallop refer to the same gait performed at different speeds: the canter is a slow speed, 3 beat gait (Fig. 4.8) and the gallop is a 4 beat gait performed at a higher speed (Fig. 4.9). At the canter, the stance phases of the diagonal limb pair (leading hind and trailing fore) are synchronized while at the gallop the footfalls of the diagonal are dissociated, with the leading hindlimb contacting the ground before the trailing forelimb. The gallop is the fastest equine gait, and is the racing gait of Thoroughbreds and Quarter Horses.

The canter and gallop show asymmetric movements of both the hind and forelimbs. There are two possible footfall sequences: right lead canter or gallop and left lead canter or gallop. Horses at liberty prefer to canter or gallop through a turn with the inside limbs leading.

The *lead change* is the transition between the footfall sequences of the right and left leads. Racehorses usually change the forelimb lead before the hindlimb lead. However, in dressage the rider can elicit the canter lead change during the suspension phase so the change is initiated in the hindlimbs. In racing the horses change leads eight or more times per mile to avoid excessive muscular fatigue due to the asymmetric work of the limbs and also to minimize the centrifugal forces as they accomodate to the curve (Leach, 1987).

At the gallop, there are two ways of coordinating the hind or fore footfalls. These are called the *transverse gallop* and the *rotary gallop* (Fig. 4.10). The transverse gallop is more frequently used by horses than the rotary gallop but the rotary sequence is observed temporarily during a lead change initiated by the forelimbs or when muscular fatigue occurs during racing. The disunited canter has the same footfall sequence as the rotary gallop except that stance phase of the lateral limbs is synchronized. It can be observed for one or more strides after a bad lead change in dressage or landing after jumping.

Jump

The jump is a gallop stride in which the airborne phase is a long dissociation of the diagonal. The footfalls of the jump stride are trailing hind and leading hind at take-off, jump suspension, then trailing fore and leading fore at landing. At take-off, the hindlimb stance phases are more synchronized than in a normal gallop stride to produce a powerful push-off. The footfalls of the forelimbs at landing are not synchronized (Leach *et al.*, 1984b). A lead change can take place during the airborne phase and, in this case, the change of forelimb placement order occurs before that of the hindlimbs. A disunited canter can be observed after the jump if the lead change of the hindlimbs does not occur immediately after the landing phase.

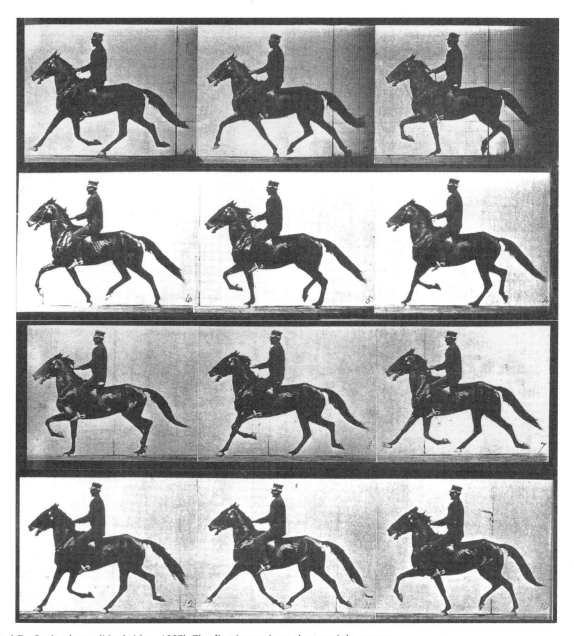

Fig. 4.7 Pacing horse (Muybridge, 1887). The first image is on the top right corner.

Gait transitions

In order to increase its velocity, the horse can switch gaits from walk to trot, from trot to canter and then extend the canter into a gallop. Each gait can be extended by changing the spatial and temporal characteristics of its strides. Ponies were shown to have a preferred speed for the trot to gallop transition and this particular speed was related to an optimal metabolic cost of running (Hoyt & Taylor, 1981). However, another experiment demonstrated that the trot–gallop transition was triggered when the peak of ground reaction force reached a critical level of about 1 to 1.25 times the body weight (Farley & Taylor, 1991). Carrying additional weight reduced the speed of the trot–gallop transition.

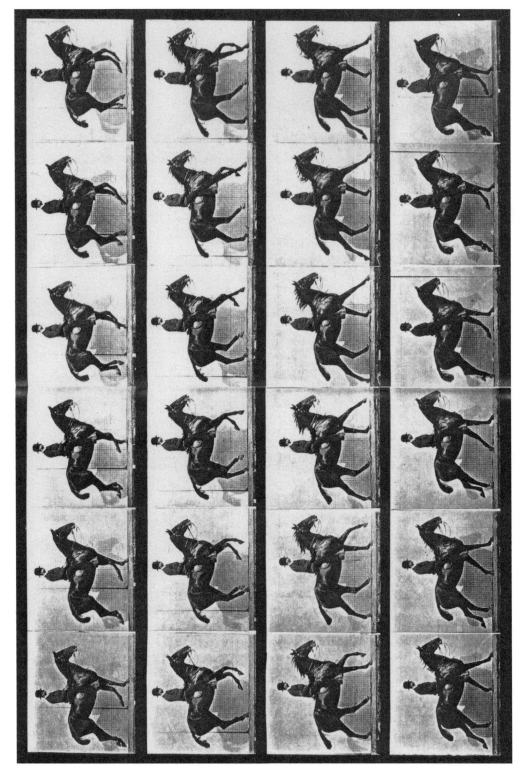

Fig 4.8 'Daisy' cantering, right lead (Muybridge, 1887). First image on the top left corner.

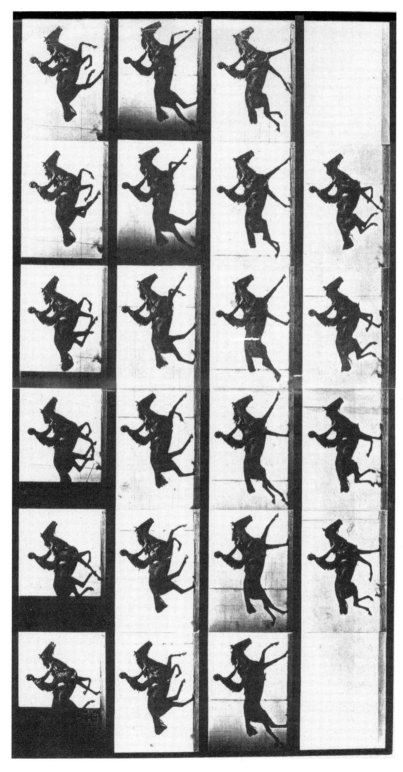

Fig. 4.9 'Bouquet' galloping, right lead (Muybridge, 1887). First image on the top left corner.

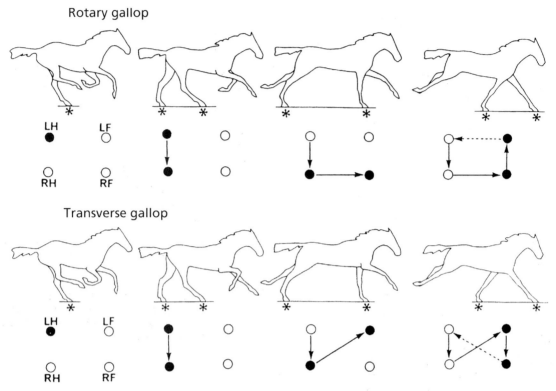

Fig. 4.10 Differences of the footfall sequences of transverse and rotary gallops (Leach, 1984b). In the rotary gallop the limbs are placed down in one of the following orders: left hind (LH), right hind (RH), right fore (RF), left fore (LF) (counterclockwise rotary gallop); RH, LH, LF, RF (clockwise rotary gallop). The term rotary is derived from the circular order in which the limbs are placed on the ground. In the counterclockwise rotary gallop illustrated the right hindlimb and left forelimb are the lead legs. In the transverse gallop the placement of limbs, and therefore the support pattern of the limbs, is transferred from the lead hindlimb diagonally to the forelimb of the opposite side, thereby transversing the body axis. As in the rotary gallops two forms of this gallop also exist, depending on the order of limb placement: LH, RH, LF, RF (right lead transverse gallop); or RH, LH, RF, LF (left lead transverse gallop). In the right lead transverse gallop illustrated the right forelimb and right hindlimb are the lead legs. The less precise terms right lead and left lead gallops are also acceptable for the right and left transverse gallops, repectively.

The footfall sequence of various gait transitions has been described by Marey (1873), Barroil (1887) and Lenoble du Teil (1893) (Fig. 4.11). Kinematic studies have described alternative footfall sequences observed in dressage horses during transitions between the walk and trot transition (Argue & Clayton, 1993a) and during the transitions between trot and canter (Argue & Clayton, 1993b).

Velocity-related changes in stride variables

To increase speed at a particular gait, the amplitude of the steps becomes larger and the duration of the limb cycle is reduced in order to repeat the limb movements more frequently. The stride frequency (SF) and stride length (SL) are the two main components of speed. The mean speed can be estimated by the product of the stride frequency and stride length:

$$\text{Speed} = \text{SF} \times \text{SL}$$

The speed-related changes in stride parameters have been studied in many horse breeds and disciplines. Stride length increases linearly with the speed of the gait (Fig. 4.12).

Stride frequency increases nonlinearly and more slowly (Dusek et al., 1970; Leach & Cymbaluk, 1986; Ishii et al., 1989) (Fig. 4.13). During rapid acceleration, such as that occuring at the start of a gallop race, the stride frequency reaches its maximum value very rapidly to produce the initial acceleration, while the maximum stride length increases more slowly to its maximum value (Hiraga et al., 1994) (Fig. 4.14).

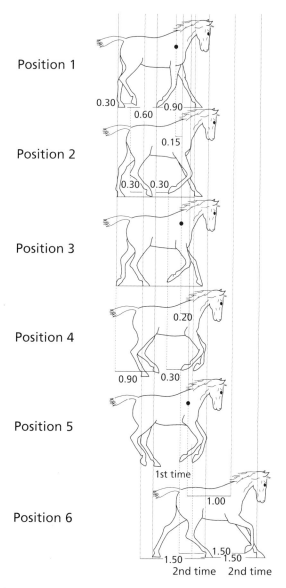

Fig. 4.11 Example of limb placement sequence during a transition from walk to canter (Barroil, 1887).

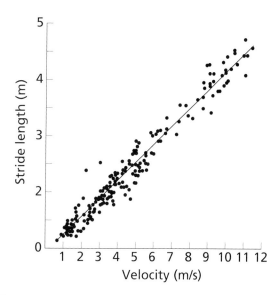

Fig. 4.12 Linear relationship between the stride length and velocity of the gaits. Data are from 6-month-old Quarter Horse foals (Leach & Cymbaluk, 1986, © American Veterinary Medical Association).

When the rider stimulated the horse with a whip, there was a reduction in the stride length and an increase in the stride frequency corresponding to a reduction of the forelimb stance phase duration. However, the velocity was not significantly influenced (Deuel & Lawrence, 1987).

GAIT DEVELOPMENT AND TRAINING EFFECT

Gait patterns are influenced by the age of the horse, but little is known about gait development. Studies in different breeds of foals have analyzed the relationship between the conformation and the stride variables in foals aged 6–8 months. In Quarter Horse foals, speed increases were obtained by a longer stride length in heavier foals and a higher stride frequency in taller foals (Leach & Cymbaluk, 1986). In Dutch Warmblood foals, the elbow, carpal and fetlock joint angle flexions were the most significant differences between the stride kinematics of individual foals (Back *et al.*, 1993). The stride and stance duration increased with age as a consequence of the increase in height but the swing duration and the protraction and retraction angles were consistent over time. The joint angle patterns recorded at 4 months and

In Thoroughbred race horses, the effects of fatigue include increases in the overlap time between the leading hindlimb and the trailing forelimb, the stride duration and the suspension phase duration (Leach & Springings, 1979). The compliance of the track surface can also influence the stride parameters when the horse is trotting or galloping at high speed. At the gallop, the stride duration tends to be reduced on a harder track surface (Fredricson *et al.*, 1983b). There is a slight increase in the stride duration on a wood-fiber track in comparison with a turf track at the same speed.

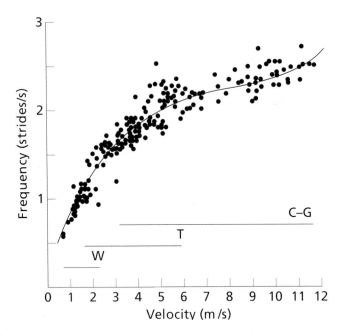

Fig. 4.13 Nonlinear relationship between the stride frequency of the gaits (Leach & Cymbaluk, 1986, © American Veterinary Medical Association). Data from 6-month- old foals. W: walk; T: trot; C–G: canter–gallop.

26 months of age were very similar. The duration of the trot swing phase, the maximal range of protraction–retraction of the limbs and the maximal flexion of the hock joint were well correlated between 4 and 26 months of age (Back *et al.*, 1994a).

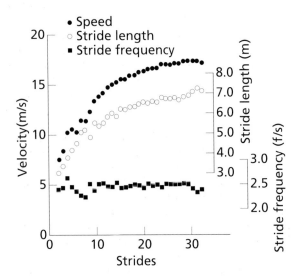

Fig. 4.14 Changes in velocity, stride frequency and stride length at the start dash in a galloping horse (Hiraga *et al.*, 1994).

The good correlations between the kinematic parameters measured in the foals and adults make it possible to assess these parameters in young horses in order to predict the gait quality of adult horses. According to the correlations with the judge scores, there are some objective indicators of good trot. A slow stride frequency with a long swing phase, a large amplitude of the scapula rotation, a maximal forelimb retraction and a maximal hindlimb protraction lead to a long stride length with a good trot. The vertical elasticity of the trot was associated with a maximal fetlock extension, a maximal stifle and tarsal flexion (Back *et al.*, 1994b). In race horses, the influence of training has been investigated in Standardbreds and Throughbreds. After 3 years of training, Standardbreds showed increases in stride length, stride duration and swing phase duration (Drevemo *et al.*, 1980). In Thoroughbreds, stride duration and stride length increased (Leach & Springings, 1979). After 8 weeks of high-intensity training on a treadmill, the stance phase duration of the Thorougbred gallop stride was reduced by 8 to 20% (Corley & Goodship, 1994).

In young saddle horses (2.5 years old), some kinematic changes were observed on a treadmill at trot after a 70-day training period for dressage and jumping (Back *et al.*, 1995). The protraction and retraction range of the forelimbs decreased and the stance duration and the flexion of the hindlimbs decreased. The engagement

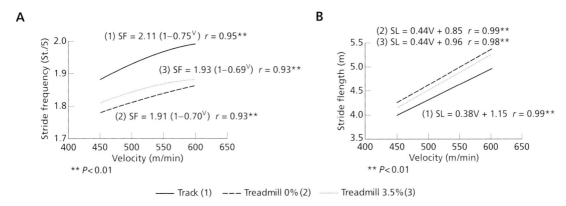

Fig. 4.15 Relationship of velocity with stride frequency (**A**) and stride length (**B**) for locomotion on a track, a flat treadmill and a treadmill with a 3.5% inclination (Barrey *et al.*, 1993b © Karger, Basel.)

increased with a maximal protraction of the hindlimbs that took place earlier in the stride cycle. The stride frequency kept constant. During the same 70-day period, the stride frequency in the control group (in pasture day and night) was reduced with a longer swing phase. The trained horses were trotting with impulsion 'on the bit' with the same stride frequency while the pastured horses were trotting in a more relaxed way with a lower stride frequency.

Dressage requires a high level of locomotor control by the rider, which is obtained progressively through exercise and collecting the gaits. A horse's ability for collection seems to be one of the main limiting factors for dressage because it is impossible to execute correctly the more complex exercises without having attained a good collected gait at trot and canter. Some locomotor parameters were identified as favoring collection ability, extended gaits and the expressiveness of the gait (Back *et al.*, 1994b; Holmström *et al.*, 1994). A slow stride frequency including a long swing phase is required for good trot quality. The elapsed time between the hindlimb contact and the diagonal forelimb contact defines the diagonal advanced placement and should be positive and high at the trot. The diagonal hindlimb should touch the ground about 30 milliseconds before the diagonal forelimb. In space, a good engagement is required: the hindlimb footfall should be placed as far as possible under the body for a good propulsion activity.

Influence of the treadmill on gait characteristics

Under laboratory conditions it is possible to study the locomotion of horses running on an experimental track or on a treadmill. The latter provides an excellent means of controlling the regularity of the gaits because the speed and slope of the treadmill belt are determined by the operator. In order to analyze the gaits without stress, some pre-experimental exercise sessions are required to accustom the horse to this unusual exercise condition (Buchner *et al.*, 1994). The horse adapts rapidly at trot, and stride measurements can be undertaken at the beginning of the third session. For the walk, however, adaptation occurs more slowly and many stride parameters are not stable even after the ninth training session. Within a session, a minimum of 5 min of walking or trotting is required to reach a steady-state locomotion.

Many locomotion studies have been performed on high-speed treadmills, since the development of the first installation of this type of machine at the Swedish University of Agricultural Science in Uppsala (Fredricson *et al.*, 1983). However, it was demonstrated experimentally that the stride length was longer on the treadmill at the trot and canter than at the same speed on a track (Barrey *et al.*, 1993a; Couroucé *et al.*, 1998) (Fig. 4.15).

The mechanical reasons for these differences are not entirely known, but some explanations have been suggested by the experimental and theoretical results. The speed of the treadmill belt fluctuates in relationship to the hoof impact on the belt (Savelberg *et al.*, 1994). The energy transfer between the hooves and the treadmill belt are not exactly the same as in overground locomotion because the belt and the hooves are driven backwards by the engine of the treadmill. During level treadmill exercise, the horse receives some mechanical energy from the treadmill. This assumption is based on the fact that the heart rate response and blood lactate concentration, which reflect the horse's workload, were lower on a tread-

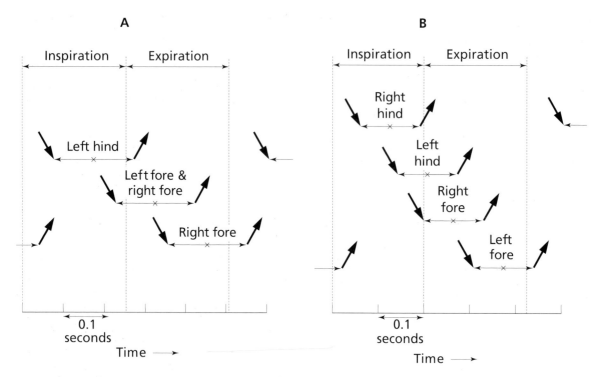

Fig. 4.16 Schematic diagrams showing the relationship between the limb cycle and the respiratory cycle at the canter (**A**) and gallop (**B**) (Attenburrow, 1982). The distances, x, represent the periods of ground contact of the feet.

mill than overground during a standardized exercise test (Valette *et al.*, 1992; Barrey *et al.*, 1993a). At a slow trot, a treadmill inclination of 6% tends to increase the stride duration and significantly increases the stance duration, more so in the hindlimbs than the forelimbs (Sloet *et al.*, 1997). Maximal fetlock extension was reduced in the forelimbs and increased in the hindlimbs on the incline, which indicated that the hindlimbs generate more propulsion on the inclined than on the flat treadmill. The inclination of the treadmill did not change stride length nor did it change the stance, swing or stride duration in a cantering Thoroughbred (Kai *et al.*, 1997).

Locomotion and respiratory coupling

Some relationships have been established between stride parameters and other physiological variables. At the canter and gallop, the respiratory and limb cycle are synchronized. Inspiration starts at the beginning of the suspension phase and ends when the trailing forelimb contacts the ground. Expiration then occurs during the forelimb stance phases (Attenburrow, 1982) (Fig. 4.16). Expiration is facilitated by compression of the rib cage between the weight-bearing forelimbs. This functional coupling of respiration to the stride cycle might be a limiting factor for

ventilation at maximal exercise intensity. At the walk, trot and pace there is no consistent coupling between the locomotor and respiratory cycles. At trot, the ratio between locomotor and respiratory frequency ranged between 1 and 3 depending on speed, duration of exercise and breed of horse (Hörnicke *et al.*, 1987; Art *et al.*, 1990). A similarly variable coupling mechanism was observed at the pace where the ratio between the stride and respiratory frequencies ranged from 1.0 to 1.5 (Evans *et al.*, 1994).

REFERENCES

Alexander, R. McN. (1984) The gait of bipedal and quadrupedal animals. *Int. J. Robotics Res*, **3**: 49–59.

Argue, C.K. and Clayton, H.M. (1993a) A preliminary study of transitions between the walk and trot in dressage horses. *Acta Anat.* **146**: 179–182.

Argue, C.K. and Clayton, H.M. (1993b) A study of transitions between the trot and canter in dressage horses. *J. Equine Vet. Sci.* **13**: 171–174.

Art, T., Desmecht, D., Amory, H. and Lekeux, P. (1990) Synchronization of locomotion and repiration in trotting ponies. *J. Vet. Med. A* **37**: 95–103.

Attenburrow, D.P. (1982) Time relationship between the respiratory cycle and limb cycle in the horse. *Equine Vet. J.* **14**: 69–72.

Back, W., van den Bogert, A.J., van Weeren, P.R., Bruin, G. and Barneveld, A. (1993) Quantification of the locomotion of Dutch Warmblood foals. *Acta Anat.* **146**: 141–147.

Back, W., Barneveld, A., Schamhardt, H.C., Bruin, G. and Hartman, W. (1994a) Longitudinal development of the kinematics of 4-, 10-, 18- and 26-month-old Dutch Warmblood horses. *Equine Vet. J.* **17**(Suppl.): 3–6.

Back, W., Barneveld, A., Bruin, G., Schamhardt, H.C. and Hartman, W. (1994b) Kinematic detection of superior gait quality in young trotting warmbloods. *Vet. Quart.* **16**: S91–96.

Back, W., Hartman, W., Schamhardt, H.C., Bruin, G. and Barneveld, A. (1995). Kinematic response to a 70 day training period in trotting Dutch Warmbloods. *Equine Vet. J.* **18** (Suppl.): 127–131.

Barebeau, H. and Rossignol, S. (1987). Recovery of locomotion after chronic spinalisation in the adult cat. *Brain Res.* **412**: 84–95.

Barrey, E. and Desbrosse, F. (1996) Lameness detection using an accelerometric device. *Pferdeheilkunde* **12**: 617–622.

Barrey, E., Galloux, P., Valette, J.P., Auvinet, B. and Wolter, R. (1993a). Stride characteristics of overground versus treadmill locomotion in the saddle horse. *Acta Anat.* **146**: 90–94.

Barrey, E., Auvinet, B. and Couroucé, A. (1995) Gait evaluation of race trotters using an accelerometric device. *Equine Vet. J.* **18**(Suppl.): 156–160.

Barrey, E., Galloux, P., Valette, J.P.., Auvinet, B. Wolter, R. (1993b) Determination of the optimal treadmill slope for reproducing the same cardiac response in saddle horses as overground exercise conditions. *Vet Rec.* **133**: 183–185

Barroil, E. (1887) L'art équestre de haute école d'équitation: traité pratique. J. Rothschild Ed., fig. 31.

Buchner, H.H.F., Savelberg, H.H.C.M., Schamhardt, H.C., Merkens, H.W. and Barneveld, A. (1994) Habituation of horses to treadmill locomotion. *Equine Vet. J.* **17**(Suppl.): 13–15.

Burns, T.E. and Clayton, H.M. (1997), Comparison of the temporal kinematics of the canter pirouette and collected canter. *Equine Vet. J.* **23**(Suppl.): 58–61.

Cazalets, J.R., Borde, M. and Clarac, F. (1996) The synaptic drive from the spinal locomotor network to motoneurons in the newborn rat. *J. Neuroscience* **16**: 298–306.

Clayton, H. (1997) Classification of collected trot, passage and piaffe based on temporal variables. *Equine Vet. J.* **23** (Suppl.): 54–57.

Clayton, H.M. (1989) Terminology for the description of equine jumping kinematics. *J. Equine Vet. Sci.* **9**: 341–348.

Clayton, H.M. (1994). Comparison of the collected, working, medium and extended canters. *Equine Vet. J.* **17** (Suppl.): 16–19.

Clayton, H.M. (1995) Comparison of the stride kinematics of the collected, medium and extended walks in horses. *Am. J. Vet. Res.* **56**: 849–852.

Clayton, H.M. and Bradbury, J.W. (1995) Temporal characteristics of the foxtrot: a symmetrical equine gait. *Appl. Anim. Behav. Sci.* **42**: 153–159.

Collins, J.J. and Stewart, I.N. (1993) Coupled nonlinear oscillators and the symmetries of animal gaits. *J. Nonlinear Sci.* **3**: 349–392.

Corley, J.M. and Goodship, A.E. (1994) Treadmill training induced changes to some kinematic variables measured at the canter in Thoroughbred fillies. *Equine Vet. J.* **17**(Suppl.): 20–24.

Couroucé, A., Geoffroy, O., Barrey, E. and Rose, R.J. (1999). Comparison of exercise tests on different tracks and on an uninclined treadmill in French trotters. *Equine Vet. J.* **30**(Suppl.): 528–532.

Deuel, N.R. and Lawrence, L.M. (1984) Computer-drawn gait diagrams. *J. Equine Vet. Sci.* **4**: 228–229.

Deuel, N.R. and Lawrence, L.M. (1987) Individual variation in the quarter horse gallop. In: Gillespie, J.R. and Robinson, N.E. (eds) *Equine Exercise Physiology*, 2nd edn. J. Davis: ICEEP Publications, pp. 564–573.

Deuel, N.R. and Lawrence, L.M. (1987) Effect of urging by the rider on equine gallop stride limb contacts. *Proc. 10th Equine Nutrit. Physiol. Symp.*, pp. 487–492.

Drevemo, S., Dalin, G., Fredricson, I. and Hjerten, G. (1980) Equine locomotion 3: the reproducibility of gait in Standardbred trotters. *Equine Vet. J.* **12**: 71–73.

Dusek, J., Ehrlein, H.J., von Engelhardt, W. and Hornicke, H. (1970) Beziehungen zwischen trittlange, trittfrequenz und geschwindigkeit bei Pferden. *Zeitschrift fur Tierzuechtung und Zuechtungsbiologie* **87**: 177–188.

Evans, D.L., Silverman, E.B., Hodgson, D.R., Eaton, M.D. and Rose, R.J. (1994). Gait and respiration in Standardbred horses when pacing and galloping. *Res. Vet. Sci.* **57**: 233–239.

Farley, C.T., Taylor, C.R. (1991) A mechanical trigger for the trot-gallop transition in horses. *Sciences* **253**: 306–308

Forssberg, H., Grillner, S., Halbertsma, J. and Rossignol, D. (1980a) The locomotion of low spinal cat. 1. Coordination within a hindlimb. *Acta Physiol. Scand.* **108**: 269–281.

Forssberg, H., Grillner, S., Halbertsma, J. and Rossignol, D. (1980b) The locomotion of low spinal cat. 2. Interlimb coordination. *Acta Physiol. Scand.* **108**: 282–295.

Fredricson, I., Drevemo, S., Dalin, G. *et al.* (1983a) Treadmill for equine locomotion analysis. *Equine Vet. J.* **15**: 111–115.

Fredricson, I., Hellander, J., Hjertén, J., Drevemo, S., Björne, K., Dalin, G. and Eriksson, L.E. (1983b) Galloppaktion II – Basala gangartsvariabler i relation till banunderlag. *Svensk Veterinärtidning* **35**(Suppl. 3): 83–88.

Grasselli, A., Grasselli, R. and Iotti, P. (1991) Quantitative analysis of 4-beat leral gaits. In: *Proc. 42nd Ann. Meet. EAAP*, 8–12 September, Berlin, H4–2, pp. 558–559.

Habib, M. (1989) Organisation de la motricité. In: Habib, M. *Bases neurologiques des Comportements.* (ed.) Paris: Masson, pp. 63–80.

Hildebrand, M. (1965) Symmetrical gaits of horses. *Science* **191**: 701–708.

Hiraga, A., Yamanobe, A. and Kubo, K. (1994) Relationships between stride length, stride frequency, step length and velocity at the start dash in a racehorse. *J. Equine Sci.* **5**: 127–130.

Holmström, M., Fredricson, I. and Drevemo, S. (1994). Biokinematic differences between riding horses judged as good and poor at the trot. *Equine Vet. J.* **17**(Suppl.): 51–56.

Holmström, M., Fredricson, I. and Drevemo, S. (1995). Variation in angular pattern adaptation from trot in hand to passage and piaffe in the Grand Prix dressage horse. *Equine Vet. J.* **17**(Suppl.): 51–56.

Hörnicke, H., Meixner, R. and Pollmam, U. (1987) Respiration in exercising horses. In: Snow, D.H., Persson, S.G.B. and Rose, R.J. (eds) *Equine Exercise Physiology*. Cambridge: Granta Editions, pp. 7–16.

Hoyt, D.F. and Taylor, C.R. (1981). Gait and energetics of locomotion in horses. *Nature* **292**: 239.

Ishii, K., Amano, K., and Sakuraoka, H. (1989). Kinetics analysis of horse gait. *Bull. Equine Res. Inst.* **26**: 1–9.

Kai, M., Hiraga, A., Kubo, K. and Tokuriki, M. (1997). Comparison of stride characteristics in a cantering horse on a flat and inclined treadmill. *Equine Vet. J.* **23**(Suppl.): 76–79.

Leach, D.H. (1987). Locomotion of the athletic horse. In: Gillespie, J.R. and Robinson, N.E. (eds) *Equine Exercise Physiology*, 2nd edn. Davis: ICEEP Publications, pp. 516–535.

Leach, D.H. (1993) Recomended terminology for researchers in locomotion and biomechanics of quadrupedal animals. *Acta Anat.* **146**: 130–136.

Leach, D.H. and Cymbaluk, N.F. (1986) Relationship between stride length, stride frequency, velocity and morphometrics of foals. *Am. J. Vet. Res.* **47**: 2090–2097.

Leach, D.H. and Springings, E.J. (1979) Gait fatigue in the racing Thoroughbred. *J. Equine Med. Surg.* **3**: 436–443.

Leach, D.H., Ormrod, K. and Clayton, H.M. (1984a). Standardised terminology for the description and analysis of equine locomotion. *Equine Vet. J.* **16**: 522–528.

Leach, D.H., Ormrod, K. and Clayton, H.M. (1984b) Stride characteristics of horses competing in Grand Prix jumping. *Am. J. Vet. Res.* **45**: 888–892.

Leach, D.H., Springings, E.J. and Laverty, W.H. (1987). Multivariate statistical analysis of stride-timing measurements of nonfatigued racing Thoroughbreds. *Am. J. Vet. Res.* **48**: 880–888.

Lenoble du Teil (1893). *Les Allures du Cheval Dévoilées par la Méthode Expérimentale.* Paris and Nancy: Berger Levrault, pp. 192–211.

Massion, J. (1997) Locomotion. In: Massion, J. (ed.) *Cerveau et Motricité?* Paris: Presses Universitaires de France, Collections Pratiques corporelles, pp. 67–87.

Marey, E.J. (1873) In: Marey, E.J. (ed.) *La Machine Animale: Locomotion Terrestre et Aérienne,* 2nd edn. Paris: Coll. Bibliothèque Science Internationale, Librairie Gerner Baillère et Cie, pp. 145–186.

Muybridge, E. (1887) *Muybridge's Complete Human and Animal Locomotion,* Vol. 3. (Republication of *Animal Locomotion*). New York: Dover Publications.

Savelberg, H.H.C.M., Vostenbosch, M.A.T.M., Kamman, E.H., van de Weijer, J. and Schamhardt, H.C. (1994) The effect of intra-stride speed variation on treadmill locomotion. *Proc. 2nd World Congr. Biomechan.,* Amsterdam.

Sloet van Oldruitenborgh-Oosterbaan, M.M., Barneveld, A. and Schamhardt, H.C. (1997) Effect of treadmill inclination on kinematics of the trot in Dutch Warmblood horses. *Equine Vet. J.* **23**(Suppl.): 71–75.

Valette, J.P., Barrey, E., Auvinet, B., Galloux, P. and Wolter, R. (1992) Comparison of track and treadmill exercise tests in saddle horses: a preliminary report, *Annale de Zootechnie* **41**: 129–135.

Wilson, B.D., Neal, R.J., Howard, A. and Groenendyk, S. (1988a) The gait of pacers: I. Kinematics of the racing stride. *Equine Vet. J.* **20**: 341–346.

Wilson, B.D., Neal, R.J., Howard, A. and Groenendyk, S. (1988b) The gait of pacers: II. Kinematics of the racing stride. *Equine Vet. J.* **20**: 347–351.

5

Intra-limb Coordination: the Forelimb and the Hindlimb

Willem Back

INTRODUCTION

Since the 1960s, horses have become increasingly popular for use in sport and recreation and there are a wide range of equestrian sports that test various aspects of the horse's athletic ability. The movements of the four limbs are coordinated to produce the recognizable gaits. During each stride the fore and hindlimbs act to absorb concussion, to overcome the effects of gravity and to provide propulsion. This is achieved through alternating stance and swing phases. During the stance phase, the limbs push against the ground to create the forces that are necessary for support and propulsion of the body mass. During the swing phase the limbs are protracted in preparation for the next stance phase. This chapter reviews the locomotor functions of the fore and hindlimbs.

Man domesticated *Equus* to benefit from the capabilities of the equine locomotor apparatus. Several types of horses have been produced by selective breeding. Heavy draught horses were selected to haul heavy guns and to carry medieval knights with their cumbersome and extremely bulky armour, whereas slender, faster Arabians and Thoroughbreds were selected for their speed and endurance. The invention of the steam engine at the end of the 18th century marked the beginning of the industrial revolution and the decline of the horse's importance as a source of power. One and a half centuries later the horse was definitively overtaken as an essential element of warfare, agriculture and civil transport, and after World War II the number of horses markedly declined. As farms became more mechanized, horses were replaced by tractors and it is symbolic that mechanical power, until very recently, was expressed as horsepower. However, in the 1960s the horse regained popularity, particularly for riding purposes in sport

and leisure, a development that was favored by the growing economies and relative wealth of the post-war era. Since then, horse breeders have primarily produced performance horses that have been selected for an elegant gait and efficient jumping technique. These horses, which are referred to as Warmbloods, are used in dressage and jumping competitions. Today's sport horses are described as 'equine athletes' which again emphasizes the importance of their locomotor apparatus.

QUANTIFICATION

The locomotor performance of the horse can be quantified using modern computerized gait analysis equipment (Clayton, 1991). Force plates are used to study the external load on the limb (kinetics) during the stance phase (Merkens & Schamhardt, 1994), whereas joint motion (kinematics) is evaluated not only during the stance but also during the swing phase. Markers are glued to the skin overlying certain anatomical landmarks to facilitate the analysis by representing different limb segments. The movements of the limbs can then be evaluated from the excursions of these markers and the error introduced by skin displacement over the anatomical landmarks should be taken into account (van Weeren, 1989). Videographic and optoelectronic systems use special hardware and computer programs to automate much of the analysis (see chapter 3 for more details).

The most representative evaluations of sport horses are made when the horses are performing over ground in their normal manner. However, speed affects both the kinematics and kinetics (Leach & Drevemo, 1991; Peham *et al.*, 1998). The treadmill is a useful tool for evaluating limb movement under controlled conditions and at constant speed. The treadmill also enables the investigator to record many strides without moving the recording equipment. Therefore, the intra-individual variation between strides is minimal. After three sessions, the horse becomes just more or less habituated to the treadmill, but should be 'warmed up' on the device before every recording session (Buchner *et al.*, 1994a). Although in theory, treadmill and overground locomotion should be similar when the speed is constant (van Ingen Schenau, 1980), treadmill locomotion appears to differ slightly, both kinematically (Buchner *et al.*, 1994b) and metabolically (Barrey *et al.*, 1993; Sloet & Barneveld, 1995b). The stance duration (expressed as a percentage of total stride) is longer and the maximal retraction angle of the limbs is greater in treadmill than in overground locomotion (Buchner *et al.*, 1994b). The horizontal hoof velocity is not constant during the stance phase (Buchner *et al.*, 1994b; Back *et al.*, 1995e), and treadmill locomotion appears to be slightly less energy consuming for horses than overground locomotion. Similar heart rate and lactate levels as during overground exercise can be achieved by inclining the treadmill (Barrey *et al.*, 1993) or increasing speed (Sloet & Barneveld, 1995b). Psychological factors and the lack of air resistance also affect recordings on a treadmill.

The most important gait for selection of sport horses is the trot (Podhajsky, 1981; Clayton, 1994a). At the speed of 4 m/s horses of all ages move on a treadmill at a comfortable though demanding trot that can be used to evaluate the stride characteristics (Back *et al.*, 1994a). Podhajsky (1981) suggested that the ideal gait and speed to train a horse overground under saddle is the trot at 3.75 m/s, which is between the speeds recorded for the working and medium trot in dressage competition (Clayton, 1994a; Sloet & Clayton, 1999). The same speed has also been used to analyze the gait of Standardbreds and Thoroughbreds (Drevemo *et al.*, 1987; Herring *et al.*, 1992).

Kinematic and ground reaction force data provide useful information describing the limb movements and the forces responsible for those movements, but they do not describe the internal forces in the limbs. This type of information can be calculated using a link segment model of the limb. In a two-dimensional link segment model, each limb segment is represented as a solid bar with its center of mass being located relative to the co-ordinates that define the segment. The input for the model comprises kinematic and force data that are synchronized in time and space. They are combined with segment morphometric data using an inverse dynamics solution to compute net joint moments and joint powers (Colborne *et al.*, 1997a,b). The net joint moment represents the net torque acting around a joint, which is pro-

duced primarily by the soft tissues (muscle, tendon and ligament). Joint power measures the rate of mechanical energy generation and absorption across a joint. Discrete bursts of positive and negative work can be quantified as the area under the positive and negative phases, respectively, of the power curve. The joint power is calculated as the product of the joint moment and that joint's angular velocity. The value is positive, indicating mechanical energy generation, when the net joint moment acts in the same direction as the angular velocity of the joint. Power generation occurs when the muscle shortens as it generates tension (concentric contraction). The joint power is negative and mechanical energy is absorbed when the net joint moment acts in the opposite direction to the angular velocity of the joint, so the muscle lengthens as it generates tension (eccentric contraction). During power absorption the muscles restrain joint movement in opposition to gravity or an other external force.

This chapter gives a detailed description of the motions and functions of the limbs during trotting. The findings for the trot are compared with those for the walk and the canter. To aid in visualizing equine intra-limb coordination patterns, the fore and hindlimbs are graphically represented using stick figures and joint angle–time diagrams, which have been extracted from the kinematic recordings of riding horses, Standardbreds and Thoroughbreds (Fredricson & Drevemo, 1972; Fleiss *et al.*, 1984; Martinez-del Campo *et al.*, 1991; Holmström *et al.*, 1994a, Back *et al.*, 1994a; Degueurce *et al.*, 1997). Back *et al.* (1995a) used standardized procedures to make graphical representations of fore and hindlimb kinematic data from a large group of warmblood horses (Fig. 5.1, Table 5.1) The variability between individual horses was evaluated, and the effect of correcting for skin displacement on joint angle–time diagrams was illustrated. The joint angle–time diagrams were analysed simultaneously with corresponding stick figures and marker diagrams to create a complete picture of equine forelimb and hindlimb motion at the trot that could be related to limb function (Back *et al.*, 1995a). Net joint moments and power that were recently described to calculate the mechanical work and energy transfer (Colborne *et al.*, 1997a,b; Clayton *et al.*, 1998), will also be discussed in this chapter.

FORELIMB COORDINATION

The joints of the horse's forelimb from the elbow distally are more or less constrained to move in a sagittal plane. Only limited information is available describing movements of the forelimb in directions other than the sagittal plane (Thompson *et al.*, 1992; Degueurce *et al.*, 1996).

Table 5.1A Anatomical locations of the markers on the forelimb and the hindlimb as depicted in Fig. 5.1.

Marker	Anatomical location
1	Hoof at heel region
2	Hoof at toe region
3	Hoof at coronary band
4	Distal metacarpus
5	Proximal metacarpus
6	Distal radius at lateral styloid process
7	Proximal radius at collateral ligament elbow
8	Distal humerus at lateral epicondyle
9	Proximal humerus at caudal greater tubercle
10	Distal scapular spine
11	Proximal scapular spine
12	Tuber coxae
13	Proximal femur at cranial greater trochanter
14	Distal femur at lateral epicondyle
15	Proximal tibia at fibular head
16	Distal tibia at lateral malleolus
17	Proximal metatarsus
18	Distal metatarsus
19	Hoof at coronary band
20	Hoof at toe region
21	Hoof at heel region

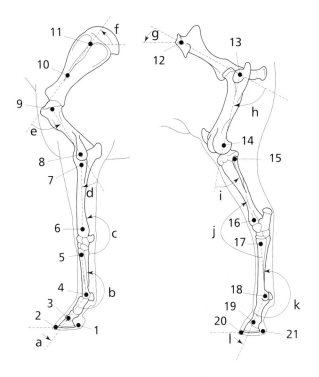

Fig. 5.1 Schematic representation of the anatomical locations of markers on the skin and the calculations of forelimb and hindlimb joint angles. The arrows indicate the positive direction of movement (Back *et al.*, 1995a,b).

Table 5.1B Calculation of the joint angles of the forelimb and the hindlimb as depicted in Fig. 5.1.

Angle	Joint representation
a	Fore coffin
180 – b	Fore fetlock
180 – c	Carpus
d	Elbow
e	Shoulder
f	Scapula rotation
g	Pelvis rotation
h	Hip
i	Stifle
180 – j	Tarsus
180 – k	Hind fetlock
l	Hind coffin

Moments of force in joints of the forelimb have been calculated during the stance phase at the trot for the distal joints (Hjertén & Drevemo, 1993) and for all the joints of the forelimb during the stance (Clayton *et al.*, 1998) and swing (Lanovaz *et al.*, 1999) phases. Therefore the following section describes the sagittal plane motion and power flow of the forelimb in detail (Figs 5.2A, 5.3A, 5.4A, 5.5A, 5.6A and Table 5.2A).

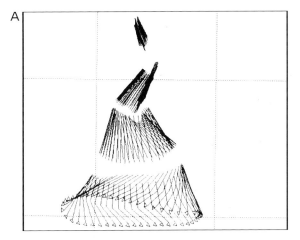

Fig. 5.2A Stick figure of a complete stride of the forelimb of an individual horse trotting on a treadmill at a speed of 4 m/s (Back *et al.*, 1995a).

Table 5.2A Characteristic timing points in the mean joint angle–time curves of the forelimb of a group of horses at the trot (4m/s, Back et al., 1995a).

Code[*]	Characteristic joint action	Time (% of total stride)
	STANCE	
a	Maximal carpal extension	7.6
b	Maximal coffin stance flexion	15.2
c	Maximal fetlock extension	21.5
d	Maximal coffin extension (= heel lift)	36.6
e	Fetlock angle at i.g.c.[**] (= toe lift)	40.3
	SWING	
f	1st maximal fetlock flexion	46.8
g	1st maximal fetlock extension	56.3
h	Maximal carpal flexion	62.1
i	2nd maximal fetlock flexion	73.7
j	2nd maximal fetlock extension	84.6
k	3rd maximal fetlock flexion	87.0

[*] codes a–k correspond with the events illustrated in Fig. 5.5A

[**] i.g.c.: initial ground contact

Description of limb motion

Scapula

The *scapular* rotation shows a sinusoidal pattern during protraction and retraction. Maximal protraction of the forelimb precedes initial ground contact, and maximal retraction occurs just after the end of the stance phase. Angle–time curves before and after correction for skin displacement are similar, except for an inflection in the curve at mid-swing before correction; this dip appeared to represent a moment of maximal protraction after correction for skin displacement.

Shoulder

The *shoulder* joint is almost fully extended at initial ground contact, but during loading the joint flexes maximally. This flexion peak was visible before and after correction for skin displacement, but in the later parts of the stride, skin movement completely dominates joint motion characteristics. Therefore, it is not possible to describe in detail the various peaks in the angle–time curve of this joint at the end of the stance phase and during the swing phase. The net joint moment at the shoulder joint shows peaks on the cranial and caudal aspects in early stance, followed by a cranial (flexor) moment that is sustained until lift-off. The long head of the triceps brachii is biarticular, exerting an extensor moment

at the elbow and a flexor moment at the shoulder. The latter is more than compensated by the biceps brachii and other extensors of the shoulder to produce a net extensor moment at the shoulder throughout most of the stance phase. The power profile suggests elastic energy storage and release in early stance, followed by active propulsion in terminal stance. Early in the swing phase, an extensor moment at the shoulder joint brings the brachial segment (and possibly the entire limb) forward. As the shoulder starts to extend just before mid swing, the joint moment moves to the flexor side. The flexor moment at the shoulder then works to slow the extension of the shoulder joint and to decelerate the rotation of the proximal limb.

Elbow

At the beginning of the stance phase, the *elbow* joint extends, then flexes until just after mid stance, after which it extends to its maximum near the end of the stance phase. During the swing phase it undergoes a flexion cycle. The amplitudes of maximal flexion and extension of the elbow do not appear to be influenced much by skin displacement, but the flexion peak occurs somewhat earlier in the swing phase. The net joint moment at the elbow joint acts predominantly on the caudal (extensor) side during most of the stance phase, to resist collapse of the joint under the influence of gravity. This is probably due to the action of the triceps brachii which shows electromyographic activity at this time (Korsgaard 1982; Tokuriki et al., 1989). The net joint moment shifts to the cranial side of the elbow in the second half of stance. The power profile shows a phase of power absorption peaking in early stance, followed by an almost equal phase of power generation peaking around mid stance, which appears to represent elastic energy storage and release. In the swing phase, the elbow joint shows a different pattern from all other joints. During the first half of swing, elbow flexion is primarily responsible for folding the limb, and during most of this time the net joint moment is on the flexor side of the joint. Therefore, elbow flexors such as the brachialis muscle (Tokuriki et al., 1989) are working to actively flex the joint during the first half of swing. There is a short period at mid swing when the elbow is still flexing after the net joint moment has moved to the extensor side coinciding with the activation of the triceps brachii (Korsgaard, 1982; Tokuriki et al., 1989) and, later, the flexor carpi ulnaris (Korsgaard, 1982; Jansen et al., 1992). The action of the extensors slows flexion of the joint and then reverses its direction of motion. In the later part of swing, the extensor moment at the elbow actively extends the limb in preparation for ground contact.

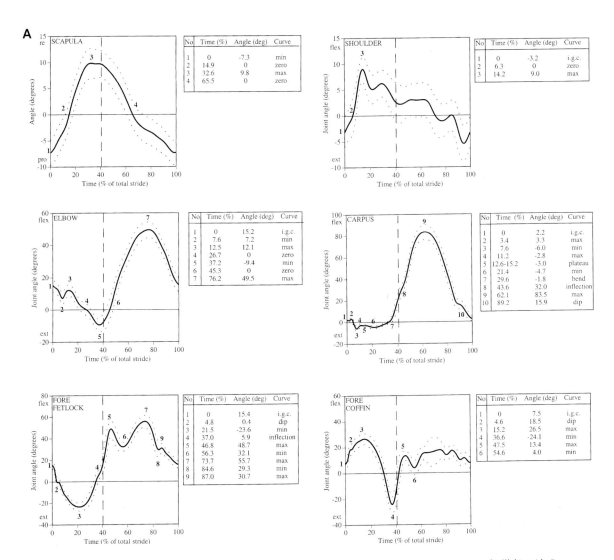

SCAPULA

No	Time (%)	Angle (deg)	Curve
1	0	-7.3	min
2	14.9	0	zero
3	32.6	9.8	max
4	65.5	0	zero

SHOULDER

No	Time (%)	Angle (deg)	Curve
1	0	-3.2	i.g.c.
2	6.3	0	zero
3	14.2	9.0	max

ELBOW

No	Time (%)	Angle (deg)	Curve
1	0	15.2	i.g.c.
2	7.6	7.2	min
3	12.5	12.1	max
4	26.7	0	zero
5	37.2	-9.4	min
6	45.3	0	zero
7	76.2	49.5	max

CARPUS

No	Time (%)	Angle (deg)	Curve
1	0	2.2	i.g.c.
2	3.4	3.3	max
3	7.6	-6.0	min
4	11.2	-2.8	max
5	12.6-15.2	-3.0	plateau
6	21.4	-4.7	min
7	29.6	-1.8	bend
8	43.6	32.0	inflection
9	62.1	83.5	max
10	89.2	15.9	dip

FORE FETLOCK

No	Time (%)	Angle (deg)	Curve
1	0	15.4	i.g.c.
2	4.8	0.4	dip
3	21.5	-23.6	min
4	37.0	5.9	inflection
5	46.8	48.7	max
6	56.3	32.1	min
7	73.7	55.7	max
8	84.6	29.3	min
9	87.0	30.7	max

FORE COFFIN

No	Time (%)	Angle (deg)	Curve
1	0	7.5	i.g.c.
2	4.6	18.5	dip
3	15.2	26.5	max
4	36.6	-24.1	min
5	47.5	13.4	max
6	54.6	4.0	min

Fig. 5.3A Mean joint angle–time diagrams of the forelimb of a group of horses trotting on a treadmill (4 m/s). Data are presented as mean ±SD (···). The horizontal zero line indicates the joint angle of the square standing horse. The vertical dashed line marks the transition from stance to swing phase (i.g.c.: initial ground contact; re: retraction; pro: protraction; flex: flexion; ext: extension. Back *et al.*, 1995a).

Carpus

The *carpal* joint, which is slightly flexed at initial ground contact, rapidly extends in early stance. After a plateau and a second extension peak at mid stance, it starts to flex and before the end of the stance phase initiates a rapid flexion that reaches its maximum via a slight inflection. There is a flexion cycle during the swing phase and as the joint extends in preparation for initial ground contact, the curve shows another deviation. Correction for skin displacement did not significantly alter the curve. A palmar (flexor) moment is present at the carpus throughout most of stance, peaking around mid stance. There are small bursts of positive and negative power during the stance phase but, compared with the other forelimb joints, the carpus plays only a small role in energy generation and absorption in the stance phase. A functional similarity between the equine carpus and the human knee has been identified (Colborne *et al.*, 1997a,b). During the early swing phase, carpal flexion is slowed by an extensor moment that is most likely due to a combination of passive structures and activation

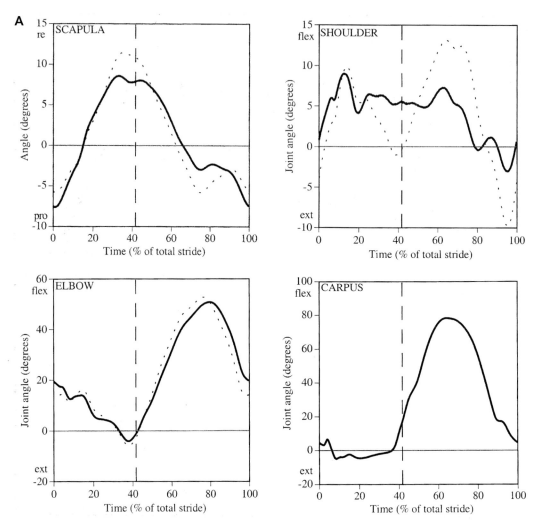

Fig. 5.4A Mean joint angle–time diagrams of the forelimb of an individual horse recorded at trot at a speed of 3 m/s on a treadmill before (–) and after (···) correction for skin displacement (Back *et al.*, 1995a).

of the extensor carpi radialis (Korsgaard 1982; Jansen *et al.*, 1992). In mid swing, the moment at the carpus moves to the flexor side and the joint begins to extend. The flexor moment increases during the last one-third of swing as the flexor carpi ulnaris is activated (Korsgaard, 1982). The net action of both the flexor and extensor joint moments at the carpus during the swing phase is to control, rather than initiate, the joint motion.

Fetlock

Just after initial ground contact, the *fetlock* joint rapidly extends to a plateau, then extends again during early

stance to reach its maximal value at mid stance. Just before hoof lift there is an inflection. During the swing phase the joint shows two flexion peaks separated by a slight extension, but towards the end of the swing phase its rapid extension is abruptly stopped. Correction for skin displacement does not change the fetlock joint pattern. The net joint moment at the fetlock joint acts on the palmar (flexor) side of the joint during the entire stance phase peaking around mid stance. This reflects the supporting role of the palmar soft tissues as the fetlock joint extends during weight acceptance then flexes for push off. The superficial digital flexor tendon, deep digital flexor tendon and suspensory ligament experience peak strains around mid stance (Riemersma *et al.*,

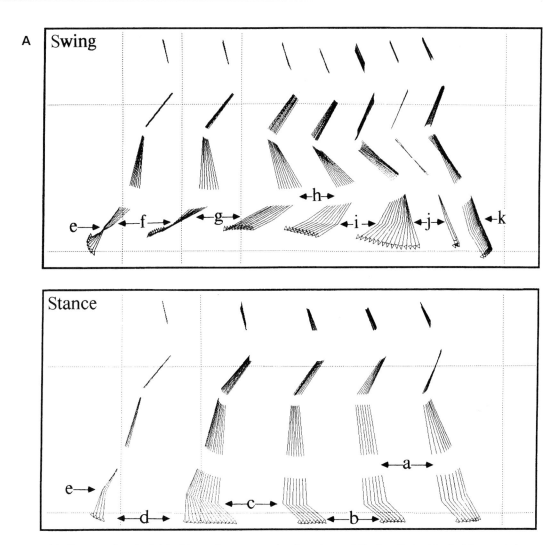

Fig. 5.5A Stick diagram of an individual horse in stance and swing phase of the forelimb at typical time points characterized a–k (see Table 5.2A; Back *et al.*, 1995a).

1988a,b), which corresponds with the time of maximal extension of the fetlock joint and its maximal palmar moment. Both the superficial and deep digital flexor muscles contract actively in the first half of the stance phase (Korsgaard, 1982) to increase tension in their tendons and provide a palmar moment at the distal joints. The proximal and distal accessory ligaments provide mechanisms for passive support, generating a palmar moment in the later part of stance.

The power profile of the fetlock during stance shows almost equal amounts of negative and positive work, which is typical of elastic energy storage and release. Energy is absorbed in the first half of stance as the flexor tendons and suspensory ligament store elastic energy

and is later released as a result of elastic recoil. During the swing phase, the fetlock joint initially has a small dorsal moment, which moves to the palmar aspect in mid swing. Like the coffin joint, the fetlock appears to be inertially driven in early swing, with input from the deep and superficial digital flexor muscles and tendons in late swing.

Coffin

The *coffin* joint curve shows an inflection during the rapid loading of the limb at the beginning of the stance phase, with maximal flexion occurring just before mid stance. At the end of the stance phase, the joint flexes

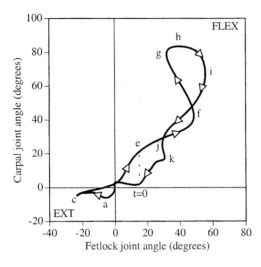 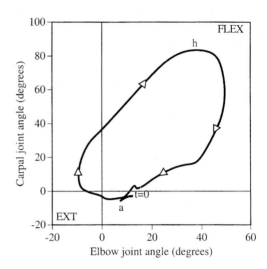

Fig. 5.6A Angle–angle diagrams of the forelimb of a group of horses trotting on a treadmill (4 m/s). The characters a–k indicate typical time points (see Table 5.2A; Back *et al.*, 1995a).

rapidly from its maximally extended position at heel lift to a flexion peak at the beginning of the swing phase. The rest of the swing phase consists of some oscillatory movements, which are highly individual and variable. Peaks during mid swing can be caused by markedly out-of-plane movements (Back *et al.*, 1995a). The net coffin joint moment acts on the palmar (flexor) side of this joint throughout the stance phase, peaking at 63% stance. The net palmar moment is due to tension in the deep digital flexor tendon acting through its distal accessory ligament combined with tension in the navicular system. The extensor branches of the suspensory ligament are taut to control hoof placement and prevent buckling of the interphalangeal joints in the early 25% stance, and this contributes to a balancing force on the dorsal side of the joint in early stance. The palmar moment at the coffin joint is responsible for hoof rotation during breakover. In the early swing phase there is a small extensor moment at the coffin joint. Since there is little evidence of activity in the extensor muscles at this time (Korsgaard, 1982; Jansen *et al.*, 1992), this can be interpreted as a passive effect of the tendinous and ligamentous structures working to slow the flexion of the joints after lift off. As the limb extends during the later part of the swing phase, the coffin joint extends under the influence of a flexor moment, which can be attributed to activation of the deep digital flexor muscles during the last half of swing (Korsgaard, 1982; Jansen *et al.*, 1992). The flexor moment slows joint extension prior to initial ground contact.

The predominant feature of the power curve at the coffin joint is a burst of power beginning one-third of the way through the stance phase and continuing into breakover as the coffin joint extends against a palmar moment and acts as an energy damper. Peak power absorption coincides with the maximal longitudinal ground reaction force (GRF). Strain gauge studies have indicated that strain in the distal accessory ligament increases as the coffin and fetlock joints extend, peaking at the start of breakover (Riemersma *et al.*, 1988a,b), which also coincides with peak power absorption at the coffin joint.

Functional interpretation

The body is lower than its standing height throughout the trot stride which decreases the necessary potential energy and results in a more efficient gait. The forelimb can be considered as moving like a pendulum with a rotation point in the proximal part of the scapula, as was previously reported by Krüger (1938). The muscles acting on the proximal segments initiate the protraction and retraction of the forelimb and the distal part of the limb follows passively. At mid swing phase the proximal limb reduces velocity and even temporarily stops rotating, while the distal limb advances to maximal protraction. Then the proximal limb completes its forward swing. In this way, by changing angular momentum between proximal and distal segments, energy is conserved (Hildebrand, 1987).

Another way the horse increases the efficiency of gait is by using its tendons as elastic springs (Dimery *et al.*, 1986). The weight of the horse on the forelimb results in extension of the fetlock joint (Schauder, 1952), which loads the suspensory ligament, the superficial and deep flexor tendons, and their respective accessory ligaments. Elastic energy is stored during loading, which can be used later in the stride, thereby conserving energy. In trotting horses, the fetlock is the main site of elastic energy storage and release during the stance phase, with the shoulder, elbow and carpal joints showing some elastic behavior (Clayton *et al.*, 1998).

It has even been suggested that the swing of the forelimb is mainly passive due to the release of elastic energy stored in tendon springs. This view is supported by the finding that EMG signals are low during the majority of this period (Korsgaard, 1982; Tokuriki *et al.*, 1989; Jansen *et al.*, 1992). In man, it has been calculated that when the limb gains an initial velocity at the beginning of the swing phase, the remaining part of the swing phase is completed under the action of inertia (Mochon & McMahon, 1980). These phenomena (tendons acting as springs, role of inertia) increase the efficiency of locomotion.

At the end of the stance phase, unloading of the flexor tendons in the distal limb causes an upward movement of the distal metacarpus which initiates carpal flexion. Maximal flexion of the carpal and fetlock joints occurs synchronously. When the limb further retracts, the extending elbow joint passes its angle value at square stance and thereby increases the load on the biceps brachii muscle. After hoof lift the elastic rebound of the biceps brachii assists the brachialis muscle in producing elbow flexion. Similarly, the elastic rebound of the serratus ventralis muscle may support protraction of the scapula (Smythe *et al.*, 1993). These phenomena can be reproduced in a horse under general anaesthesia in lateral recumbency. When the forelimb is pulled caudally with a fully extended carpal joint, a complete, passive swing similar to the normal protraction follows, after lifting the hoof artificially. Moreover, from clinical experience it is known that a horse with a low radial nerve paralysis is able to walk by using this passive pendulum capacity. However, a horse suffering from a rupture of the extensor carpi radialis tendon will stumble and fall at the trot, because it is not able to protract its forelimb in time. Indeed, EMG activity of the extensor carpi radialis muscle is concentrated at the beginning of the swing phase (Jansen *et al.*, 1992). This suggests that this muscle, due to its biarticular nature, has an important function in supporting the flexion of the elbow joint and in initiating the forward swing of the limb during the swing phase. Furthermore, the extensor carpi radialis muscle acts to control carpal flexion in early swing

(Colborne *et al.*, 1997a,b): a horse with a ruptured extensor carpi radialis tendon, when walking, will hyperflex its carpal joint during swing. Again this can be illustrated in a horse under general anaesthesia in lateral recumbency: an artificially flexed carpal joint always snaps back into its stable extended position.

Fetlock flexion just after toe-off may be principally seen as an elastic phenomenon due to the loading of the flexor tendons. After this phase, fetlock flexion can be fully explained by inertial forces: the dip in the joint flexion is merely but a relative extension of the fetlock due to the rapid flexion of the carpal joint. When the carpal flexion decelerates, fetlock flexion increases again.

The extension of the carpal joint in the second half of the swing phase can also be attributed at least in part to inertia. The abrupt manner in which both the carpal, but even more strikingly the fetlock joint curve, show an abrupt cessation of extension at the end of the swing phase, illustrates the passive motion properties of the distal forelimb once again. The passive swing caused by inertial forces is halted by anatomical constraints.

Just before initial ground contact, the extension of the elbow joint leads to synchronous extension of the carpal and fetlock joints. This is more than a merely passive phenomenon, because EMG activity of the extensor carpi radialis and common digital extensor muscle at that time has been recorded by Jansen *et al.* (1992). However, this phenomenon can also be reproduced *in vitro*. There is a certain passive component because the common digital extensor tendon extends the distal joints when the elbow is extended. The spring-like action of tendons results in a 'smooth' gait, but also serves as a shock absorber in the coffin, fetlock, elbow and shoulder joints at the time of ground contact at the beginning of the stance phase (Schauder, 1952).

At the same time, however, the carpal joint seems to be important in supporting the forelimb, which acts like a propulsive strut (Smythe *et al.*, 1993). At initial ground contact the carpal joint is still slightly flexed at slow trotting speeds, but then quickly snaps into its overextended position and remains with minimal oscillations in this stable position during the majority of the stance phase. At higher speeds the carpal joint snaps into a stable position at the end of the swing phase just before initial ground contact (Back *et al.*, 1993a 1995a; Johnston *et al.*, 1997). The rapid transition from slight flexion to overextension in the slow trot is also visible as a marked dip in the elbow joint angle and a change in the slope of the shoulder joint angle, while the course of the fetlock and coffin joint curves also change sharply.

Some researchers have found a corresponding deviation from the regular build-up of force in the pattern of the vertical GRF at the trot (Merkens & Schamhardt,

1994), while others have described shortening of the limb at the distal radius and the proximal metacarpus (Hjertén & Drevemo, 1993). All these phenomena are closely connected to the above-mentioned changes in joint angles, which cause limb length to be reduced, thereby damping the rapid build-up of force at impact (Back *et al.*, 1995e; Johnston *et al.*, 1995). Moreover, extension of the carpal joint invariably leads to extension of the elbow and flexion of the fetlock joint, assuming that the humerus and hoof are fixed. In normal loading situations, the deep palmar carpal ligament prevents the carpal joint from hyperextension. However, it is generally accepted that at the end of the race, the fatigued Thoroughbred is at serious risk of developing chip fractures of the carpal bones due to hyperextension of the carpal joint (Johnston *et al.*, 1999).

Some authors stressed the importance of the so-called clicking phenomenon (Alexander & Trestik, 1989). *In vitro* experiments on dissection specimens have shown that the eccentric attachments of the collateral ligaments relative to their rotation axis makes the joint bistable: it springs either into full extension or strong flexion. Functions attributed to this phenomenon include storage of elastic energy (Rooney, 1990) and the damping of oscillations (Mosimann & Micheluzzi, 1969). The moments required to produce this phenomenon *in vitro* are so small compared to those occurring *in vivo* that if clicking plays a role at all, it must be during the swing phase when the limb is not loaded. We can only speculate whether the inflection in the carpal joint curve at the onset of swing and synchronous with the first fetlock flexion peak is related to this phenomenon and thus enables rapid movement (Palmgren, 1929) contributing to the elegance of gait (Alexander & Trestik, 1989).

During most of stance at the trot the net joint moment is on the caudal/palmar side of all joints except the shoulder (Clayton *et al.*, 1998). Both the elbow and shoulder joints show phases of elastic energy storage and release in the middle part of the stance phase, followed by a propulsive function at the shoulder in the later part of stance. The carpus does not appear to play an important role in energy absorption or propulsion. The fetlock acts as a spring, showing energy storage in the first half of stance followed by an almost equal amount of energy generation in the second half of stance. The coffin joint acts as an energy damper. Interestingly energy absorption at the coffin joint is almost equal to energy generation at the shoulder joint. During the swing phase (Lanovaz *et al.*, 1999), all the forelimb joints initially have the net joint moment on the cranial/dorsal side of the joint, which is the extensor side for all joints except the elbow. The cranial/dorsal moments gradually decrease and move to the caudal/palmar between

Summary

Thus, the kinematics of the equine forelimb at the trot can be analyzed and presented as joint angle–time curves, angle–angle curves, stick figures and marker displacement diagrams. Characteristic peak amplitudes in the joint angle–time diagrams can be related to the motion and power flow of the whole limb, which can be applied in studies that try to quantify objectively gait quality and the effect of training, for example.

35–52% of the swing phase in the various joints. The peak magnitudes of the net joint moments decrease in a proximal to distal direction, with those at the shoulder and elbow joints being several times larger than those at the more distal joints. The moments in the proximal limb are indicative of muscular activity accelerating the limb forward during the first 30 to 40% of the swing phase, then decelerating the forward swing of the upper limb segments. At the elbow the net joint moments actively flex and extend the joint during swing, which has the effect of raising and lowering the distal limb. The large magnitude of the moments in the proximal joints suggests muscular input. The low net joint moments at the distal joints are consistent with their motion being primarily a result of inertial forces during the first half of swing augmented by flexor muscle activity during the latter part of swing as the limb is prepared for ground contact. All of the net joint moments, except those at the elbow, act to slow the motion of the joint (eccentric muscular activity). Therefore, the elbow joint drives the forelimb movements during the swing phase at the trot.

HINDLIMB COORDINATION

Although kinematic gait analysis of the equine hindlimb has been performed since the early part of this century (Walter, 1925; Krüger, 1938), the development of the computer gave new impetus to this field of research, both in the area of clinical applications (Fleiss *et al.*, 1984; Kobluk *et al.*, 1989; Martinez-del Campo *et al.*, 1991; Back *et al.*, 1995b) and in computer simulation studies (van den Bogert & Schamhardt, 1993). The reciprocal apparatus, which couples the stifle and tarsal joint motion, has been one of the main subjects of study (Strubelt, 1928; Molenaar, 1983; Wentink, 1978b; van Weeren *et al.*, 1990). Back *et al.* (1995b) standardized the graphical presentation of kinematic data of the equine hindlimb by use of joint angle–time diagrams in a large group of horses. The kinematic information can be combined with ground reaction forces and morphometric data to calculate net joint moments and joint powers to give a more complete description of the functional aspects of the equine hind limb. (Figs 5.2B, 5.3B, 5.4B, 5.5B, 5.6B and Table 5.2B).

Description of limb motion

Hip

The *hip* joint shows a more or less sinusoidal flexion and extension pattern. Maximal extension occurs just before the end of the stance phase, and maximum flexion near the end of the swing phase. After correction for skin displacement, the pattern hardly changes but the range of motion is twice as high as that deduced from skin markers only.

Stifle

At initial ground contact the *stifle* joint is rapidly flexed during loading. At the end of the stance phase the joint seems to be flexed, but this is an artifact due to skin displacement. Correction for skin displacement also reveals that maximal flexion of the stifle joint appears somewhat later and is more pronounced than suggested by the skin marker data.

Tarsus

The *tarsal* joint is also rapidly flexed at the beginning of the stance phase and reaches a flexion peak. Just before the end of the stance phase, the tarsal joint is maximally extended. In the swing phase, there is a flexion peak approximately at mid swing via an inflection just after passing its angle value at square stance in early swing. Correction for skin displacement reveals only minor differences between the curves before and after correction.

Fetlock

Just after initial ground contact, the *fetlock* joint is rapidly extended via a typical inflection to reach its maximal extension at mid stance. The slope changes just before lift-off, and the joint reaches its first maximal flexion peak early in the swing phase. There is a slight extension in mid swing, followed by a second flexion peak. At the end of the swing phase, the joint extends towards initial ground contact. No differences are found between the curves before and after correction for skin displacement.

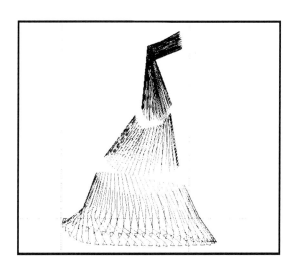

Fig. 5.2B Stick figure of a complete stride of the hindlimb of an individual horse trotting on a treadmill at a speed of 4 m/s (Back *et al*., 1995b).

Table 5.2B Characteristic timing points in the mean joint angle–time curves of the hindlimb of a group of horses at the trot (4 m/s, Back *et al*., 1995b).

Code[*]	Characteristic joint action	Time (% of total stride)
	STANCE	
a	Maximal tarsal stance flexion	9.6
b	Maximal coffin stance flexion	17.0
c	Maximal fetlock extension	23.7
d	Maximal coffin extension (= heel lift)	35.8
e	Fetlock angle at i.g.c.[**] (= toe lift)	40.6
	SWING	
f	Maximal fetlock flexion	53.9
g	Maximal stifle flexion	69.1
h	Maximal tarsal flexion	73.2

[*] codes a–k correspond with the events illustrated in Fig. 5.5B
[**] i.g.c.: initial ground contact

Coffin

The *coffin* joint curve demonstrates a typical inflection during the rapid loading phase of the limb at the beginning of the stance phase. Peak flexion occurs just before mid stance. Maximal extension occurs at heel lift. In the swing phase the joint flexes rapidly via a small flexion peak to reach peak flexion at mid swing. It then extends to initial ground contact (Back *et al*., 1995b).

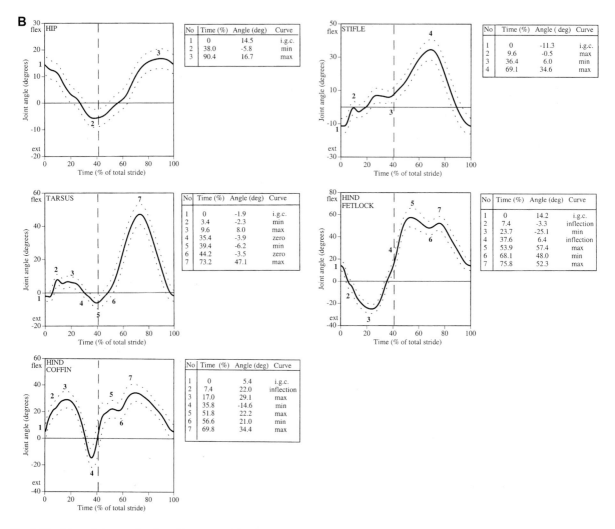

Fig. 5.3B Mean joint angle–time diagrams of the hindlimb of a group of horses trotting on a treadmill (4 m/s). Data are presented as mean ±SD (···). The horizontal zero line indicates the joint angle of the square standing horse. The vertical dashed line marks the transition from stance to swing phase (i.g.c.: initial ground contact; re: retraction; pro: protraction; flex: flexion; ext: extension. Back *et al.*, 1995b).

Limited information is available at the present time describing the net joint moments and joint powers for the hindlimb at the trot. During the stance phase the net joint moment is on the flexor (plantar) aspect of the coffin and fetlock joints, peaking around mid stance. At the tarsal joint the extensor (plantar) moment peaks around or just before mid stance, and moves to the flexor aspect during breakover. Both the stifle and hip joints have a flexor moment that peaks in the first half of stance and changes to an extensor moment in the second half of stance. At the coffin joint the joint power is close to zero during the first one third of stance, after which power is

absorbed on the flexor aspect as the joint extends against a flexor moment. During breakover, energy is generated on the plantar aspect as the joint is actively flexed. The fetlock joint shows elastic behavior during stance with a period of energy absorption followed by energy generation on its flexor side. The tarsal joint also behaves elastically during the stance phase, but the power profile is close to zero during breakover. The stifle and hip joints generate energy on their flexor aspects during much of the stance phase. However, the stifle shows a period of energy absorption on its extensor aspect that controls flexion of the joint during breakover.

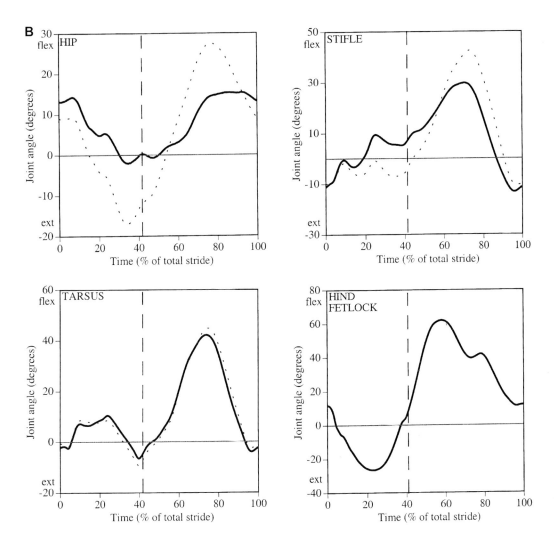

Fig. 5.4B Mean joint angle–time diagrams of the hindlimb of an individual horse recorded at trot at a speed of 3 m/s on a treadmill before (–) and after (···) correction for skin displacement (Back *et al.*, 1995b).

Functional aspects

The stick figure of a horse trotting on a treadmill shows that the hindlimb, like the forelimb, can be considered to move like a pendulum with a rotation point in the acetabulum, because the hip joint–time curve and the cranio-caudal movement of the marker on the distal metatarsus during a complete stride are similar. The latter curve is similar to that of the distal metacarpus (Back *et al.*, 1995a), although the maximal protraction in the hindlimb occurs almost 10% later in the stride than in the forelimb. This phenomenon is in accordance with the results of Holmström *et al.* (1994a) in four Swedish Warmbloods ridden overground at the trot. The involve-

ment of pelvic rotation in hindlimb motion is minimal in the sagittal plane as the pelvis maintains a fairly constant angle relative to the horizon. However, pelvic rotation in the transverse plane is considerable in the stance and swing phases. During a complete stride the body remains below its level when the horse is standing squarely, which is similar to findings in the forelimb (Back *et al.*, 1995a). This decreases the necessary potential energy and thus results in a more efficient gait.

In the hindlimb the horse increases its efficiency of gait by using its tendons as energy-conserving elastic springs (Dimery *et al.*, 1986). The stored elastic energy is released during the second half of the stance phase, contributing to propulsion and flexion of the joints during

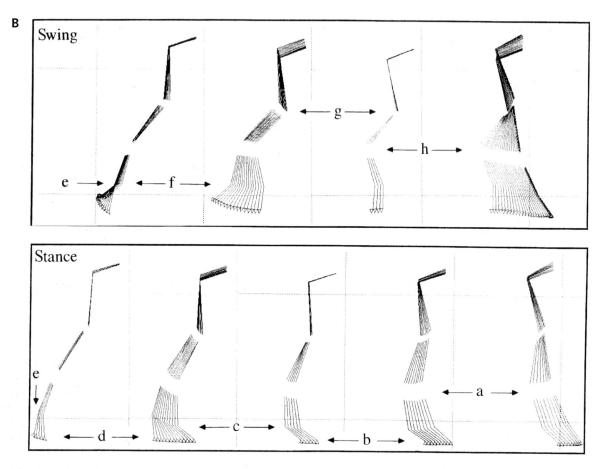

Fig. 5.5B Stick diagram of an individual horse in stance and swing phase of the hindlimb at typical time points characterized a–k (see Table 5.2B; Back *et al.*, 1995b).

the swing phase. The stifle and tarsal joints, with their synchronous flexion peaks, also contribute to the shock absorbing capacities of the hindlimb. At the same time there is an inflection in the curves of the fetlock and coffin joint. These events correspond with the interruption in the build-up of the vertical ground reaction force at the trot (Merkens & Schamhardt, 1994), though it is much less pronounced in the hindlimb than in the forelimb. The net effect of these changes in joint angles is to reduce the distance from hip to hoof (Hjertén *et al.*, 1994). In computer simulations of hindlimb movement, the dip in the fetlock angle just after initial ground contact could be reproduced by integrating the natural oscillating movements of the masses of the body and the limb (van den Bogert & Schamhardt, 1993).

It has been suggested that the swing of the hindlimb is merely passive due to the release of elastic energy stored in these tendons. This view is supported by the finding that EMG signals are low during the swing phase (Wentink, 1978a; Jansen *et al.*, 1992; Tokuriki & Aoki, 1995). Only at the beginning of the swing phase is fetlock flexion actively supported by the deep digital flexor, while the long digital extensor flexes the tarsus, and the gastrocnemius flexes the stifle (Jansen *et al.*, 1992). As in the forelimb, loading of the suspensory ligament and the deep and superficial digital flexor tendons during the stance phase is important for fetlock flexion. In the hindlimb the strain build-up in the superficial flexor tendon during the stance phase contributes to stifle flexion, while the loaded interosseus facilitates the upward movement of the distal part of the metatarsal bone at the end of the stance phase. At that time the distal metatarsus acts as a moment arm that further extends the tarsal joint and increases the loading of the peroneus tertius/tibialis cranialis muscle. This is similar to the mechanism described for the biceps brachii tendon,

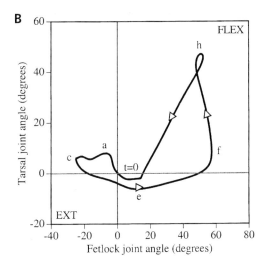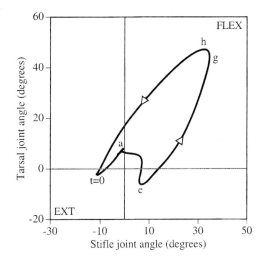

Fig. 5.6B Angle–angle diagrams of the hindlimb of a group of horses trotting on a treadmill (4 m/s). The characters a–k indicate typical time points (see Table 5.2B; Back *et al.*, 1995b).

when the elbow joint passes its zero value at the end of the stance phase (Back *et al.*, 1995a). At the beginning of the swing phase, the release of elastic energy greatly supports tarsal and stifle flexion (Wentink, 1978b), which occur synchronously, since these joints are coupled by the reciprocal apparatus. Van Weeren *et al.* (1990) showed that correction for skin displacement could explain the discrepancies between the *in vitro* coupling of stifle and tarsal joint and the *in vivo* kinematic measurements. Some minor discrepancies had to be explained by stretching of the tendons especially at faster gaits. In attempting to explain these discrepancies, Molenaar (1983) assigned functional significance to the various insertions of the peroneus tertius in shifting of tension between axial and abaxial insertions.

It is known that experimental cutting of only the peroneus tertius does not influence the function of the reciprocal apparatus and thus does not visually affect the walking ability of the horse (Strubelt, 1928; Schamhardt *et al.*, 1985), although Wentink (1978b) recorded some slight hyperextension at the end of stance and less flexion of the tarsal joint at swing. Locomotor disturbance only becomes visible when both peroneus tertius and tibialis cranialis tendons are cut (Wentink, 1978b and personal communication).

Besides the coupling of stifle and tarsal joints, this study also demonstrated a coupling between flexion and extension of tarsal and fetlock joints in the swing phase. The second flexion peak of the fetlock and coffin joints

is synchronized with maximal stifle and tarsal flexion. Furthermore, constant rate of extension in the angle–angle diagram of tarsal and fetlock joints suggests that these joints are also coupled during extension. The fetlock has to flex when the stifle and tarsal joints flex because the action of the entirely tendinous superficial digital flexor tendon is passive (Molenaar, 1983). At the end of the swing phase, when the stifle and tarsal joints are extended, the fetlock joint is also extended due to the action of the long digital extensor tendon and the lengthening of the limb. This is in contrast to what was found in the forelimb, where the fetlock joint was extended by the force of inertia (Back *et al.*, 1995a). The spring action and coupling mechanism in the hindlimb can be reproduced in a horse under general anesthesia in lateral recumbency. After the hindlimb is flexed, it jumps back to its initial fully extended position as soon as the limb is released. During the synchronous flexion of the joints in the hindlimb, the motion of the fetlock joint appears to be stabilized by the extensor and flexor tendons. Alexander and Trestik (1989) stated that the typical inflections found in joint angle–time curves of the tarsal joint *in vitro* indicated the time at which a labile equilibrium was passed and the joint clicked out of this equilibrium to rapidly flex or extend. It remains to be proven whether the inflection found in the first part of the swing phase of the tarsal joint, which coincided with the first flexion peak of the fetlock, is really the result of this clicking phenomenon and thus contributes to an elegant gait (Alexander & Trestik, 1989).

Summary

As in the forelimb, characteristic peaks in the hindlimb joint angle–time diagrams were related to the motion of the whole limb as represented by the stick figures. The joint angle and angle–angle diagrams of the tarsal and fetlock joints are considered to give the most reliable description of equine hindlimb motion in kinematic studies aimed at objectively quantifying gait.

FORE vs HIND DISTAL LIMB COORDINATION

In today's sport horses, more lameness develops in the forelimbs than in the hindlimbs (3:1), and 95% of forelimb lameness is localized in the carpus or distal to that joint (Stashak, 1987). The greater concussion of the forelimb at impact, as subjectively evaluated with the clinical eye, has been suggested to be a mechanical predisposing factor for development of chronic lameness in the distal portion of the forelimb (Stashak, 1987). High-frequency oscillations at the beginning of the stance phase have been recorded, using a force plate in the forelimbs and hindlimbs of walking and trotting horses (Schamhardt & Merkens, 1994). These impact oscillations are dampened by the hoof and transmitted proximally through structures of the distal portion of the limb. Horses with signs of pain in the distal forelimbs and shod with orthopedic 'damping' shoes appear to trot more comfortably and have decreased peak vertical impact oscillations, as recorded by an accelerometer (Benoit at al., 1993).

Back et al. (1995e) found that, although the fore and hind distal limb are anatomically similar, they have different angles, velocities and accelerations at the beginning of the stance phase (Fig. 5.7A,B,C). Hoof accelerations can be measured directly or calculated by double differentiation of positional data, which has the advantage that correction for differences in the orientation of the accelerometers, as occurring during the stance and swing phase, is not necessary. The absolute value of the peak vertical acceleration of the fore hoof at the beginning of the stance phase determined from the kinematics (Back et al., 1995e) was similar to the value recorded by use of a calibrated accelerometer on a treadmill surface (Barrey et al., 1991). Therefore, both methods appear to be valid for studying hoof impact.

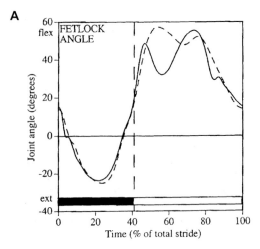

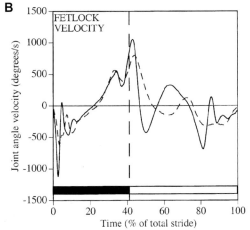

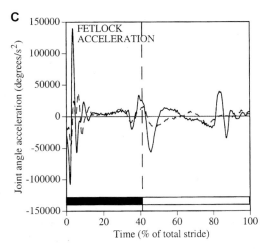

Fig. 5.7 Diagrams of fetlock joint angle–time **(A)**, fetlock joint angular velocity–time **(B)** and angular acceleration-time **(C)** of the fore and hindlimb fetlock joints of a group of treadmill trotting horses ■ stance phase, □ swing phase (Back et al., 1995e).

It appears that the front hoof becomes flat on the ground earlier than the hind hoof, because the hind hoof has a greater angle at impact than the fore hoof during both overground and treadmill locomotion (Merkens & Schamhardt, 1993; Schamhardt & Merkens, 1994; Back et al., 1995e). The metacarpus has a significantly larger impact angle than the metatarsus (Clayton, 1994a; Back et al., 1995e), but the fetlock angle at impact is similar between the forelimbs and hindlimbs.

The timing of the horizontal and vertical oscillations of the hoof at the beginning of the stance phase shows differences in force plate as well as in optoelectronic tracings (Merkens & Schamhardt, 1993; Schamhardt & Merkens, 1994; Back et al., 1995e). Within approximately 3% of total stride duration, the hoof angle of both the forelimb and hindlimb is zero, and the vertical velocity and acceleration of the hoof are stationary. However, it is not until approximately 6% of the total stride duration that the horizontal velocity and acceleration of the hoof reach zero. The vertical and horizontal accelerations of the hooves at impact result in oscillations in the fetlock acceleration–time diagram, which are visible until 14% of stride duration in the forelimbs and hindlimbs.

The amplitude of the vertical velocity at impact and the peak acceleration are significantly greater in the fore hoof than in the hind hoof both on the treadmill and overground (Back et al., 1995e; Johnston et al., 1995, 1996). However, on the treadmill the hoof landing phenomenon in the horizontal direction is more difficult to understand owing to the cranio-caudally moving belt. It might be easier for interpretation to add the treadmill speed to the observed hoof velocity data. The horizontal deceleration appears to be greater in the hindlimb than in the forelimb. In normal movements, the maximal friction force is proportional to the vertical force. Transposing this phenomenon to the sliding of the hoof, the positive horizontal hoof acceleration peak, immediately after the vertical hoof acceleration peak, is related to the moment at which the vertical acceleration or force starts to decrease. At that time, friction temporarily decreases, allowing the hoof to slide a little faster over the ground surface before the horizontal hoof acceleration is reduced to zero. This interaction between vertical and horizontal accelerations of the hoof, as suggested by kinematics, was also found between F_z and F_y forceplate tracings at the trot (Dow et al., 1991). Thus, the landing velocity of the hoof seems to be related to these differences in acceleration: the front hoof, with a higher vertical hoof velocity, bounces more at impact, whereas the rear hoof, with a higher horizontal velocity, shows more sliding (Back et al., 1995e; Johnston et al., 1995, 1996).

During the stance phase, the fetlock angle can be considered as a kinematic expression of the load on the limb (Riemersma et al., 1988a,b; Johnston et al., 1999). In the forelimb, the fetlock extends more rapidly at the beginning of the stance phase than in the hindlimb, because the angular velocity is significantly higher in the forelimb (Back et al., 1995e; Johnston et al., 1996). During this rapid extension, the fetlock curve of the forelimb has a sharp dip, whereas in the hindlimb the dip had a smoother appearance. This discontinuity in fetlock extension is related to the rapid maximal extension of the carpal joint in the forelimb and stance flexion of the tarsal joint in the hindlimb (Back et al., 1995a,b; Johnston et al., 1995, 1996). These angular movements begin at about the same time as the friction force peaks in the front and rear hooves. This phenomenon is also connected with a rapid decrease in limb length to reduce impact (Hjérten & Drevemo, 1993; Hjérten et al., 1994), which is evident from the considerable decrease in angular acceleration in the fetlock between the first and second set of minimal and maximal acceleration peaks. It has been reported that, in horses with subclinical tendon lameness, the slope of a similar inflection in the vertical ground reaction force curve was higher, probably to smooth force build up in the fetlock (Dow et al., 1991). Similarly, this dip became less pronounced when a coir mat, instead of a stiffer and less flexible rubber treadmill belt, was used (Roepstorff et al., 1994). Also the slopes of the vertical and horizontal force curves at the beginning of the stance phase are less steep on the coir mat treadmill. Apparently, ground reaction force (F_z) and friction force (F_y) interactions at the hoof are reflected in the smoothness of the fetlock curve.

Concussion can be seen in the fetlock as the combination of rapid joint loading and peak oscillations in joint movement. Both variables are significantly higher in the forelimb than in the hindlimb in almost all horses. Apparently, this phenomenon already occurs when horses are young, probably starting just after birth and is repeated every time the hoof hits the ground. When the horse enters a more intense training program, normal shoeing, which usually protects the hooves against excessive wear, and riding on hard surfaces amplify the accelerations of the hoof at impact (Barrey et al., 1991; Benoit et al., 1993). However, the higher accelerations recorded at the hoof wall may not be transmitted to the bones of the limb (Willemen et al., 1999) perhaps because the hoof tissues act as a low pass filter (Lanovaz et al., 1998). In addition, the weight of the rider increases the impulsive loading, especially on the forelimb at the beginning of the stance phase (Schamhardt et al., 1991; Sloet et al., 1995a).

Repetitive impulsive loading in combination with rapid oscillations in the joint, even within physiologic limits, plays a mechanical role in the development of osteoarthrosis (Radin *et al.*, 1991). Therefore, the kinematic differences between the distal forelimb and hindlimb might be related to the higher incidence of chronic lameness in the forelimbs.

The Walk

When the locomotor apparatus of a horse has to be judged for a purchase examination or studbook selection sales, locomotion both at walk and trot on a loose shank are evaluated. The walk and trot are both symmetrical gaits, but they differ in inter-limb coordination. The walk is a 4 beat gait with a lateral sequence of limb placements in which there is always at least one fore and one hind foot on the ground. The trot is a 2 beat gait with the limbs moving by diagonal pairs. The diagonal support phases are separated by periods in which all feet are off the ground (Alexander & Jayes, 1978).

In the literature stick figures and joint angle–time diagrams for the walk have been reported for individual horses (Walter, 1925; Krüger, 1937, 1938; Fleiss *et al.*, 1984) and groups of Warmblood and Andalusian horses at walk and trot (Back *et al.*, 1996b, Galisteo *et al.*, 1996). Back *et al.* (1996b) objectively evaluated whether kinematics of the walk (1.6 m/s) are related to the locomotor characteristics at the trot (4 m/s) (Fig. 5.8A,B, Table 5.3A,B).

Apparently, walk and trot kinematics are similar with regard to the intra-limb coordination pattern, stance distance and swing duration (Back *et al.*, 1996b). Kinematic differences, however, are caused by the fact that the trot is a faster gait than walk, so the limb shows the same movements in a shorter time. The less powerful push off in the walk is reflected by decreased fore and hindlimb fetlock extension combined with less carpal extension and tarsal flexion during the stance phase, leading to less retraction in the hindlimbs. Force plate recordings show smaller vertical ground reaction forces at the walk compared to the trot (Ueda *et al.*, 1981; Merkens & Schamhardt, 1994; Schamhardt & Merkens, 1994).

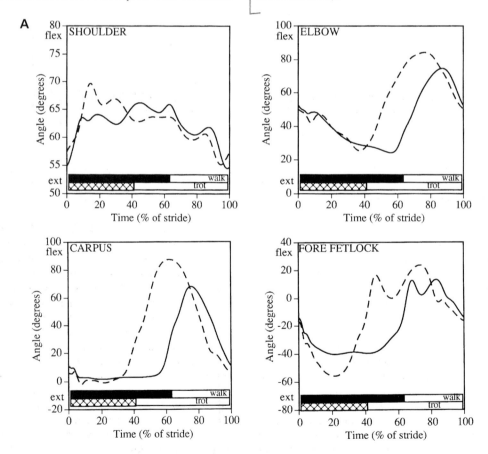

Fig. 5.8A Mean joint angle–time diagrams of the forelimb joints of a group of horses at walk (treadmill, 1.6 m/s, ——) and trot (treadmill, 4 m/s, ------). The joint angles are defined zero when the adjacent bone segments are aligned ■ stance phase at walk ▨ stance phase at trot □ swing phase at walk and trot (Back *et al.*, 1996b).

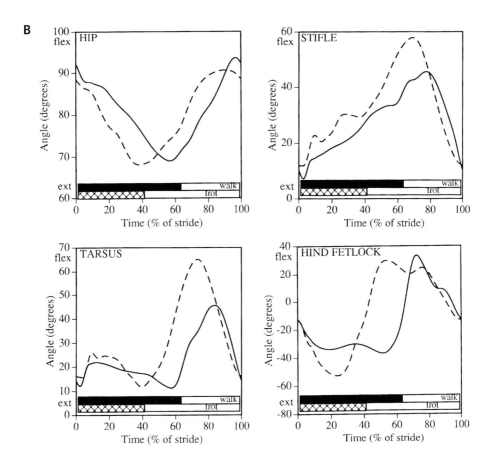

Fig. 5.8B Mean joint angle–time diagrams of the hindlimb joints of a group of horses at walk (treadmill, 1.6 m/s, ——) and trot (treadmill, 4 m/s, ------). The joint angles are defined zero when the adjacent bone segments are aligned ■ stance phase at walk ▨ stance phase at trot □ swing phase at walk and trot (Back *et al.*, 1996b).

There is also a striking difference in fetlock extension pattern between walk and trot. The two extension peaks are more pronounced at a faster walk and 'melt' into one extension peak at the trot, similar to vertical ground reaction force recordings at walk and trot (Back *et al.*, 1996b; Niki *et al.*, 1982). Schryver *et al.* (1978) explained this phenomenon as a result of the transition from a double to a single limb support. Alexander and Jayes (1978) presented a mathematical model which is capable of describing both possibilities and the gradation between them. They proposed that this phenomenon was related to mechanical properties of the distal limb. At a stiff walk the deceleration forces at landing and acceleration forces at take off are generated by the exchange of kinetic and potential energy (inverted pendulum mechanism).

In normal locomotion, however, the support limb saves energy by acting as a mass-spring mechanism with a natural frequency determined by the elastic properties of the limb and the amount of body mass supported by the limb (Alexander & Bennet-Clark, 1977). This involves an exchange between kinetic and elastic energy. Computer simulation experiments show that oscillations in the vertical GRF had roughly (not exactly, since muscle stiffness depends on muscle activation) the same frequency in walk and trot (van den Bogert, 1989). Thus, in the trot only one peak occurs since the limb is lifted before the second peak.

The increased forward velocity at the trot is accomplished by moving a longer distance during the swing phase, which has the same duration as at the walk, as a result of a greater impulse from the hindlimbs which showed a larger increase in maximal fetlock extension than in the forelimb. In the walk, the elbow, carpal, stifle and tarsal joints were less flexed during the swing phase, which resulted in a longer pendulum and a slower forward motion, leading to less protraction. The similarity in stance distance and swing time at different speeds and in different gaits has also been noted in cats and dogs (Grillner, 1975). Apparently, fore and hindlimbs have to

Table 5.3A Kinematic differences and correlation between the walk (1.6 m/s) and trot (4 m/s) of the forelimb of a group of horses (Back et al., 1996b).

Forelimb	Mean ± sd			Difference		Correlation	
	Walk (W)	Trot (T)		W → T		W-T	W w/score
Stride duration (s)	1.09 ± 0.06	0.67 ± 0.03	*	-0.42	**	0.68 †	-0.42 ††
Stance duration (s)	0.69 ± 0.04	0.27 ± 0.01	*	-0.42	**	0.52 †	-0.36
Stance duration (%)	63.2 ± 1.7	40.3 ± 1.7	*	-23.0	**	0.45 †	0.06
Swing duration (s)	0.40 ± 0.03	0.40 ± 0.03		0.0		0.68 †	-0.34
Max scapula rotation range (deg)	19.4 ± 1.9	17.8 ± 1.7	*	-1.6	**	0.65 †	-0.39
Angle of max protraction (deg)	20.2 ± 1.6	21.5 ± 1.5	*	1.3	**	0.56 †	-0.64 ††
Angle of max retraction (deg)	-22.5 ± 1.7	-22.8 ± 1.5		-0.3		0.65 †	0.11
Max pro-/retraction range (deg)	42.8 ± 2.5	44.4 ± 1.7	*	1.6	**	0.61 †	-0.49 ††
SHOULDER							
Angle at i.g.c. (deg)	54.9 ± 5.9	57.4 ± 5.9	*	2.6	**	0.94 †	0.08
Angle of max extension (deg)	53.8 ± 5.9	54.6 ± 4.2		0.8		0.94 †	0.10
Angle of max flexion (deg)	66.9 ± 4.2	69.9 ± 5.1	*	3.0	**	0.94 †	0.11
Range of motion (deg)	13.1 ± 1.9	15.3 ± 1.8	*	2.2	**	0.77 †	0.04
ELBOW							
Angle at i.g.c. (deg)	52.4 ± 4.9	50.1 ± 3.8	*	-2.3		0.66 †	-0.31
Angle of max extension (deg)	23.4 ± 3.1	24.5 ± 3.1	*	1.1		0.82 †	0.30
Angle of max flexion (deg)	75.2 ± 3.6	84.7 ± 4.3	*	9.5	**	0.70 †	-0.23
Range of motion (deg)	51.8 ± 3.6	60.2 ± 4.0	*	8.4	**	0.62 †	-0.49 ††
CARPUS							
Angle at i.g.c. (deg)	11.0 ± 3.9	6.0 ± 3.1	*	-5.0	**	0.63 †	-0.44 ††
Angle of max extension (deg)	1.3 ± 2.3	-2.9 ± 2.6	*	-4.2	**	0.77 †	-0.11
Angle of max flexion (deg)	69.9 ± 6.2	87.9 ± 7.4	*	18.0	**	0.78 †	-0.38
Range of motion (deg)	68.7 ± 5.7	90.8 ± 7.1	*	22.2	**	0.67 †	-0.36
FETLOCK							
Angle at i.g.c. (deg)	-14.1 ± 4.5	-16.8 ± 4.9	*	-2.7	**	0.86 †	0.28
Angle of max extension (deg)	-41.1 ± 6.1	-55.9 ± 6.2	*	-14.8	**	0.98 †	0.58 ††
Angle of max flexion (deg)	16.5 ± 6.4	21.3 ± 6.8	*	4.8	**	0.80 †	0.26
Range of motion (deg)	60.2 ± 1.4	80.6 ± 7.1	*	20.4	**	0.73 †	-0.38

* indicates a significant difference between W and T kinematics in Student's paired t-test at $p<0.05$
** indicates a significant difference between W and T kinematics in Bonferroni's post-hoc test at $p <0.0020$
☐: indicates that the difference between the means at W and T is larger than the sd at W
† indicates a significant correlation between W and T kinematics at $p<0.05$
†† indicates a significant correlation between W kinematics and W score at $p<0.05$
i.g.c.: initial ground contact

be more flexed during swing and more loaded during stance to enable a faster locomotion. However, the elbow and tarsal joints maintain a similar maximal extension level probably due to anatomical constraints.

This higher 'operating' velocity at the trot also leads to a higher impact peak at the beginning of the stance phase, which results in a sharper dip in the curves of the fetlock, carpal and elbow joints together with an increased maximal flexion of the shoulder joint in the stance phase. For the same reason a more pronounced dip and inflection can be seen in the fore fetlock and carpal joint curves at the end of the swing phase when the hoof is maximally protracted. In the hindlimb a similar though less pronounced dip can be seen in the fetlock, tarsal and stifle joints only at the beginning of the stance phase. Also the forelimb fetlock extension at impact increased more than that of the hindlimb (2.7° vs 0.8°). This phenomenon is more apparent in the forelimbs, because the passive forward swing of the distal limbs is controlled primarily by inertia in the forelimbs, and by tendons in the hindlimbs (Back et al., 1995a,b).

Most of the kinematic variables show a significant correlation between walk and trot, and the variables indicative of gait quality at the walk behave similarly to those at

Table 5.3B   Kinematic differences and correlation between the walk (1.6 m/s) and trot (4 m/s) of the hindlimb of a group of horses (Back *et al.*, 1996b).

Hindlimb	Mean ± sd			Difference	Correlation	
	Walk (W)	Trot (T)		W → T	W-T	W w/score
Stride duration (s)	1.09 ± 0.06	0.67 ± 0.03	*	-0.42 **	0.41 †	-0.20
Stance duration (s)	0.69 ± 0.04	0.27 ± 0.01	*	-0.42 **	0.46 †	-0.15
Stance duration (%)	63.4 ± 1.4	40.5 ± 1.9	*	-22.9 **	0.50 †	0.07
Swing duration (s)	0.40 ± 0.03	0.40 ± 0.03		0.0	0.44 †	-0.20
Max pelvis rotation range (deg)	8.2 ± 1.4	9.1 ± 1.3	*	0.9	0.14	-0.24
Angle of max protraction (deg)	23.1 ± 1.8	21.6 ± 1.3	*	-1.5 **	0.69 †	-0.35
Angle of max retraction (deg)	-23.6 ± 1.6	-26.6 ± 1.5	*	-2.9 **	0.33	0.41 ††
Max pro-/retraction range (deg)	46.7 ± 2.9	48.1 ± 1.6	*	1.4	0.40	-0.45 ††
HIP						
Angle at i.g.c. (deg)	92.1 ± 3.2	88.4 ± 3.4	*	-3.7 **	0.88 †	-0.05
Angle of max extension (deg)	68.9 ± 3.8	67.8 ± 3.9	*	-1.1 **	0.95 †	0.10
Angle of max flexion (deg)	93.7 ± 3.2	91.1 ± 3.6	*	-2.6 **	0.93 †	-0.09
Range of motion (deg)	24.8 ± 1.9	23.3 ± 1.8	*	-1.5 **	0.72 †	-0.35
STIFLE						
Angle at i.g.c. (deg)	10.3 ± 5.4	12.0 ± 4.1	*	1.7	0.85 †	-0.19
Angle of max extension (deg)	7.0 ± 4.9	11.0 ± 4.0	*	3.9 **	0.87 †	-0.24
Angle of max flexion (deg)	46.1 ± 5.9	58.3 ± 5.1	*	12.1 **	0.69 †	-0.37
Range of motion (deg)	39.1 ± 3.7	47.3 ± 3.8	*	8.2 **	0.33	-0.27
TARSUS						
Angle at i.g.c. (deg)	14.3 ± 4.4	16.1 ± 3.4	*	1.8 **	0.90 †	0.02
Angle of max extension (deg)	10.4 ± 3.5	10.3 ± 2.9		-0.1	0.94 †	0.19
Angle of max flexion (deg)	46.0 ± 0.1	65.7 ± 5.1	*	19.7 **	0.73 †	-0.23
Range of motion (deg)	35.6 ± 4.5	55.4 ± 5.3	*	19.9 **	0.70 †	-0.45 ††
FETLOCK						
Angle at i.g.c. (deg)	-12.7 ± 3.7	-13.5 ± 3.1	*	-0.8	0.93 †	0.22
Angle of max extension (deg)	-37.0 ± 4.2	-53.0 ± 4.0	*	-16.0 **	0.76 †	0.48 ††
Angle of max flexion (deg)	34.8 ± 9.1	32.0 ± 7.5	*	-2.8	0.77 †	0.29
Range of motion (deg)	71.8 ± 9.0	85.0 ± 7.7	*	13.2 **	0.70 †	0.07

 *   indicates a significant difference between W and T kinematics in Student's paired t-test at *p*<0.05
 ** indicates a significant difference between W and T kinematics in Bonferroni's post-hoc test at *p* <0.0020
 ☐ : indicates that the difference between the means at W and T is larger than the sd at W
 † indicates a significant correlation between W and T kinematics at *p*<0.05
 †† indicates a significant correlation between W kinematics and W score at *p*<0.05
 i.g.c.: initial ground contact

the trot: stride duration, protraction and retraction range, maximal fetlock extension and tarsal range of motion (Back *et al.*, 1996b). This similarity may reflect the influence of conformation on kinematics (Back *et al.*, 1997). At the walk, protraction is important for gait quality in the forelimb and retraction in the hindlimb, and these two variables are increased at the trot. This phenomenon might facilitate the transition from walk to trot, which is a prerequisite for a good performance.

In conclusion, the kinematics recorded at the walk are very similar to and show a good correlation with those at the trot when the effect of the higher speed on the intra-limb coordination is taken into consideration. Therefore the quality of the walk is a good predictor of the quality of the trot.

The canter

The canter is an asymmetrical gait in which the footfalls of both the fore and hindlimbs occur as couplets. The first limb of the couplet to contact the ground is defined as the trailing limb, the second is the leading limb. The sequence of footfalls is trailing hindlimb, leading hind and trailing forelimbs together, then the leading

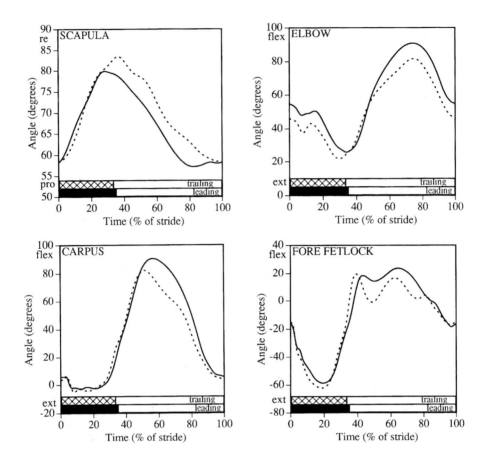

Fig. 5.9A Mean joint angle–time diagrams of the leading and trailing forelimb at the canter of a group of horses (treadmill, 7 m/s). The joint angles are defined zero when the adjacent bone segments are aligned. ▨ stance phase of trailing limb, ■ stance phase of leading limb (Back *et al.*, 1995d).

forelimb. An airborne phase follows lift off of the leading forelimb. The transition from a slow speed canter to the higher speed gallop involves a dissociation of the footfalls of the diagonal limb pair (leading hind and trailing fore) that can be perceived by the human eye.

In literature canter has been described at speeds ranging from 3 to 11 m/s. The recordings were made under various circumstances from a collected canter of a mounted horse overground to an extended canter of an unmounted horse on a treadmill (Clayton, 1994b; Corley & Goodship, 1994; Deuel & Park, 1990b). Kinematic studies used stick diagrams to describe canter (Walter, 1925; Krüger, 1937, 1938), report inter-limb timing variables (Deuel & Park, 1990b; Clayton, 1993, 1994b) or evaluate changes in temporal and linear kinematics induced by training (Corley & Goodship, 1994). None of these studies looked at the asymmetry in intra-limb coordination. Since the canter is an essential component at all levels of dressage and jumping compe-

titions, an understanding of limb kinematics and ground reaction forces is required.

Back *et al.* (1997) focused on the kinematics of the leading and trailing fore and hindlimbs of Dutch Warmbloods, cantering on a treadmill at a speed of 7 m/s, and found that the leading limb is more protracted. Furthermore, it appeared that the trailing limb is more retracted (Fig. 5.9A,B, Table 5.4A,B). This is achieved in the leading limbs by a greater flexion of the elbow and hip joints. As the leading limb has a somewhat larger total range of maximal protraction and retraction, the carpal and tarsal joints have to be more flexed to allow the distal limb to reach further in the same swing time. This principle was also found as an effect of training in six young Thoroughbreds at the canter (Corley & Goodship, 1994) and in four mounted Quarter horses at the gallop (Deuel, 1994). In the more retracted trailing limb, however, the scapula is more rotated caudally and moreover the fetlocks are more extended and thus more

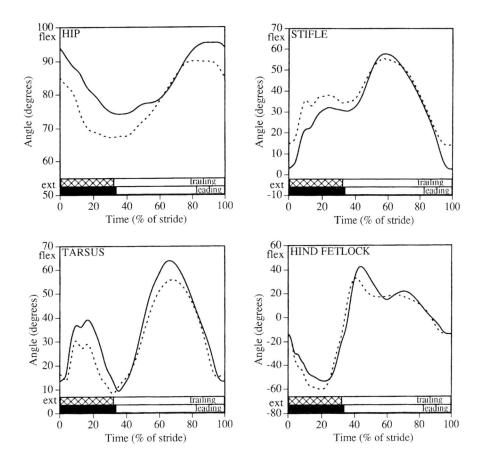

Fig. 5.9B Mean joint angle–time diagrams of the leading and trailing hindlimb at the canter of a group of horses (treadmill, 7 m/s). The joint angles are defined zero when the adjacent bone segments are aligned. ▓ stance phase of trailing limb, ■ stance phase of leading limb (Back *et al.*, 1995d).

loaded (Sloet *et al.*, 1995a), which is in accordance to force plate studies in mounted horses at the canter recorded overground (Niki *et al.*, 1984; Merkens *et al.*, 1993). In conclusion, the difference in inter-limb timing between left and right limbs at canter also leads to an asymmetry in intra-limb coordination of these limbs. The leading limb is the swinging limb, while the trailing limb is the – more loaded – supporting limb.

QUALITY OF MOVEMENT

Performance horses are selected by horsemen on the basis of their gait patterns, with selections often being made at a young age. However, the definition of 'good gait' or 'good action' is rather subjective (Smythe, 1957), and always leads to discussion between experts (Oliver &

Langrish, 1992). Observational gait analysis seems to be a convenient technique to quantify gait (Krebs *et al.*, 1985), but it should be standardized by using a uniform scoring list to improve reliability between judges (Eastlack *et al.*, 1991). In the second half of this century people began to breed warmblood horses for their elegance of gait and for performance under saddle in dressage and jumping. Good gait or action became a prerequisite for good performance. The high performance level of warmbloods in today's competitions is actually the historical proof of the expertise of horse breeding and selection in the past. Recently, the Royal Warmblood Studbook of the Netherlands developed a gait score to quantify gait quality in horses (van Veldhuizen, 1991). Modern kinematic analysis equipment has also been used to assess the quality of gait of elite dressage and show-jumping horses during competition (Leach *et al.*, 1984; Deuel & Park, 1990a, 1991;

Table 5.4A Kinematic differences between the leading and trailing forelimb of a group of horses at the canter (7 m/s, Back et al., 1997).

Forelimb	Limb		
	Leading	Trailing	L vs T
Stride duration (s)	0.556 ± 0.04	0.545 ± 0.02	
Stance duration (s)	0.192 ± 0.02	0.183 ± 0.01	
Stance duration (%)	34.5 ± 2.4	33.6 ± 1.4	
Swing duration (s)	0.364 ± 0.03	0.362 ± 0.02	
Max shoulder range of motion (deg)	23.3 ± 4.9	22.1 ± 2.9	
Angle of max protraction (deg)	33.4 ± 3.2	24.9 ± 2.1	*L
Angle of max retraction (deg)	-24.7 ± 1.7	-31.6 ± 1.8	*L
Max pro-/retraction range (deg)	58.1 ± 3.2	56.5 ± 1.6	
SCAPULA			
Angle at i.g.c. (deg)	58.3 ± 2.7	58.4 ± 2.9	
Angle at max rotation (deg)	80.2 ± 4.4	83.7 ± 3.9	
Max rot angle rel to i.g.c. (deg)	21.9 ± 3.3	25.3 ± 2.8	*T
Angle at min rotation (deg)	56.3 ± 3.9	57.9 ± 1.6	
Min rot angle rel to i.g.c. (deg)	-2.0 ± 2.2	-0.5 ± 0.8	*T
Max scapula rotation range (deg)	23.9 ± 2.3	25.8 ± 1.6	*T
ELBOW			
Angle at i.g.c. (deg)	54.6 ± 3.0	46.1 ± 3.0	*L
Angle of max extension (deg)	23.5 ± 3.8	20.1 ± 2.1	*L
Max ext rel to i.g.c. (deg)	-31.2 ± 3.8	-26.0 ± 3.3	*T
Angle of max flexion (deg)	91.2 ± 6.7	81.9 ± 4.6	*L
Max flexion rel to i.g.c. (deg)	36.5 ± 5.6	35.8 ± 6.5	
Range of motion (deg)	67.7 ± 5.6	61.8 ± 4.8	*L
CARPUS			
Angle at i.g.c. (deg)	5.7 ± 3.1	3.8 ± 2.9	
Angle of max extension (deg)	-4.4 ± 2.8	-6.7 ± 3.6	
Max ext rel to i.g.c. (deg)	-10.1 ± 1.7	-10.5 ± 1.6	
Angle of max flexion (deg)	91.2 ± 8.3	83.0 ± 7.9	*L
Max flex rel to i.g.c. (deg)	85.5 ± 7.1	79.1 ± 6.5	*L
Range of motion (deg)	95.6 ± 8.1	89.7 ± 7.0	
FETLOCK			
Angle at i.g.c. (deg)	-16.6 ± 7.3	-15.3 ± 4.1	
Angle of max extension (deg)	-59.0 ± 8.1	-62.4 ± 4.7	
Max ext rel to i.g.c. (deg)	-42.4 ± 4.0	-47.1 ± 3.8	*L
Angle of max flexion (deg)	29.1 ± 6.1	22.8 ± 7.3	*L
Max flex rel to i.g.c. (deg)	45.7 ± 6.4	38.0 ± 5.6	*L
Range of motion (deg)	88.1 ± 7.5	85.2 ± 8.0	

*L indicates that the variable has a significantly higher value in the leading limb group while
*T indicates a significantly higher value in the trailing limb group ($p<0.05$)

Clayton & Barlow, 1991; Holmström et al., 1994b) and to compare the quality of the overground trot scored by a judge with kinematic variables recorded on a treadmill (Back et al., 1994b). In the latter study the judge used a linear scoring system, in which trot was rated on three criteria: length, strength and suppleness. The measured kinematic variables included forelimb and hindlimb stride and swing duration, scapula rotation, forelimb maximal fetlock extension, forelimb maximal retraction, hindlimb maximal protraction, maximal stifle flexion and maximal tarsal flexion. The kinematic variables correlated very well with the judged score and allowed the subjective terms used by horsemen to be quantified.

Table 5.4B Kinematic differences between the leading and trailing hindlimb of a group of horses at the canter (7 m/s, Back *et al.*, 1997).

Hindlimb	Limb		
	Leading	Trailing	L vs T
Stride duration (s)	0.547 ± 0.02	0.553 ± 0.02	
Stance duration (s)	0.185 ± 0.01	0.177 ± 0.01	*L
Stance duration (%)	33.9 ± 1.3	32.1 ± 1.3	*L
Swing duration (s)	0.362 ± 0.02	0.376 ± 0.02	
Max pelvis rotation range (deg)	21.6 ± 2.2	19.6 ± 2.3	*L
Angle of max protraction (deg)	35.8 ± 1.7	22.7 ± 1.4	*L
Angle of max retraction (deg)	-29.7 ± 1.0	-37.6 ± 1.2	*L
Max pro-/retraction range (deg)	65.5 ± 1.6	60.3 ± 1.7	*L
HIP			
Angle at i.g.c. (deg)	93.9 ± 4.0	85.0 ± 3.5	*L
Angle of max extension (deg)	73.8 ± 3.2	66.7 ± 4.4	*L
Max ext rel to i.g.c. (deg)	-20.1 ± 2.5	-18.4 ± 2.1	*T
Angle of max flexion (deg)	96.3 ± 3.2	91.0 ± 3.6	*L
Max flexion rel to i.g.c. (deg)	2.4 ± 1.3	6.0 ± 1.9	*T
Range of motion (deg)	22.5 ± 1.8	24.3 ± 1.9	*T
KNEE			
Angle at i.g.c. (deg)	3.0 ± 4.4	14.7 ± 2.8	*T
Angle of max extension (deg)	2.3 ± 5.1	13.5 ± 4.6	*T
Max ext rel to i.g.c. (deg)	-0.7 ± 5.0	-1.2 ± 4.2	
Angle of max flexion (deg)	57.9 ± 4.3	55.5 ± 3.0	
Max flexion rel to i.g.c. (deg)	54.9 ± 0.6	40.8 ± 1.3	*L
Range of motion (deg)	55.5 ± 4.7	42.0 ± 3.9	*L
TARSUS			
Angle at i.g.c. (deg)	13.6 ± 4.9	16.3 ± 3.1	
Angle of max extension (deg)	8.1 ± 3.0	7.0 ± 2.6	
Max ext rel to i.g.c. (deg)	-5.5 ± 3.7	-9.4 ± 1.9	*L
Angle of max flexion (deg)	64.5 ± 8.6	56.0 ± 8.0	*L
Max flexion rel to i.g.c. (deg)	51.0 ± 8.2	39.7 ± 7.9	*L
Max stance flexion	39.5 ± 4.6	31.3 ± 4.4	
Max stance flexion rel to i.g.c.	26.0 ± 3.0	15.0 ± 2.0	
Range of motion (deg)	56.5 ± 7.6	49.0 ± 8.3	*L
FETLOCK			
Angle at i.g.c. (deg)	-13.9 ± 3.4	-14.3 ± 3.7	
Angle of max extension (deg)	-53.9 ± 3.8	-60.6 ± 3.4	*L
Max ext rel to i.g.c. (deg)	-40.0 ± 4.0	-46.2 ± 3.3	*L
Angle of max flexion (deg)	43.8 ± 7.3	35.6 ± 8.9	*L
Max flexion rel to i.g.c. (deg)	57.7 ± 6.0	49.9 ± 6.9	*L
Range of motion (deg)	97.7 ± 7.0	96.1 ± 9.1	

*L indicates that the variable has a significantly higher value in the leading limb group while
*T indicates a significantly higher value in the trailing limb group ($p<0.05$)

Stride and swing duration

At the same velocity, stride length and duration are inversely related: the longer the stride, the lower the stride frequency. Horses with good gaits use longer strides and a lower frequency (Knopfhart, 1966). The longer stride duration in horses with a better trot was associated with longer stance and swing phases, whereas in the hindlimb, a long stride duration was achieved as a result of having a long swing phase (Back *et al.*, 1994b; Morales *et al.*, 1998a,b). This might indicate the 'strength' or 'impulsion', which should come from the hindlimbs in a horse with a good gait (Knopfhart, 1966; Spooner, 1977; Oliver & Langrish, 1992). In connection to this horses with a good quality trot show a positive diagonal advanced placement (Holmström *et al.*, 1994b; Morales *et al.*, 1998a,b): the hoof of the hindlimb lands on the ground before that of the diagonal forelimb.

Scapula rotation, forelimb retraction and hindlimb protraction

If the forelimb is likened to a pendulum, rotation of the scapula is representative of the translation of the lower limb (Fig. 5.10A,B).

To increase stride length, an increased scapular movement is obligatory (Spooner, 1977). Therefore Smythe (1957) and Spooner (1977) both stressed the importance of having enough space between the elbow and the ribs to facilitate the sliding movement of the proximal forelimb over the rib cage. Better moving horses show more retraction in the forelimbs and more protraction of the hindlimbs (Fig. 5.11). A superior synchronous ipsilateral retracting forelimb and protracting hindlimb at the trot might also indicate the increased 'suppleness' in lateral bending of the body found in horses with a good gait (Back *et al.*, 1994b).

Maximal fetlock extension, and maximal stifle and tarsal flexion

The spring-like action of the fetlock joint is essential for horses to reduce the shock at limb–ground contact (Smythe, 1957; Alexander, 1988; Gray, 1993), to give smoothness of action (Gray, 1993) and to store elastic energy (Clayton *et al.*, 1998). This feature of the equine locomotor apparatus allows the horse to move in a graceful, floating manner (Oliver & Langrish, 1992). Although the maximal stance phase flexion of the shoulder represents energy absorption in the shoulder joint (Clayton *et al.*, 1998), the maximal fetlock extension has been found to be the most crucial variable for this purpose in the forelimb (Back *et al.*, 1994b). In the hindlimb, the stifle and tarsal joint also act as dampers during the stance phase together with the fetlock joint, in contrast with the situation in the forelimb, where the fetlock joint mainly acts as shock absorber. Maximal flexion of the elbow and carpal joints do not seem to be important variables to indicate good gait in warmblood horses. However, it appears that stifle and tarsal joint flexion, which are closely related through the reciprocal apparatus (van Weeren, 1990), support protraction and thus result in superior action in the hindlimb (Spooner, 1977; Alexander & Trestik, 1989; Oliver & Langrish, 1992; Back *et al.*, 1994b; Morales *et al.* 1998a,b; Fig. 5.12).

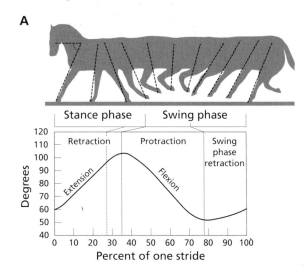

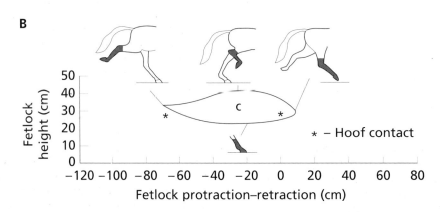

Fig. 5.10 Illustration of protraction and retraction of **(A)** the forelimb (Holmström *et al.*, 1994a) and **(B)** the hindlimb (Kobluk *et al.*, 1989, © EVJ Ltd.)

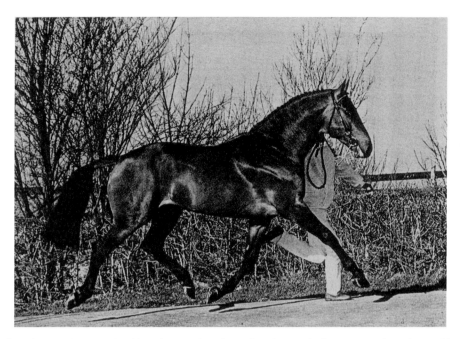

Fig. 5.11 Good quality trot is recognized by a long swing phase duration and a long suspension phase with more retraction of the forelimb and more protraction of the hindlimb (photo by Ellen van Leeuwen, NL).

TRAINING

Training is defined as a program of exercise to improve the horse's physical performance in a particular task (Blood & Studdert, 1990). Most of the literature on training involves the effect on the respiratory and cardiovascular systems and on blood chemistry. This section mainly focuses on the influence of training on kinematics of riding horses. Clayton (1993) found differences in stride variables of the extended canter under a rider between nine horses trained for dressage and seven horses trained for racing. The most salient of these was the longer stance durations and overlap periods in the dressage horses. Argue and Clayton (1993a,b) demonstrated that the level of training determined the sequence of footfalls in the transitions between walk and trot, but not between trot and canter in 16 dressage horses.

In young Dutch warmbloods a training period of 70 days is used to select young horses, and the outcome of testing during this period appears to correlate well with the future performance of the tested horses (Huizinga, 1991). Back *et al.* (1995d) objectively evaluated the influence of such a 70-day training period compared with turn out on pasture on the temporal, angular and segmental kinematics of the fore and hindlimbs in riding horses. In the hindlimbs of the trained horses the same stride duration was achieved with a significantly shorter stance duration (s) after the 70-day period, illustrating the development of 'impulsion' (Fig. 5.12). Horses pastured for 70 days also decreased their stance percentage, but this was associated with an increase in swing and stride duration (Back *et al.*, 1995d). Similarly, Schwarz (1971) analyzed some temporal kinematic variables of eight Hannoverian stallions walking and trotting overground and found that the swing duration expressed as a percentage of total stride duration increased after one year of training. Corley and Goodship (1994) also reported a decrease in stance duration in cantering Thoroughbred racehorses trained on a treadmill, as did Drevemo *et al.* (1980) in four young Standardbreds that were trained over a 3-year period. Training changes the relation between the stance and swing durations (Clayton, 1997) and between stride duration and stride frequency (Muñoz *et al.*, 1997), but the definition and effects of 'training' appear to be rather relative. 'Engagement of the hind quarters,' which is one of the primary goals of training the young sport horse (Crossley, 1993), might thus be visible as an earlier maximal protraction of the hindlimb with respect to the retracting ipsilateral forelimb, as a consequence of the ability to generate the impulsion needed from the hindlimbs over a shorter period of time (Fig. 5.12).

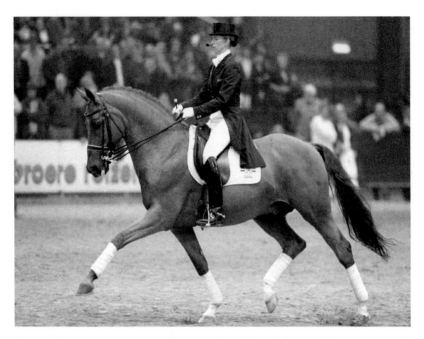

Fig. 5.12 Positive advanced placement and increase of impulsion with training contribute to the collected appearance in good-moving Warmbloods (photo of 'Cocktail' with Anky van Grunsven by Jacob Melissen, NL).

In trained horses the load seems to shift from the forelimbs towards the hindlimbs, in which maximal fetlock extension increases. When the weight shifts to the hindlimbs the horse is said to 'carry itself' (Crossley, 1993). Back *et al.* (1995d) hypothesized that the increased impulsion in the trained horses might be visible as increased extension of the tarsal and fetlock joints, in the hindlimb, which is the opposite reaction to that seen in pastured horses, in which there is increased extension of the carpal and fetlock joints in the forelimbs. Young Standardbreds that were trained for 5 months showed both phenomena: increased carpal and fetlock extension in the forelimb and increased tarsal and fetlock extension in the hindlimb (van Weeren *et al.*, 1993).

Greater flexion of the joints in the hindlimbs of the trained horses during swing phase might also indicate that the movement is directed more forward instead of upward, leading to the earlier occurrence of maximal protraction. It is well known that when horses are broken-in and ridden under saddle at the beginning of their career, their movement becomes 'shorter in the front.' After a period of training, young horses find their balance, and are able to carry a rider 'on the bit.' These changes are accompanied by re-establishment of movement of the proximal segments, which is reflected by gradual increases in cranio-caudal movement of the distal segments of the forelimb similar to pastured horses (Back *et al.*, 1995d; Table 5.5).

Rose and Evans (1990) defined six criteria that should be the aims of training. One of these is the development of biomechanical skills. Kinematic studies have shown that the stride characteristics change under the influence of training (Back *et al.*, 1995d; Muñoz *et al.*, 1997). A shorter stance duration and reduced flexion in the hindlimb cause maximal protraction to occur earlier, so the hindlimb reaches the retracting ipsilateral forelimb earlier, which is seen as being more engaged in the hindquarters (Table 5.6). At the same time, increased fetlock extension illustrates more weight carrying by the hindlimbs (Table 5.7).

In the early stages of training, young horses show less cranio-caudal movement of the distal forelimb through less elbow joint movement. The combination of the hindlimbs generating 'impulsion' by operating faster in a more forward directed movement with less limb flexion and the forelimbs 'trotting shorter' gives the trained horse the appearance of being more collected, and moving 'on the bit.' However, when horses are put at pasture the swing and stride durations increase in both fore and hindlimbs. These horses have a larger range of protraction and retraction and an increase in maximal carpal and fetlock extension of the forelimb. So, in contrast to the trained horses, horses kept on pasture actually give the impression of moving more on the forehand and in a more relaxed manner, with the forelimb acting as a passive strut. The hindlimb acts as an engine that shows more power.

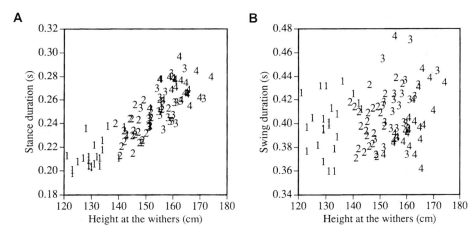

Fig. 5.13 Correlation **(A)** between height at the withers and stance duration, and **(B)** between height at the withers and swing duration recorded at trot in a group of horses at four different ages ('1': 4 months; '2': 10 months; '3': 18 months; '4': 26 months of age. Back *et al.*,1994a).

Table 5.5 Maximal cranial and caudal movement in centimeters of the forelimb segments relative to the proximal scapula before and after 70 days in training or 70 days at pasture (Back *et al.*, 1995d).

Forelimb segment	Training (n = 12)		Pasture (n = 12)		ANOVA
	Before	After	Before	After	(post hoc)
SCAPULA					
Distal	5.1	5.6*	4.7	5.3*	
HUMERUS					
Proximal	11.4	12.3*	11.1	12.2*	
Distal	22.7	23.6*	22.4	24.0*	
RADIUS					
Proximal	27.9	29.2*	27.2	29.1*	
Distal	62.1	62.4	61.2	62.7*	†
METACARPUS					
Proximal	75.6	75.1	74.3	76.3*	† (**)
Distal	93.9	92.9	92.2	93.9*	†(**)
HOOF					
Coronet	112.2	111.2	110.3	112.6*	†(**)
Heel	113.5	112.7	111.3	114.2*	† (**)
Toe	116.2	115.8	113.9	116.5*	† (**)

* indicates that the values before and after 70 days are significantly different (*p* <0.05) within the training or pasture groups (Student's t-test)

† indicates that the changes in the values over the period of 70 days are significantly different (*p* <0.05) between the training and pasture groups (ANOVA)

** indicates that the changes in the values over the period of 70 days are also significantly different between the training and pasture groups after a Bonferroni post-hoc test (*p* ≤ 0.05)

There was a statistically significant interaction between 'time' (before/after) and 'group' (training/pasture), and between 'segment' (marker no. 1–10), 'time' and 'group' (*p* <0.05; ANOVA)

Table 5.6 Time relative to initial ground contact ($t = 0$) of the maximal protraction of the different segments of the hindlimb before and after 70 days in training or 70 days at pasture. Time is expressed as % of total stride duration (Back et al., 1995d).

Hindlimb segment	Training ($n = 12$)		Pasture ($n = 12$)		ANOVA
	Before	After	Before	After	(post hoc)
FEMUR					
Distal	-1.9	-3.2*	-2.7	-2.9	
TIBIA					
Proximal	-2.4	-3.8*	-3.0	-3.5	
Distal	-1.4	-2.4*	-1.6	-1.8	†
METATARSUS					
Proximal	-1.6	-2.5*	-1.7	-1.9	†
Distal	-2.1	-2.8*	-2.1	-2.0	†
HOOF					
Coronet	-2.0	-2.7*	-1.8	-1.9	
Heel	-1.9	-2.6*	-1.8	-1.8	
Toe	-1.8	-2.5*	-1.7	- 1.8	

* indicates that the values before and after 70 days are significantly different ($p < 0.05$) within the training or pasture groups (Student's t-test)

† indicates that the changes in the values over the period of 70 days are significantly different ($p < 0.05$) between the training and pasture groups (ANOVA)

** indicates that the changes in the values over the period of 70 days are also significantly different between the training and pasture groups after a Bonferroni post-hoc test ($p < 0.05$)

There was a statistically significant interaction between 'time' (before/after) and 'group' (training/pasture), but not between 'segment' (marker no. 1–10), 'time' and 'group' ($p < 0.05$; ANOVA)

ONTOGENY OF GAIT

Horse breeders are interested in identifying gait characteristics of young animals that are predictive for future performance. Using modern automated kinematic

Table 5.7 Response to 70 days in training or 70 days at pasture detected in the change in maximal fetlock extension of the forelimb and the hindlimb (Back et al., 1995d).

No. of horses	Forelimb			
	Training ($n = 12$)		Pasture ($n = 12$)	
	Decrease	Increase	Decrease	Increase
HINDLIMB				
Decrease	3	2	1	6
Increase	5	2	2	3
Total	8	4	3	9††

†† indicates that the ratio of the number of horses that showed an increased and decreased value after 70 days is significantly different ($p < 0.05$) between the training and pasture groups (Chi square test)

analysis equipment, Back et al. 1994a, 1995c) compared the gaits of foals with those of adults.

There have been few longitudinal studies on the locomotion of the same horses recorded at different ages (Drevemo et al., 1987). Drevemo et al. (1987) analyzed temporal kinematic variables in ten Standardbreds trotting at 4 m/s on a treadmill at the age of 8, 12 and 18 months. After scaling the data to height at the withers, a decrease in relative stride length was found. Back et al. (1994a) recorded 24 Warmblood horses at the ages of 4, 10, 18 and 26 months at the walk, trot and canter on the treadmill. He found that in horses, as in primates, stride and stance duration increased with age as a result of an increase in height (Beck et al., 1981; Vilensky et al., 1990a,b). A treadmill was used to record the horses at the same velocity, because Dusek (1974) was not able to find any correlations between height and temporal gait variables during overground locomotion when the individuals selected their own, preferred walking or trotting speed. Galisteo et al. (1998) concluded that there was a closer relationship with linear than temporal variables.

If the forelimb is regarded as a pendulum that moves the body forward at constant horizontal velocity with the same pro-/retraction angles and stance durations, the

Table 5.8A Recorded and predicted temporal kinematics of the forelimb and the hindlimb of a group of horses trotting on a treadmill at foal and adult age (Back *et al.*, 1995c).

Variable	Foal	Adult									
	Mean	Not corrected predicted		Linearly predicted			Dynamically predicted			Recorded	
		(Range)	Correlation	Value	(Range)	Correlation	Value	(Range)	Correlation	Mean	
FORELIMB											
Stance duration (%)	34.7	(33.4–36.0)	0.10	42.9	(41.0–44.9)	0.82†	38.6	(37.1–40.1)	0.95†	40.3*	
Stance duration (s)	0.21	(0.20–0.22)	0.43†	0.26	(0.25–0.28)	0.89†	0.24	(0.22–0.25)	0.97†	0.27*	
Swing duration (s)	0.40	(0.38–0.42)	0.65†	0.50	(0.47–0.53)	0.90†	0.45	(0.42–0.47)	0.97†	0.40	
Stride duration (s)	0.62	(0.59–0.65)	0.83†	0.76	(0.72–0.80)	0.86†	0.68	(0.65–0.72)	0.96†	0.67*	
HINDLIMB											
Stance duration (%)	34.3	(32.1–36.5)	0.63†	42.3	(39.7–44.9)	0.92†	38.1	(35.8–40.4)	0.98†	40.5*	
Stance duration (s)	0.21	(0.20–0.22)	0.65†	0.26	(0.25–0.27)	0.61†	0.23	(0.22–0.25)	0.66†	0.27*	
Swing duration (s)	0.41	(0.38–0.44)	0.77†	0.50	(0.46–0.54)	0.68†	0.45	(0.42–0.49)	0.73†	0.40	
Stride duration (s)	0.62	(0.59–0.65)	0.86†	0.76	(0.72–0.80)	0.71†	0.68	(0.65–0.72)	0.80†	0.67*	

☐ : recorded adult variable outside the predicted range at foal age
*, † $p < 0.05$: significant difference and correlation between foal and adult
Predicted range is based on foal kinematics +/- SD

distance moved during the stance phase will increase almost linearly with height. During the swing phase the limb must move over a greater distance in the same time. Since the forward swing is initiated from the proximal part of the limb, the resulting inertial forces on the lower limb lead to increased limb flexion.

Models found in the literature that would compensate for the influence of height on temporal kinematic variables, like trot–gallop transitions (elastic similarity) and Froude numbers (dynamic similarity), showed inconclusive results (Vilensky & Gankiewicz, 1986; Drevemo *et al.*, 1987). The principle of Günther (1975), in which frequencies are related to linear dimensions, showed a decrease in relative stride duration with age, which is in accordance with Back *et al.* (1995d) that younger animals take relatively longer strides (Fig. 5.13).

Angle–angle diagrams are indicative of intra-limb coordination (Kobluk *et al.*, 1989; Martinez-del Campo *et al.*, 1991). Their use in longitudinal studies shows that some horses accelerate their carpal joint flexion during the swing phase ('spike' pattern) and some maintain a constant joint flexion during the same period ('straight' pattern), demonstrating a smoother type of carpal flexion ('convex' pattern, Fig. 5.14).

These typical intra-limb coordination features can be recognized as early as 4 months of age (Back *et al.*, 1993a, 1994a). Since the variability of the kinematic variables was similar at 4 months of age and when the horses were older, kinematics appear to be already mature at a young age. Remarkable resemblance between angle–angle diagrams recorded in the foal compared with the adult can be observed. There is a better resemblance in intra-limb coordination when the pattern of the individual horse is more typical ('spike' versus 'convex'). At the present time, the interpretation of similarities in patterns is subjective, and a standardized quantitative pattern recognition technique needs to be developed to allow an objective assessment. Neural networks could play a crucial role in this type of research (Holzreiter & Köhle, 1993; Dalin, 1994).

PREDICTION

The gait of the horse is one of the main factors determining its future level of performance. Dressage horses must have an elegant gait, while jumping horses need to have a good jumping technique. Horsemen would like to be able to pick out potential winners at an early age to avoid investing time and money in horses that are incapable of succeeding in the competitive arena. Such a selection effectively implies a prediction of adult gait. Therefore there is a need for objective criteria to select performance horses at a young age.

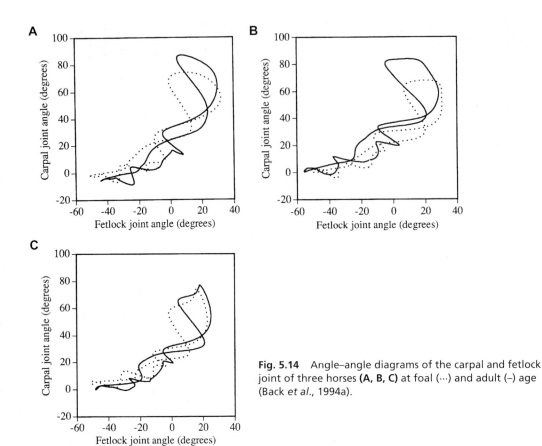

Fig. 5.14 Angle–angle diagrams of the carpal and fetlock joint of three horses **(A, B, C)** at foal (···) and adult (–) age (Back *et al.*, 1994a).

The intra-limb coordination pattern of warmblood foals and adult horses has been objectively quantified (Back *et al.*, 1993a) and appears to be qualitatively similar (Back *et al.*, 1994a), despite considerable differences in height at the withers and body weight. Gait timing variables in differently sized animals of the same breed can be made comparable after a transformation based on linear and dynamic similarity principles (Günther, 1975; Alexander & Jayes, 1983; Alexander, 1984). Back *et al.* (1995c) hypothesized that, after normalization for differences in conformation, foal and adult kinematics are similar within a certain range (Table 5.8A,B,C).

Normalization of temporal variables

Differences in height at the withers between foals and adult horses influence temporal kinematics. In the literature two different models to compare the kinematics of

differently sized animals have been published. These techniques were applied to the temporal kinematic variables of the foals to evaluate whether *linear* or *dynamic* similarity standardization improved the predicted adult variables.

Linear similarity

Consider a small and a large horse, in which the dimensions of the large one are a simple multiplication of the dimensions of the smaller one. When the maximal protraction and retraction angles of the limbs are the same (Back *et al.*, 1994a), and the speed of the hooves is also the same (treadmill speed), the larger animal moves with a longer stride length and a slower stride frequency. Normalization can be achieved by multiplying the quotient of the height at the withers of the larger and smaller horse with, for example, the stride duration of the smaller horse (Günther, 1975).

Table 5.8B Recorded and predicted kinematics of the forelimb of a group of horses trotting on a treadmill at foal and adult age (Back *et al.*, 1995c).

Forelimb variable	Foal Recorded	Adult Predicted range	Adult Recorded	Foal–adult correlation
PRO & RETRACTION (deg)				
Max protraction	23.0	21.1–24.9	21.5[*]	0.44†
Max retraction	-21.7	-23.0– -20.4	-22.8[*]	0.03
Range of max pro- and retraction	44.7	42.8–46.6	44.4	0.50†
SCAPULA (deg)				
Range of max rotation	15.5	13.8–17.2	17.8[*]	0.47†
ELBOW (deg)				
At i.g.c.	53.6	50.1–57.1	50.1[*]	0.12
Max extension rel to i.g.c.	-25.7	-28.7– -22.7	-25.6	0.36
Max flexion rel to i.g.c.	30.9	26.6–35.2	34.6[*]	0.48†
Range of movement	56.6	52.1–61.1	60.2[*]	0.44†
CARPUS (deg)				
At i.g.c.	4.4	1.8–7.0	6.0	0.03
Max extension rel to i.g.c.	-7.6	-9.9– -5.3	-9.0	0.36
Max flexion rel to i.g.c.	70.0	64.9–75.1	81.9[*]	0.42†
Range of movement	77.5	73.2–81.8	90.8[*]	0.47†
FETLOCK (deg)				
At i.g.c.	-15.3	-18.4– -12.2	-16.8	0.01
Max extension rel to i.g.c.	-36.9	-40.4– -33.4	-39.1[*]	0.37
Max flexion rel to i.g.c.	42.2	37.8–46.6	41.5	0.47†
Range of movement	79.1	73.6–84.6	80.6	0.36

☐ : recorded adult variable outside the predicted range at foal age
*, † p<0.05: significant difference and correlation between foal and adult
Predicted range based on foal kinematics +/ -SD
i.g.c.: initial ground contact

Dynamic similarity

Forces occurring in a pendular locomotor system are considered dynamically similar when the ratio of kinetic energy ($1/2\ mv^2$) and potential energy (mgh, where $g = 9.81$ m/s^2) is the same in the smaller and a larger horse. The ratio between these energy variables has been introduced earlier and was called the Froude number (v^2/gh). When the substitution of $v = h/t$ is used, the Froude number equals h/gt^2. This relationship leads to the following scaling procedure, if dynamic similarity conditions are fulfilled: the stride duration of the smaller horse is multiplied by the square root of the quotient of the height at the withers of the larger and the smaller horse (Alexander & Jayes, 1983; Alexander, 1984).

Most of the recorded kinematic variables of the young adult fell within the range of one standard deviation around the mean data at foal age (Back *et al.*, 1995c). As joint angles become more extended during growth (Krüger, 1939; Green, 1961; Campbell & Lee, 1981; Magnusson, 1985), it was not surprising that the

tarsal and hindlimb fetlock joint angles at impact were predicted to be more flexed than they were found to be. The femur tends to grow faster than the tibia (Krüger, 1939), implying that retraction of the hindlimb decreases and protraction increases. However, the total range of pro- and retraction remain the same in both fore and hindlimbs of foals and adults.

Due to the increased limb length in adult horses, the distance between the position of maximal protraction and retraction of the hoof is longer and, thus, the stance duration is longer in adult horses trotting at the same velocity because the body moves forward over a greater distance during the stance phase (Back *et al.*, 1994a). Compensation for the difference in stance duration was achieved by multiplying stance duration by the ratio of the height at the withers, assuming linear similarity. In contrast, stride duration of foals became similar to adults after dynamic correction. When using linear similarity principles to correct stride duration, it was found that adult horses take shorter strides than foals (Back *et al.*, 1994a, 1995c; Drevemo *et al.*, 1987).

Table 5.8C Recorded and predicted kinematics of the hindlimb of a group of horses trotting on a treadmill at foal and adult age (Back *et al.*, 1995c).

Hindlimb variable	Foal	Adult		Foal–adult
	Recorded	Predicted range	Recorded	correlation
PRO & RETRACTION (deg)				
Max protraction	18.1	17.1–19.1	21.6*	0.28
Max retraction	-29.7	-30.9– -28.5	-26.6*	0.48†
Range of max pro- and retraction	47.8	46.5–49.1	48.1	0.58†
PELVIS (deg)				
Range of max rotation	7.6	5.9–9.3	9.1*	0.77†
HIP (deg)				
At i.g.c.	91.7	87.5–95.9	88.4*	0.07
Max extension rel to i.g.c.	-20.9	-23.4– -18.4	-20.6	0.70†
Max flexion rel to i.g.c.	2.0	0.9–3.1	2.7*	0.55†
Range of movement	22.9	20.9–24.9	23.3	0.59†
STIFLE (deg)				
At i.g.c.	15.9	11.7–20.1	12.0*	0.08
Max extension rel to i.g.c.	-0.8	- 1.6–0.0	-1.0	0.19
Max flexion rel to i.g.c.	48.4	43.8–53.0	46.3*	0.48†
Range of movement	49.2	44.4–54.0	47.3*	0.55†
TARSUS (deg)				
At i.g.c.	21.4	18.0–24.8	16.1*	0.42†
Stance flexion rel to i.g.c.	9.6	6.8–12.4	10.6*	0.52†
Max extension rel to i.g.c.	-6.1	-8.2– -4.0	-5.8	0.17
Max flexion rel to i.g.c.	47.3	42.3–52.3	49.7*	0.65†
Range of movement	53.4	48.3–58.5	55.4*	0.70†
FETLOCK (deg)				
At i.g.c.	-8.8	-12.9– -4.7	-13.5*	0.27
Max extension rel to i.g.c.	-37.8	-42.0– -33.6	-39.5*	0.53†
Max flexion rel to i.g.c.	44.8	38.9–50.7	45.5*	0.61†
Range of movement	82.6	75.6–89.6	85.0	0.56†

□ : recorded adult variable outside the predicted range at foal age
*, † $p<0.05$: significant difference and correlation between foal and adult
Predicted range based on foal kinematics +/-SD
i.g.c.: initial ground contact

From the latter study it became clear that as the swing duration at foal age was already similar to that at adult age, the limbs were less flexed in the foals than in adults, because a shorter distance had to be covered in the same time. This is nicely illustrated in the forelimb, in which the carpal joint showed greater flexion in adult horses. The extension dip in the fetlock joint at the end of the swing phase in the fore and hindlimbs is more pronounced in adults compared with foals, because mass and speed of the hoof are higher. In the hindlimb, the pendular response in tarsal joint flexion to the increase in limb length is minimal. This fact, together with the remarkably high correlation coefficient, illustrates the 'adult-like' capacities of this joint at foal age.

Prediction aims to select horses with a good gait quality at an early age. It has been shown that the swing duration, the maximal angle of protraction–retraction, and the maximal flexion of the tarsal joint are similar and show a good correlation between foals and adults. Since these kinematic variables are indicative of gait quality (Back *et al.*, 1994b), it is not surprising that the variables scored by the judge also show a good correlation between foals and adults. Gifted horse breeders are said to be able to predict future gait performance at a young age (Clayton, 1989a; Grant, 1989). Back *et al.* (1995c) proved that, by the age of 4 months, locomotor variables can also be predicted quantitatively.

From locomotion prediction to performance prediction . . .

Prediction of good gait at a young age seems to be possible, but the question remains as to whether good gait also results in good performance when ridden. Researchers from Sweden found that when dressage horses were ridden under saddle, the stride duration was longer in horses that were good movers compared to poor movers (Holmström *et al.*, 1994b). Furthermore, they calculated that the judgment of conformation and locomotion accounted for 43% of the variation of their gaits under saddle (Holmström & Philipsson, 1993). In selection procedures, dressage and jumping performance are increasingly considered separately. It seems reasonable, nonetheless, to believe that a good gait is an absolute prerequisite for superior performance as a dressage horse.

Performance under saddle also depends on the way the individual horse responds to being ridden, since kinematics change when horses carry a rider (Sloet *et al.*, 1995a). The intra-limb coordination pattern, however, as illustrated by the angle–angle diagram seems to be established already as a foal (Back *et al.*, 1994a). In dressage horses this pattern might be related to the ability to perform gait transitions or piaffe and passage, while in jumping horses this might be related to the technique of how to clear fences. Jumping technique has become a more substantial part of selection procedures and it seems that horsemen can detect the typical jumping characteristics to enable future superior jumping performance in the young horses. This knowledge can be quantified using gait analysis equipment, while neural networks can be developed to automate pattern recognition in the data (Holzreiter & Köhle, 1993; Dalin, 1994). In this way, more specific selection criteria for dressage or jumping can be defined and objectively measured. Finally, it should be remembered that horses can be trained to perform well, but for élite performance in competition the mental capacities of rider and horse might be the crucial factor.

REFERENCES

Alexander, R.McN. (1984) *Animal Mechanics*, 2nd edn. Oxford: Blackwell Scientific Publications, pp. 33–36.

Alexander, R.McN. (1988) *Elastic Mechanisms in Animal Movement*. Cambridge: Cambridge University Press.

Alexander, R.McN. and Bennet-Clark, H.C. (1977) Storage of elastic strain energy in muscle and other tissues. *Nature* **265**: 114–117.

Alexander, R.McN. and Jayes, A.S. (1978) Vertical movements in walking and running. *J. Zool.* **185**: 27–40.

Alexander, R.McN. and Jayes, A.S. (1983) A dynamic similarity hypothesis for the gaits of quadrupedal mammals. *J. Zool. London* **201**: 135–152.

Alexander, R.McN. and Trestik, C.L. (1989) Bistable properties of the hock joint of horses (*Equus* spp.). *J. Zool.* **218**: 383–391.

Argue, C.K. and Clayton, H.M. (1993a) A preliminary study of transitions between the walk and trot in dressage horses. *Acta Anat.* **146**: 179–182.

Argue, C.K. and Clayton, H.M. (1993b) A study of transitions between the trot and canter in dressage horses. *J. Equine Vet. Sci.* **13**: 171–174.

Back, W., Bogert, A.J. van den, Weeren, P.R. van, Bruin, G. and Barneveld, A. (1993a) Quantification of the locomotion of Dutch Warmblood foals. *Acta Anat.* **146**: 141–147.

Back, W., Barneveld, A., Weeren, P.R. van and Bogert, A.J. van den (1993b) Kinematics of equine carpal lameness. *Acta Anat.* **146**: 86–89.

Back, W., Schamhardt, H.C., Barneveld, A. and Hartman, W. (1993c) Correction of joint angle-time diagrams to standardize equine kinematic data. *Proc. 14th Congr. Inter. Soc. Biomech.*, Paris, France, pp. 132–133.

Back, W., Barneveld, A., Schamhardt, H.C., Bruin, G. and Hartman, W. (1994a) Longitudinal development of the kinematics in 4-, 10-, 18-, and 26-month-old Dutch Warmblood horses. *Equine Vet. J.* **17**(Suppl.): 3–6.

Back, W., Barneveld, A., Schamhardt, H.C., Bruin, G. and Hartman, W. (1994b) Kinematic detection of superior gait quality in young trotting warmbloods. *Vet. Quart.* **16**: S91–96.

Back, W., Schamhardt, H.C., Savelberg, H.H.C.M., *et al.* (1995a) How the horse moves: significance of graphical representations of equine forelimb kinematics. *Equine Vet. J.* **27**: 31–38.

Back, W., Schamhardt, H.C., Savelberg, H.H.C.M. *et al.* (1995b) How the horse moves: significance of graphical representations of equine hind limb kinematics. *Equine Vet. J.* **27**: 39–45.

Back, W., Schamhardt, H.C., Hartman, W., Bruin, G. and Barneveld, A. (1995c) Predictive value of foal kinematics for adult locomotor performance. *Res. Vet. Sci.* **59**: 64–69.

Back, W., Hartman, W., Schamhardt, H.C., Bruin, G. and Barneveld, A. (1995d) Kinematic response to a 70-day training period in trotting Dutch Warmbloods. *Equine Vet. J.* **18** (suppl.): 127–131.

Back, W., Schamhardt, H.C., Hartman, W. and Barneveld, A. (1995e) Repetitive loading and oscillations in the distal fore and hind limb as predisposing factors for equine lameness. *Am. J. Vet. Res.* **56**: 1522–1528.

Back, W., Schamhardt, H.C. and Barneveld, A. (1996a) The influence of conformation on fore and hind limb kinematics of the trotting Dutch warmblood horse. *Pferdeheilkunde* **12**: 647–650.

Back, W., Schamhardt, H.C. and Barneveld, A. (1996b) Are kinematics of the walk related to the locomotion of a warmblood horse at the trot? *Vet. Quart.* **18**: S79–84.

Back, W., Schamhardt, H.C. and Barneveld, A. (1997) Kinematic comparison of the leading and trailing limb at the canter. *Equine Vet. J.* **23**(Suppl.): 80–83.

Barrey, E., Landjerit, B. and Wolter, R. (1991) Shock and vibration during the hoof impact on different track surfaces. *Equine Exerc. Physiol.* **3**: 97–106.

Barrey, E., Galloux, P., Valette, J.P., Auvinet, B. and Wolter, R. (1993) Determination of optimal treadmill slope for reproducing the same cardiac response in saddle horses as overground conditions. *Vet. Rec.* **133**: 183–185.

Beck, R.J., Andriacchi, T.P., Kuo, K.N., Fermier, R.W. and Galante, J.O. (1981) Changes in the gait patterns of growing children. *J. Bone Joint Surg.* **63a**: 1452–1456.

Benoit, P., Barrey, E. and Regnault, J.C. (1993) Comparison of the damping effect of different shoeing by measurement of hoof acceleration. *Acta Anat.* **46**: 109–113.

Blood, D.C. and Studdert, V.P. (1990) *Ballière's Comprehensive Veterinary Dictionary*, 2nd edn. London: Ballière Tindall, p. 927.

Bogert, A.J. van den. (1989) Computer simulation of locomotion in the horse. *Thesis, Utrecht.*

Bogert, A.J. van den and Schamhardt, H.C. (1993) Multi-body modelling and simulation of animal locomotion. *Acta Anat.* **146**: 95–102.

Buchner, H.H.F., Savelberg, H.H.C.M., Schamhardt, H.C., Merkens, H.W. and Barneveld, A. (1994a) Habituation of horses to treadmill locomotion. *Equine Vet. J.* **17**(Suppl.): 13–15.

Buchner, H.H.F., Savelberg, H.H.C.M., Schamhardt, H.C., Merkens, H.W. and Barneveld, A. (1994b) Kinematics of treadmill versus overground locomotion. *Vet. Quart.* **16**: S87–90.

Campbell, J.R. and Lee, R. (1981) Radiological estimation of the different growth rates of the long bones of foals. *Equine Vet. J.* **13**: 247–250.

Clayton, H.M. (1989a) Gait analysis as a predictive tool in performance horses. *J. Equine Vet. Sci.* **9**: 335–336.

Clayton, H.M. (1989b) Locomotion. In: Jones, W.E. (ed) *Equine Sports Medicine*. Philadelphia: Lea & Febiger, pp. 149–187.

Clayton, H.M. (1993) The extended canter: a comparison of the stride kinematics of horses trained for dressage and for racing. *Acta Anat.* **146**: 183–187.

Clayton, H.M. (1994a) Comparison of the stride kinematics of the collected, working, medium, and extended trot in horses. *Equine Vet. J.* **26**: 230–234.

Clayton, H.M. (1994b) Comparison of the stride kinematics of the collected, working, medium and extended canter in horses. *Equine Vet. J.* **17**(Suppl.): 16–19.

Clayton, H.M. (1997) Classification of collected trot, passage and piaffe based on temporal variables. *Equine Vet. J.* **23**(Suppl.): 54–57.

Clayton, H.M. and Barlow, D.A. (1991) Stride characteristics of 4 Grand Prix jumping horses. *Equine Exerc. Physiol.* **3**: 151–157.

Clayton, H.M., Lanovaz, J.L., Schamhardt, H.C., Willemen, M.A., and Colborne, G.R. (1998) Net joint moments and powers in the equine forelimb during the stance phase at the trot. *Equine Vet. J.* **30**: 384–389.

Colborne, G.R., Lanovaz, J.L., Sprigings, E.J., Schamhardt, H.C. and Clayton, H.M. (1997a) Joint moments and power flow in equine gait: a preliminary study. *Equine Vet. J.* **23**(Suppl.): 33–36.

Colborne, G.R., Lanovaz, J.L., Sprigings, E.J., Schamhardt H.C. and Clayton, H.M. (1997b) Power flow in the equine forelimb. *Equine Vet. J.* **23**(Suppl.): 37–40.

Corley, J.M. and Goodship, A.E. (1994) Treadmill training induced changes to some kinematic variables measured at the canter in Thoroughbred fillies. *Equine Vet. J.* **17**(Suppl.): 20–24.

Crossley, A. (1993) *Training the Young Horse: the First Two Years*, 10th edn. London: Stanley Paul & Co. Ltd.

Dalin, G. (1994) Pattern recognition in equine locomotion. *Equine Vet. J.* **26**: 173–174.

Degueurce, C., Dietrich, G., Pourcelot, P., Denoix, J.M. and Geiger, D. (1996) Three dimensional kinematic technique for evaluation of horse locomotion in outdoor conditions. *Med. Biol. Engineering Comp.* **5**: 249–252.

Degueurce, C., Pourcelot, P., Audigie, F., Denoix, J.M. and Geiger, D. (1997) Variability of the limb joint patterns of sound horses at the trot. *Equine Vet. J.* **23**(Suppl.): 89–92.

Deuel, N.R. (1994) Coordination of equine forelimb motion during the gallop. *Equine Vet. J.* **17**(Suppl.): 29–34.

Deuel, N.R. and Park, J-J. (1990a) The gait patterns of Olympic dressage horses. *Int. J. Sport Biomech.* **6**: 198–226.

Deuel, N.R. and Park, J-J. (1990b) Canter leads change kinematics of superior dressage horses. *J. Equine Vet. Sci.* **10**, 287–298.

Deuel, N.R. and Park, J-J. (1991) Kinematic analysis of jumping sequences of Olympic showjumping horses. *Equine Exerc. Physiol.* **3**: 158–66.

Dimery, N.J., Alexander, R.McN. and Ker, R.F. (1986) Elastic extension of leg tendons in the locomotion of horses (*Equus caballus*). *J. Zool.* **210**: 415–425.

Dow, S.M., Leendertz, J.A., Silver, I.A. *et al.* (1991) Identification of subclinical tendon injury from ground reaction force analysis. *Equine Vet. J.* **23**: 266–272.

Drevemo, S., Dalin, G., Fredricson, I. and Björne, K. (1980) Equine locomotion 3: The reproducibility of gait in Standardbred trotters. *Equine Vet. J.* **12**: 71–73.

Drevemo, S., Fredricson, I., Hjertén, G. and McMiken, D. (1987) Early development of gait asymmetries in trotting Standardbred colts. *Equine Vet. J.* **19**: 189–191.

Dusek, J. (1974) Beitrag zur Problem der Beziehung zwischen der Höhe und der Bewegungsmechnik bei den Hannoveraner Hengsten. *Bayer. Landwirtsch. Jahrb.* **51**: 209–213.

Eastlack, M.E., Arvidson, J., Snyder-Mackler, L., Danoff, J.V. and McGarvey, C.L. (1991) Interrater reliability of videotaped observational gait-analysis assessments. *Phys. Therapy* **71**: 465–472.

Fleiss, O., Edl, M. and Schubert, P. (1984) Intra und interlimbkoordination bei verschiedenen Ganggeschwindigkeiten des Pferdes. *Arch. Tierärztl. Fortbild.* **8**: 116–128.

Fredricson, I. and Drevemo, S. (1972) Methodological aspects of kinematics of the joints in the forelimbs of fast-moving horses. In: Fredricson, I. (ed) A photogrammetic study applying high speed cinematography. *Acta Vet. Scand.* **37**(Suppl.): 1–136.

Fredricson, I., Drevemo, S., Dalin, G. *et al.* (1983). Treadmill for equine locomotion analysis. *Equine Vet. J.* **15**: 111–115.

Galisteo, A.M., Cano, M.R., Miro, F., Vivo, J., Morales, J.L. and Aguera, E. (1996) Angular joint parameters in the Andalusian horse at walk, obtained by normal videography. *J. Equine. Vet. Sci.* **16**: 73–77.

Galisteo, A.M., Cano, M.R., Morales, J.L., Vivo, J. and Miro, F. (1998). The influence of speed and height on the kinematics of sound horses at the hand trot. *J. Equine. Vet. Sci.* **16**: 73–77.

Goiffon and Vincent (1779) *Mémoire artficielle des principes relatifs à la fidelle représentation des animaux tant en peinture, qu'en sculpture. I Partie concernant le cheval*. Alfort, France.

Goslow, G.E. (1985) Neural control of locomotion. In: Hildebrand, M. *et al.* (eds) *Functional Vertebrate Morphology*, 1st edn. Cambridge, Massachusetts: Harvard University Press, pp. 338–365.

Grant, B.D. (1989) Performance prediction. *The Equine Athlete* **2**: 1–2.

Gray, P. (1993) *Smythe and Goody's Horse Structure and Movement*. London: Allen, pp. 152–202.

Green, D.A. (1961) A review of studies on the growth rate of the horse. *British Vet. J.* **117**: 181–191.

Grillner, S. (1975) Locomotion in vertebrates: central mechanisms and reflex interaction. *Physiol. Rev.* **55**: 247–304.

Grillner, S. and Zangger, P. (1975) How detailed is the central pattern generation for locomotion? *Brain Res.* **88**: 367–371.

Günther, B. (1975) Dimensional analysis and theory of biological similarity. *Physiol. Rev.* **55**: 659–699.

Herring, L., Thompson, K.N. and Jarret, S. (1992) Defining normal three-dimensional kinematics of the lower forelimb in the horse. *J. Equine Vet. Sci.* **12**: 172–176.

Hildebrand, M. (1977) Analysis of asymmetrical gaits. *J. Mamm.* **58**: 131–156.

Hildebrand, M. (1987) The mechanics of the horse leg. *American Scientist* **75**: 594–601.

Hjertén, G. and Drevemo, S. (1993) Shortening of the forelimb in the horse during the stance phase. *Acta Anat.* **146**: 193–195.

Hjertén, G., Drevemo, S. and Eriksson, L.-E. (1994) Shortening of the hind limb in the horse during the stance phase. *Equine Vet. J.* **17**(Suppl.): 48–50.

Hof, A.L. (1996) Scaling gait data to body size. *Gait and Posture* **4**: 222–223.

Holmström, M. and Philipsson, J. (1993) Relationship between conformation, performance and health in 4-year-old Swedish Warmblood riding horses. *Livestock Prod. Sci.* **33**: 293–312.

Holmström, M., Fredricson, I. and Drevemo, S. (1994a) Biokinematic analysis of the Swedish Warmblood riding horse at trot. *Equine Vet. J.* **26**: 235–240.

Holström, M., Fredricson, I. and Drevemo, S. (1994b) Biokinematic differences between riding horses judged as good and poor at the trot. *Equine Vet. J.* **17**(Suppl.): 51–56.

Holt, K.G., Hamill, J. and Andres, R.O. (1991) Predicting the minimal energy costs of human walking. *Med. Sci. Sports and Exerc.* **23**: 491–498.

Holzreiter, S.H. and Köhle, M.E. (1993) Assessment of gait patterns using neural networks. *J. Biomech.* **26**: 645–651.

Huizinga, H.A. (1991) Genetic studies on the performance of Dutch Warmblood riding horses. *Thesis, Utrecht.*

Ingen Schenau, G.J. van (1980) Some fundamental aspects of the biomechanics of overground versus treadmill locomotion. *Med. Sci. Sports and Exerc.* **12**: 257–261.

Jansen, M.O., Raaij, J.A.G.M. van, Bogert, A.J. van den, Schamhardt, H.C. and Hartman, W. (1992) Quantitative analysis of computer-averaged electromyographic profiles of intrinsic limb muscles in ponies at the walk. *Am. J. Vet. Res.* **53**: 2343–2349.

Jeffcott, L.B., Rossdale, P.D., Freestone, J., Frank, C.J. and Towers-Clark, P.F. (1982) An assessment of wastage in Thoroughbred racing from conception to 4 years of age. *Equine Vet. J.* **14**: 185–198.

Johnston, C., Roepstorff, L. and Drevemo, S. (1995) Kinematics of the distal forelimb during the stance phase in the fast trotting Standardbred. *Equine Vet. J.* **18**(Suppl.): 170–174.

Johnston, C., Roepstorff, L. and Drevemo, S. (1996) Kinematics of the distal hind limb during the stance phase in the fast trotting Standardbred. *Equine Vet. J.* **28**: 263–268.

Johnston, C., Drevemo, S. and Roepstorff, L. (1997) Kinematics and kinetics of the carpus. *Equine Vet. J.* **23**(Suppl.): 84–88.

Johnston, C., Gottlieb-Vedi, M., Drevemo, S. and Roepstorff, L. (1999) The kinematics of loading and fatigue in the Standardbred trotter. *Equine Vet. J.* **30**(Suppl.): 249–253.

Knopfhart, A. (1966) *Het rijpaard: beoordeling en keuze.* Amsterdam: Veen 's Uitgeversmaatschappij, pp. 70–77.

Kobluk, C.N., Schnurr, D., Horney, F.D. *et al.* (1989) Use of high speed cinematography and computer generated gait diagrams for the study of equine hind limb kinematics. *Equine Vet. J.* **21**: 48–58.

Korsgaard, E. (1982) Muscle function in the forelimb of the horse. An electromyographical and kinesiological study. *Thesis, Copenhagen.*

Krebs, D.E., Edelstein, J.E. and Fishman, S. (1985) Reliability of observational kinematic gait analysis. *Phys. Therapy* **65**: 1027–1033.

Krüger, W. (1937) Ueber den Bewegungsablauf an dem oberen Teil der Vordergliedmaße des Pferdes im Schritt, Trab and Galopp. *Tierärztl. Rundsh.* **43**: 1–24.

Krüger, W. (1938) Ueber den Bewegungsablauf an dem oberen Teil der Hintergliedmaße des Pferdes im Schritt, Trab und Galopp. *Tierärztl. Rundsh.* **44**: 549–557.

Krüger, W. (1939) Über Wachstumsmessungen an den Skelettgrundlagen der Gliedmaßen – und Rumpfabschnitte beim lebenden Trakehner Warmblut – und Mecklenburger Kaltblutpferd mittels eines eigenen Meßverfahrens. *Zeitschr. für Tierzüchtk. und Zuchtüngsbiol.* **43**: 145–163.

Lanovaz, J.L., Clayton, H.M. and Watson, L.H. (1998) In vitro attenuation of impact shock in equine digits. *Equine Vet. J.* **26**(Suppl.): 96–102.

Lanovaz, J.L., Clayton, H.M., Colborne, G.R. and Schamhardt, H.C. (1999) Forelimb kinematics and net joint moments during the swing phase of the trot. *Equine Vet. J.* **30**(Suppl.): 235–239.

Lanyon, L.E. (1971) Use of an accelerometer to determine support and swing phase of a limb during locomotion. *Am. J. Vet. Res.* **32**: 1099–1101.

Leach, D.H. and Crawford, W.H. (1983) Guidelines for the future of equine locomotion research. *Equine Vet. J.* **15**: 103–110.

Leach, D.H. and Cymbaluk, N.F. (1986) Relationships between stride length, stride frequency, and morphometrics of foals. *Am. J. Vet. Res.* **47**: 2090–2097.

Leach, D.H. and Drevemo, S. (1991) Velocity-dependant changes in stride frequency and length of trotters on a treadmill. *Equine Exerc. Physiol.* **3**: 136–140.

Leach, D.H., Omrod, K. and Barlow, D.A. (1984) Stride characteristics of horses competing Grand Prix jumping. *Am. J. Vet. Res.* **45**: 888–892.

Magnusson, L.-E. (1985) Studies on the conformation and related traits of Standardbred trotters in Sweden. *Thesis, Uppsala.*

Marey, E.J. (1882) *La Machine Animale. Locomotion terrestre et aérienne,* 3rd edn. Paris: Ballière & Co.

Martinez-del Campo, L.J., Kobluk, C.N., Greer, N. *et al.* (1991) The use of high-speed videography to generate angle-time and angle-angle diagrams for the study of equine locomotion.*Vet. Comp. Orthop. Traum.* **4**: 120–131.

Merkens, H.W. and Schamhardt, H.C. (1994) Relationship between ground reaction force patterns and kinematics in the walking and trotting horses. *Equine Vet. J.* **17**(Suppl.): 67–70.

Merkens, H.W., Schamhardt, H.C., Osch, G.J.V.M. van and Bogert, A.J. van den (1993) Ground reaction force patterns of Dutch Warmbloods at the canter. *Am. J. Vet. Res.* **54**: 670–674.

Mitchelson, D.L. (1988) Automated three dimensional movement analysis using the CODA-3 system. *Biomed. Tech.* **33**: 179–182.

Mochon, S. and McMahon, T.A. (1980) Ballistic walking. *J. Biomech.* **13**: 49–57.

Molenaar, G.J. (1983) Kinematics of the reciprocal apparatus in the horse. *Zbl. Vet. Med. C/Anat. Histol. Embryol.* **12**: 278–287.

Morales, J.L., Manchado, M., Cano, M.R., Miro, F. and Galisteo, A.M. (1998a) Temporal and linear kinematics in elite and riding horses at the trot. *J. Equine Vet. Sci.* **18**: 835–839.

Morales, J.L., Manchado, M., Vivo, J., Galisteo, A.M., Agûera, E. and Miro, F. (1998b) Angular kinematics in elite and riding horses at the trot. *Equine Vet. J.* **30**: 528–533.

Morris, E., Seeherman, H. and O'Callaghan, M.W. (1990) The Equisport program: a comprehensive clinical evaluation of the Equine Athlete. *The Equine Athlete* **3**: 3–10.

Mosimann, W. and Micheluzzi, P. (1969) Die Bewegung im Cubitus des Pferdes als gedampfte, erzwungene Schwingung. *Zentbl. Vet. Med. Reihe A* **16**: 180–184.

Muir, G.D., Leach, D.H., Cymbaluk, N.F. and Dyson, S. (1991) Velocity-dependent changes in intrinsic stride timing variables of Quarterhorse foals. *Equine Exerc. Physiol.* **3**: 141–145.

Muñoz, A., Santisteban, R., Rubio, M.D., *et al.* (1997) Training as an influential factor on the locomotor pattern of Andalusian horses. *J. Vet. Med. A* **44**: 473–480.

Niki, Y., Ueda, Y., Yoshida, K. and Masumitsu, H. (1982) Force plate study of equine biomechanics. 2. The vertical and fore-aft components of floor reaction forces and motion of equine limbs. *Bull. Equine Res. Inst.* **19**: 1–17.

Niki, Y., Ueda, Y. and Masumitsu, H. (1984) A forceplate study in equine biomechanics 3. The vertical and fore aft components of floor reaction forces and motion of equine limbs at canter. *Bull. Equine Res. Inst.* **21**: 8–18.

Oliver, R. and Langrish, B. (1992) *A Photographic Guide to Conformation*, 2nd edn. London: Allen, pp. 114–124.

Palmgren, A. (1929) Zur Kenntnis der sogenannten Schnappgelenke. II Die Physiologische Bedeutung des Federungsphänomens. *Zeitschr. anat. entwickl. Gesch.* **89**: 194–200.

Peham, C., Licka, T., Mayr, A., Scheidl, M. and Girtler, D. (1998) Speed dependency of motion pattern consistency. *J. Biomech.* **31**: 769–772.

Podhajsky, A. (1981) *The Complete Training of Horse and Rider*, 10th edn. London: Harrap, p. 34.

Quddus, M.A., Kingsbury, H.B. and Rooney, J.T. (1978) A force and motion study of the foreleg of a Standardbred trotter. *J. Equine Med. Surg.* **2**: 233–242.

Radin, E.L., Yang, K.H., Riegger, C., Kish, V.L. and O'Connor, J.J. (1991) Relationship between lower limb dynamics and knee joint pain. *J. Orthop. Res.* **9**: 398–405.

Ratzlaff, M.H., Wilson, P.D., Hyde, M.L., Balch, O.K. and Grant, B.D. (1993) Relationships between locomotor forces, hoof position and joint motion during the support phase of the stride of galloping horses. *Acta Anat.* **146**: 200–204.

Riemersma, D.J., Schamhardt, H.C., Hartman, W. and Lammertink, J.L.M.A. (1988a) Kinetics and kinematics of the equine hind limb: in vivo tendon loads and force plate measurements in ponies. *Am. J. Vet. Res.* **49**: 1344–1352.

Riemersma, D.J., Bogert, A.J. van den, Schamhardt, H.C. and Hartman, W. (1988b) Kinetics and kinematics of the equine hind limb: in vivo tendon strain and joint kinematics *Am. J. Vet. Res.* **49**: 1353–1359.

Roepstorff, L., Johnston, C. and Drevemo, S. (1994) The influences of different treadmill constructions on ground reaction forces as determined by the use of a force-measuring horseshoe. *Equine Vet. J.* **17**(Suppl.): 71–74.

Rooney, J.R. (1990) The jump behaviour of the humeroradial and tarsocrural joints of the horse. *J. Equine Vet. Sci.* **4**: 311–314.

Rose, R.J. and Evans, D.L. (1990) Training – art or science? *Equine Vet. J.* **9**(Suppl.): 2–4.

Schamhardt, H.C. and Merkens, H.W. (1994) Objective determination of ground contact of the limbs of the horse at the walk and trot: comparison between ground reaction forces, accelerometer data and kinematics. *Equine Vet. J.* **17**(Suppl.): 75–79.

Schamhardt, H.C., Hartman, W. and Lammertink, J.M.L.A. (1985) In vivo bone strain in the equine tibia before and after transection of the peroneus tertius muscle. *Res. Vet. Sci.* **39**: 139–144.

Schamhardt, H.C., Merkens, H.W. and Osch, G.J.V.M. van (1991) Ground reaction force analysis of horses ridden at the walk and trot. *Equine Exerc. Physiol.* **3**: 120–127.

Schamhardt, H.C., Bogert, A.J. van den, Lammertink, J.L.M.A. and Markies, H. (1992) Measurement and analysis of equine locomotion with the CODA-2 kinematic analysis system. *Proceedings 8th Meeting ESB, June 21–24, Rome, Italy*, p. 270.

Schamhardt, H.C., Bogert, A.J. van den, Lammertink, J.L.M.A. and Markies, H. (1993) Measurement and analysis of equine locomotion using a modified CODA-3 kinematic analysis system. *J. Biomech.* **26**: 861.

Schwarz, H.G. (1971) Bewegungsanalyse beim Pferd und Untersuchung der Trainingseinwirkung auf den Bewegungsablauf im Schritt und Trab. *Thesis Giessen, Germany.*

Schauder, W. (1952) Die besonderen stoßbrechenden Einrichtungen an den Gliedmaßen des Pferdes. *Dtsch. tierärztl. Wschr.* **59**: 35–38.

Schmaltz, R. (1906) Konstruktion und Größe der Standwinkel an den Beinen des Pferdes. *Berl. Tierärztl. Wschr.* **14**: 257–261.

Schryver, H.F., Bartel, D.L., Langrana, N. and Lowe, J.E. (1978) Locomotion in the horse: kinematics and external and internal forces in the normal equine digit in the walk and trot. *Am. J. Vet. Res.* **39**: 1728–1733.

Sloet van Oldruitenborgh-Oosterbaan, M.M. van, Schamhardt, H.C. and Barneveld, A. (1995a) Effects of weight and riding on workload and locomotion during treadmill exercise. *Equine Exerc. Physiol.* **4**: 413–417.

Sloet van Oldruitenborgh-Oosterbaan, M.M. and Barneveld, A. (1995b) The workload of ridden Dutch Warmblood horses: a comparison of overground and treadmill exercise. *Vet. Rec.* **137**: 136–139.

Sloet van Oldruitenborgh-Oosterbaan, M.M. and Clayton, H. M. (1999) Advantages and disadvantages of track vs. treadmill tests. *Equine Vet. J.* **30**(Suppl.): 645–647.

Smythe, R.H. (1957) What makes a good horse: its structure and performance. London: Country Life Ltd, pp. 86–102.

Smythe, R.H., Goody, P.C. and Gray, P. (1993) *Horse Structure and Movement.* London: Allen & Co.

Spooner, G. (1977) *The Handbook of Showing.* London: Allen, pp. 50–58.

Stashak, T.S. (1987) *Adams' Lameness in Horses*, 4th edn. Philadelphia: Lea & Febiger, pp. 76, 88, 102.

Strubelt (1928) Uber die Bedeutung des Lacertus Fibrosus und des Tendo Femorotarsicus fur das stehen und die Bewegung des Pferdes. *Arch. Tierheilk.* **57**: 575–585.

Taylor, B.M., Tipton, C.M., Adrian, M. and Karpovich, P.V. (1966) Action of certain joints in the legs of the horse recorded electrogoniometrically. *Am. J. Vet. Res.* **27**: 85–89.

Thompson, K.N., Herring, L. and Shapiro, R. (1992) A three dimensional kinematic study of the metacarpophalangeal joint in horses. *J. Equine Vet. Sci.* **12**: 172–176.

Tokuriki, M. and Aoki, O. (1991) Neck muscle activity in horses during locomotion with and without a rider. *Equine Exerc. Physiol.* **3**: 146–150.

Tokuriki, M. and Aoki, O. (1995) Electromyographic activity of hind limb joint muscles during walk, trot and canter. *Equine Vet. J.* **18**(Suppl.): 152–155.

Tokuriki, M., Aoki, O., Niki, Y., Kurakawa, Y., Hataya, M. and Kita, T. (1989) Electromyographic activity of cubital joint muscles in horses during locomotion. *Am. J. Vet. Res.* **50**: 950–957.

Ueda, Y., Niki, Y., Yoshida, K. and Masumitsu, H. (1981) Force plate study of equine biomechanics: floor reaction forces of normal walking and trotting horses. *Bull. Equine Res. Inst.* **18**: 28–41.

Veldhuizen, A.E. van (1991) Nogmaals uitleg over het lineair scoren. *In de Strengen* **58**: 34–35.

Vilensky, J.A. and Gankiewicz, E. (1986) Effect of size on vervet *(Cercopithecus aethiops)* gait parameters: a preliminary analysis. *Am. J. Phys. Anthrop.* **46**: 104–117.

Vilensky, J.A. and Gankiewicz, E. (1990) Effects of growth and speed on hind limb joint angular displacement patterns in vervet monkeys *(Cercopithecus aethiops)*. *Am. J. Phys. Anthropol.* **81**: 441–449.

Vilensky, J.A., Gankiewicz, E. and Townsend, D.W. (1990a) Effects of size on vervet *(Cercopithecus aethiops)* gait parameters: a longitudinal approach. *Am. J. Phys. Anthropol.* **81**: 429–439.

Vilensky, J.A., Gankiewicz, E. and Townsend, D.W. (1990b) Effect of growth and speed on hind limb joint angular displacement patterns in vervet monkeys *(Cercopithecus aethiops)*. *Am. J. Phys. Anthrop.* **81**: 441–449.

Walter, K. (1925) Der Bewegungsablauf an den freien Gliedmassen des Pferdes im Schritt, Trab und Galop. *Arch. Wiss. Pract. Tierheilk.* **53**: 316–352.

Wentink, G.H. (1978a) Biokinetical analysis of the movement of the pelvic limb of the horse and the role of the muscles in the walk and trot. *Anat. Embryol.* **152**: 261–272.

Wentink, G.H. (1978b) An experimental study on the role of the reciprocal tendinous apparatus of the horse at walk. *Anat. Embryol.* **154**: 143–151.

Weeren, P.R. van (1989) Skin displacement in equine kinematic gait analysis. *Thesis, Utrecht, The Netherlands.*

Weeren, P.R. van, Bogert, A.J. van den, Barneveld, A., Hartman, W. and Kersjes, A.W. (1990) The role of the reciprocal apparatus in the hind limb of the horse investigated by a modified CODA-3 opto-electronic kinematic analysis system. *Equine Vet. J.* **9** (Suppl.): 95–100.

Weeren, P.R. van, Bogert, A.J. van den and Barneveld, A. (1992) Correction models for skin displacement in equine kinematic gait analysis. *J. Equine Vet. Sci.* **12**: 178–192.

Weeren, P.R. van, Bogert, A.J. van den, Back, W., Bruin, G. and Barneveld, A. (1993) Kinematics of the Standardbred trotter measured at 6, 7, 8, and 9 m/s on a treadmill, before and after 5 months of prerace training. *Acta Anat.* **146**: 154–161.

Willemen, M.A., Jacobs, M.W.H. and Schamhardt, H.C. (1999) In vitro attenuation of impact vibrations in the distal forelimb. *Equine Vet. J.* **30** (Suppl.): 245–248.

Woltring, H.J. (1986) A Fortran package for generalized, cross-validatory spline smoothing and differentiation. *Adv. Eng. Software* **8**: 104–113.

6
The Role of the Hoof and Shoeing

Willem Back

INTRODUCTION

To deliver maximal performance it is essential that a horse has good balance. A part of the required balance comes from factors connected to the hoof (Balch *et al.*, 1991a; Curtis, 1999). 'No foot, no horse' is a well-known saying that emphasizes the important role of the hoof.

After domestication of the horse 5000–6000 years ago, man assumed much of the responsibility for the balance between hoof growth and hoof wear. The Greek horse people (hippiaters) were in favor of breeding horses with good hoof quality that did not need shoes. The Romans invented the hipposandal that was attached to the hoof with straps and was used to protect the feet of the horse en route to the battlefield, where they were removed. The first iron horseshoes with nails were made by the Celts 2000 years ago and were similar to the ones we use today (Fig. 6.1).

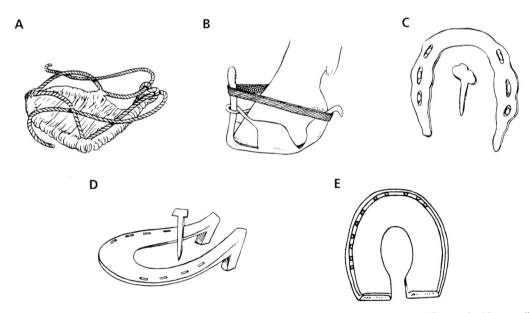

Fig. 6.1 The development of the horseshoe. (**A**) Ancient grass sandal; (**B**) Roman iron hipposandal fastened without nails; (**C**) Celtic horseshoe with oval nailholes; (**D**) Medieval shoe with square nail holes; (**E**) Renaissance shoe with fullering (Butler, 1995).

During locomotion every stride involves forces at the hoof–ground interface that load the locomotor apparatus. Repeated application of forces that have a high magnitude and/or an abnormal direction of action, overload the limb and may lead to the development of pathological processes. When we have an insight how these forces work, we can modulate them by corrective hoof trimming and optimal shoeing as rational measures to treat and prevent lameness. That is the basic theme of this chapter.

FUNCTIONAL ANATOMY OF THE FOOT

General anatomy

The equine foot has evolved from the third digit, which has been greatly elongated and strengthened. The hoof wall has developed from the nail of the third digit. The hoof of the first digit is still present, though rudimentary, in the form of the chestnut on the medial side of the radius (forelimb) or metatarsus (hindlimb), while that of the fifth digit, especially in coldbloods, persists as the ergot on the palmar/plantar side of the metacarpo-/metatarsophalangeal joint.

The hoof capsule consists of several parts: the coronet, the horny wall, the sole, the frog and the heels (Fig. 6.2).

The horn of each part of the hoof is produced by a corresponding area of dermis (corium). The estimated horn regeneration time based on a growth rate of 8–10 mm/month is 12 months for the toe, 6–8 months for the quarters, and 4–5 months for the heels. The coronet separates and connects the skin above from the hoof wall below. Deep to the coronet lies the dermis that produces the horn tubules of the hoof wall via the horn papillae, which project distally into the horn of the hoof wall. The horn tubules are responsible for the striated appearance of the hoof wall.

Projecting from the inner surface of the hoof wall are the primary epidermal lamellae (600/hoof) and secondary epidermal lamellae (100–200/primary lamella). The insensitive horn of these epidermal lamellae interdigitates with the sensitive dermal lamellae to form the functional connection between the hoof wall and P3. The horn that forms the epidermal lamellae is unstructured (non-tubular). As the hoof wall grows, it moves distally by a mechanism that allows the primary epidermal lamellae to slide past the stationary secondary epidermal lamellae. On the solar surface, the white zone demarcates the junction between sensitive and insensitive tissues. When shoes are nailed in place, the nails should enter peripheral to the white zone.

The bony skeleton of the hoof consists of the distal phalanx (P3) or coffin bone, the navicular bone and

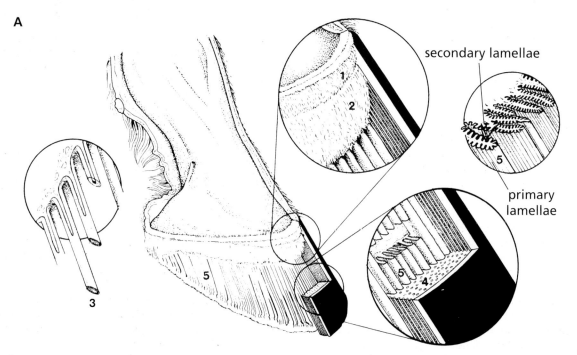

Fig. 6.2 The hoof capsule and its parts. (**A**) Lateral view. 1: Coronary band epidermal layer; 2: coronary band germinative layer; 3: horn papillae and tubulae; 4: unstructured horn; 5: primary and secondary epidermal lamellae. (Dyce & Wensing, 1980).

B

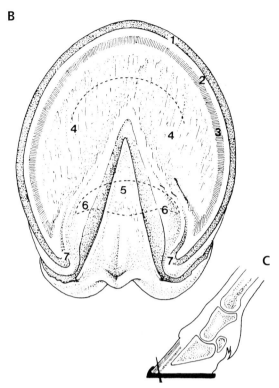

C

Fig. 6.2 (**B**) Ventral view. 1: Pigmented outer hoofwall; 2: unpigmented inner hoofwall; 3: white line; 4: sole; 5: frog; 6: sulcus; 7: heels. (The interrupted lines indicate the projected location of the navicular bone and the third phalanx.) (**C**) Schematic drawing of the correct location of a hoof nail (Dyce & Wensing, 1980).

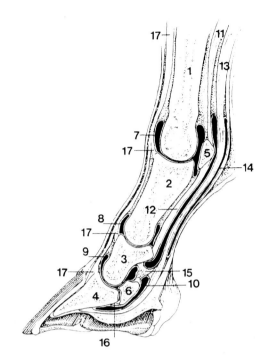

Fig. 6.3A Sagittal section of the equine distal lower limb. 1: Metacarpal bone (McIII); 2: first phalanx (P1); 3: second phalanx (P2); 4: third phalanx (P3); 5: proximal sesamoid bone; 6: navicular bone; 7: fetlock joint; 8: pastern joint; 9: coffin joint; 10: navicular bursa; 11: suspensory ligament; 12: straight sesamoidean ligament; 13: deep digital flexor tendon; 14. superficial digital flexor tendon; 15: synovial membrane of coffin joint, navicular bursa and tendon sheath with connective tissue; 16: distal navicular 'impar' ligament; 17: common digital extensor tendon (Dyce & Wensing, 1980).

part of the middle phalanx (P2) or short pastern bone. All three of these bones take part in the formation of the distal interphalangeal or coffin joint (Fig. 6.3).

The medial and lateral hoof cartilages (ungual cartilages) are square-shaped structures located on either side of P3 and connected to P1 and P2 by connective tissue. They are large and flexible. Between them lie the digital cushion and a venous plexus. Compression of these structures during locomotion assists the return of venous blood to the heart. The navicular bone is connected to P3 by the distal navicular or 'impar' ligament, to P2 by connective tissue and the synovial membranes of the coffin joint, navicular bursa and tendon sheath, and to P1 by the proximal navicular ligaments. The navicular bone is covered on one side by hyaline cartilage and on the opposite side by fibrocartilage. Its hyaline cartilage side is in contact with the palmar/plantar aspect of P2 and P3. The deep digital flexor tendon (DDFT) curves around the palmar/plan-

tar aspect of the navicular bone before attaching to the flexor surface of P3. The navicular bursa is interposed between the DDFT and the fibrocartilage of the navicular bone.

Vascular supply

The blood supply enters the hoof via the palmar/plantar digital arteries, which run through the terminal arch within P3 (Fig. 6.4). A network of arteries perforates the dorsal surface of P3 and ramifies in the lamellar dermis. Some branches from this plexus are directed proximally to supply the coronet, where they anastomose with branches of the circumflex artery of the coronet. The dorsal branches leave the palmar/plantar digital arteries just before they enter the terminal arch of P3. The

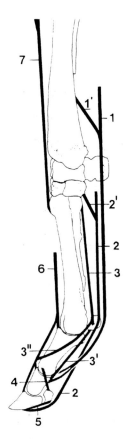

Fig. 6.3 B Schematic drawing of tendons and ligaments of the equine lower limb. 1: Superficial digital flexor tendon; 1ᴵ: proximal accessory ligament; 2: deep digital flexor tendon; 2ᴵ: distal accessory ligament; 3: suspensory ligament; 3ᴵ: straight sesamoideum ligament; 3ᴵᴵ: rami extensori; 4: proximal navicular ligament; 5: distal navicular 'impar' ligament; 6: common digital extensor tendon; 7: extensor carpi radialis tendon (Dyce & wensing, 1980).

palmar/plantar branches run to the heel region where they form the venous plexus and anastomose with the circumflex artery of the sole.

Nerve supply

The hoof is innervated by the palmar/plantar digital nerves, which are located caudal to the vein and artery in the pastern region (Fig. 6.5). The nerves can be blocked by injection of a local anesthetic at the proximal pastern level where the nerves are crossed by the ligament of the ergot (low palmar block) or more distally as the nerve passes deep to the hoof cartilage (palmar

digital block). Palmar digital nerve blocks anesthetize the caudal third of the hoof and its contents; low palmar nerve blocks just distal to the fetlock joint anesthetize the entire hoof.

Proprioception

Bowker *et al.* (1993, 1995) described the concentration of nociceptors in the palmar/plantar part of the frog and in the proximal navicular area. It is hypothesized that these so-called lamellar bodies supply the central nervous system and the brain with proprioceptive information describing the location of the body in space. This information is needed to control the central pattern generator (CPG) and thus intra- and inter-limb coordination (Fig. 6.6).

Studies of the effects of local anesthesia in sound horses have yielded conflicting results. Keg *et al.* (1996) demonstrated no effect of a low palmar nerve block on gait symmetry as evaluated kinetically, whereas Kübber *et al.* (1994) did detect some kinematic effects. It is not known whether the differences between these studies were due to the sensitivity of the analytic equipment or to the (un-) soundness of the horses.

HOOF MECHANICS IN THE STANDING HORSE

Hoof–pastern axis

Ideally, hoof trimming optimizes the interaction between the hoof and the ground during locomotion. Since the hoof is a three-dimensional structure, it should be balanced in both the craniocaudal and mediolateral planes. Forces at the toe, medial and lateral heels collectively are the lowest when the hoof and pastern angles are aligned (Balch *et al.*, 1997).

Hoof balance

Craniocaudal balance

Craniocaudal balance evaluates the hoof in a lateral view (Fig. 6.7). It is assessed with the horse standing square on a level surface. Alignment of the dorsal hoof wall with the pastern axis is achieved by adjusting the absolute and relative lengths of the heels, the quarters and the toe. A hoof that is balanced in this manner usually contacts the ground flat-footed or slightly heel first. When the hoof has a more acute angle than the pastern, the hoof–pastern axis is said to be broken backward. Conversely, when the angle of the hoof is more upright than that of the pastern, the hoof–pastern axis is said to

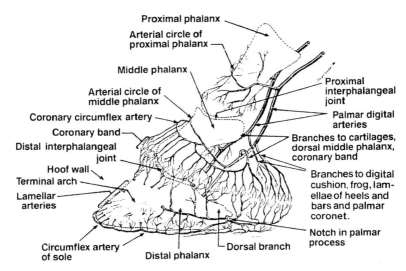

Fig. 6.4A The main arteries of the foot: lateral view (Pollitt, 1995).

be broken forward. Radiographic studies have shown that P1 is always a little more upright (vertical) than P2 and P3 with the three phalanges being most closely aligned when the hoof is trimmed with the dorsal hoof wall parallel to the pastern axis (Bushe *et al.*, 1987). Under these circumstances the angle between the solar surface of P3 and the ground is approximately 5°. The dorsal face of P3 is parallel to the dorsal hoof wall at a distance of about 19 ± 0.5 mm in warmbloods (K.J. Dik, personal communication, 1999).

There is a difference between the shape of the fore and hind hooves: the fore hoof is wider and usually has a smaller (more acute) hoof angle, while the hind hoof is narrower and has a larger hoof angle. In farriery books (Hermans, 1984; Hertsch *et al.*, 1996; Ruthe *et al.*, 1997) angles ranging from 45–50° for the forelimbs and

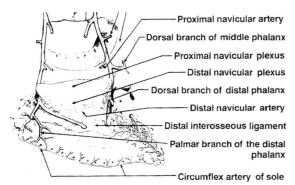

Fig. 6.4B The main arteries of the foot: caudal view (Pollitt, 1995).

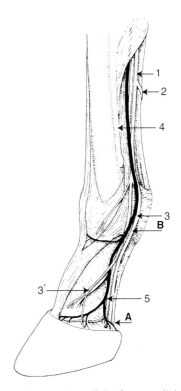

Fig. 6.5 Sensory innervation of the foot, medial view. 1: Medial palmar nerve; 2: ramus communicans; 3: digital medial palmar nerve; 3′: ramus dorsalis; 4: medial palmar artery and vein; 5: medial digital palmar artery and vein; (**A**) site of digital nerve block; (**B**) site of low palmar (abaxial) nerve block (Dyce & Wensing, 1980).

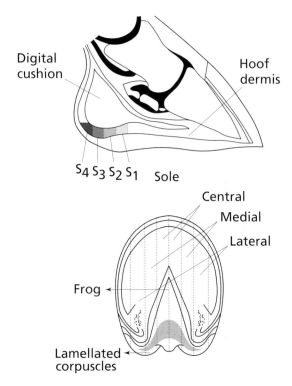

Fig. 6.6A Sensory receptors in the foot. In the sagittal view the four zones of the sole (S1–S4) represent locations of the lamellated corpuscles with the relative density being indicated by the dots in zones S1–S4. S4 shows the highest density. In the ventral view the lamellated corpuscles were obtained from the shaded areas (Bowker *et al.*, 1993).

50–55° for the hindlimbs have been reported, but more recently the average angles have been reported to be over 50° in the fore and over 55° in the hindlimbs (Clayton, 1988; Kobluk *et al.*, 1990; Balch *et al.*, 1991a; Butler, 1995; Hickman & Humphrey, 1997).

The second component of craniocaudal balance is the location of the bearing surface of the hoof relative to the weight-bearing axis through the cannon bone. The bulbs of the heel should lie vertically below the central axis of the cannon bone in the sagittal plane. In some horses, although the hoof–pastern axis is aligned, the whole hoof capsule is located too far forward so that the bulbs of the heels are ahead of the central axis of the cannon bone. The resulting caudal concentration of the weight bends the hoof tubules at the heels, which reduces their ability to withstand compression, and leads to underrun heels (Stashak, 1987; Balch *et al.*, 1997). Normally, the dorsal toe wall and caudal heel wall should run parallel to each other and the toe wall length relative to heel wall length should be 2:1.0 in the fore hooves and 2:1.5 in the hind

hooves (Hermans, 1984). Underrun heels have been defined as having a difference between the angles of the toe and heels that is more than 5° (Balch *et al.*, 1997).

Mediolateral balance

Mediolateral balance evaluates the hoof in a frontal plane and attempts to optimize hoof balance by either a static or a dynamic evaluation (Seeherman, 1991; Balch *et al.*, 1997). Static balance seeks to achieve symmetry in the square standing horse so that a line that bisects the limb longitudinally is intersected at 90° by a transverse line drawn across the heels (geometric limb axis). Caudron *et al.* (1997a,b, 1998) used radiographs to evaluate and correct this balance. In the dynamic method, the hoof is trimmed so that the medial and lateral sides contact the ground simultaneously, which adds a new dimension to the equation and makes the solution even more elusive. In a horse with ideal conformation, static and dynamic balancing will show a rather similar result, but when conformational defects are present the two methods produce different results.

When a horse is standing quietly, the force due to gravity is compensated by the ground reaction force (GRF) acting near the geometric centre of pressure (CP) of the foot, which lies around the apex of the frog (Barrey, 1990; Balch *et al.*, 1997; Ovnicek 1997). The hoof rotates around the instantaneous center of rotation of the coffin joint, which is located in the distal part of P2. Equilibrium exists when the moment (torque) of the GRF about the coffin joint ($F_{GRF} * d_{GRF}$) is equal to the moment of the DDFT ($F_{DDFT} * d_{DDFT}$). Ideally, the central reference point (CRP) should be located midway between the toe and the heels (Wright & Douglas, 1993), although in wild horses the distance from the toe to the CRP is only about one-third of the toe-to-heel distance (Ovnicek, 1997, Fig. 6.8).

Four point trimming

Ovnicek (1997) studied the hooves of 65 wild horses. From his observations he developed the natural trimming technique for unshod horses. The principles of this technique are that the heels are trimmed back to the widest point of the frog, along the sole plane. The toe is bevelled to a 15–20° angle in a manner akin to what would be done in preparation for a rockered toe shoe. The quarters are hollowed slightly by rasping so they are not weight-bearing on a firm surface. This leaves a raised area projecting downwards at the heel buttress. There is a gradual arc between the impression mark at the lateral side of the toe and the heel impression mark on each side of the foot. The hoof wall has four loading points: one at each side of the toe and one at each heel. Little to no sole, frog and bars are ever removed. Within a few

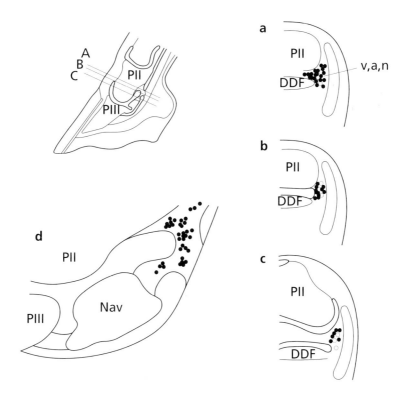

Fig. 6.6B Sensory receptors in the navicular region. Inset shows the three levels from which drawings **a–c** were obtained. Note that the lamellated corpuscles (dots) are located primarily abaxially and proximal to the collateral sesamoidean ligament (CSL) often in association with the palmar digital nerve (n), as well as with the artery (a) and vein (v). **d** is a parasagittal drawing from the abaxial region of CSL. PII: pastern bone; PIII: coffin bone; DDF: deep digital flexor tendon; Nav: navicular bone (Bowker *et al.*, 1995).

months this method of trimming should result in a stronger hoof structure with a cupped sole, spreading heels, and a well-developed frog.

HOOF MECHANICS DURING LOCOMOTION

Several techniques have been used to document the kinematics and kinetics of the hoof. One of the requirements of the recording equipment is that it should have a high enough sampling frequency to distinguish events such as initial ground contact, heel-off and toe-off with sufficient accuracy (Linford, 1994). This can be especially difficult on outdoor tracks where reflective markers disappear in the sand (Merkens & Schamhardt, 1994). See chapter 3 for more information on equipment and techniques.

Initial ground contact

When the horse is observed in the lateral view, initial ground contact is heel first, flat-footed or toe first. The hindlimbs show a greater tendency to heel first contacts than the forelimbs, and heel first contacts occur more frequently during high-speed locomotion (Back *et al.*, 1995). However, in some movements, such as piaffe, toe first contacts are normal. The frequency of toe first contacts increases when the hoof is trimmed with an acute angle (long toes and/or low heels). Conversely, when horses are trimmed with a steep hoof angle (short toe and/or long heels), heel first contacts are more numerous (Clayton, 1990a). Therefore, the manner of initial ground contact depends on speed, gait and farriery.

Impact

Immediately after initial ground contact, the hoof is rapidly decelerated by the vertical landing forces and horizontal braking forces that reduce its speed to zero during the impact phase that follows initial ground contact. The forces and decelerations associated with impact have been measured using a force plate (Merkens & Schamhardt, 1994), force shoe (Barrey, 1990; Frederick & Henderson 1970; Ratzlaff *et al.*, 1985,

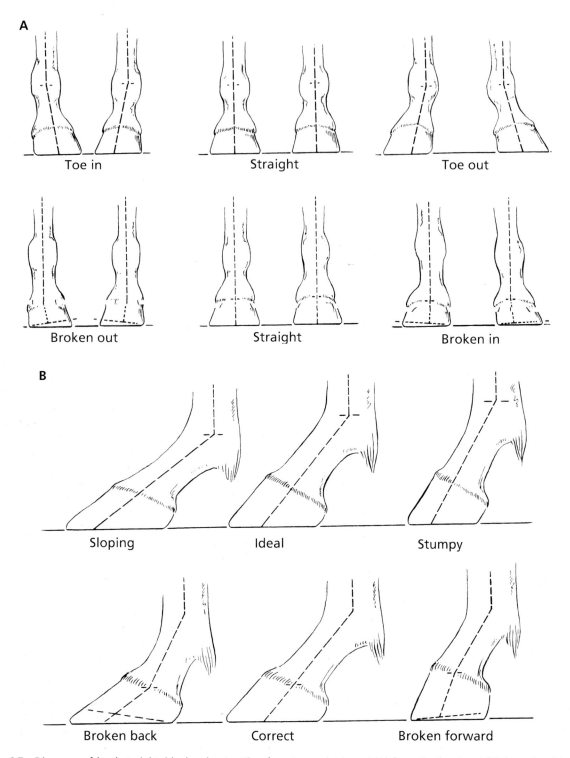

Fig. 6.7 Diagrams of (not) straight, ideal and correct hoof–pastern axis viewed (**A**) from the front and (**B**) from the side (Butler, 1995).

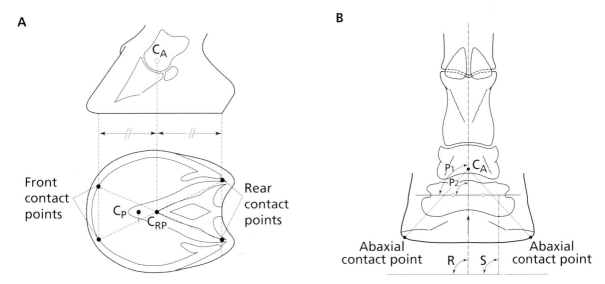

Fig. 6.8 Schematic representation of foot balance showing the ideal equilibrium of the foot relative to the center of articulation in the distal part of the second phalanx. (**A**) Craniocaudal balance: Lateral and solar view and (**B**) mediolateral balance: heel view. C_A; centre of articulation, C_P; centre of pressure, CRP; central reference point.

1993) and accelerometers (Benoit *et al.*, 1993; Burn *et al.*, 1997). The hoof and interphalangeal joints attenuate the shock wave associated with impact (Dyhre-Poulsen *et al.*, 1994; Lanovaz *et al.*, 1998; Willemen *et al.*, 1998). Nevertheless, the forces acting in different directions have the potential to damage the body (Fig. 6.9). Friction between the hoof and the ground and hardness of the ground affect the forces applied to the limb during the impact phase (Hjertén & Drevemo, 1993).

The impulsive loading that occurs during impact has been implicated as a causative factor in arthritis in animals (Radin *et al.*, 1981; Pratt, 1997; Radin 1999) and in humans (Folman *et al.*, 1986; Ker *et al.*, 1989). The time during which these forces have to be absorbed is reduced as speed increases. For example the time taken to absorb impact shock at the canter (7 m/s) is 50% of that at the walk (1.6 m/s), which is a consequence of the shorter time the foot is on the ground. Back *et al.* (1995) found that during trotting on a treadmill the hoof was flat on the ground, and the vertical speed and acceleration were zero within 3% (20 ms) of the total stride duration. However, it took 6% (40 ms) of total stride duration for the horizontal speed to reach zero. Moreover, the forelimbs appeared to land with a higher vertical velocity and the hindlimbs with a higher horizontal velocity (Back *et al.*, 1995). Thus, the forelimbs 'bounce', whereas the hindlimbs 'slide.' The sliding of the hoof in the sagittal plane has been measured for horses trotting on a treadmill: steel shoes slide for longer than rubber shoes and the hoof stops

less abruptly on a coir mat than on a rubber belt (Roepstorff *et al.*, 1994). Johnston (personal communication, 1999) found that the sliding of the hoof took 16 ms on a dirt track, whereas on a hard surface (asphalt or concrete) it took 21 ms for the unshod hoof and 32 ms for steel shoes. The active neurophysiological response time is the time required for the muscles to respond to a stimulus. It has been estimated to be around 30 ms in humans (Nigg *et al.*, 1981) and horses (Bowker *et al.*, 1993; Hjertén & Drevemo, 1993). This suggests that the forces acting on the equine lower limb during the impact phase are determined mainly by passive factors like coordination and ground properties (Hjertén & Drevemo, 1993).

Hoof mechanism

Since the hoof shows more elasticity in the heel area than at the toes or quarters, its geometry changes when it is loaded: the heels expand and sink caudally, and the toe retracts (Douglas *et al.*, 1998); this is called the hoof mechanism (Fig. 6.10).

At impact the distance between the heels is wider than at rest, while at breakover, because of increased pressure in the toe area, the distance between the heels is narrower than at rest. Thus, the foot has three functional areas: the heels for damping; the wall, frog and sole for support; and the toe for propulsion (Barrey, 1990). Deformation of the foot during the stance phase optimizes these functions, and also enables the hoof to act as a pump for the blood circulation (Ratzlaff *et al.*, 1985; Fig. 6.11).

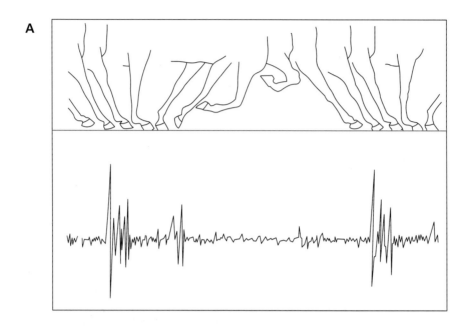

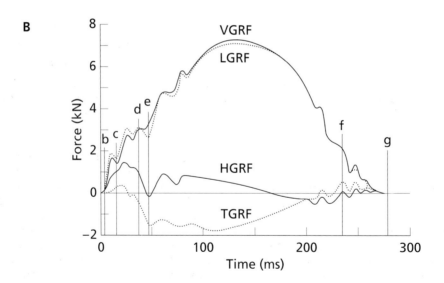

Fig. 6.9A The impact phase is the short period immediately following initial ground contact, in which the decelerating hoof is oscillating relative to the ground until hoof velocity has been reduced to zero. **B** During impact the vertical landing (VGRF) and horizontal braking (HGRF) forces acting on the hoof are transferred into longitudinal (LGRF) and transverse (TGRF) forces acting on the equine lower limb (Hjertén & Drevemo, 1994. With permission from Elsevier Science.).

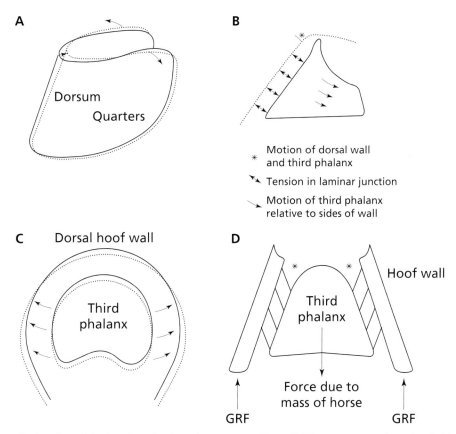

Fig. 6.10 Schematic drawing of the hoof mechanism phenomenon. The solid line represents the unloaded hoof wall, the dashed line shows the change in shape that occurs during weight-bearing. Under load the dorsal wall flattens and moves palmarly, while the heels move laterally and caudally. GRF: Ground reaction force (Douglas *et al.*, 1998. © Company of Biologists Ltd.)

The hoof mechanism has been measured using strain gauges (Knezevic, 1966; Bayer, 1973; Dyhre-Poulsen *et al.*, 1994; Summerley *et al.*, 1998; Thomason, 1998), photoelastic material (Davies, 1997; Dejardin *et al.*, 1997, 1999) and special horse boots (Barrey, 1990; Preuschoft, 1989). As hoof strain and limb loading are related, the GRF can be estimated from hoof strain data using artificial neural networks in experiments where force plates cannot be used (Savelberg *et al.*, 1997). Photoelastic materials did not show any concentrations of colored fringes in the foot of the standing horse following trimming (Davies, 1996b). Shoeing stabilized (Thomason, 1998) or even decreased hoof movements (Colles, 1989b; Dyhre-Poulsen *et al.*, 1994), but the extra frog pressure provided by heart bar shoes did not influence hoof expansion in a consistent manner (Colles, 1989a). Strains on the hoof wall are considerably higher at the trot than at the walk (Thomason, 1998) and are higher in the trailing limb than the leading limb at a gallop (Summerley *et al.*,

1998). Surprisingly, riding decreases the strain in the quarters by 30%, while hoof wall strains are 20% higher on the medial side when the rider sits in the saddle and 20% higher on the lateral side for the forward seat (Summerley *et al.*, 1998). Turning increases the hoof strain in the quarter that is on the inside of the turn by 40% (Summerley *et al.*, 1998). A larger hoof angle and a longer toe length increased the strain at the toe, even when the length of the toe was proportional to the body size of the animals (Thomason, 1998). In the medial and lateral wall this relation was reversed: more upright feet were stiffer (Thomason, 1998). Elasticity of the hoof structures, however, is also affected by the moisture content: the wall consists of 82% keratin and 16% water, while the frog is 56% keratin and 42% water (Hertsch *et al.*, 1996). Tubules are unlikely to be involved in the hydration status of the foot, but appear to have a more mechanical function in the hoof wall to redirect and resist cracks (Kasapi & Gosline, 1997, 1998).

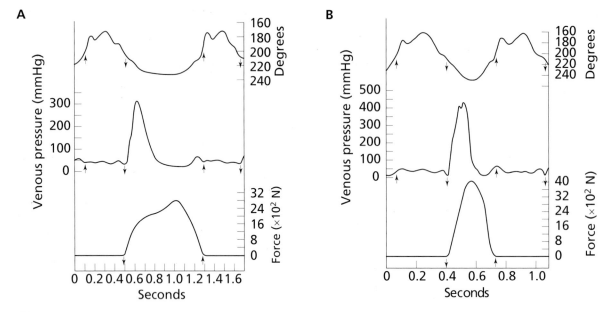

Fig. 6.11 Relationships between vertical forces, digital venous pressure and angular displacement of the fetlock joint of a horse (**A**) at a walk and (**B**) at a trot (Ratzlaff *et al.*, 1985).

Center of pressure

By tracking the path of the center of pressure in a craniocaudal plane it can be seen that immediately after initial ground contact it moves from the point of hoof contact to a position close to the apex of the frog (Barrey, 1990; Balch *et al.*, 1997; Ovnicek 1997). It remains there for most of the stance phase. At the end of the stance phase the center of pressure starts moving toward the toe. At toe-off it lies beneath the dorsal hoof wall at its breakover point (Barrey, 1990).

The location of the center of pressure in a mediolateral plane shows that when the horse is standing squarely the pressure is concentrated on the medial quarters (Colahan *et al.*, 1991). During locomotion more force is recorded on the medial hoof with force shoes (Ratzlaff *et al.*, 1993; Balch *et al.*, 1997). Transverse forces as recorded with force plates are not consistent throughout the gaits in the fore and hindlimbs (Merkens & Schamhardt, 1994).

Changes in fetlock and coffin joint angulation affect strain in the palmar soft tissues that support the limb during the stance phase (Leach 1983; Bushe *et al.*, 1987; Thompson *et al.*, 1993; Riemersma *et al.*, 1996a). The suspensory ligament (SL) and superficial digital flexor tendon (SDFT) are affected by the fetlock joint angle; strain increases as the fetlock extends. The distal accessory ligament (DAL) and deep digital flexer tendor (DDFT) are affected by the coffin joint angle: strain increases when

this joint extends. The load distribution between the tendinous structures changes with alterations in hoof balance: strain reduction in one tendon may result in an increased strain in another structure. Also the horse may compensate, to a certain extent, for hoof imbalances by adjusting the length of the muscle bellies of the SDFT and DDFT or by changing the configuration of the joint angles in the proximal limb.

Breakover

Breakover is the terminal part of the stance phase from heel-off to toe-off. Rotation of the hoof is brought about as a result of tension in the DDFT and DAL, and in the navicular ligaments (Schamhardt *et al.*, 1991; Riemersma *et al.*, 1996b). Farriery modifications that facilitate breakover may reduce tension in the DAL and in the navicular ligaments and also reduce pressure of the DDFT against the navicular bone. The onset and duration of breakover are sensitive to changes in hoof balance, especially hoof angle and toe length. Hooves trimmed with a low heel and long toe have a significantly longer breakover time, although other stride variables like stride duration do not change significantly (Clayton, 1988, 1990a,b). On the other hand, rocker, rolled and square toe shoes did not significantly alter breakover time of horses trotting on a hard surface (Clayton *et al.*, 1991) or on a rubber floor (Willemen *et al.*, 1996).

Flight arc

The flight arc of the hoof represents the summation of all the joint movements in the limb (Fig. 6.12). The highest point in the flight arc occurs soon after lift-off with a second, smaller elevation, that may coincide with an upward flip of the toe, at the time of maximal protraction. This gives a slightly biphasic flight arc (Clayton, 1990a; Balch *et al.*, 1991a, 1997; Back *et al.*, 1995).

After the hoof leaves the ground, the limb swings forward to reach its position of maximal protraction, and is then retracted prior to contact with the ground. The final retraction is important for reducing the forward velocity of the hoof relative to the ground and so decreasing hoof deceleration at ground contact and preventing the horse from stumbling. Protraction of the limb is driven by muscles in the proximal limb, with the distal limb following passively (Back *et al.*, 1995). In the forelimb the joints from the carpus proximally are driven by muscular action, while the fetlock, pastern and coffin joints move in response to inertial effects (Lanovaz *et al.*, 1999). As maximal protraction is approached, the motion of the proximal limb is slowed and reversed by muscular action, while the distal limb continues moving forward until resisted by the passive structures (bones, ligaments, tendons). Swinging the limbs back and forth uses considerable energy, and a number of energy-saving mechanisms have evolved. One of the most important is the use of elastic structures as springs; energy is stored when elastic tissues are stretched as the limb is loaded during the stance phase, then released during unloading to bounce the limb off the ground and assist in flexing the joints. At the trot the SDFT, DDFT and SL are maximally stretched at midstance which corresponds with the time of maximal weight-bearing. Thus, the elbow, carpal and fetlock joints behave elastically during the stance phase at the trot (Clayton *et al.*, 1998).

Below the elbow and stifle joints the horse's limbs are designed to move in a sagittal plane, which is another energy-saving strategy. The distal limbs sometimes deviate from this ideal pattern by being abducted (winging) or adducted (plaiting) during protraction as a result of slight asymmetries in the articular surfaces, which also have a tendency to cause breakover to occur on the medial or lateral side of the toe. If horses that naturally show these deviations are shod in a manner that forces them to breakover the center of the toe, it creates torsional forces before and after breakover. As the hoof leaves the ground, these torsional forces cause it to deviate medially or laterally, depending on the type of asymmetry. Careful observation of the horse in motion, together with an examination of the wear pattern on the ground surface of the shoe or hoof, will reveal the preferred side of breakover. If the horse is shod to facilitate breakover at the preferred location, there will often be a

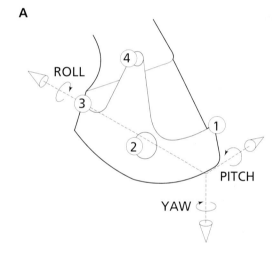

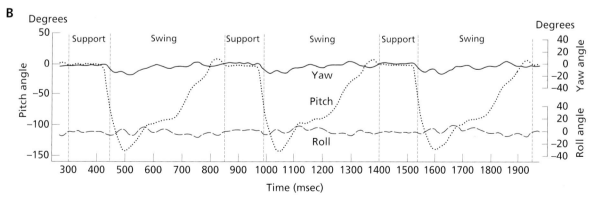

Fig. 6.12 The pitch, yaw and roll motions of a set of shoes with special glass-fiber moulds mounted to a trotter (**A**) were recorded using high-speed kinematic analysis equipment and could be illustrated in (**B**) a three-dimensional hoof coordination diagram (Fredricson & Drevemo, 1971).

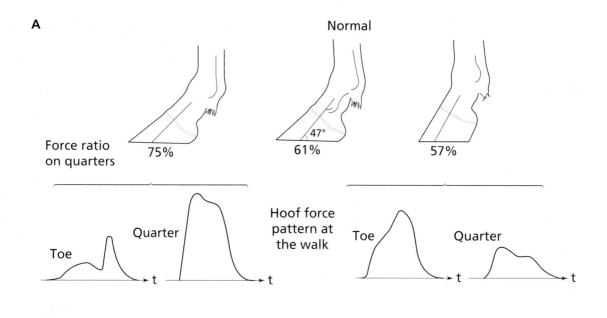

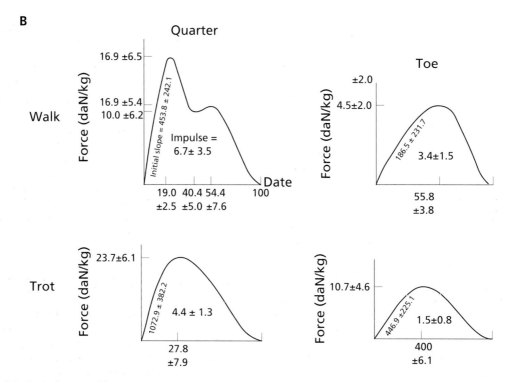

Fig. 6.13 **(A)** The influence of foot axis on the individual vertical hoof force distribution at the toe and at the quarters (Barrey, 1990). **(B)** Forces experienced at the medial toe and quarters at walk and trot in a group of 10 horses (Barrey, 1990).

marked reduction in winging or plaiting and this, in turn, affects the hoof's angle of approach to, and contact with, the ground.

EFFECTS OF HOOF MANIPULATIONS

Hoof angle

When a horse is trimmed with relatively long toes and/or short heels the hoof angle becomes more acute or sloping, while the pastern becomes more upright creating a broken-back hoof pastern axis (Bushe *et al.*, 1987). Conversely, when horses are trimmed with a short toe and/or long heels, the hoof angle becomes more upright and the pastern angle becomes more sloping. Raising the heels decreases strain in the DDFT and DAL (Leach, 1983; Bushe *et al.*, 1987; Thompson *et al.*, 1993; Riemersma *et al.* 1996a), but increases strain in the SDFT and SL (Willemen *et al.*, 1999). One of the goals of hoof trimming is to achieve a flat landing with the objective of disseminating the forces on the foot as much as possible. When the hoof angle is more upright, the hoof has a more exaggerated heel first landing (Clayton, 1988; Back *et al.*, 1995).

Barrey (1990) looked at the relation between hoof angle and force distribution: 75% of the weight was borne by the heels when the hoof angle was 39°, and this was reduced to 57% when the hoof angle was increased to 55° (Fig. 6.13). This agrees with the finding that a larger toe angle results in more strain of the hoof wall at the toe (Thomason, 1998). Nevertheless, the quarters experience higher forces during stance than the toe (Barrey, 1990).

Many racehorses are trimmed with an acute hoof angle because it is believed that the long toe low heel conformation enhances performance by increasing stride length. Comparison of the trot stride for a normal hoof angle versus an acute hoof angle showed no significant changes in stride length or suspension, and the flight arc of the hoof was almost identical with the two angulations (Clayton, 1990a; Balch *et al.*, 1997; Girtler *et al.*, 1995). However, the acute hoof angle was associated with an increased frequency of toe-first contacts, which was thought to be a consequence of the proprioceptive reflexes ensuring a fairly flat placement of P3 regardless of the shape of the hoof capsule (Clayton, 1990a). Since toe-first contacts are associated with a tendency to trip or stumble, this may be an undesirable effect.

The duration of breakover was prolonged with the acute hoof angulation and the orientation of the limb segments at the start of breakover suggested an increased tension in the DAL and navicular ligaments (Fig. 6.14). The effects of an acute hoof angle on breakover may be mitigated on a softer surface that allows penetration of the toe during the terminal part of the stance phase, since flexion of the coffin joint reduces tension in the DAL and navicular ligaments.

The hoof wall grows approximately 1 cm per 6 weeks, with the wall at the toe growing faster than at the heels (Hertsch *et al.*, 1996). When a horse is shod the hoof wears mainly in the heel region. Consequently, the hoof angle changes between farriery treatments and this is associated with alterations in the pressure on the navicular area (Hermans, 1984). Willemen *et al.* (1999) calculated a decrease in force on the navicular bone of 24% when the angle was 6° more upright. The mean toe angle of the forelimbs of the 12 horses used in that study was 55°. Therefore, horses should receive regular farrier treatment every 6–8 weeks or earlier when considerable changes in hoof angle can be expected in a particular horse.

Hoof length

Long hooves, often augmented by pads, are a feature of some gaited breeds in which they are used to give a showy, exaggerated elevation of the distal limbs during the swing phase (Fig. 6.15).

In a study designed to investigate the effects of overall hoof length on the flight arc of the hoof, pads were applied to increase hoof length by 5 cm without changing the total weight of the shoe-pad combination (Balch *et al.*, 1994). Compared with a normal hoof length, the long hooves were associated with a prolongation of stride duration, swing duration and breakover, but overall stride length and stance duration did not change. The flight arc of the hoof peaked earlier and higher with the longer hooves, but the normal movement pattern was re-established in the later part of the swing phase. Although stride length did not change, the prolongation of the swing phase may be esthetically pleasing. However, longer toes also lead to more strain on the dorsal hoof wall, which predisposes to hoof wall pathology (Thomason, 1998).

EFFECTS OF SHOE MANIPULATIONS

Shoes are applied to protect against too much wear of the hoof wall, to improve performance and to provide additional support for the horse on slippery surfaces. On the other hand, shoes restrict the hoof mechanism, increase the weight of the distal limb and increase the impact shock (Hermans, 1984). When good quality shoes are put on correctly, with the least number of nails and not too far backwards, and when adequate hoof care by a farrier takes place on a regular basis, then the aforementioned objections can be more or less compensated (Moyer, 1975).

Shoe weight

The distal limb of the horse has evolved to become very light in weight. One of the goals when shoeing a horse is to keep the weight of the shoe as low as possible (Balch

et al., 1997). This decreases its inertia, which reduces energy expenditure in protracting and retracting the limbs. When weight is added to the horse's limb, for example by the application of shoes or protective boots, the effect depends on the location of the weight (Fig. 6.16). The effect is greater with a more distal placement. The weight of a shoe is likely to affect both the energetics and the kinematics of locomotion. Therefore in race horses steel training shoes are replaced by aluminum plates for racing (Curtis, 1999). The increase in energy expenditure has been estimated to be the same for 1 oz at the foot as for 30 oz at the withers; the maximal weight that should added be to the hoof is 5–10 oz (1 oz = 28.4 g) (Butler, 1995).

Willemen *et al.* (1997) investigated the influence of shoeing on stride kinematics of young horses that were shod the first time (Table 6.1). The average weight of the horses was 516 kg and the average weight of the shoes was 478 g. With shoes there was an increase in the maximal height of the flight arc of the hoof and greater flexion of the coffin, fetlock and carpal joints during the swing phase, which improved the quality or 'animation' of the trot. Stride duration and the relative swing phase duration were longer in the shod horses, but stride length was not significantly different. During the stance phase the load on the navicular bone increased by 14% when shod, probably as a consequence of these swing phase adaptations which were achieved with a less protracted

A

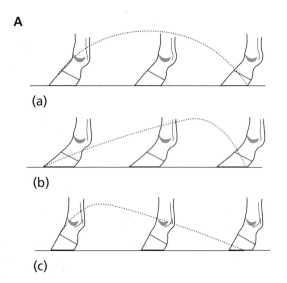

(a)

(b)

(c)

B

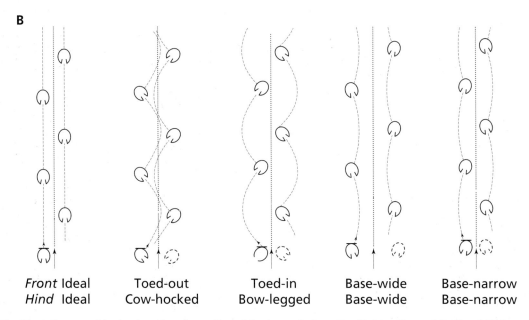

Front Ideal	Toed-out	Toed-in	Base-wide	Base-narrow
Hind Ideal	Cow-hocked	Bow-legged	Base-wide	Base-narrow

Fig. 6.14 The influence of foot axis and conformation of the lower limb on the flight pattern of the hoof (**A**) from the side and (**B**) from above (Stashak, 1987; Butler, 1995).

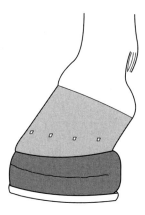

Fig. 6.15 The hoof length of Tennessee Walking Horses is artificially increased by nailing special wooden blocks under the feet (Hermans, 1984).

forelimb. The increase in maximal vertical ground reaction force when shod was also found by Roepstorff *et al.* (1999).

Balch *et al.* (1996) doubled the weight of the shoe from 348–417 g to 724–869 g, and did not find any changes in stride length, stride duration or breakover time, but again there were increases in the maximal heights of the hoof, fetlock and carpus during the swing phase, with the peak height of the flight arc tending to occur later in the swing phase. The hoof and pastern segments had a more acute angle at initial ground contact,

probably as a result of the increased momentum of the distal limb during the swing phase.

The location of the weight on the hoof may also have an influence on its effect.

Butler (1995) stated that toe weight would improve fold and heel weight would improve reach. Willemen *et al.* (1994) applied 88 g toe weights to the fore hooves of Standardbreds. During trotting on the treadmill the flight arc was elevated with the extra weight. Interestingly, the effects of toe weights on stride kinematics varied with the individual locomotion pattern: horses that initially showed too little carpal flexion showed more flexion, whereas those with adequate carpal flexion did not show a significant change. The effect on stride length was doubtful and there were no significant changes in stride duration or relative stance duration.

When egg bar shoes were put on young horses, the increased 'animation' effect was less than that found in horses wearing flat shoes. It has been speculated that it might be an effect of the increased weight distribution over the heels of this bar shoe (Willemen *et al.* 1997).

The Seattle shoe was designed to increase the energetic efficiency of locomotion but its main effect appeared to be due to its weight of 310–325 g compared with control shoes weighing 76–85 g (Wilson *et al.* 1992).

Weight attached to the feet increases the height to which the feet are lifted from the ground through greater limb flexion. This is a well known effect used to improve the performance of gaited, carriage horses. Effects related to the location of the weight on the foot

Table 6.1 Kinetic comparison of unshod versus shod conditions in a group of 12 horses trotting on a treadmill at 4 m/s (Willemen *et al.*, 1997. With permission from Elsevier Science). Values are mean ± SD.

Variable	Unshod	Shod
Stride length (cm)	2.78 ± 0.12	2.82 ± 0.12
Stride duration (msec)	694 ± 31	706 ± 28[*]
Stance phase duration (%)	37.0 ± 1.3	36.0 ± 1.2[*]
Range of pro/retraction (degrees)	43.5 ± 1.6	42.7 ± 1.3[*]
Max protraction (degrees)	112.0 ± 1.3	111.2 ± 0.8[*]
Max retraction (degrees)	68.5 ± 1.8	68.5 ± 1.5
Swing phase retraction (%)	9.8 ± 3.7	6.9 ± 3.4[*]
Range of carpal motion (degrees)	86.7 ± 7.1	98.2 ± 6.1[*]
Max carpal flexion (degrees)	80.6 ± 6.5	92.5 ± 6.0[*]
Range of fetlock motion (degrees)	81.2 ± 8.3	91.5 ± 8.8[*]
Max fetlock extension (degrees)	25.5 ± 2.7	24.3 ± 3.5
Max fetlock flexion (degrees)	55.6 ± 8.3	67.2 ± 8.5[*]
Range of vertical displacement hoof (cm)	10.0 ± 3.6	17.4 ± 4.5[*]
Range of vertical displacement fetlock (cm)	18.0 ± 3.9	20.0 ± 3.7[*]
Range of vertical displacement carpus (cm)	11.0 ± 3.4	13.9 ± 3.0[*]
Max total moment coffin joint (N m)	158 ± 30	175 ± 48
Max total moment fetlock joint (N m)	862 ± 124	835 ± 148

[*] indicates a statistically significant difference between unshod and shod ($p<0.05$); N m: Newton metres

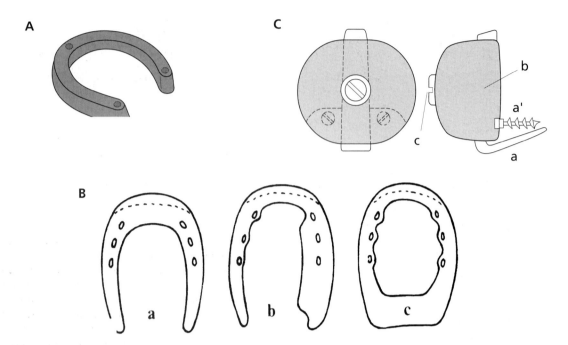

Fig. 6.16 Basic principles to increase the weight of the shoe–foot combination: (**A**)Double shoe, (**B**) toe (a), side (b) and heel (c) weighted shoes (**C**) extra toe or heel weight attached to hoof wall.

(heel/toe) or direct beneficial influence on stride length remain speculative. Empirically, young trotters can find their balance more easily using weights, and interference can be prevented (see also the section on interference p. 157).

Shoe length

The hoof is more elastic in the heel area and its geometry changes when loaded: the heels expand and sink caudally, while the toe retracts (Douglas *et al.*, 1998). Lengthening the heels of the shoe depending on foot conformation in routine shoeing automatically allows for this change in shape (Balch *et al.*, 1997).

The extended heel of an egg bar shoe does not change the position of the center of pressure within the hoof during the stance phase. Compared with flat shoes, however, it reduces the torque at the fetlock joint by changing the orientation of the GRF vector so that its line of action is closer to the fetlock joint on its dorsal side (Auer & Butler, 1986; Willemen *et al.* 1999; Table 6.2). The net effect is that egg bar shoes have a negligible effect on tendon strain patterns in sound ponies at a walk (Riemersma *et al.*, 1996a). Bouley shoes, which have a lengthened heel, may be effective, however, in cases of severed tendons, especially if the DDFT or DAL is involved (Figs 6.17 & 6.18).

In the absence of tension in the DDFT, the hoof rotates to such an extent that the point of application of the GRF vector is directly below the center of rotation of the coffin joint. The tip of the toe lifts up and the hoof rolls back onto the heels, which puts the hoof in an unstable position. In these cases egg bar shoes stabilize the hoof, and provide pain relief in horses with injury of the DDFT or DAL, laminitis or navicular disease (Auer & Butler, 1986). Bar shoes may also be useful to prevent lifting of the tip of the toe on soft ground (Wright & Douglas, 1993).

In horses trotting on a rubber floor there was no significant difference in limb loading between egg bars and flat shoes (Willemen *et al.*, 1999), although the 'animation' effect was more pronounced with flat shoes. Egg bar shoes, as a result of having more ground support and stability, should prevent the heels from sinking into the ground and allow reestablishment of heel growth leading to an increased toe angle. Furthermore, it has been proven indirectly that the dorsal laminar blood flow is enhanced by egg bar or heart bar shoes in laminitic horses, as a result of distributing the weight more caudally and thus protecting the toe region of the foot (Ritmeester *et al.*, 1998). It should be remembered that egg bars on the fore hooves are more likely to be stepped on and torn off by overreaching. Bell boots can be applied to the forelimbs to prevent this.

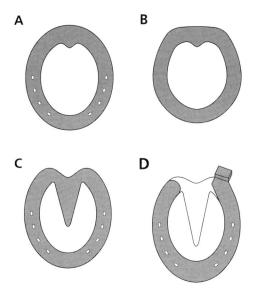

Fig. 6.17 Bar shoes to support the caudal heel at stance. (**A**) Egg bar; (**B**) straight bar; (**C**) (adjustable) heart bar; or (**D**) the lateral heel using a trailer with caulk.

Bar shoes in general provide more ground support and thus might reduce limb rotation and pain in horses that are lame due to bone spavin. This effect can also be achieved using a unilateral trailer (heel extension) at an angle of 45° (Stashak, 1987; Balch *et al.*, 1997; Martinelli & Ferrie, 1997). Trailers are also supposed to give more medial or lateral support and to change the mediolateral landing pattern depending on whether they are applied on the inside or outside. In foals with contracted flexor tendons toe extensions are used to stretch the DAL and DDFT at the end of the stance phase (see also the section on flexural limb deformities, p. 161).

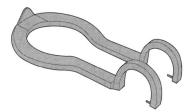

Fig. 6.18 The longer heels of a so-called Bouley shoe support a dropped fetlock joint caused by severe flexor tendon lacerations.

Shoe width

As mentioned previously, the geometry of the hoof changes when the hoof is loaded: the heels expand and sink caudally, and the toe retracts (Douglas *et al.*, 1998). Increasing the width of the shoe accommodates for these movements (Balch *et al.*, 1997). Another application for widening the shoes is in foals with angular limb deformities. The goal is to bring the weight-bearing surface of the limb, and thus the point of application of the GRF, under the fetlock joint as opposed to under the hoof capsule (see also the section on angular limb deformities, p. 162).

Hoof pads

Shoes increase pressure on the navicular region (Willemen *et al.*, 1997, 1999). Compared with horses that are bare-footed, shod horses have less damping of the impact forces and both the median and maximal amplitudes of the frequencies are higher (Balch *et al.* 1991b; Benoit *et al.*, 1993; Dyhre-Poulsen *et al.*, 1994).

Benoit *et al.* (1993) explored the shock damping effect on the hoof wall of different combinations of

Table 6.2 Kinetic comparison of three shoe manipulations of a group of 12 horses trotting on a treadmill at 4 m/s (Willemen *et al.*, 1999). Values are mean ± SD.

Variable	Unshod	Flat shoe	Egg bar
Maximum GRF (N)	6364 ± 600	6421 ± 647	6477 ± 699
Vertical displacement at scapular spine (cm)	7.2 ± 1.8	8.0 ± 1.5	7.9 ± 1.5
Maximal total moment at coffin joint (N m)	158 ± 30	175 ± 48	175 ± 46
Maximal total moment at fetlock joint (N m)	862 ± 124	835 ± 148	829 ± 100
Maximal moment at fetlock joint of DDFT (N m)	211 ± 40	231 ± 67	231 ± 63
Maximal moment at fetlock joint of SDFT and SL (N m)	726 ± 115[*]	676 ± 110	674 ± 97
Force on navicular bone by DDFT (N)	3060 ± 438[*]	3546 ± 526	3504 ± 459

[*] indicates a statistically significant difference with the value of the flat shoe ($p<0.05$); N m: Newton metres; GRF: ground reaction force; DDFT: deep digital flexor tendon; SDFT: superficial digital flexor tendon; SL: suspensory ligament.

shoes and pads. For unshod hooves the impact shock wave had a velocity of 450 m/s² and this increased to 800 m/s² when steel shoes were applied, which is in accordance with Hertsch *et al.* (1996). Various shock-absorbing pads have been developed to decrease the amount of shock transmitted to the limb (Marks *et al.*, 1971). Good attenuation of the impact shock was achieved using an aluminium Equisoft shoe combined with a polyurethane Easy-Glu pad, which had a value of 200 m/s². Benoit *et al.* (1993) recommended using a shoe with a pad of rubber or polyurethane and working the horse on soft footing to reduce the risk of lameness. A polyurethane / elastomer / viscoelastic hoof pad is a much better shock absorber than rubber (Marks *et al.*, 1971; Vasko & Farr, 1984; Rööser *et al.*, 1988). For an optimal effect, hoof pads or silicone should be put under pressure to prevent it from moving and to show increased shock damping (Jörgensen & Ekstrand, 1988). This is also ideal for increasing the surface area to disseminate high-frequency oscillations at impact. An additional benefit is that increased deformation of the hoof also leads to an increase in the hoof mechanism and thus circulation.

It should be noted that most of the studies of the effects of shoes and pads on impact shock have evaluated the effects at the level of the hoof wall. Little information is available regarding attenuation of the amplitude or frequency of the vibrations within the hoof. *In vitro* studies have suggested that the hoof acts as a filter to protect the more proximal bones and joints from the potentially damaging effects of impact shock (Dyhre-Poulsen *et al.*, 1994; Lanovaz *et al.*, 1998; Willemen, 1998).

Toe of the shoe

Breakover is defined as the time from the moment of heel lift to toe-off. In theory, the speed of breakover can be enhanced by shoes that facilitate the movement of the hoof in rolling over the toe or by raising the heel (Fig. 6.19). For horses trotting even on a hard surface, however, the duration of breakover was no different for a rolled toe, a rocker toe or a square toe, compared with a flat shoe (Clayton *et al.*, 1991; Willemen *et al.*, 1996). A possible disadvantage, particularly with the square-toed shoes, is that they direct the breakover point to the middle of the toe, which is not the natural position in all horses. This might enhance the likelihood of lameness, especially at high speeds when rapid movements of the hoof occur (Clayton, 1990a; Wilson *et al.*, 1992). Therefore, Caudron *et al.* (1997b) successfully used a full roller motion (Equi+) shoe to provide easy

breakover in all directions for horses with poorly balanced hooves.

Wedges

Wedges are applied to one or both heels for specific reasons. In horses with bone spavin, a lateral wedge is used to relieve pressure from the medial, affected side. In horses with upward fixation of the patella, lateral wedges enhance inward rotation and rolling over the medial toe. In both cases, the overall effect may result from the fact that raising the heels leads to less overextension and thus diminishes the chance of developing these phenomena.

Side wedges

Colahan *et al.* (1991) and Wilson *et al.* (1998) found that lateral wedges shifted the center of pressure to the lateral side of the hoof. Firth *et al.* (1988) put lateral wedges under the feet of foals and found a rapid compensation of bone strain to this alteration. Lateral corrective trimming restored the mediolateral balance of 15 chronically digital lame horses using a radiological protocol to assess the imbalance of the foot (Caudron *et al.*, 1998).

Heel/toe wedges

Heel wedges facilitate rolling over the toe and are used to relieve pressure from the heels, as in navicular disease. A wedge of 6° resulted in a 24% load reduction on the navicular bone in trotting horses (Willemen *et al.*, 1999). Heel wedges caused only slight changes in strain of the SDFT, DDFT and SL during walking (Riemersma *et al.*, 1996a,b), though a larger increase in SDFT strain has been recorded at the trot (Stephens *et al.*, 1989). With heel wedges there is an earlier shift of the center of pressure from the mid-hoof to the toe and the unloading of the heels is enhanced, whereas toe wedges delay the forward shift of the center of pressure and the unloading of the heels is delayed (Riemersma *et al.*, 1996a,b; Wilson *et al.*, 1998).

With a toe wedge, strain in the DAL increases, whereas strain in the SDFT and SL decreases (Thompson *et al.*, 1993). Since the DAL has no muscular component that can actively change its length, strain in this structure is totally dependent on limb configuration, especially the angle of the coffin joint. The DAL is normally maximally strained at the start of breakover, which is when heel wedges have their greatest effect on the GRF (Fig. 6.20). This emphasizes the importance of the DAL in influencing

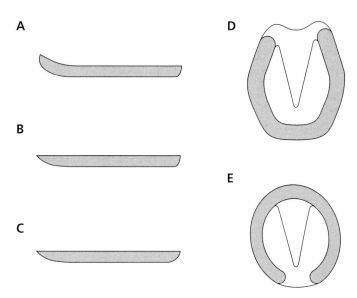

Fig. 6.19 Toe manipulations of shoes to reduce breakover time. (**A**) Rolled shoe; (**B**) rocker toed shoe; (**C**) full roller motion shoe; (**D**) square toe shoe; (**E**) reversed shoe.

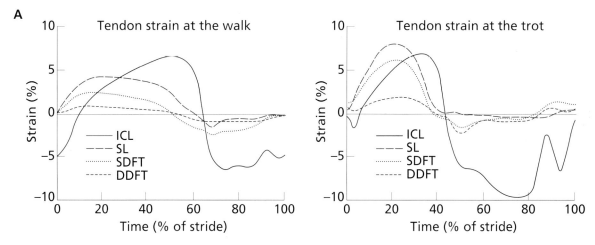

Fig. 6.20A The strain in the distal accessory ligament and DDFT combination determines the force on the navicular bone at the end of the stance phase (Schamhardt *et al.*, 1991); SL; suspensory ligament, ICL; inferior check ligament, SDFT; superficial digital flexor tendon, DDFT; deep digital flexor tendon.

limb forces and movements in the final part of the stance phase. Raising the heels seems appropriate in DAL injury, though this may slightly increase SDFT loading. During recuperation from DAL injury, however, the limitations on exercise make it unlikely that the safety margin of the SDFT will be exceeded even with heel wedges in place. Toe wedges are used clinically as a passive flexion test in lameness examination.

Toe grabs and heel caulks

On a soft, slippery surface, caulks are screwed into the horse's shoes, where they act in a similar manner to spikes in a runner's shoes (Thompson & Herring, 1994). Toe grabs are used in racing Thoroughbreds with the objective of increasing the propulsion at the toe. There have not been any studies to prove these beneficial effects, but a correlation has been shown between the presence of toe grabs

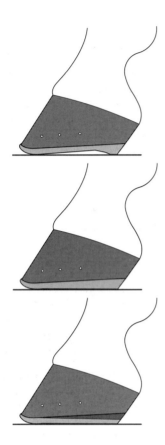

Fig. 6.20B Some examples of wedged shoes (Wright and Douglas 1993).

and the incidence of breakdowns involving the suspensory-sesamoidean apparatus (Kane *et al.*, 1996). The higher the toe grab, the greater the risk of injury. Thompson & Herring (1994) found also a decrease in the dorsal metacarpophalangeal, and an increase in the dorsal phalangeal joint excursion in the sagittal plane during stance, while in the transverse plane the distal limbs appeared to take a limb conformation similar to a varus limb.

Rims, clips and nails

A minimum number of nails should be used, usually 6–8, to minimize damage to the hoof wall and to reduce blocking the hoof mechanics to a minimum (Balch *et al.*, 1997). Therefore nailing should be done from the toe to the widest part of the hoof,

with the clinches being formed one-third of the way up in a line parallel to the ground. Clips and rims reduce the shearing stress upon the nails especially when more traction is needed, for example in barrel racing and polo (Stashak, 1987; Balch *et al.*, 1997; Martinelli & Ferrie, 1997).

EFFECT OF FOOTING

Properties of the ground

The hoof–ground interaction has been found to be the major determinant in studies relating track properties to limb pathology, both in horses (Kane *et al.*, 1996) and in humans (Folman *et al.*, 1986). Two important phenomena play a role: the banking and the surface type.

Fredricson *et al.* (1975 a,b) made three recommendations for banking to improve racetracks for trotters: increase the banking of the curve, incorporate a transition curve and eliminate slopes in the straight part of the track. Davies (1997) also stressed the importance of the track shape to prevent shin soreness. She found a considerable increase in dorsal bone strain when horses gallop through turns.

Most tracks and arenas are constructed with two layers: a looser cushion on top of a firmer base. Variations in the depth and quality of the base and the cushion affect both performance and soundness of the horses. Hard surfaces absorb little energy, which leads to fast race times, but they are associated with a high incidence of lameness (Cheney *et al.*, 1973; Pratt, 1997). The hardness of the ground is related to the impact time: the harder the surface, the shorter the impact time (Drevemo & Hjertén, 1991). Running on a rough instead of a smooth track surface changed the vertical hoof force and balance of the resultant hoof forces (Kai *et al.*, 1999).

A loose top layer of 5 cm or more can give dynamic response values that reduce impact by 40 to 60% (Cheney *et al.*, 1973). Reduction of impact forces and enhancement of energy absorption can be achieved using a layer of wood shavings (Barrey *et al.*, 1991; Drevemo & Hjertén, 1991). Wood products are effective shock absorbers but are sufficiently resilient that little impulse is lost. Wood products (shavings, mulch, chips) mixed with sand give good shock damping with lower vibration frequencies (Barrey *et al.*, 1991). Rubber chips from recycled tires can also be mixed with sand to reduce impact shock without losing much impulse. Differences were found for horses trotting on a concrete track compared with a rubber or a sand track: stride and

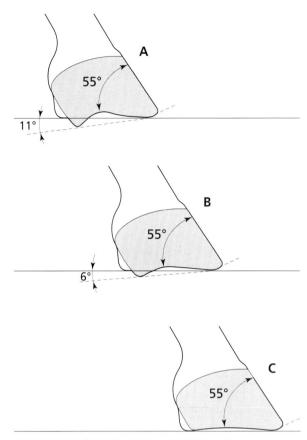

Fig. 6.21 Hoof conformation of wild horses living on different ground surfaces. (**A**) Soft; (**B**) medium; and (**C**) hard surfaces (Ovnicek, 1997).

swing duration were longer on the softer track due to the lower impact shock combined with more elastic rebound (Buchner *et al.*, 1994; Riemersma *et al.*, 1996b). Barrey *et al.* (1991) categorized the damping properties into three types: no damping (asphalt), friction damping (sand) and structural damping (wood). Sand tracks can have different properties depending on the moisture content, dry density and depth of the layers (Ratzlaff *et al.*, 1997).

In wild horses hoof growth appeared to be related well to hoof wear. By natural selection only horses with good hoof quality survive. Ovnicek *et al.* (1995, 1997) found differences between the hooves of the wild horses that had lived for a prolonged period on one of three surfaces: sand, gravel or firm soil (Fig. 6.21).

The form of the hoof was adapted to the surface. On sand less shock damping was needed so the hoof wall carried more weight. The hooves did not show more

wear as one would have expected, but on both sides of the wall spikes were formed at the quarters to give more grip in the sand ('natural caulks'). The hoof angle was about 55°. On a firmer surface of gravel, the hoof angle was more upright at the toe but the spikes at the quarters were lower, so the angle was again 55°. On firm soil the hoof wall was worn flat without a heel spike which would not be useful in this type of ground. Again the hoof angle was 55°. Regardless of the type of surface the horse moved over, the toe was always rolled.

PRACTICAL APPLICATIONS TO PERFORMANCE

Interference

Horses trimmed with normal angles in their fore hooves and acute angles in their hind hooves showed a prolonged breakover time and delayed lift off in the hind hooves (Hermans, 1984; Clayton, 1990b). However, the hindlimbs were protracted more rapidly to re-establish the normal sequence of limb placements by the time of ground contact (Clayton, 1990a,b). Therefore, delaying breakover in the hind hooves seems unlikely to have a beneficial effect in horses that interfere (Curtis, 1999, Fig. 6.22).

A more effective solution to interference problems may be to hasten breakover and lift off in the fore hooves. Furthermore, another solution is to put on square toe shoes more towards the heels of the hind hooves so that the hoof wall instead of the shoe hits the forelimbs (toe preventer shoe). Also, weights are used to balance horses moving at high speed and thus prevent interference (see section on action below).

Action

It is recognized among horse trainers that heavier shoes give horses more action. Double shoes are applied in trotters just before the race to encourage them to lift the limbs higher, in spite of the fact that heavier shoes require greater energy expenditure to overcome inertia at the start of the swing phase and to overcome momentum at the end of the swing phase. Young trotters are shod with heavier shoes in the forelimb than in the hindlimb to improve their balance (Hermans, 1984; Butler, 1995; Ruthe *et al.*, 1997). Too little folding of the forelimb allows interference by the hindlimbs; too much folding results in elbow hitting. Mediolateral imbalances leads to knee hitting by the contralateral limb, which

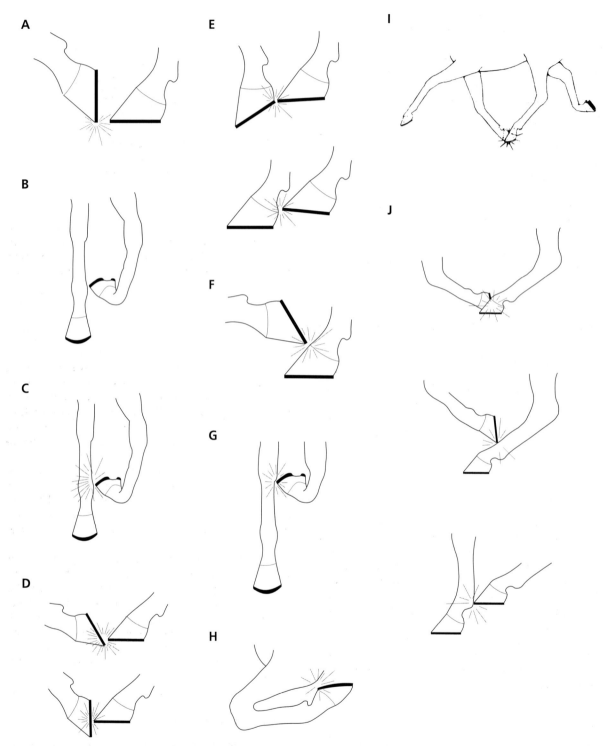

Fig. 6.22 Interference injuries. At walk: (**A**) stumbling; (**B**) brushing. At trot: (**C**) interfering; (**D**) forging; (**E**) overreaching; (**F**) scalping; (**G**) knee hitting; (**H**) elbow hitting. At pace: (**I**) crossfiring. At gallop: (**J**) speedy cutting (Butler, 1995).

can also be compensated for by lateral weights on the hindlimbs so that their forward swing is outside the forelimbs.

Willemen *et al.* (1994) found that the effect of toe weights on the flight arc dependent on the individual locomotion pattern of the horse. Horses that normally trotted with too little carpal flexion showed more action with toe weights. Stride duration and relative stance duration did not change at high speeds (10 and 11 m/s), and it is doubtful whether there was any effect on stride length.

In young horses shod for the first time the weight of the shoes increased the maximal heights of the hoof, fetlock and carpus during the swing phase, which thus resulted in a longer, more 'animated' swing phase at the trot (4 m/s). This is the desired effect of double shoes applied in harness horses just before the race (Balch *et al.*, 1996; Wilson *et al.*, 1992; Willemen *et al.*, 1997).

PRACTICAL APPLICATION TO LAMENESS

Lameness is caused by pain, a mechanical deficit, a shortage of oxygen or a neurological problem. Therapeutic trimming and shoeing can be used to improve lameness by reducing pain or influencing limb mechanics (Stashak, 1987). This section highlights some practical applications to treat specific lameness conditions, thereby illustrating the aforementioned principles.

Hoof cracks

Hoof wall defects can be very painful in the acute stages, which makes the horse reluctant to bear weight on the affected foot. Cracks should be relieved from hoof wall pressure and should be repaired with the objective of minimizing movement (Fig. 6.23) and propagation of the crack using mechanical or composite material (Wilson & Pardoe, 1998). Cracks are stress raisers and can be detected using photoelastic material (Davies, 1997). The hoof wall tubules seem to play a major mechanical role in resisting and redirecting these hoof cracks (Kasapi & Gosline, 1998).

P3 fracture

Fractures of P3 can be stabilized successfully by reducing hoof movements during weight-bearing. Heel expansion can be stabilized by using a full bar shoe with quarter and heel clips (Hermans, 1984;

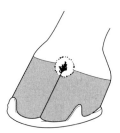

Fig. 6.23 Clips reduce shearing forces on the nails and restrict lateral movement of the hoof wall to treat hoof cracks and P3 fractures (Hermans, 1984).

Colles, 1989a,b; Thomason, 1998), and the effect can be enhanced by applying a rigid cast over the clip shoe (Kersjes *et al.*, 1985). However, frequent trimming does not help to prevent P3 fractures from developing in foals (Kaneps *et al.*, 1998).

Laminitis

Laminitis, an aseptic pododermatitis mainly caused by endotoxins and gastrointestinal disorders, affects the laminae primarily on the dorsal aspect of the foot. The avascular damage to those laminae and thus to the connection between P3 and the hoof wall can lead to rotation and sinking of P3 within the hoof capsule. Basic principles of shoeing treatment are to protect the foot and damp impact shock, to facilitate breakover and thus relieve tension on the dorsal laminae, and to prevent sole pressure in the toe region by posterior support of the frog and heels (Goetz, 1987). In a chronic founder it is also important to restore normal hoof conformation by corrective trimming (Fig. 6.24).

A reversed shoe laid back from the toe facilitates breakover, relieves pressure from the dorsal laminae and gives caudal heel support. The use of a pad protects the sole and damps oscillations (White & Bagget, 1983; O'Grady, 1997). Dorsal hoof wall resection and the use of adjustable heart bar shoes, however, still remain somewhat controversial (Eustace & Caldwell, 1989a,b; Peremans *et al.*, 1991; Jurga, 1997).

Navicular syndrome

Navicular syndrome comprises pathological changes to the navicular bone, its ligaments and the DDFT caused by mechanical overloading and/or vascular obstruction (Wright *et al.*, 1998). Recent histological examination

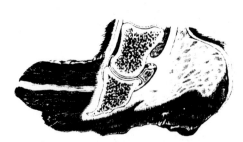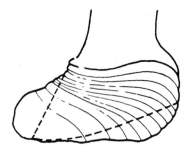

Fig. 6.24 Functional trimming of chronically foundered hooves fascilitates breakover to reduce stress on the dorsal hoof wall and restore the angle of P3 with the ground (Ruthe *et al.*, 1997).

has proved that lesions in the navicular bone occur predominantly on the fibrocartilage side and are comparable to osteoarthritis (Wright *et al.*, 1998). Pain is due to pressure of the DDFT on the navicular bursa and bone, tension in the navicular ligaments, and elevated intramedullary bone pressure in the navicular bone (Pleasant *et al.*, 1993). The navicular bone in the forelimb is significantly larger than in the hindlimb, probably to compensate for the larger forces in the forelimb (Gabriel *et al.*, 1997). Smaller feet seem to have a higher risk of developing navicular disease (Balch *et al.*, 1997). Shoeing principles for horses with navicular syndrome aim to reduce concussion and facilitate breakover by elevating the heels and rolling the toe.

When the horse is bare-foot, pressure of the DDFT on the navicular bone is 14% lower than when flat shoes are applied (Willemen *et al.*, 1999). Therefore, it might be beneficial for shod horses suffering for navicular pain to the shoes have temporarily removed; this will also decrease concussion. Elevation of the heels using heel wedges may be beneficial (Wintzer, 1971; Leach, 1983; Turner, 1986, 1988; Bushe *et al.*, 1987; Ratzlaff & White, 1989; Wright & Douglas, 1993; Keegan *et al.*, 1998) due to the reduced net joint moment at the coffin joint (Willemen *et al.*, 1999, Table 6.3). Empirically, the use of a rolled toe/rocker toe shoe is promoted, although this type of shoeing did not reduce breakover time in sound horses (Clayton *et al.*, 1991; Willemen *et al.*, 1996). Egg bar shoes may prevent hyperextension of the coffin joint on a soft surface and rotation of the foot, thus avoiding high stresses on the navicular region (Østblom *et al.*, 1984; Auer & Butler, 1986; Wright & Douglas, 1993).

Arthrosis and arthritis

The high-frequency oscillations together with rapid loading of the joints experienced at impact promote the

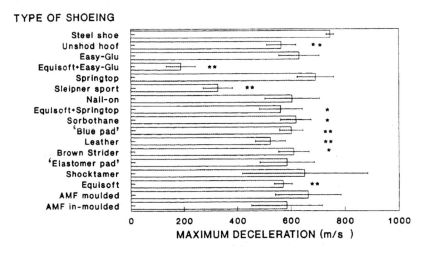

Fig. 6.25A The maximum decelerations at hoof impact of horses trotting on an asphalt road with different types of shoeing. *$p<0.05$ and **$p<0.01$ to reference steel shoe (Benoit *et al.*, 1993).

TYPE OF SHOEING

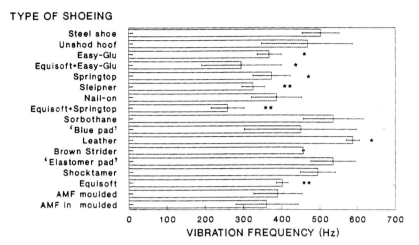

Fig. 6.25B The vibration frequencies at hoof impact of horses trotting on an asphalt road with different types of shoeing. *$p<0.05$ and **$p<0.01$ to reference steel shoe (Benoit *et al.*, 1993).

development of osteoarthrosis (Radin *et al.*, 1981, 1999). Prevention and treatment aim to reduce these impact oscillations with a shock absorbing pad (Marks *et al.*, 1971; Benoit *et al.*, 1993, Fig. 6.25). In vitro tests, however, revealed that the hoof capsule (Willemen, 1998) and the distal limb were able to attenuate impact shock quite considerably (Dyhre-Poulsen *et al.*, 1994; Lanovaz *et al.*, 1998). A polyurethane/elastomer/viscoelastic pad is a much better shock absorber than rubber (Marks *et al.*, 1971; Vasko & Farr, 1984; Rööser *et al.*, 1988). A leather pad is more susceptible to variations in moisture content of the ground (Stashak, 1987). For arthritis of the distal interphalangeal joint, Caudron *et al.* (1997a,b, 1998) used a special full roller motion shoe (Equi+) to facilitate breakover and to reduce stress and thus pain from the ligaments and the joint capsule while adapting to the breakover path of the particular horse.

Spavin

Bone spavin is an aseptic osteoarthritis on the dorsomedial aspect of the distal intertarsal joint or the tarsometatarsal joint (Stashak, 1987). The rationale behind treating bone spavin by lowering the medial side of the hoof or elevating the lateral heel is that it may relieve pressure from the medial side (Firth *et al.*, 1988; Colahan *et al.*, 1991). It has also been suggested that heel wedges and rolled toes prevent the hindlimb from hyperextending the distal intertarsal and/or tarsometatarsal joints. Trailers have been used in selected cases to reduce rotation of the distal limb, but this can also exacerbate the symptoms (Stashak, 1987; Balch *et al.*, 1997; Martinelli & Ferrie, 1997).

Patellar fixation

In horses with patellar fixation, lateral heel wedges and rolled toes prevent hyperextension and outward rotation of the stifle and thus avoid locking the patella (Stashak, 1987). Most affected horses are aged 3–5 years. When corrective trimming and shoeing are combined with training of the appropriate muscles, symptoms often disappear. Empirically, some horses, especially trotters, respond better to a medial wedge than a lateral wedge, this also prevents them from interfering.

Flexural limb deformities

The greatest threat to the young foal's locomotor system is the foal itself. In the first 4–5 months of its life a foal grows as much as during the rest of its life. Just recently, it has been hypothesized that foals from older mares, that are

A

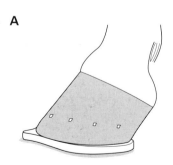

Fig. 6.26A Shoeing principles for flexural deformities in foals. A contracted deep digital flexor tendon.

B

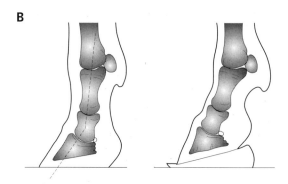

Fig. 6.26B a contracted superficial digital flexor tendon.

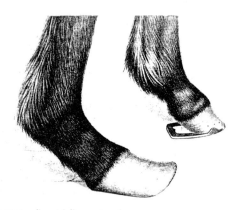

Fig. 6.26C flaccid flexor tendons.

poorly developed at birth because of the smaller placenta but then receive a surplus of milk, are prone to develop pathology in their locomotor system. Asynchronous bone–tendon growth results in flexural deformities.

Table 6.3 Growth plate closure times and periods of rapid growth for equine long bones (Curtis, 1999).

Growth plate	Age at closure	Rapid growth period
Distal radius	24–30 months	< 8 months
Distal tibia	24 months	< 6 months
Distal McIII/MtIII	12 months	< 3 months
Proximal Ph I	6 months	< 3 months
Mc: metacarpal; Mt: metatarsal; Ph: phalanx		

Contraction of the DDFT is responsible for a hyper-flexed coffin joint found at 1–6 months of age, while at 1 year of age SDFT contraction leads to a hyperflexed fetlock joint (Fig. 6.26). Treatment options depend on the severity of the contraction. Possible treatments for DDFT contraction include lowering the heels, extending the toe of the shoe using a cast, and desmotomy of the distal accessory (check) ligament. For SDFT contraction a wedged pad would be an option. So-called 'weak' flexor tendons are often seen in premature foals and lead to hyperextension of the distal limb. If this does not have a traumatic origin, the initial treatment can be supported by shoes with longer heels (Curtis, 1992a; Ellis, 1998).

Angular limb deformities

In the rapidly growing young foal asymmetric bone growth, caused by congenital or acquired factors can lead to angular limb deformities. They should be corrected at the fetlock joint before 3 months of age, while in those at the carpus/tarsus region this should be corrected before 6–8 months of age (Table 6.3). At that time the growth plates start to close. Treatment options of first choice are corrective wall/toe rasping, a medial/lateral extension shoe (Dallric, Dallmer Salzhausen-Putensen, Germany; Baby Glu, Mustad Hoofcare SA, Bulle, Switzerland) and a limited exercise regime (Curtis, 1992b, 1999). The objective is to center the hoof-bearing surface under the fetlock joint (Fig. 6.27).

CONCLUSION

The major effects of farriery are similar in most horses of a group, but there are likely to be minor differences in

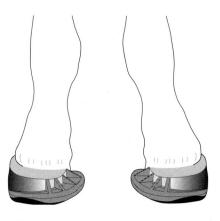

Fig. 6.27 Diagram of a foal with a fetlock valgus deviation treated with a medial extension glue-on shoe.

the response of individual horses. Basic farriery considerations that influence locomotion are toe angle and weight of the shoe, which interact with the type of footing. The mechanisms by which trimming and shoeing affect locomotion and lameness involve relieving pain, altering the mechanics of the stance phase and influencing inertia during the swing phase. In experimental studies the mean effect of a particular modification on the kinetics and kinematics is often smaller than the differences between individuals. Therefore, as much as possible, test objects have to be measured when trying to prove farriery effects.

In young foals, regular trimming is necessary from 1 month of age (every 4–6 weeks). If pathological deformities start to develop, then therapeutic trimming should be performed at least every 2 weeks. Prevention of these deformities is the best option, of course, because forced correction of conformation by trimming and corrective shoeing at an older age will lead to lameness sooner or later.

REFERENCES

Anderson, G.F. (1992) Evaluation of the hoof and foot relevant to purchase. *Vet. Clin. North Am. Equine Pract.* **8**: 303–318.

Auer, J. and Butler, K.D. (1986) An introduction into the Kaegi equine gait analysis system in the horse. *Proc. Ann. Conv. Am. Assoc. Equine Pract.* **31**: 209–226.

Back, W., Schamhardt, H.C., Hartman, W. and Barneveld, A. (1995) Kinematic differences between the distal portions of the forelimbs and hindlimbs of horses at the trot. *Am. J. Vet. Res.* **56**: 1522–1528.

Balch, O., White, K. and Butler, D. (1991a) Factors involved in the balancing of equine hooves. *J. Am. Vet. Med. Ass.* **198**: 1980–1989.

Balch, O., Ratzlaff, M. and Hyde, M. (1991b) The effects of different pads on locomotion forces exerted by a horse exercising on a high speed treadmill. *Proc. Ann. Meet. Assoc. Equine Sports Med.* **10**: 3–7.

Balch, O.K., Clayton, H.M. and Lanovaz, J.L. (1994) Effects of increasing hoof length on limb kinematics of trotting horses. *Proc. Ann. Conv. Am. Assoc. Equine Pract.* **40**: 40–43.

Balch, O.K., Clayton, H.M. and Lanovaz, J.L. (1996) Weight- and length-induced changes in limb kinematics in trotting horses. *Proc. Ann. Conv. Am. Assoc. Equine Pract.* **42**: 218–219.

Balch, O.K., Butler, D. and Collins, M.A. (1997) Balancing the normal foot: hoof preparation, shoe fit and shoe modification in the performance horse. *Equine Vet. Educ.* **9**: 143–154.

Barrey, E. (1990) Investigation of the vertical hoof force distribution in the equine forelimb with an instrumented horseboot. *Equine Vet. J.* **9**(Suppl.): 35–38.

Barrey, E., Landjerit B. and Wolter, R. (1991) Shock and vibration during the hoof impact on different track surfaces. *Equine Exerc. Physiol.* **3**: 97–106.

Bayer, A. (1973) Bewegungsanalysen an Trabrennpferden mit Hilfe der Ungulographie. *Zbl. Vet. Med. A* **20**: 209–221.

Benoit, P., Barrey, E., Regnault, J.C. and Brochet, J.L. (1993) Comparison of the damping effect of different shoeing by

the measurement of hoof acceleration. *Acta Anat.* **146**: 109–113.

Bowker, R.M., Breuer, A.M., Vex, K.B. *et al.* (1993) Sensory receptors in the equine foot. *Am. J. Vet. Res.* **54**: 1840–1844.

Bowker, R.M., Linder, K.E., Sonea, I.M. and Guida, L.A. (1995) Sensory nerve fibers and receptors in the equine distal forelimbs and their potential role in locomotion. *Equine Vet. J.* **18**: 141–146.

Buchner, H.H.F., Savelberg, H.H.C.M., Schamhardt, H.C. and Merkens, H.W. (1994) Kinematics of treadmill versus overground locomotion in horses. *Vet. Quart.* **16**: S87–90.

Burn, J.F., Wilson, A. and Nason, G.P. (1997) Impact during equine locomotion: techniques for measuring and analysis. *Equine Vet. J.* **23**(Suppl.): 9–12.

Bushe, T., Turner, T.A., Poulos, P.W. and Harwell, N.M. (1987) The effect of hoof angle on coffin, pastern and fetlock joint angles. *Proc. Am. Assoc. Equine Pract.* **33**: 729–738.

Butler, D. (1995) *The Principles of Horseshoeing II – Farrier Science and Craftmanship*, 4th edn. LaPorte: Walsworth Co. Inc., 6

Caudron, I., Miesen, M., Grulke, S., Vanschepdael, P. and Serteyn, D. (1997a) Clinical and radiological assessment of corrective trimming in lame horses. *J. Equine. Vet. Sc.* **17**: 375–379.

Caudron, I., Miesen, M., Grulke, S., Vanschepdael, P. and Serteyn, D. (1997b) Radiological assessment of the effect of a full roller motion shoe during asymmetrical weightbearing. *Equine Vet. J.* **23**(Suppl.): 20–22.

Caudron, I., Grulke, S., Farnir, F., Vanschepdael, P. and Serteyn, D. (1998) Clinical and radiological assessment of corrective trimming in lame horses. *Vet. Quart.* **20**:131–135.

Cheney, J.A., Shen, C.K. and Wheat, J.D. (1973) Relationship of track surface to lameness in the Thoroughbred racehorse. *Am. J. Vet. Res.* **34**: 1258–1289.

Clayton, H.M. (1988) Comparison of the stride of trotting horses trimmed with a normal and a broken-back hoof axis. *Proc. Ann. Conv. Am. Assoc. Equine Pract.* **33**: 289–298.

Clayton, H.M. (1990a) The effect of an acute hoof angulation on the stride kinematics of trotting horses. *Equine Vet. J.* **9** (Suppl.): 86–90.

Clayton, H.M. (1990b) The effect of an acute angulation of the hind hooves on diagonal synchrony of the trotting horse. *Equine Vet. J.* **9**(suppl.): 91–94.

Clayton, H.M., Sigafoos, R. and Curle, R.D. (1991) Effect of three shoe types on the duration of breakover in sound trotting horses. *J. Equine Vet. Sci.* **11**: 129–132.

Clayton, H.M., Lanovaz, J.L., Schamhardt, H.C., Willemen, M.A. and Colborne, G.L. (1998) Net joint moments and powers in the equine forelimb in the stance phase of the trot. *Equine Vet. J.* **30**: 384–389.

Colahan, P., Leach, D. and Muir, G. (1991) Center of pressure location of the hoof with and without hoof wedges. *Equine Exerc. Physiol.* **3**: 113–119.

Colles, C.M. (1989a) The relationship of frog pressure to heel expansion. *Equine Vet. J.* **21**: 13–16.

Colles, C.M. (1989b) A technique for assessing hoof function in the horse. *Equine Vet. J.* **21**: 17–22.

Curtis, S.J. (1992a) Farriery in the treatment of flexural deformities and a discussion on applying shoes to young horses. *Equine Vet. Educ.* **4**: 193–197.

Curtis, S.J. (1992b) The assessment and farriery treatment of mediolateral deformities in foals. *Equine Athlete* **9**:15–19.

Curtis, S.J. (1999) *From Foal to Racehorse*, 1st edn. Newmarket: R and W Publications.

Davies, H.M.S. (1996a) The effect of different exercise conditions on metacarpal strains in Thoroughbred racehorses. *Pferdeheilkunde* **12**: 666–670.

Davies, H.M.S. (1996b) A technical report on the distribution of strain in the hoof wall of a standing horse before and after trimming. *Pferdeheilkunde* **12**: 679–680.

Davies, H.M.S. (1997) Non invasive photoelastic method to show distribution of strain on the hoof wall of a living horse. *Equine Vet. J.* **23**: 13–15.

Dejardin, L.M., Arnoczky, S.P., Fox, D.B., Ciavelli, M.J. and Makidon, P.E. (1997) The use of photoelastic technology in the analysis and localization of strain on the loaded equine hoof – an in vitro pilot study. *Vet. Surg.* **26**: 413.

Dejardin, L.M., Arnoczky, S.P. and Cloud, G.L. (1999) A method for determination of equine hoof strain patterns using photoelasticity. *Equine Vet. J.* **31**: 232–237.

Douglas, J.E., Biddick, T.L., Thomasson, J.J. and Jofriet, J.C. (1998) Stress/strain behaviour of the equine laminar junction. *J. Exp. Biol.* **201**: 2287–2297.

Drevemo, S. and Hjertén, G. (1991) Evaluation of a shock absorbing woodchip layer on a harness race-track. *Equine Exerc. Physiol.* **3**: 107–112.

Dyce, K.M. and Wensing, C.J.G. (1980) *De Anatomie Van Het Paard.* Utrecht: Uitgeverij Bohn, Scheltema, Holkema.

Dyhre-Poulsen, P., Smedegaard, H.H., Roed, J. and Korsgaard, E. (1994) Equine hoof function investigated by pressure transducers inside the hoof and accelerometers mounted on the first phalanx. *Equine Vet. J.* **26**: 326–366.

Ellis, D.R. (1998) Conditions of the hoof wall in young horses and corrective farriery with regard to limb deformities. *Equine Vet. Educ.* **10**: 155–160.

Eustace, R. and Caldwell, M.N. (1989a) The construction of the heart bar shoe and the technique of dorsal wall resection. *Equine Vet. J.* **21**: 367–369.

Eustace, R.J. and Caldwell, M.N. (1989b) Treatment of solar prolapse using the heart bar shoe and dorsal hoof wall resection technique. *Equine Vet. J.* **21**: 370–372.

Firth, E.C., Schamhardt, H.C. and Hartman, W. (1988) Measurements of bone strain in foals with altered foot balance. *Am. J. Vet. Res.* **49**: 261–265.

Folman, Y., Wosk, J., Voloshin, A. and Liberty, S. (1986) Cyclic impact on heel strike: a possible biomechanical factor in the etiology of degenerative disease of the human locomotor system. *Acta. Orthop. Trauma. Surg.* **104**: 363–365.

Frederick, F.H. and Henderson, J.M. (1970) Impact force measurement using preloaded transducers. *Am. J. Vet. Res.* **31**: 2279–2283.

Fredricson, I. and Drevemo, S. (1971) A new method of investigating equine locomotion. *Equine Vet. J.* **3**: 137–140.

Fredricson, I., Dalin, G., Drevemo, S. and Hjertén, G. (1975a) Ergonomics of poor racetrack design. *Equine Vet. J.* **7**: 63–65.

Fredricson, I., Dalin, G., Drevemo, S. and Hjertén, G. (1975b) A biotechnical approach to the design of racetracks. *Equine Vet. J.* **7**: 91–96.

Gabriel, A., Youshi, S., Detilleux, J., Dessy-Doizè, C. and Bernard, C. (1997) Bone morphometric study of the equine navicular bone: comparison between fore and rear limbs. *J. Vet. Med. A.* **44**: 579–594.

Girtler, D., Kübber, P., Kastner, Ch. and Scheidl, M. (1995) Kinematische Untersuchungen des Vorführbogen bei Pferden mit unterschiedlichen Dorsalwandwinkel des Hufes. *Wien Tier. Arztl. Mschr.* **82**: 145–151.

Goetz, Th. (1987) Anatomic hoof and shoeing considerations for the treatment of laminitis in horses. *J. Am. Vet. Med. Assoc.* **190**: 1323–1332.

Hermans, W.A. (1984) *Hoefverzorging en Hoefbeslag. Groene Reeks.* Zutphen: Uitgeverij Terra Zutphen.

Hertsch, B., Höppner, S. and Dallmer, H. (1996) *The Hoof and How To Protect It Without Nails*, 1st edn. Salzhauzen-Putensen: Dallmer Publications.

Hickman, J. and Humphrey, M. (1997) *Hickman's Farriery*, 2nd edn. London: J.A. Allen.

Hjertén, G. and Drevemo, S. (1993) Shortening of the forelimb in the horse during the stance phase. *Acta Anat.* **146**: 193–195.

Hjertén, G. and Drevemo, S. (1994) Semi-quantitative analysis of hoof strike in the horse. *J. Biomech.* **17**: 997–1004.

Jörgensen, U. and Ekstrand, J. (1988) Significance of heel pad confinement for the shock absorption at heel strike. *Int. J. Sports* **9**: 468–471.

Jurga, F. (1997) Progress in laminitis therapy. *Hoofcare and Lameness* **68**: 16–23.

Kai, M., Takahashi, T., Aoki, O. and Oki, H. (1999) Influence of rough track surfaces on components of vertical forces in cantering Thoroughbred horses. *Equine Vet. J.* **30**(Suppl.): 214–217.

Kane, A.J., Stover, S., Gardner, I.A. *et al.* (1996) Horseshoe characteristics as possible risk factor in fatal musculoskeletal injury of Thoroughbred racehorses. *Am J. Vet. Res.* **37**: 1147–1152.

Kaneps, A.J., O'Brien, T.R., Willits, N.H., Dykes, J.E. and Stover, S.M. (1998) The effect of hoof trimming on the occurrence of distal phalangeal palmar process fractures in foals. *Equine Vet. J.* **26**(Suppl.): 36–45.

Kasapi, M.A. and Gosline, J.M. (1997) Design complexity and fracture control in the equine hoof wall. *J. Exp. Biol.* **200**: 1639–1659.

Kasapi, M.A. and Gosline, J.M. (1998) Exploring the possible functions of equine hoof wall tubulus. *Equine Vet. J.* **26**(Suppl.): 10–14.

Keegan, K.G., Wilson, D.J., Wilson, D.A., Barnett, C.D. and Smith, B. (1998). Effects of balancing and shoeing of the forelimb feet on kinematic gait analysis in five horses with navicular disease. *J. Equine Vet. Sci.* **18**: 522–528.

Keg, P.R., Schamhardt, H.C., Weeren, P.R. van and Barneveld, A. (1996) The effect of diagnostic nerve blocks in the forelimb on the locomotion of clinically sound horses. *Vet. Quart.* **18**: S106–109.

Ker, R.F., Bennett, M.B., Alexander, R.M.c.N. and Kester, R.C. (1989) Foot strike and the properties of the human heel pad. *Proc. Inst. Mech. Engrs.* **203**: 191–196.

Kersjes, A.W., Németh, F. and Rutgers, L.J.E. (1985) *Atlas of Large Animal Surgery*. Utrecht: Uitgeverij Bunge, p. 133.

Knezevic, P. (1966) Measuring of strain in the hoof capsule of the horse. *Proc. Ann. Conv. Am. Assoc. Equine Pract.* **12**: 293–304.

Kobluk, C., Robinson, R., Gordon, B., Clanton, C., Trent, A. and Ames, T. (1990) The effect of conformation and shoeing: a cohort study of 95 thoroughbred racehorses. *Proc. Ann. Conv. Am. Assoc. Equine Pract.* **35**: 259–274.

Kübber, P., Kastner, J., Girtler, D. and Knezevic, P.F. (1994) Erkenntnisse über den Einfluss der tiefen Palmarnervanästhesie auf das Gangbild des lahmheitsfreien Pferdes mit Hilfe einer kinematischen Messmethode. *Pferdeheilkunde* **10**: 11–21.

Lanovaz, J.L., Clayton, H.M. and Watson, L.G. (1998) In vitro attenuation of impact shock in equine digits. *Equine Vet. J.* (Suppl. **26**): 96–102.

Lanovaz, J.L., Clayton, H.M., Colborne, G.R. and Schamhardt, H.C. (1999) Forelimb kinematics and joint moments during the swing phase of the trot. *Equine Vet. J.* **30**(Suppl.) 235–239.

Leach, D.H. (1983) Biomechanical considerations in raising and lowering the heel. *Proc. Ann. Conv. Am. Assoc. Equine Pract.* **28**: 333–342.

Linford, R.L. (1994) Camera speeds for optoelectronic assessment of stride timing characteristics in horses at the trot. *Am. J. Vet. Res.* **55**: 1189–1195.

Marks, D., Mackay-Smith, M.P., Cushing, L.S. and Leslie, J.A. (1971) Use of an elastomer to reduce concussion to horses' feet. *J. Am. Vet. Med. Assoc.* **158**: 1361–1365.

Martinelli, M.J. and Ferrie, J.W. (1997) Farrier primer for the student and practising veterinarian. *Equine Vet. Educ.* **9**: 89–97.

Merkens, H.W. and Schamhardt, H.C. (1994) Relationship between ground reaction force patterns and kinematics in the walking and trotting horse. *Equine Vet. J.* (Suppl. **17**): 67–70.

Merkens, H.W., Schamhardt, H.C., Osch, G.J.V.M., van and Bogert, A.J. van den (1994) Ground reaction force patterns of Dutch warmblood horses at normal trot. *Equine Vet. J.* **25**: 134–137.

Moyer, W. (1975) Lameness caused by improper shoeing. *J. Am. Vet. Med. Assoc.* **1**: 47–52.

Nigg, B.M., Denoth, J. and Neukomm, P.A. (1981) Quantifying the load on the human body: problems and some possible solutions. In: Morecki, A., Fideliu, K., Kedzior, K. and Wit, A. (eds) *Biomechanics VII*. Baltimore: University Park Press, pp. 88–99.

O'Grady, S. (1997) Shoeing the laminitic horse. *Am. Farriers J.* **3**: 33–38.

Østblom, L.C., Lund, C. and Meslen, F. (1984) Navicular bone disease: results of treatment using egg bar shoeing principle. *Equine Vet. J.* **16**: 203–206.

Ovnicek, G., Erfle, J.B. and Peters, D.F. (1995) Wild horse hoof patterns offer a formula for preventing and treating lameness. *Proc. Ann. Conv. Am. Assoc. Equine Pract.* **41**: 258–260.

Ovnicek, G. (1997) *New Hope for Soundness*. Columbia Falls: EDSS Publishers.

Pollit, C. (1995) *Color Atlas of the Horse's Foot*. London: Mosby–Wolfe.

Peremans, K., Verschooten, F., de Moor, A. and Desmet, P. (1991) Laminitis in the pony: conservative treatment versus dorsal hoof wall resection. *Equine Vet. J.* **23**: 243–246.

Pleasant, R.S., Baker, G.J., Foreman, J.H., Eurell, J.C. and Losonsky, J.M. (1993) Intraosseous pressure and pathologic changes in horses with navicular disease. *Am. J. Vet. Res.* **54**: 7–12.

Pratt, G.W. (1997) Model for injury to the foreleg of the Thoroughbred racehorse. *Equine Vet. J.* **23** (Suppl.): 30–32.

Preuschoft, H. (1989) The external force and internal stresses in the feet of dressage and jumping horses. *Z. Säugetierkunde* **54**: 172–190.

Radin, E.L., Parker, H.G., Pugh, J.W., Steinberg, R.S., Paul, I.L. and Rose, R.M. (1981) Response of joints to impact loading III. Relationship between trabecular microfractures and cartilage degeneration. *J. Biomech.* **6**: 51–57.

Radin, E.L. (1999) Subchondral bone changes and cartilage damage. *Equine Vet. J.* **31**: 94–95.

Ratzlaff, M.H. and White, K.K. (1989) Some biomechanical considerations concerning navicular disease. *J. Equine Vet. Sci.* **9**: 149–153.

Ratzlaff, M.H., Shindell, R.M. and Debowes, R.M. (1985) Changes in digital venous pressures of horses moving at the walk and trot. *Am. J. Vet. Res.* **46**: 1545–1549.

Ratzlaff, M.H., Wilson, P.D., Hyde, M.L., Balch, O.K. and Grant, B.D. (1993) Relationships between locomotor forces, hoof position and joint motion during the support phase of the stride of galloping horses. *Acta Anat.* **146**: 200–204.

Ratzlaff, M.H., Hyde, M.L., Hutum, D.V., Rathgeber, R.A. and Balch, O.K. (1997) Interrelationships between moisture content of the track, dynamic properties of the track and the locomotor forces exerted by galloping horses. *J. Equine Vet. Sci.* **17**: 35–42.

Riemersma, D.J., van den Bogert, A.J., Jansen, M.O. and Schamhardt, H.C. (1996a) Influence of shoeing on ground reaction forces and tendon strains in the forelimbs of ponies. *Equine Vet. J.* **28**: 126–132.

Riemersma, D.J., van den Bogert, A.J., Jansen, M.O. and Schamhardt, H.C. (1996b) Tendon strain in the forelimbs as a function of gait and ground characteristics and in vitro limb loading in ponies. *Equine Vet. J.* **28**: 133–138.

Ritmeester, A.J., Blevins, W.E., Ferguson, D.W. and Adams, S.B. (1998) Digital perfusion, evaluated scintigraphy and hoof wall growth in horses with chronic laminitis treated with egg bar heart bar shoeing and coronary grooving. *Equine Vet. J.* **26** (Suppl.): 111–118.

Roepstorff, L., Johnston, C. and Drevemo, S. (1994) The influence of different treadmill constructions on ground reaction forces as determinant by the use of a force measuring horseshoe. *Equine Vet. J.* **17** (Suppl.): 71–74.

Roepstorff, L., Johnston, C. and Drevemo, S. (1999) The effect of shoeing on kinetics and kinematics during the stance phase. *Equine Vet. J.* **30** (Suppl.): 279–285.

Rööser, R., Ekbladh, R. and Lidgren, L. (1988) The shock absorbing effect of soles and insoles. *Int. Orthop.* **12**: 335–338.

Ruthe, H., Müller, H. and Reinhard, F. (1997) *Der Huf*. Stuttgart: Ferdinand Enke Verlag.

Savelberg, H.H.C.M., Loon, T. van and Schamhardt, H.C. (1997) Ground reaction forces in horses assessed from hoof wall deformation using artificial neural networks. *Equine Vet. J.* **23** (Suppl.): 6–8.

Schamhardt, H.C., Hartman, W., Jansen, M.O. and Back, W. (1991) Biomechanics of the thoracic limb of the horse. *Swiss Vet.* **8**: 7–10.

Seeherman, H.J. (1991) The use of high speed treadmills for lameness and hoof balance evaluation in the horse. *Vet. Clin. North Am.: Equine Pract.* **7**: 271–309.

Stashak, T.S. (1987) *Adam's Lameness in Horses*. Philadelphia: WB Saunders, pp. 786–833.

Stephens, P.R., Nunamaker, D.M. and Butterweck, D.M. (1989) Application of Hall-effect transducer for measurement of tendon strains in horses. *Am. J. Vet. Res.* **50**: 1089–1095.

Summerley, H.L., Thomason, J.J. and Bignell, W.W. (1998) Effect of rider style on deformation of the front hoof wall in Warmblood horses. *Equine Vet. J.* **26** (Suppl.): 81–85.

Thompson, K.N. and Herring, L.S. (1994) Metacarpophalangeal and phalangeal joint kinematics in horses shod with hoof caulks *J. Equine Vet. Sci.* **14**: 319.

Thomason, J.J. (1998) Variation in surface train on the equine hoof wall at the midstep with shoeing, gait, substrate, direction of travel, and hoof angle. *Equine Vet. J.* **26** (Suppl.): 86–95.

Thompson, K.H., Cheung, T.K. and Silverman, M. (1993) The effect of toe angle on tendon, ligament, band and hoofwall strains. *J. Equine Vet. Sci.* **13**: 651–654.

Turner, T.A. (1986) Shoeing principles for the management of navicular disease. *J. Am. Vet. Med. Assoc.* **189**: 298–301.

Turner, T.A. (1988) Proper shoeing and shoeing principles for the management of navicular syndrome. *Proc. Ann. Conv. Am. Assoc. Equine Pract.* **33**: 299–305.

Vasko, K.A. and Farr, D. (1984) A viscoelastic polymer as an aid in injury management and prevention in equine athletes. *J. Equine. Vet. Sci.* **4**: 278–280.

White, N.A. and Baggett, N. (1983) A method of corrective shoeing for laminitis in horses. *Vet. Med. Small Anim. Clin.* **5**: 775–778.

Willemen, M.A. (1998) Een onderzoek naar de biomechanische effecten van hoefbeslag. *Tijdschr. Diergeneesk* **123**: 408–410.

Willemen, M.A., Savelberg, H.C.C.M., Bruin, G. and Barneveld, A. (1994) The effect of toe weights on linear and temporal stride characteristics of Standardbred trotters. *Vet. Quart.* **16**: S97–100.

Willemen, M.A., Savelberg, H.C.C.M., Jacobs, M.W.H. and Barneveld, A. (1996) Biomechanical effects of rocker-toed shoes in sound horses. *Vet. Quart.* **18**: S75–78.

Willemen, M.A., Savelberg, H.C.C.M. and Barneveld, A. (1997) The improvements of the gait quality of sound trotting warmblood horses by normal shoeing and its effect on the load on the lower forelimb. *Livestock. Prod. Sci.* **52**: 145–153.

Willemen, M.A., Savelberg, H.C.C.M. and Barneveld, A. (1999) The effect of orthopaedic shoeing on the force exerted by the deep digital flexor tendon on the navicular bone in horses. *Equine Vet. J.* **31**: 25–30.

Wilson, A.M. and Pardoe, C.H. (1998) Equine hoof cracks: mechanical considerations and repair techniques. *Equine. Vet. Educ. Manual.* **4**: 52–56.

Wilson, P.D., Ratzlaff, M.H., Grant, B.D., Hyde, M.L. and Balch, O.K. (1992) The effects of a compressible plastic – the Seattle-shoe on the kinematics of the strides of galloping Thoroughbred horses. *J. Equine Vet. Sci.* **12**: 374–381.

Wilson, A.M., Seelig, T.J., Shield, R.A. and Silverman, B.W. (1998) The effect of foot imbalance on point of force application in the horse. *Equine. Vet. J.* **30**: 540–545.

Wintzer, H.J. (1971) Besitzen der Hufbeslag und die Hufpflege eine Bedeutung bei der Behandlung und Verhutung der Podotrochleose. *Wien Tierärtzl. Mschr.* **58**: 148–151.

Wright, I.M. and Douglas, J. (1993) Biomechanical considerations in the treatment of navicular disease. *Vet. Rec.* **7**: 109–114.

Wright, I.M., Kidd, L. and Thorp, B.H. (1998) Gross, histological and histomorphometric features of the navicular bone and related structures in the horse. *Equine Vet. J.* **30**: 220–234.

7
The Neck and Back

Jean-Marie Denoix and Fabrice Audigié

INTRODUCTION

Back flexibility and active mobility are essential to the accomplishment of sport exercises and are the subject of constant observation and concern for trainers and riders. Back pathology, inducing pain and reducing the amount of motion, has been identified as an important cause of poor performance (Jeffcott, 1975, 1980; Denoix, 1998). Kissing spines, vertebral spondylosis (Jeffcott, 1980) and osteoarthrosis of the dorsal synovial intervertebral joints between the articular processes (Denoix, 1998) are the most significant vertebral lesions responsible for back discomfort and clinical manifestations in horses.

Several *in vitro* studies have been performed on the biomechanics of the back and neck (Jeffcott & Dalin, 1980; Townsend *et al.*, 1983; Denoix, 1987; Clayton & Townsend, 1989a,b) but our knowledge of these areas is still incomplete. *In vitro* studies were mainly performed to evaluate the nature and maximal amount of regional or intervertebral movements of flexion and extension, rotation and lateral bending. With the different protocols used, wide displacements were studied (Denoix, 1999), but mobility of the vertebral column rarely reaches its maximal limits during locomotion and sporting performance, although back pain due to pressure, tension and/or shearing on vertebral structures (Denoix, 1999) can alter locomotion of sport and race horses (Jeffcott *et al.*, 1982; Denoix, 1998; Jeffcott, 1998).

A general geometric approach to the biomechanics of the back in relation to vertebral pathology has been presented (Rooney, 1982). Recently, an anatomo-functional synthesis of the behavior of the osteoarticular components of the equine thoracolumbar vertebral column mainly based on *in vitro* investigations has been performed (Denoix, 1999). Three major movements

take place in the equine intervertebral joints (Jeffcott, 1980; Townsend *et al.*, 1983; Clayton & Townsend 1989a; Denoix, 1999). They are:

- flexion (ventral bending inducing a dorsal convexity) and extension (dorsal bending inducing a ventral convexity) movements, occurring in the median plane, around a transverse axis
- lateral bending (lateroflexion) to the left and right sides, developed in the horizontal plane, around a dorsoventral axis
- left rotation (left deviation of a vertebral body with respect to the following one) or right rotation, occurring around a longitudinal axis.

Movements of minor amplitude take place in a vertical transverse plane:

- vertical shearing (dorsoventral translation) is associated with flexion and extension movements
- transverse shearing (left to right displacement) is associated with lateroflexion and rotation.

Longitudinal compression and tension occur in some parts of the intervertebral joints for every major movement of the vertebral column.

Considering the complete equine vertebral column, the movements of the neck and trunk and an anatomo-functional description of the behavior of the axial muscles during different gaits and sport exercises has been published previously (Denoix, 1988, Denoix & Pailloux 1996). At present, few *in vivo* studies have been published. A kinematic method to evaluate back flexibility on standing horses was presented (Licka & Peham, 1998). Neck and back motion and coordination are very different according to the gait and movement that are being performed and there is a need for a better knowledge of the nature and amplitude of *in vivo* equine vertebral mobility.

The purpose of this chapter is to present a synthesis of the current and still partial knowledge on *in vivo* neck and back motion and coordination at walk, trot, gallop as well as during lameness and jumping. The data presented are mainly based on kinematic analysis, accelerometric studies and electromyographic (EMG) investigations. Descriptions of coordination are limited to the relative displacements of different axial regions of the horse (mainly neck *versus* back), as visualized using kinematic analysis techniques. As these displacements are induced and controlled by long muscle chains, co-ordination of muscular activity was investigated via electromyographic studies.

WALK

Kinematic and accelerometric data

Kinematic and accelerometric studies of head and trunk movement at walk and trot on treadmills have been performed (Barrey *et al.*, 1994; Buchner *et al.*, 1996). At the walk, the vertical displacement, velocity and acceleration of the head, withers and tuber sacrale showed a sinusoidal pattern with two similar oscillations during each stride. The height of the withers and tuber sacrale was minimal at the beginning of the stance phase and maximal at about mid stance of both thoracic or pelvic limbs (Buchner *et al.*, 1996). The acceleration signal recorded over the sternum showed also two similar dorsoventral deviations corresponding to each half-stride (Barrey *et al.*, 1994).

A complementary analysis of the walk on a treadmill using three-dimensional accelerometers fixed to the front of a saddle (Galloux *et al.*, 1994) showed that, at the walk, the amplitude of movement was higher in the vertical axis than in the transverse or longitudinal axes; rotation around the transverse axis (pitching motion) was higher than rotation around the longitudinal axis (rolling) and vertical axis (twisting). Furthermore, the twisting movement was greater in the walk than in the other gaits.

Head movement adaptations associated with a supporting forelimb lameness induced by pressure on the hoof sole resembled those of the trot: the amplitude of the dorsoventral oscillation decreased during the stance phase of the lame limb and increased during the contralateral limb stance phase (Buchner *et al.*, 1996). Similarly, the maximum acceleration amplitude over the sternum was reduced during the stance phase of the lame forelimb (Barrey *et al.*, 1994). For induced hindlimb lameness, elevation of the tuber sacrale was slightly reduced during the lame stance phase while head and withers movements were not significantly altered (Buchner *et al.*, 1996).

Electromyographic data

EMG activity of neck and trunk muscles of horses walking on a treadmill or on hard surfaces, using skin contact surface electrodes, is presented in Fig. 7.1.

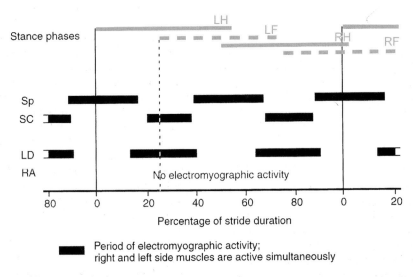

Fig. 7.1   Electromyographic activity of neck and trunk muscles at walk (1.8 m/s) on a hard surface. **Limbs**: LF: left forelimb; RF: right forelimb; LH: left hindlimb; RH: right hindlimb. **Muscles**: Sp: splenius; SC: sternocephalicus; LD: longissimus dorsi; RA: rectus abdominis. (Courtesy of Céline Robert, Maison-Alfort, France)

This figure shows that:

- the left and right splenius muscles act simultaneously before the landing of each forelimb (or during the second half of the opposite forelimb stance phase) to elevate the head and neck and facilitate forelimb protraction by the elongated brachiocephalicus muscle
- the sternocephalicus muscles had reciprocal activity to splenius muscles and act before and during the first half of each forelimb stance phase
- the longissimus dorsi muscles act during the intermediate part of each hindlimb stance phase to facilitate propulsion
- the rectus abdominis muscles do not show any significant EMG activity during the walk (Tokuriki *et al.*, 1997; Robert *et al.*, 1998), and this is correlated to the limited vertical acceleration of the abdominal visceral mass in this gait, which has no suspension phase.

A previous study performed with intramuscular wire electrodes on four horses with and without a rider reported that the multifidus lumborum muscle was active in the intermediate part of the stance phase of the ipsilateral hindlimb and the obliquus externus abdominis muscle had intermittent activity (Tokuriki *et al.*, 1991). On the standing horse, in the neck region, the splenius muscle showed some activity, while the sternocephalicus and brachiocephalicus muscles were silent (Tokuriki & Aoki, 1991).

Clinical observation

Clinical observation shows that it is probably during walking that the mobility of the thoracolumbar vertebral column is most diversified, with association of rotation and lateroflexion combined with limited movements of flexion and extension.

TROT

Kinematic and electromyographic data of neck and trunk motion and coordination have been established on sound horses with a three dimensional (3-D) kinematic analysis system allowing simultaneous recording of the left and right sides of the horse (Audigié *et al.*, 1998; Robert *et al.*, 1998; Pourcelot, 1999). Lame horses have also been investigated using kinematic analysis (Buchner *et al.*, 1996; Audigie *et al.*, 1998; Audigié, 1999).

Sound horses

Kinematic data

The vertical displacement versus time of the head, withers and tuber sacrale at trot shows a sinusoidal pattern (Buchner *et al.*, 1996) with two symmetrical oscillations during a stride. The general orientation of the neck and trunk and their alignment vary during the stride (Fig. 7.2). With respect to the tuber sacrale position, the withers elevate during the first and intermediate parts of each diagonal stance phase (upward rotation of the trunk) and descend during the last part of the stance phase as well as during the suspension phase (downward rotation of the trunk). Additionally, the croup presents wider dorsoventral movements (lowering and elevation) than the withers.

In sound trotting horses, the head position is highest in the first half of each diagonal stance phase (Vorstenbosch *et al.*, 1997). During the major part of the stance phase (Fig. 7.2), the neck rotates downward and becomes closer to the horizontal, with the head reaching its lowest point before the end of this phase. During the suspension and beginning of the following stance phase the neck becomes more oblique (Fig. 7.2), and the head is elevated again (upward rotation of the neck).

In early stance both the neck and trunk undergo an upward rotation; during the middle part of the stance phase the angle between the neck and trunk flexes (Fig. 7.2) and during the last part of the stance phase, the neck and trunk rotate downward to become closer to the horizontal. During the suspension phase, extension between the trunk and neck occurs (Fig. 7.2).

A 3-D *in vivo* kinematic study of flexion and extension movements of the thoracolumbar spine was performed at the trot in 13 sound horses using five skin markers placed on the median plane of the back over the 6th and 13th thoracic spinal processes as well as at the thoracolumbar, lumbosacral and sacrocaudal junctions (Pourcelot *et al.*, 1998; Audigié *et al.*, 1998). This study showed that maximal thoracic extension occurs near mid stance (Fig. 7.3). This passive movement is produced by the visceral mass inertia. The maximal thoracolumbar extension occurs in the second half of each stance phase, followed by the maximal lumbosacral extension at the end of the stance phase (Audigié *et al.*, 1998).

The maximal thoracic flexion takes place during the swing phase and is concomitant to an elevation of the neck (Figs 7.3 & 7.4). It is followed by the maximal thoracolumbar flexion. Finally, the maximal flexion of the lumbosacral junction occurs at the end of the swing

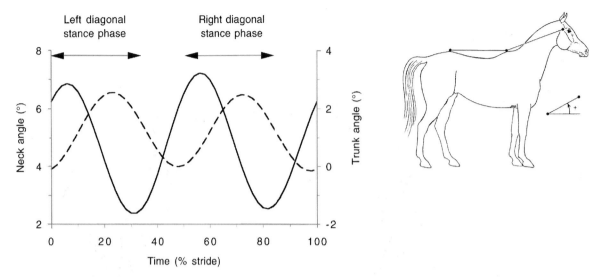

Fig. 7.2 Neck and trunk orientation in sound horses guided by hand on hard track at trot (3.1 m/s). Markers are placed over the zygomatic arch, withers (6th thoracic spinal process) and tuber sacrale. The straight line between the first two markers represents the neck orientation; the line between the last two markers represents the trunk orientation. The figure shows the angle variations occurring between these lines and the horizontal plane during one stride. A positive angle indicates an upward angulation. (——) Neck angle (°) with respect to the horizontal plane; (-----) trunk angle (°) with respect to the horizontal plane; diagonal stance phase: full fore hoof–ground contact.

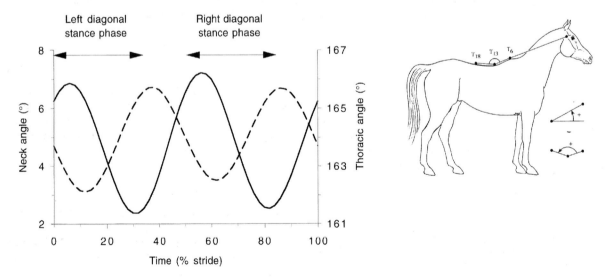

Fig. 7.3 Coordination between the neck orientation and thoracic spine dorsoventral movements in sound horses guided by hand on a hard track at trot (3.1 m/s). Markers are placed over the zygomatic arch, withers (6th thoracic spinal process), 13th and 18th thoracic spinal processes. The straight line between the first two markers represents the neck orientation. The thoracic angle is drawn between the last three markers. The figure shows the angle variations occurring between the neck orientation and the horizontal plane as well as the thoracic angle variations during one stride. For the neck, an increasing angle indicates an upward rotation; the thoracic angle increases during flexion of the back and decreases during extension. (——) Neck angle (°) with respect to the horizontal plane; (----) thoracic angle (°); diagonal stance phase: full fore hoof–ground contact.

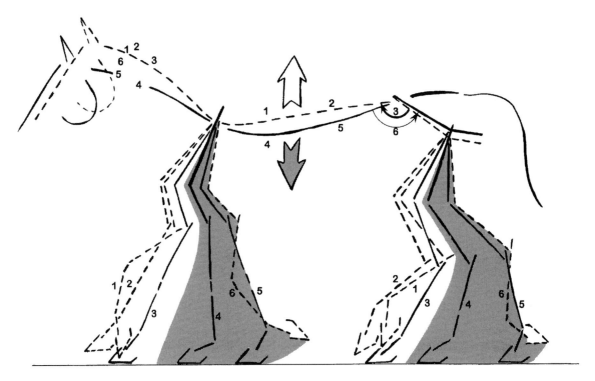

Fig. 7.4 Schematic representation of the trunk movements and neck positions during half a stride with reference to the vertebral column dorsoventral peaks of mobility. 1: Maximal thoracic flexion; 2: maximal thoracolumbar flexion; 3: maximal lumbosacral flexion; 4: maximal thoracic extension; 5: maximal thoracolumbar extension; 6: maximal lumbosacral extension. The same numbers indicate the respective positions of the neck and limbs (left diagonal).

phase at the time of maximal protraction of the hindlimb (Audigié *et al.*, 1998).

The influence of the neck orientation on the thoracic spine dorsoventral mobility has been investigated in cadaver specimens (Denoix, 1987). The results showed that elevation of the neck facilitates thoracic flexion (Fig. 7.4).

Accelerometric data

An accelerometric device fixed over the sternum area by an elastic girth (Barrey *et al.*, 1994) showed that, for horses trotting on a treadmill, the dorsoventral acceleration curves had a deviation corresponding to each half-stride. The height of the dorsoventral acceleration signal was linearly correlated with speed. Longitudinal accelerations were less repetitive than dorsoventral ones; their magnitude increased with the increasing speed of the gait.

Analysis of the trot on a treadmill using three-dimensional accelerometers fixed to the saddle (Galloux *et al.*, 1994) showed that the linear movements along the three axes (longitudinal, transverse and vertical) were similar in amplitude. Rotation around the transverse axis (pitching motion) was smaller in comparison with the other two gaits (walk and canter).

Electromyographic data

The electromyographic activity of neck and trunk muscles at trot has been investigated on hard track surfaces, with or without riders, as well as on a treadmill (Tokuriki & Aoki, 1991; Tokuriki *et al.*, 1991, 1997; Robert *et al.*, 1998).

Neck muscle activity and neck orientation Comparison of neck muscle activity and neck orientation demonstrates that:

- the splenius muscle acts before and during the first part of the stance phase of each forelimb (Figs 7.5 & 7.6) to limit lowering of the neck (antigravitational activity). As mentioned by Tokuriki and Aoki (1991),

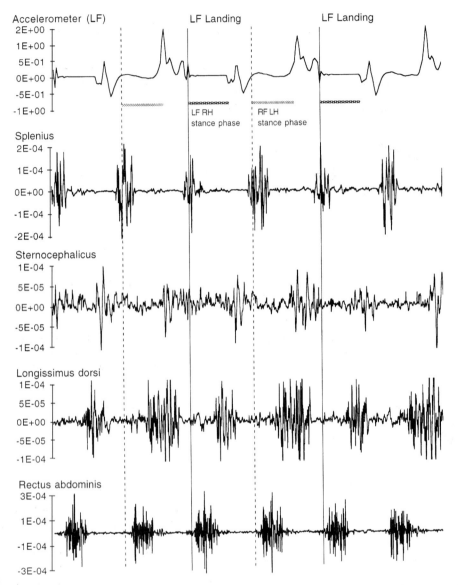

Fig. 7.5 Electromyographic activity of two neck and two trunk muscles (left side) at trot on a treadmill (4 m/s) on three consecutive strides. An accelerometer was placed on the left forelimb. LF: left forelimb; RF: right forelimb; LH: left hindlimb; RH: right hindlimb. (Courtesy of Céline Robert, Maisons-Alfort, France)

muscle activity tends to be higher during the stance phase of the contralateral forelimb than for the ipsilateral one (Fig. 7.5)

- the sternocephalicus muscles have a reciprocal activity during the suspension phase to control neck elevation (Figs 7.5 & 7.6)
- the brachiocephalicus muscle activity is high during the later part of the ipsilateral forelimb stance phase and during the suspension phase (Fig. 7.6) to

achieve protraction of the ipsilateral forelimb; this muscle is inactive during most of the stance phase of the ipsilateral forelimb in order to avoid limiting forelimb propulsion.

Effect of neck orientation on neck muscle activity Lowering of the neck using the reins induces a reduction of splenius muscle activity during the first half of the stance phase of each diagonal (Fig. 7.7). These data can be

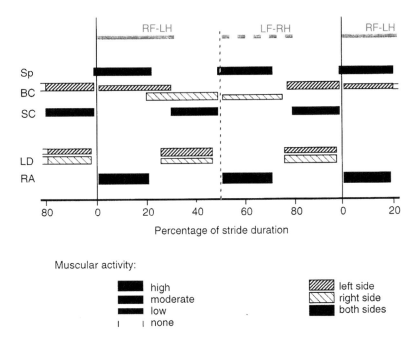

Fig. 7.6 Electromyographic activity of neck and trunk muscles at trot (4 m/s) on a treadmill (mean periods for five horses). **Limbs:** LF: left forelimb; RF: right forelimb; LH: left hindlimb; RH: right hindlimb. **Muscles:** Sp: splenius; BC: brachiocephalicus; SC: sternocephalicus; LD: longissimus dorsi; RA: rectus abdominis. (Courtesy of Céline Robert, Maisons-Alfort, France)

explained by the lower amplitude of the neck displacement as well as by increased tension in passive anatomical structures that support the head and neck, such as the nuchal ligament.

Trunk muscle activity and thoracolumbar movements
Comparison of trunk muscle activity and thoracolumbar movements shows that:

- the rectus abdominis muscle acts during the stance phase (Figs 7.5 & 7.6) to limit the passive thoracolumbar extension induced by the visceral mass acceleration
- the longissimus dorsi muscles act at the end of each stance phase and during the suspension phase (Figs 7.5 & 7.6) to induce lumbosacral extension and facilitate hindlimb propulsion as well as to stabilize the thoracolumbar spine undergoing flexion.

A previous study (Tokuriki *et al.*, 1991) showed that the multifidus lumborum and longissimus lumborum were active before and after lift off of each hindlimb, with the activity being higher for the ipsilateral hindlimb. According to this study the obliquus externus abdominis and rectus abdominis had roughly reciprocal activity to these epiaxial muscles. In another study (Tokuriki *et al.*, 1997) the longissimus lumborum was thought to play a

role in limiting lateral bending of the trunk during symmetrical gaits.

Lame horses (see also chapter 10)

Neck and trunk orientation and coordination

Neck and trunk orientation and coordination are altered in lame horses (Cadiot & Almy 1924).

Forelimb lamenesses Under clinical conditions, it has been known for a long time that forelimb lamenesses are associated with a higher elevation of the head during the stance phase of the affected limb, whereas the head is lowered during the stance phase of the sound forelimb (Cadiot & Almy 1924). This was confirmed experimentally for induced forelimb lameness in horses trotting on a treadmill (Buchner *et al.*, 1996). It was also shown that during the stance phase of the lame limb the amplitude of the head oscillation decreased, while it increased during the contralateral stance phase. The amplitude of the displacements was greater for the head than for the tuber sacrale or the withers (Buchner *et al.*, 1996).

In horses with a moderate or severe forelimb lameness trotting on a hard track (Figs 7.8 & 7.9), neck orientation is severely altered with a downward orientation

173

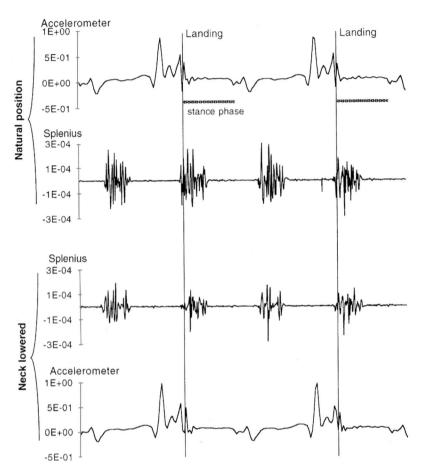

Fig. 7.7 Influence of the neck position on the electromyographic activity of the splenius at trot (4 m/s) (left side muscle with reference to the left front limb). (Courtesy of Céline Robert, Maisons-Alfort, France)

during the sound diagonal stance phase. Only one oscillation per stride takes place (Fig. 7.9). The same downward orientation of the trunk during the sound diagonal stance phase is also observed but two oscillations per stride persist for the trunk even for severe forelimb lameness (Figs 7.8 & 7.9). These modifications are correlated with an increased weight-bearing on the sound forelimb compared with the painful opposite limb. Dynamic aspects of the asymmetric head and neck movements were shown to play a major role in lameness compensation which can be explained by inertial interaction between the neck and trunk (Vorstenbosch *et al.*, 1997).

Hindlimb lamenesses Under clinical conditions, it has been known for a long time that when horses with hindlimb lamenesses are examined at the trot, there is an elevation of the croup during the stance phase of the

affected limb, and lowering of the croup during the stance phase of the sound hindlimb (Cadiot & Almy 1924). Moreover, during the stance phase of the lame hindlimb and opposite forelimb (lame diagonal), there is a lowering of the head that simulates a lameness of the forelimb ipsilateral to the affected hindlimb (Cadiot & Almy 1924; Uhlir *et al.*, 1997). These observations are correlated with severe modifications of neck and trunk orientation observed when hindlimb lamenesses are present (Figs 7.10 & 7.11). The increasing *trunk angle* during the lame diagonal stance phase is correlated with lowering of the croup during weight-bearing on the lame hindlimb (Figs 7.10 & 7.11). Because of reduced elevation of the croup by the lame hindlimb (lack of propulsion), the trunk angle inflexion during the suspension phase is reduced for moderate hindlimb lamenesses (Fig. 7.10) and disappears for severe lamenesses

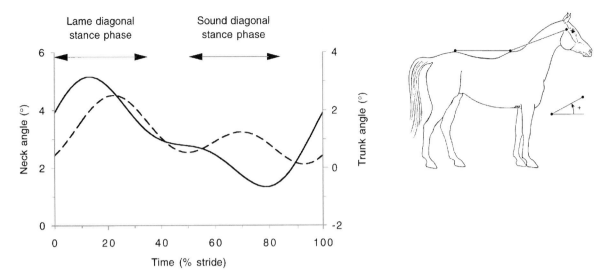

Fig. 7.8 Neck and trunk orientation of a horse with a moderate unilateral forelimb lameness (superficial digital flexor tendinitis combined with desmopathy of the palmar ligament) trotting on a hard track (compare with Fig. 7.2). Markers are placed over the zygomatic arch, withers (6th thoracic spinal process) and tuber sacrale. The straight line between the first two markers represents the neck orientation; the line between the last two markers represents the trunk orientation. The figure shows the angle variations occurring between these lines and the horizontal plane during one stride. An increasing angle indicates an upward rotation; a decreasing angle indicates a downward rotation. (——) Neck angle (°) with respect to the horizontal plane; (-----) trunk angle (°) with respect to the horizontal plane; diagonal stance phase: full fore hoof–ground contact.

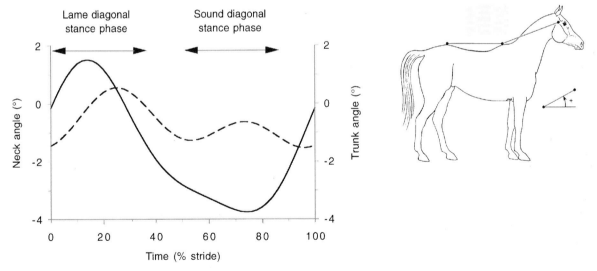

Fig. 7.9 Neck and trunk orientation of a horse with a severe unilateral forelimb lameness due to injury of the third interosseus muscle (suspensory ligament) trotting on a hard track (compare with Fig. 7.2). Markers are placed over the zygomatic arch, withers (6th thoracic spinal process) and tuber sacrale. The straight line between the first two markers represents the neck orientation; the line between the last two markers represents the trunk orientation. The figure shows the angle variations occurring between these lines and the horizontal plane during one stride. An increasing angle indicates an upward rotation; a decreasing angle indicates a downward rotation. (——) Neck angle (°) with respect to the horizontal plane; (------) trunk angle (°) with respect to the horizontal plane; diagonal stance phase: full fore hoof–ground contact.

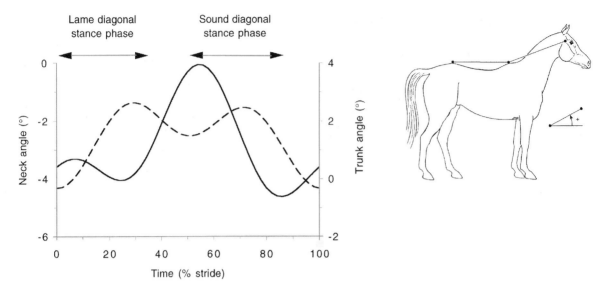

Fig. 7.10 Neck and trunk orientation of a horse with a moderate unilateral hindlimb lameness (bone spavin) trotting on a hard track (compare with Fig. 7.2). Markers are placed over the zygomatic arch, withers (6th thoracic spinal process), and tuber sacrale. The straight line between the first two markers represents the neck orientation; the line between the last 2 markers represents the trunk orientation. The figure shows the angle variations occurring between these lines and the horizontal plane during one stride. An increasing angle indicates an upward rotation; a decreasing angle indicates a downward rotation. (——) Neck angle (°) with respect to the horizontal plane; (-----) trunk angle (°) with respect to the horizontal plane; diagonal stance phase: full fore hoof–ground contact.

(Fig. 7.11). Consequently, the trunk angle makes only one oscillation per stride.

Hindlimb lamenesses also induce alteration of *neck movements:* lowering of the neck during the lame diagonal stance phase (Figs 7.10 & 7.11) contributes to reducing the weight on the painful hindlimb. However, this neck position and the acceleration required to elevate the neck at the end of the lame diagonal stance phase induce more stresses on the diagonal forelimb. These alterations are exacerbated for severe hindlimb lamenesses and, unlike the normal biphasic sinusoidal pattern of neck and trunk movements in sound horses (Fig. 7.2), there is only one peak elevation of both neck and trunk which occurs at the beginning of the sound diagonal stance phase. Synchronization of the neck and trunk orientation also occurs (Fig. 7.11). These trunk displacements participate in compensatory movements between the hindlimbs and forelimbs, which recently have been documented with kinematic analysis (Uhlir *et al.*, 1997).

Back mobility

Forelimb and hindlimb lamenesses do not have the same impact on back mobility. In sound horses a thoracic extension and a thoracolumbar extension occur successively during the stance phase (Audigié *et al.*, 1998).

During the suspension phase thoracic flexion precedes thoracolumbar flexion. EMG data demonstrate that these movements occur passively (C. Robert, Personal Communication, 1999).

With moderate forelimb lamenesses there is little modification of the dorsoventral mobility of the back (Fig. 7.12), and the sinusoidal pattern of the curve remains symmetrical between successive diagonal stance phases. Conversely, symmetry of the flexion and extension vertebral angle curves is altered with hindlimb lamenesses (Pourcelot *et al.*, 1998). Thoracic and thoracolumbar extension are reduced during the lame diagonal stance phase and increased during the sound diagonal stance phase (Fig. 7.13). This is correlated with the lower weight-bearing and propulsion of the painful hindlimb. Furthermore, there is a synchronization of the thoracic and thoracolumbar angle curves compared with sound horses and forelimb lamenesses.

Dorsoventral movements of flexion and extension have been quantified in sound horses (Audigié *et al.*, 1998; Pourcelot *et al.*, 1998). The maximal range of vertical displacements occurred near the 13th thoracic vertebra and, with respect to the tuber sacrale, reached an average value of 1.5 ± 0.2 cm. In clinical cases with intervertebral osteoarthrosis a significant reduction of this

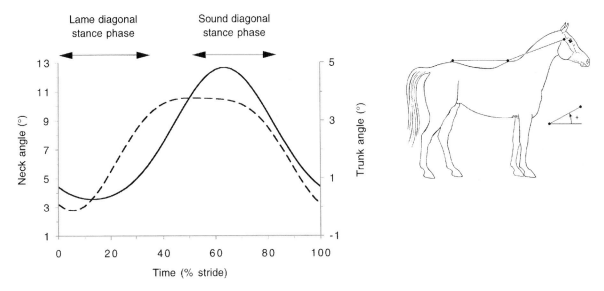

Fig. 7.11 Neck and trunk orientation of a horse with a severe unilateral hindlimb lameness (superficial digital flexor tendinitis just below the tuber calcanei) trotting on a hard track (compare with Fig. 7.2). Markers are placed over the zygomatic arch, withers (6th thoracic spinal process) and tuber sacrale. The straight line between the first two markers represents the neck orientation; the line between the last two markers represents the trunk orientation. The figure shows the angle variations occurring between these lines and the horizontal plane during one stride. An increasing angle indicates an upward rotation; a decreasing angle indicates a downward rotation. (——) Neck angle (°) with respect to the horizontal plane; (-----) trunk angle (°) with respect to the horizontal plane; diagonal stance phase: full fore hoof–ground contact.

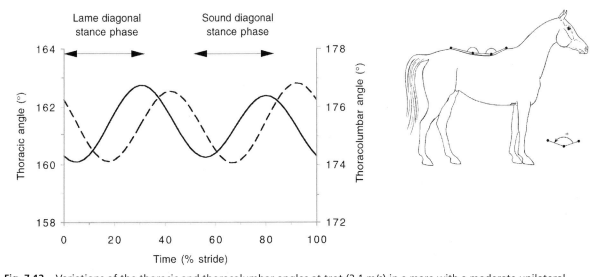

Fig. 7.12 Variations of the thoracic and thoracolumbar angles at trot (3.1 m/s) in a mare with a moderate unilateral forelimb lameness (distal enthesopathy of the biceps brachii). Markers are placed over the withers (6th thoracic spinal process), 13th and 18th thoracic spinal processes as well as over the tuber sacrale. The thoracic angle is drawn between the first three markers; the thoracolumbar angle is drawn between the last three markers. The figure shows these angle variations occurring during one stride. Each angle increases during vertebral column flexion and decreases during extension. (——) Thoracic angle (°); (------) thoracolumbar angle (°); diagonal stance phase: full fore hoof–ground contact.

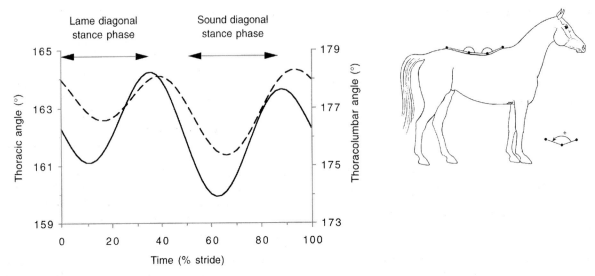

Fig. 7.13 Variations of the thoracic and thoracolumbar angles at trot (3.1 m/s) in a gelding with a moderate unilateral hindlimb lameness (bone spavin). Markers are placed over the withers (6th thoracic spinal process), 13th and 18th thoracic spinal processes as well as over the tuber sacrale. The thoracic angle is drawn between the first three markers; the thoracolumbar angle is drawn between the last three markers. The figure shows these angle variations occurring during one stride. Each angle increases during vertebral column flexion and decreases during extension. (——) Thoracic angle (°); (----) thoracolumbar angle (°); diagonal stance phase: full fore hoof–ground contact.

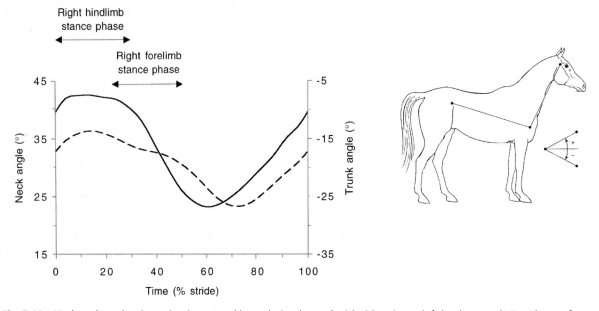

Fig. 7.14 Neck and trunk orientation in a sound horse being lunged with side reins at left lead canter (4.5 m/s) on soft ground (sand) in competitive conditions (vaulting gymnastics). Markers are placed over the zygomatic arch, point of shoulder and tuber coxae. The straight line between the first two markers represents the neck orientation; the line between the last two markers represents the trunk orientation. The figure shows the angle variations occurring between these lines and the horizontal plane during one stride. An increasing angle indicates an upward rotation; a decreasing angle indicates a downward rotation. (——) Neck angle (°) with respect to the horizontal plane; (-----) trunk angle (°) with respect to the horizontal plane.

178

range of motion was observed (F. Audigié, personal communication, 1999).

GALLOP

Kinematic data.

Kinematic analysis was performed in nine high-level vaulting horses cantering at 4–5 m/s on a circle. As no markers could be placed on the back, markers indicative of neck and trunk movements were placed over the zygomatic arch, shoulder joint and tuber coxae (Fig. 7.14). The head and neck were positioned with side reins and the horses were filmed under competitive conditions at a left lead canter from outside of the circle.

The neck and trunk angle curves showed that the cranial part of the neck and trunk becomes lower during the intermediate part of the support phase (downward rotation) and elevates (upward rotation) during the leading forelimb stance phase and the suspension phase (Fig. 7.14). The orientation changes of the neck angle occur before those of the trunk.

Accelerometric data

An analysis of the canter using three-dimensional accelerometers fixed to the saddle (Galloux *et al.*, 1994) showed higher amplitudes of motion than for the other gaits (walk and trot), especially along the longitudinal and vertical axes. Rotation around the transverse axis (pitching motion) and around the longitudinal axis (rolling) were greater than in the other gaits, while twisting around the vertical axis was lower.

Electromyographic data

EMG activity of trunk and neck muscles was recorded with skin contact electrodes at the canter (Figs 7.15 & 7.16). Recording of neck muscle activity showed that the splenius muscles were active once in the stride cycle, during the trailing diagonal stance phase (Fig. 7.15). These muscles limit neck lowering and cause the neck to extend during the leading forelimb stance phase and the suspension phase. The sternocephalicus muscles had a reciprocal activity and were active from the end of the leading forelimb stance phase to the first part of the trailing hindlimb stance phase (Fig. 7.15). The brachiocephalicus muscle moving the trailing forelimb was mainly active during the stance phase of the leading forelimb. The brachiocephalicus muscle on the side of the leading forelimb was mainly active during the suspension phase. This left to right dissociation is correlated to the asymmetry of the gait

and to the respective chronology of each forelimb protraction.

The longissimus dorsi muscles were active once per stride at the end of the leading forelimb stance phase, during the suspension phase and during the trailing hindlimb stance phase (Figs 7.15 & 7.16). The function of these muscles was to prepare the landing of both hindlimbs and to extend the trunk before forelimb landing. The rectus abdominis muscles had reciprocal activity during the support phase of the non-leading diagonal; they act to support the visceral mass and to initiate thoracolumbar flexion during the leading forelimb stance phase (Fig. 7.17) and the suspension phase. Bursts of activity were observed simultaneously in the longissimus and rectus abdominis muscles on the side opposite to the leading forelimb during the stance phase of the trailing hindlimb.

The obliquus internus abdominis muscle corresponding to the leading forelimb was active during most of the intermediate part of the support phase (Figs 7.15 & 7.16), contributing to visceral support and trunk lateroflexion. The opposite obliquus internus abdominis muscle had a burst of activity at the end of the support phase and beginning of the swing phase.

During the canter, the use of intramuscular wire electrodes has shown that the multifidus lumborum and longissimus lumborum are active during the swing phase of the trailing hindlimb. The rectus abdominis and obliquus externus abdominis have reciprocal activity (Tokuriki *et al.*, 1991).

JUMPING (see also chapter 8)

Based on high-speed cinematography (250 pictures per second), a wonderful description of several types of jumps was performed at the beginning of this century (De Sévy, no date). Several kinematic and accelerometric studies of show jumping horses jumping over fences or over a water jump have analysed the stride characteristics and velocities (Leach *et al.*, 1984; Clayton & Barlow 1991, 1995; Deuel *et al.*, 1991; Barrey & Galloux 1997). A review of these studies is presented in chapter 8. The following data are focused on the movements of the axial regions during jumping and complete a detailed anatomo-functional analysis of the neck and trunk behavior during the different phases of a jump (Denoix, 1988).

Kinematic data (see also chapter 3)

The data presented in this section were obtained from two kinematic studies of the axial regions in the median

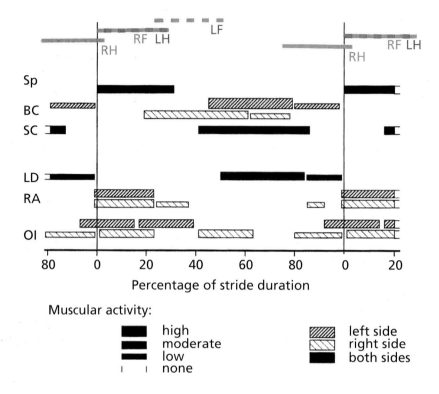

Fig. 7.15   Electromyographic activity of neck and trunk muscles at ridden left lead canter (6 m/s) on hard ground (mean values on three horses). **Limbs:** LF: left forelimb; RF: right forelimb; LH: left hindlimb; RH: right hindlimb. **Muscles:** Sp: splenius; BC: brachiocephalicus; SC: sternocephalicus; LD: longissimus dorsi; RA: rectus abdominis; OI: obliquus internus abdominis. (Courtesy of Céline Robert, Maisons-Alfort, France)

plane during jumping (Thoulon, 1991; van den Bogert *et al.*, 1994).

Study designs

In the first study (Thoulon, 1991), four horses ridden by the same rider were used. They were filmed twice over two different fences (one upright fence, 1.15–1.35 m high, and one oxer, 1.05–1.25 m high, according to the horse's capabilities). Skin markers were placed on the left side of the horse, on the nose, forehead, withers, lumbosacral junction, sacrocaudal junction as well as on the left limb joints and hooves. A high-speed 16 mm film camera was placed at 22 m from the center of the fences, so that the field of view included the take-off area, the jump and the landing. Recordings were made at 300 frames per second, but only every fifth image was used for analysis. Digitization of the coordinates of the markers allowed for calculation of kinematic variables such as orientation of trunk and croup with respect to the horizontal plane (Fig. 7.18), joint angles (e.g. lumbosacral angle), linear velocities and angular velocities.

Another study (van den Bogert *et al.*, 1994) of neck and trunk kinematics was performed in a group of 15 elite show jumping horses during the hindlimb take off before a 1.50 m upright fence. Recordings were performed at 200 frames per second with a high-speed film camera placed about 30 m from the fence. Joint centers and axial reference points were estimated on the images of the moving horse. The same kinematic parameters were analyzed.

Terminology for description of a jump has been presented (Clayton, 1989), with the five main phases (A to E) of a jump being displayed on Fig. 7.19. The same phases are indicated on Figures 7.20 to 7.24. They include:

- phase A: last approach stride before hindlimb take off (Fig. 7.19A)
- phase B: take off: stance phase of the two hindlimbs (Figs 7.19B$_1$ & B$_2$)
- phase C: jump suspension (airborne phase) (Fig. 7.19C)
- phase D: forelimb landing (Fig. 7.19D)
- phase E: after forelimb landing (first departure stride).

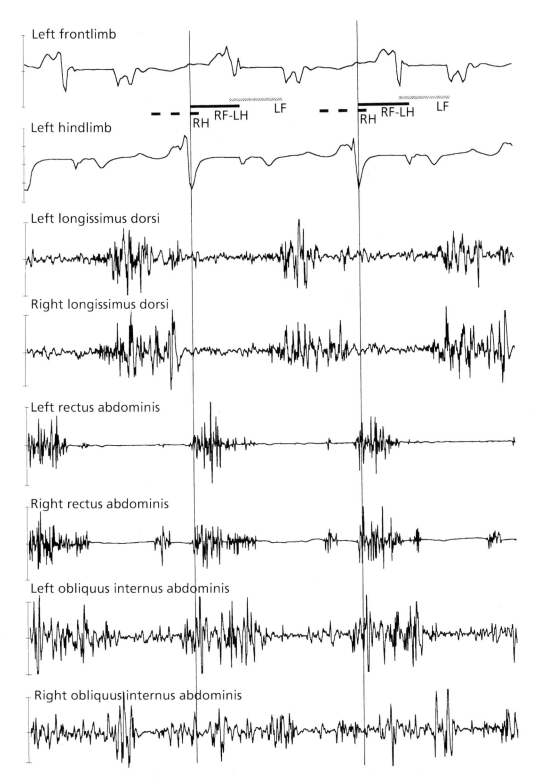

Fig. 7.16 Electromyographic activity of trunk muscles at ridden left lead canter (6 m/s) for three consecutive strides. LF: left forelimb; RF: right forelimb; LH: left hindlimb; RH: right hindlimb.

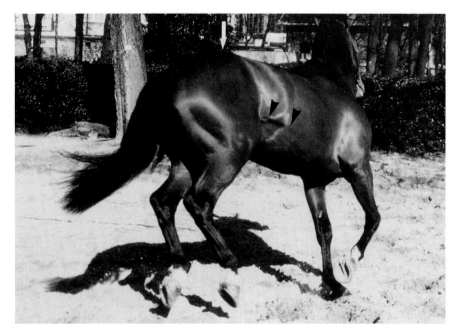

Fig. 7.17 Leading forelimb stance phase during left lead canter while lunging on a circle. See the rectus abdominis contraction (dark arrowheads) inducing lumbosacral flexion (white arrow).

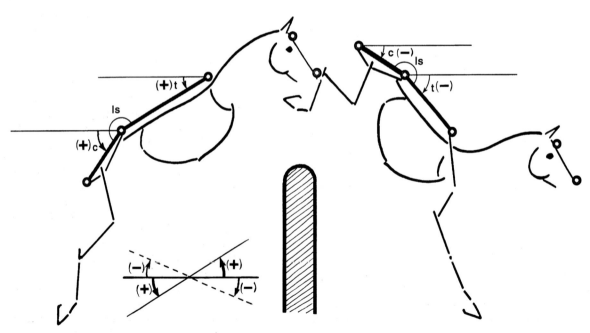

Fig. 7.18 Croup and back orientation during a jump. Five markers were placed (nose, forehead, withers, lumbosacral junction, sacrocaudal junction). Three angles were analyzed: t: trunk angle with respect to the horizontal; c: croup angle with respect to the horizontal; ls: lumbosacral angle. For the trunk and croup orientation, a 0° angle represents the horizontal line; a positive angle (+) indicates an upward angulation; a negative angle (–) indicates a downward angulation. c and t are positive during the ascendent phase and negative during the descendent phase of the jump. For the lumbosacral angle an increasing angle indicates a flexion; a decreasing angle indicates a lumbosacral extension.

Limb positions during take off

During their last stance phase before the jump (phase A) a clear dissociation of the forelimbs was observed (Fig. 7.19A), the mean distance between the two feet was 0.81 m (Thoulon, 1991). Conversely, in both studies, the position of the hindlimbs at take off (phase B) was nearly symmetrical (Fig. 7.19 B_1), the hind feet were placed at a horizontal distance of 1.80 ± 0.29 m (Thoulon, 1991) and 2.14 ± 0.18 m from the fence (van denBogert et al., 1994).

Duration

Although horses and fences were quite different in both studies, the stance phase duration of the hindlimbs (phase B, Figs. 7.19 B_1 & B_2) was similar (mean: 223 ms in the first study and 221 ms in the second). In the first study (Thoulon, 1991) the last stance phase duration of the forelimbs before take off (phase A) was significantly smaller (187 ms); the suspension phase of the forelimbs and hindlimbs during the jump (phase C) was similar (about 670 ms).

Trajectories

As the head is close to the fence during take off and far from it at landing, trajectories of the nose and forehead markers during the jump are very asymmetrical relative to the fence (Fig. 7.20). The hindfeet are placed closer to the fence during take off (1.80 ± 0.29 m) than during landing (3.58 ± 0.52 m) (Thoulon, 1991), so the trajectories of the lumbosacral and sacrocaudal junctions are slightly asymmetrical relative to the fence (Fig. 7.20). Asymmetry of the trajectory of the withers is intermediate between those of the axial extremities and shows a sudden flattening during landing (Fig. 7.20) correlated to the maximal collapse of the forelimb joint angles.

Trunk orientation

The general orientation of the trunk and croup during a jump is presented in Figures 7.19, 7.21 and 7.22. Before the hindlimb take off (phase A) there is a progressive upward rotation of the trunk (Figs 7.19 & 7.22) correlated to the elevation of the withers and a slight lowering of the lumbosacral junction. During the hindlimb take off (phase B), because of the elevation of the withers, the trunk angle progressively increases during the first half of the stance phase (Figs 7.21 & 7.22) without exceeding $40°$ in either study (Thoulon, 1991; van den Bogert et al.,

1994). Then, elevation of the lumbosacral junction, caused by the application of an eccentric impulse of the hindlimbs relative to the center of gravity (Clayton & Barlow 1991) induces a progressive reduction of the trunk angle initiating a downward rotation of the trunk (Fig. 7.22) which continues during the airborne phase. The head and neck regions were shown to have an upward action after forelimb lift off and a forward action during the hindlimb take off (Galloux & Barrey, 1997).

During the airborne phase (phase C), the trunk angle regularly decreases to become null (the trunk is horizontal), half a second after the hindlimbs contact the ground at take off (Fig. 7.22). Then, the trunk rotates downward until the forelimbs contact the ground at landing. Another study (Galloux & Barrey 1997), showed that the speed of angular rotation of the horse over a fence during the airborne phase remained nearly constant ($120 \pm 5°/s$), and that the trunk had the biggest influence on the rotation.

During landing of the forelimbs (phase D), rotation of the trunk is progressively reduced and then inverted (Fig. 7.22). In Thoulon's study (1991) the maximal negative trunk angle was about $30°$. Finally (phase E), the trunk recovers its horizontal orientation after the forelimb stance phase following the jump (Fig. 5.22).

Croup orientation and lumbosacral angle

Despite large quantitative individual variations, the lumbosacral junction progressively flexes (Figs 7.21 & 7.23) before hindlimb landing (phase A); consequently, the upright rotation of the croup (Fig. 7.24) is larger than that of the trunk (Fig. 7.22).

During the hindlimb take off (phase B) the lumbosacral junction extends (Figs 7.21 & 7.23), inducing an inversion of croup rotation (Fig. 7.24) compared with the trunk rotation (Fig. 7.22); this inversion occurs during the first half of the hindlimb take off (Fig. 7.24). During the second half of the hindlimb take off (phase B), downward rotation of the trunk combined with lumbosacral extension induces a reduction of the croup angle (Fig. 7.24).

During the most part of the airborne phase (phase C) the lumbosacral angle remains in full extension (Fig. 7.23), so the croup rotation follows the downward rotation of the trunk.

During the landing phase of the forelimbs (phase D) a progressive lumbosacral flexion, initiated during the last part of the airborne phase, occurs (Figs 7.21 & 7.24). Thus, the croup becomes horizontal before the trunk, which achieves a horizontal position (Fig.

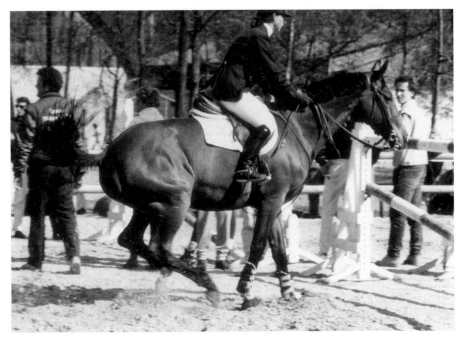

Fig. 7.19A   General presentation of the five main phases of a jump. Phase A: before hindlimb take-off, forelimb stance phase of the last approach stride. Notice the neck extension, the flexion of the lumbosacral angle and the beginning of the upward rotation of the trunk and croup.

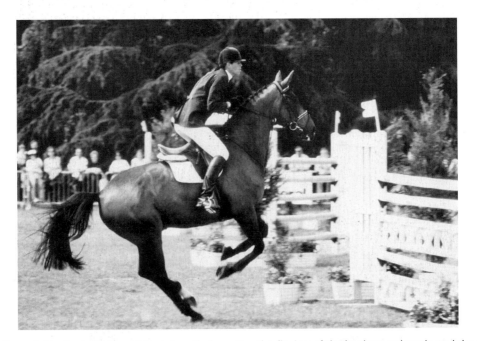

Fig. 7.19B$_1$ Phase B: hindlimb landing of the take-off phase. See the flexion of the lumbosacral angle and the upward rotation of the neck, trunk and croup.

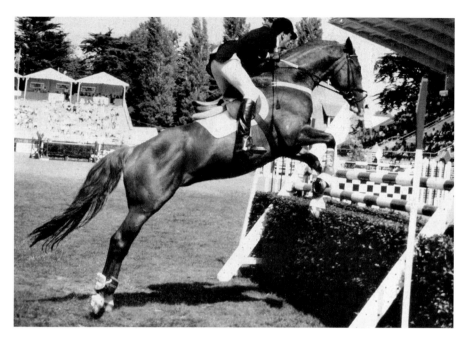

Fig. 7.19B₂ Phase B: end of the hindlimb take-off phase. Notice the extension of the lumbosacral angle, the neck flexion and the beginning of the downward rotation of the trunk and croup.

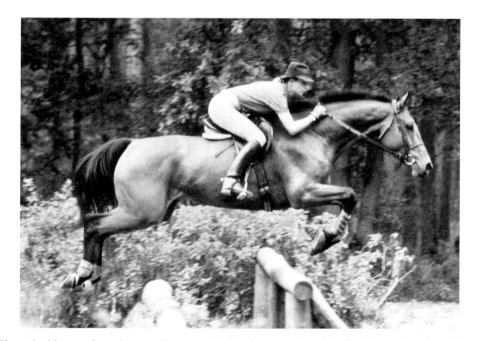

Fig. 7.19C Phase C: airborne phase, intermediate part. Notice the extension of the lumbosacral angle and the horizontalization of the trunk and croup.

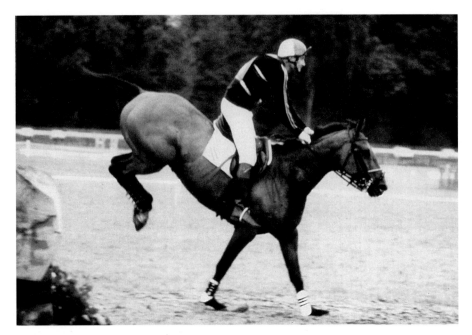

Fig. 7.19D Phase D: forelimb landing. Notice the downward rotation of the trunk, the flexion of the lumbosacral angle and the earlier horizontalization of the croup.

7.22) during the subsequent forelimb swing phase (phase E). During this latter phase, the lumbosacral angle is flexed (Fig. 7.23) and the croup is oblique (Fig. 7.24) to facilitate engagement of the hindlimbs (protraction), which is required to rebalance the horse's gait.

Angle between neck and trunk

Anatomo-functional relationships between the neck and trunk during the different phases of the jump have been analyzed (Denoix, 1988). In the last approach stride before take off, the head and neck are stretched forward and down in preparation for forelimb impulse (Clayton & Barlow 1991). Then, the upward movement of the forehand is initiated by extension of the neck and the forelimb impulse (Denoix, 1988; Clayton & Barlow 1991). During hindlimb take off (van den Bogert *et al.*, 1994) the angle between the neck and trunk flexes, as a result of the neck rotating downward with a nearly constant angular velocity.

Horizontal velocity

In the study performed by Thoulon (1991), the mean average initial horizontal velocity before hindlimb take off (phase A) was about 6 m/s. During the first half of

the hindlimb stance phase (phase B) it was reduced to about 5 m/s and, because of the hindlimb propulsion, it increased in the second part of this phase to reach a mean value of 7 m/s, which was conserved throughout the airborne phase (phase C).

In the study on elite show jumping horses (van den Bogert *et al.*, 1994), horizontal velocity was initially 4.5 m/s; it decreased during the first third of the hindlimb take off to 3.6 m/s and then increased during the last two-thirds to reach 6.5 m/s. This reduction of horizontal velocity in the last approach stride before take off has been mentioned in Grand Prix jumping horses (Clayton & Barlow 1991) and the deceleration was considered to maximize the vertical impulse during take off.

During the forelimb stance phase at landing (phase D), the horizontal velocity decreases from 7 m/s at the beginning of this phase to 6 m/s at the end (Thoulon, 1991).

Electromyographic data

Analysis of the splenius muscle EMG activity during jumping using skin contact surface electrodes was performed in five horses (Giovagnoli *et al.*, 1998). In this study, four phases of splenius muscle activity were observed during a jump:

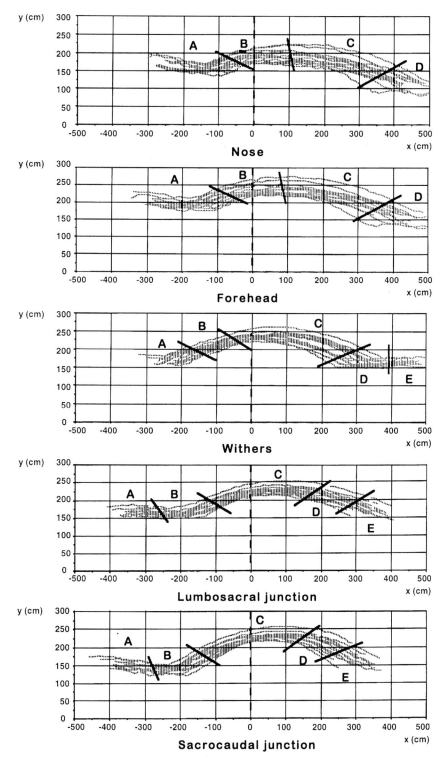

Fig. 7.20 Trajectories of five axial markers (nose, forehead, withers, lumbosacral junction, sacrocaudal junction) during 16 jumps (4 horses × 4 jumps). Phase A: before hindlimb take-off; phase B: hindlimb take off; phase C: airborne phase; phase D: landing on forelimbs; phase E: after forelimb landing; 0: position of the fence. (From Thoulon, F. (1991) Le Saut du cheval: étude cinématographique informatisée. *Veterinary doctorate thesis*, Lyon, with permission)

- before and during forelimb landing of the last stride before the fence (phase A, Fig. 7.19A), while the neck was lowered and the head was in an extended position
- during hindlimb take off and forelimb elevation (phase B, Fig. 7.19B$_1$), accompanying upward rotation of the head and neck
- during the intermediate part of the airborne phase, while the neck was lowered and the head was in extension (phase C, Fig. 7.19C)
- before and during forelimb landing (phase D, Fig. 7.19D), inducing neck extension as well as head and neck antigravitational support.

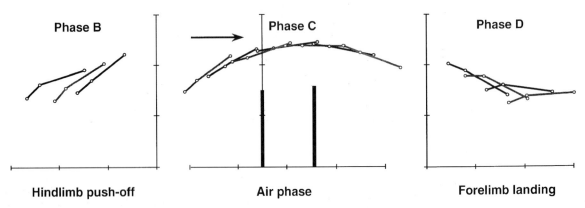

Phase B — Hindlimb push-off

Phase C — Air phase

Phase D — Forelimb landing

Fig. 7.21 Croup and back orientation during a jump. Markers are placed over the withers (6th thoracic spinal process), tuber sacrale and sacrocaudal junction. The straight line between the first two markers represents the trunk orientation; the line between the last two markers represents the croup orientation. Time duration between two positions: 5/60 s = 0.83 s; Phase B: hindlimb take off; phase C: airborne phase; phase D: landing on forelimbs. (From Thoulon, F. (1991) Le sant du cheval: étude cinématographique informatisée. *Veterinary doctorate thesis*, Lyon; with permission)

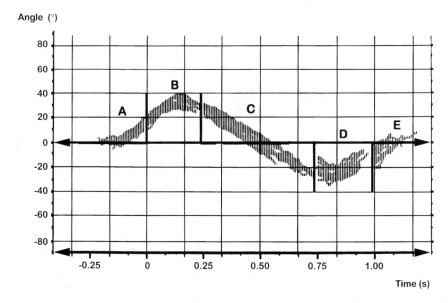

Fig. 7.22 Variations of the trunk angle during jumping; curves obtained from 16 jumps (4 horses × 4 jumps). Phase A: before hindlimb take off; phase B: hindlimb take off; phase C: airborne phase; phase D: landing on forelimbs; phase E: after forelimb landing; to: first contact of hindlimbs during take off. A positive angle indicates an upward angulation; a negative angle indicates a downward angulation. An increasing angle indicates an upward rotation; a decreasing angle indicates a downward rotation. (From Thoulon, F. (1991) Le sant du cheval: étude cinématographique informatisée. *Veterinary doctorate thesis*, Lyon; with permission)

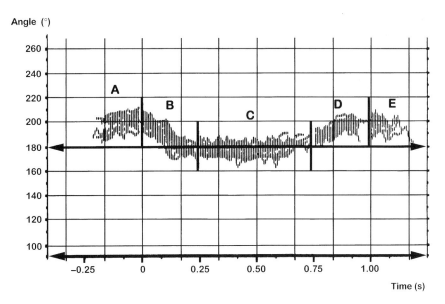

Fig. 7.23 Variations of the lumbosacral angle during jumping; curves obtained from 16 jumps (4 horses × 4 jumps). Phase A: before hindlimb take off; phase B: hindlimb take off; phase C: airborne phase; phase D: landing on forelimbs; phase E: after forelimb landing; t0: first contact of hindlimbs during take-off. An increasing angle indicates lumbosacral flexion; a decreasing angle indicates lumbosacral extension. (From Thoulon, F. (1991) Le sant du cheval: étude cinématographique informatisée. *Veterinary doctorate thesis*, Lyon; with permission)

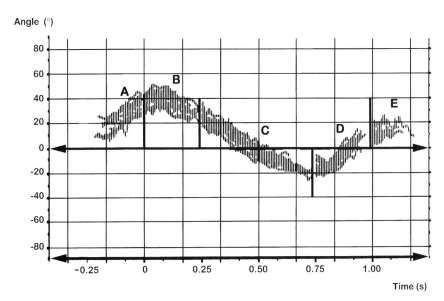

Fig. 7.24 Variations of the croup angle during jumping; curves obtained from 16 jumps (4 horses × 4 jumps). Phase A: before hindlimb take off; phase B: hindlimb take off; phase C: airborne phase; phase D: landing on forelimbs; phase E: after forelimb landing; t0: first contact of hindlimbs during take off. A positive angle indicates an upward angulation; a negative angle indicates a downward angulation. An increasing angle indicates an upward rotation; a decreasing angle indicates a downward rotation. (From Thoulon, F. (1991) Le sant du cheval: étude cinématographique informatisée. *Veterinary doctorate thesis*, Lyon; with permission)

CONCLUSION

Because of their limited mobility and heavy muscles, the axial regions of the horse are probably the most difficult to investigate with biomechanical techniques and diagnostic procedures. Nevertheless, in the recent years a lot of information has been gained on the biomechanics of the neck and back, especially with kinematic analysis and electromyographic studies. However, detailed knowledge of the functional behavior of the different structures of the axial regions is still uncomplete.

Further research is required to understand the pathogenesis of the different pathological conditions of the back as well as to identify the sources of pain in back problems. These data are essential for application of the different methods of physical therapy on equine athletes. Further investigations are needed to establish a rational basis for the training of sport and race horses in order to develop their neck and back athletic capabilities as well as to identify physical exercises helpful for the management of back problems.

ACKNOWLEDGEMENTS

The author would like to thank Patricia Perrot and Benôt Bousseau for the help in the preparation of the manuscript and figures.

REFERENCES

Audigié, F. (1999) Analyse cinématique des troubles locomoteurs de chevaux au trot. *PhD thesis, Université Paris XI - Orsay*, pp. 126–188.

Audigié, F., Pourcelot, P., Degueurce, C. *et al.* (1998) Kinematics of the equine spine: Flexion-extension movements in sound trotting horses. *Proc. 5th Int. Con. Equine Exer. Physiol.* Utsunomiya, p. 64.

Barrey, E. and Galloux, P. (1997) Analysis of the equine jumping technique by accelerometry. *Equine Vet. J.* **23**(Suppl.): 45–49.

Barrey, E., Hermelin, M., Vaudelin, J.L. *et al.* (1994) Utilisation of an accelerometric device in equine gait analysis. *Equine Vet. J.* **17**(Suppl.): 7–12.

Buchner, H.H.F., Savelberg, H.H.H.C., Schamhardt, H.C. *et al.* (1996) Head and trunk movement adaptations in horses with experimentally induced fore- and hindlimb lameness. *Equine Vet. J.* **28**: 71–76.

Cadiot, P.J. and Almy, J. (1924) *Traité de Thérapeutique Chirurgicale des Animaux Domestiques*, tome 2: Affections des Régions et des Organes, ed 3. Paris: Vigot, pp. 630–635.

Clayton, H.M. (1989) Terminology for the description of equine jumping kinematics. *J. Equine Vet. Sci.* **9**: 341–348.

Clayton, H.M. and Barlow, D.A. (1991) Stride characteristics of four Grand Prix jumping horses. *Equine Exerc. Physiol.* **3**: 151–157.

Clayton, H.M. and Townsend H.G.G. (1989a) Kinematic of the cervical spine of the adult horse. *Equine Vet. J.* **21**: 189–192.

Clayton, H.M. and Townsend, H.G.G. (1989b) Cervical spinal kinematics: a comparison between foals and adult horses. *Equine Vet. J.* **21**: 193–195.

Clayton, H.M., Colborne, R.G. and Burns, T.E. (1995) Kinematic analysis of successful and unsuccessful attempts to clear a water jump. *Equine Vet. J.* **18**(Suppl.): 166–169.

Denoix, J.M. (1987) Kinematics of the thoracolumbar spine of the horse during dorsoventral movements: A preliminary report. *Proc. 2nd Int. Conf. Equine Exerc. Physiol.*, San Diego, pp. 607–614.

Denoix, J.M. (1988) Biomécanique et travail physique du cheval L'Eperon. *Information Hippique*. Special Issue: Levallois.

Denoix, J.M. (1998) Diagnosis of the cause of back pain in horses. *Proc. Conf. Equine Sports Med. Sci.*, Cordoba, pp. 97–110.

Denoix, J.M. (1999) Spinal biomechanics and functional anatomy. *Vet. Clin. North Am.: Equine Pract.* **15**: 27–60.

Denoix, J.M and Pailloux, J.P. (1996) Anatomy and basic biomechanical concepts. In: *Physical Therapy and Massage for the Horse*. London: Manson Publishing Ltd, pp. 21–63.

Deuel, N.R. and Park, J.J. (1991) Kinematic analyses of jumping sequences of olympic show jumping horses. *Equine Exerc. Physiol.* **3**: 158–166.

De Sévy, L. (no date) *Le Cavalier sur L'obstacle*. Paris: Le Goupy.

Galloux, P. and Barrey, E. (1997) Components of the total kinetic moment in jumping horses. *Equine Vet. J.* **23**(Suppl.): 41–44.

Galloux, P., Richard, N., Dronka, T. *et al.* (1994) Analysis of equine gait using three-dimensional accelerometers fixed on the saddle. *Equine Vet. J.* **17**(Suppl.): 44–47.

Giovagnoli, C., Pieramati, G., Castellano, G. *et al.* (1998) Analysis of neck muscle (splenius) activity during jumping by surface video-electromyography technique. *Proc. Conf. Equine Sports Med. Sci.*, Cordoba, pp. 57–60.

Jeffcott, L.B. (1975) The diagnosis of diseases of the horse's back. *Equine Vet. J.* **7**: 69–78.

Jeffcott, L.B. (1980) Disorders of the thoracolumbar spine of the horse. A survey of 443 cases. *Equine Vet. J.* **12**: 197–209.

Jeffcott, L.B. (1998) Back problems in horses – their diagnosis and treatment. *Post Universitair Onderwijs (Academic dissertation), Universiteit Gent.*

Jeffcott, L.B., Dalin, G. (1980) Natural rigidity of the horse's backbone. *Equine Vet. J.* **12**: 101–108.

Jeffcott, L.B., Dalin, G., Drevemo, S. *et al.* (1982) Effect of induced back pain on gait and performance of trotting horses. *Equine Vet. J.* **14**: 129–133.

Leach, D.H., Ormrod, K. and Clayton, H.M. (1984) Stride characteristics of horses competing in Grand Prix jumping. *Am. J. Vet. Res.* **45**: 888–892.

Licka, T. and Peham, C. (1998) An objective method for evaluating the flexibility of the back of standing horses. *Equine Vet. J.* **30**: 412–415.

Pourcelot, P. (1999) Développement d'un système d'analyse cinématique 3-D. Application à l'étude de la symétrie locomotrice du cheval au trot. *PhD thesis, Université Paris XII - Val de Marne.*

Pourcelot, P., Audigié, F., Degueurce, C. *et al.* (1998) Kinematics of the equine back: a method to study the thoracolumbar flexion–extension movements at the trot. *Vet. Res.* **29**: 519–525.

Robert, C., Valette, J.P. and Denoix, J.M. (1998) Surface electromyographic analysis of the normal horse locomotion: A preliminary report. *Proc. Conf. Equine Sports Med. Science*, Cordoba, pp. 80–85.

Rooney, J.M. (1982) The horse's back: Biomechanics of lameness. *Equine Pract.* **4**: 17–27.

Thoulon, F. (1991) Le saut du cheval: étude cinématographique informatisée. *Veterinary doctorate thesis, Lyon.*

Tokuriki, M. and Aoki, O. (1991) Neck muscles activity in horses during locomotion with and without a rider. *Equine Exerc. Physiol.* **3**: 146–150.

Tokuriki, M., Nakada, A. and Aoki, O. (1991) Electromyographic activity of trunk muscles in the horse during locomotion and synaptic connections of neurons of trunk muscles in the cat. *Proc. First (ESB) Workshop Anim. Locom.,* Utrecht.

Tokuriki, M., Otsuki, R., Kai, M. *et al.* (1997) Electromyographic activity of trunk muscles during locomotion on a treadmill *(5th WEVA Congr. Abstracts: Padova). J. Equine Vet. Sci.* **17**: 488.

Townsend, H.G.G., Leach, D.H. and Fretz, P.B. (1983) Kinematics of the equine thoracolumbar spine. *Equine Vet. J.* **15**: 117–122.

Uhlir, C., Licka, T., Kübber, P. *et al.* (1997) Compensatory movements of horses with a stance phase lameness. *Equine Vet. J.* **23**(Suppl.): 102–105.

van den Bogert, A.J., Jansen, M.O. and Deuel, N.R. (1994) Kinematics of the hind limb push-off in elite show horses. *'Animal Locomotion': Equine Vet. J.* **17**(Suppl.): 80–86.

Vorstenbosch, M.A.T., Buchner, H.H.F., Savelberg, H.H.C.M. *et al.* (1997) Modeling study of compensatory head movements in lame horses. *Am. J. Vet. Res.* **58**: 713–718.

8
Performance in Equestrian Sports

Hilary M. Clayton

INTRODUCTION

Horses compete is a diverse range of sports that require many different athletic talents. For sprinting sports the prime requirements are rapid acceleration and the ability to generate a high maximum speed. Middle distance racing and endurance racing call for stamina to maintain submaximal speed over a longer distance. Other sports depend on different degrees of technical skills, visual acuity, fast reflexes or esthetics of movement. This chapter will consider the mechanical factors involved in equine athletic performance and will review the literature describing the technical aspects of different equestrian sports.

BIOMECHANICAL FACTORS INVOLVED IN EQUESTRIAN SPORTS

Speed

Speed is the determining factor in racing, and the ability to perform at high speed is a desirable characteristic in many sports. Horses change speed by altering the spatial and temporal relationships between the limbs to produce different gaits and to vary the extension within a gait. Each gait has an optimal speed at which the metabolic cost is minimized; slower and faster speeds both result in a higher metabolic cost. It has been suggested that the stimulus to changing gait is related to the energetic cost (Hoyt & Taylor, 1981) or that the forces on the limbs are the triggering factor (Farley & Taylor, 1991). Whatever the reason, horses naturally select particular speeds at which to make transitions between gaits.

Within any gait, speed is the product of stride length and stride frequency:

$$\text{Speed} = \text{stride length} \times \text{stride frequency}$$

In general, stride length shows a fairly linear increase with speed, whereas stride frequency increases more slowly and in a nonlinear manner (Dušek *et al.*, 1970; Leach & Cymbaluk, 1986). In sprinting races, a high stride frequency is the prime requirement; the ability to take longer strides becomes increasingly important as the distance of the race increases (Deuel & Park, 1990).

Stride length

Stride length increases with effective limb length. The forelimbs are generally considered to rotate around a point close to the tuber spinae scapulae, though the precise point of rotation may vary between individuals. The hindlimbs rotate around the hip joint in the symmetrical gaits (walk, trot, pace) and around the lumbosacral joint in the asymmetrical gaits (canter, gallop). The effective limb length is longer when the hindlimb rotates around the lumbosacral joint than the hip joint, and this is one of the reasons why the gallop is a faster racing gait than the trot or pace. In the symmetrical gaits lateral flexion of the vertebral column may enhance stride length, whereas in the asymmetrical gaits dorsoventral flexion and extension can make a significant contribution (Hildebrand, 1962). In horses the thoracolumbar region of the vertebral column is fairly rigid, which provides support for the large body mass and facilitates transmission of propulsive forces from the hindlimbs. Consequently, vertebral flexion and extension make a relatively small contribution to stride length in horses. This is in contrast to species that have a more flexible thoracolumbar region, such as cats. For more information on vertebral kinematics, the reader is referred to the chapter on neck and back movements (chapter 7).

Stride frequency

Stride frequency describes the rate at which the limbs are protracted and retracted. The ability to cycle the limbs rapidly is favored by having a high percentage of fast twitch fibers in the extrinsic muscles, which influences both the rapidity with which the limbs are protracted and retracted and the ability to generate large forces and impulses during the stance phase. In Standardbreds trotting at high speeds, stride length is positively correlated with the percentages of type I and type IIa muscle fibers, and negatively correlated with the percentage of type IIb muscle fibers. Stride frequency has a positive correlation with the percentage of type IIa muscle fibers (Persson *et al.*, 1991). Another study found a negative correlation between stance duration and the percentage of type IIb muscle fibers (Roneus *et al.*, 1995). A shorter stance duration is probably indicative of a better ability to generate high ground reaction forces (GRFs) and so create the necessary impulse over a shorter period of time. It has also been shown that stance duration is negatively correlated with the diameter of the muscle fibers (Rivero & Clayton, 1996).

Efficiency of movement

During locomotion energy is used to move the horse's center of mass and to cycle the limbs back and forth. For sprint races, energy expenditure is relatively unimportant, but as the distance increases beyond the capacity of the anaerobic energy production systems, energetic efficiency becomes an important determinant in the ability to maintain submaximal speed over a distance. Factors that contribute to making locomotion economical include the weights and inertial properties of the individual segments, limb kinematics, storage and release of elastic strain energy and inter-segmental transfers of kinetic energy (Cavagna *et al.*, 1977).

The weights of the limb segments as a percentage of body weight and the distribution of the mass within the segment determines its inertial properties. In horses the heavy muscular tissue is confined to the proximal limb, while the distal limb is composed of skin, connective tissue, ligament, tendon and bone, which are relatively light in weight. This proximal distribution of the weight facilitates protraction and retraction and greatly reduces the energetic expenditure.

Cycling the limbs back and forth is one of the main sources of energy expenditure during locomotion and several mechanisms are employed to reduce the energy used in protraction and retraction. The limb is folded as it is protracted, which brings the distal limb closer to the pivot point, thereby reducing its inertia, The amount of joint flexion and limb folding tend to increase with

speed. Storage and release of elastic strain energy greatly reduces the amount of metabolic energy that is used during locomotion in horses. In the first half of the stance phase, the elastic elements in the ligaments and tendons of the fore and hindlimbs are stretched, thereby storing elastic energy. As the body mass rolls over the limb, the elastic tissues recoil, releasing the stored elastic energy, which assists in raising the limb and flexing the joints. During the stance phase of the trot the fetlock, carpal, elbow and shoulder joints show elastic behavior due to the actions of the soft tissues that cross these joints (Clayton *et al.*, 1998). However, the elastic contribution is much smaller in the walk (Clayton *et al.*, 2000).

When a new motor skill is learned, the initial attempts are clumsy and inefficient. After a period of practice, efficiency in performing motor tasks improves. In human athletes, muscular activation patterns are modified by practice; champion athletes have a specific temporal and sequential order of muscle activation in the execution of their specific skill (Normand *et al.*, 1982). Sustained practice establishes an advanced level of muscular control and economy of effort. With regard to muscular control, codification that develops as a result of practice is attributed to reorganization within the CNS of the motor program required to execute the specific task. These modifications are manifest as inhibition of undesired activity in the antagonistic muscles, contributing to lower overall tension and greater economy of effort. This is an important training consideration, especially in high-intensity sports that combine speed with technical skills, such as polo, cutting and eventing.

For more information, the reader is referred to the chapters on the initiation and coordination of gait (chapters 2 and 4).

Stability and maneuverability

The properties of stability and maneuverability are at somewhat opposite ends of the spectrum. Stability is enhanced by lowering the center of mass and positioning it centrally within the horse's base of support to provide a more balanced position. Maneuverability, on the other hand, is enhanced when the center of mass lies close to the perimeter of the base of support, so that it is easily displaced outside the base of support.

An example of a sport that requires stability is roping, in which the horse must remain balanced while resisting the movement of a roped calf. Cutting demonstrates the need for maneuverability during rapid acceleration, deceleration and turning. Many sports require a combination of these properties. For example, polo requires rapid changes of direction and the ability to turn on a dime, yet the horses must also be sufficiently well-balanced to hold their line during a ride off when there is aggressive physical contact between horses. Event horses are faced with challenging obstacles on the cross country course that call for a combination of athleticism and good balance while jumping on a slope or turning between fences.

Coordination

Limb timing and coordination patterns affect many aspects of performance including locomotor efficiency, quickness of movement and esthetics. Certain basic patterns of limb coordination, which are governed by central pattern generators, give rise to the recognizable gaits. However, individual horses vary slightly in the synchronization of their limb movements, and this has a marked effect on the esthetics and energetics of sporting performance.

Reaction time

Reaction time is defined as the time that elapses between an external stimulus and the initial response to that stimulus. It is extremely important in all sports that require fast movements and quick reflexes. This includes equestrian sports like cutting and polo that have an offensive–defensive component and jumping sports (show jumping, eventing, steeplechasing) in which the horse must perceive a visual impression of a fence and respond appropriately within a short space of time.

Reaction time in response to an external stimulus is determined by the sum of the pre-motor time and the motor time. Pre-motor time is dependent on the speed of processing in the central nervous system and speed of conduction along the nerve to the motor end plate. Motor time reflects the speed of muscle contraction. In human beings, the reaction time of athletes is substantially faster than the reaction time of non-athletes (Kroll & Clarkson, 1977). Because nerve conduction velocities do not appear to differ between athletes and non-athletes (Bodine-Rees & Bone, 1976), it has been suggested that the faster reaction time of athletes may be attributed to the superior functioning of the central nervous system. Furthermore, the total reaction time is significantly correlated with pre-motor time but not with motor time (Viitsalo & Komi, 1981). In equine athletes Clayton (1989b) found that the reaction time of cutting horses in response to a visual stimulus ranged from 110 to 370 ms, with elite horses having shorter reaction times than those that were less successful in competition.

GAIT QUALITY

In warmblood sport horses the stride kinematics associated a subjective assessment of 'good' movement have been studied (Back *et al.*, 1994a; Holmström *et al.*, 1994). The characteristics described in the following section are for the trot, which is the gait used most extensively to assess gait quality. The most consistent finding is that horses rated as 'good movers' achieve a particular trotting speed using a long stride length and a slow stride frequency (Back *et al.*, 1994a; Holmström *et al.*, 1994). This type of movement, especially when it is associated with a prolonged swing phase, presents an impressive picture to the judge. Good movers tend to show more retraction in the forelimbs and more protraction in the hindlimbs. Other desirable gait qualities include a wide range of motion in the scapula, which is correlated with stride length, greater flexion of the tarsal joint and a large extension of the fetlock joints during the stance phase, which is correlated with the apparent suppleness of the movement (Back *et al.*, 1994a).

Although the trot is described as a two-beat gait in which the diagonal limb pairs make contact and lift off simultaneously, slow motion analysis has shown that there is usually a period of dissociation with either the fore or hind hoof making ground contact and lift off earlier. The time between contacts of the diagonal limbs is called the diagonal advanced placement and the time between lift offs is called diagonal advanced completion. Positive values are assigned if the hindlimb acts in advance of the forelimb, and negative values are assigned if the forelimb acts in advance of the hindlimb. A positive diagonal advanced placement is associated with good movement and a well-balanced horse (Holmström *et al.*, 1994). In horses that show a positive diagonal advanced placement, the magnitude of the dissociation tends to increase with training due to greater elevation of the forehand as the degree of collection and self-carriage improve (Clayton, unpublished).

Much of the expressiveness of the trot is judged from the limb movements during the swing phase. At the position of maximal protraction of the forelimb, good movers show a more elevated position of the carpus, with greater flexion of the elbow and carpal joints than horses classified as poor movers (Holmström *et al.*, 1994). This type of movement is indicative of the horse controlling the forward swing of the limb rather than relying on inertial forces and anatomical constraints to determine the joint position of maximal protraction. With regard to conformation, a sloping shoulder facilitates the forward and upward movement of the limb during the swing phase, so conformation of the shoulder may play a role in gait quality (Holmström *et al.*, 1990). After the limb reaches its maximally protracted position, it is retracted before making ground contact. This period, which is known as the swing phase retraction, has a longer duration in the forelimbs for horses with high trot scores (22% of stride duration) than for those with low scores (10% of stride duration).

A

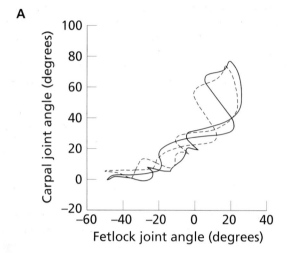

B

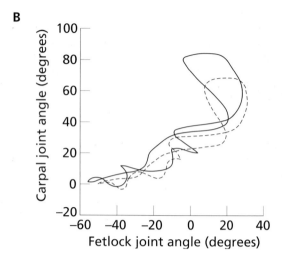

Fig. 8.1 Angle–angle diagrams for the carpal and fetlock joints of three horses (**A, B, C**) trotting on a treadmill at 4 m/s at the ages of 4 months (------) and 26 months (——). (Reprinted from Back *et al.*, 1994b, ©EVJ Ltd.)

C

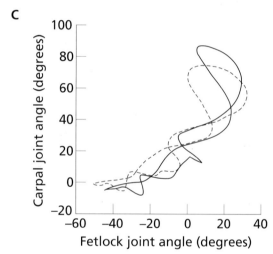

Characteristics of hindlimb motion that are associated with good movement include having a large amount of flexion of the hock and stifle joints during the swing phase, which is correlated with suppleness of movement (Back *et al.*, 1994a). In addition, the hindlimb should make ground contact in a position that is well forward beneath the horse's trunk segment. The hind hoof has a more forward placement relative to the tuber coxae in good movers, as a result of the combined actions of the joints of the hindlimb (Holmström *et al.*, 1994). During the stance phase, high scoring horses show more inclination of the pelvis and more flexion of the hock and extension of the fetlock joints as the limb bears weight. This is associated with a significantly larger angular velocity at the hock between 20 and 55% stance (negative value) and between 75 and 85% stance (positive value). During the later part of the stance phase, the limb is retracted faster in good movers (Holmström & Drevemo, 1997).

The fore hoof trajectory reaches a height of 20–25 cm during mid swing in horses with a high gait score. In horses with lower gait scores, the hoof is not raised as high and it peaks earlier in the stance phase. In the hindlimb, the maximal hoof height occurs soon after lift-off and does not differ with gait quality (Holmström *et al.*, 1994).

Development of gait

With regard to selection of horses, it is important to know what age the adult gait characteristics are acquired. Evaluation of trotting warmblood foals at a range of ages between 4 and 26 months indicated that stride and stance duration increase with age as a consequence of the increase in limb length (and overall height). However, swing duration, protraction and retraction angles, and the joint angular kinematics were consistent throughout this age range (Back *et al.*, 1994b). Within an individual animal, angle–time and angle–angle graphs for the joints of the fore- and hindlimbs were remarkably similar both visually and numerically from 4 months to 26 months (Fig. 8.1). Each animal appeared to have an inherent and characteristic intra-limb pattern that was retained from foal to adulthood, the 'gait fingerprint.'

Effect of training

The kinematic changes associated with the initial training period were studied in a group of two-and-a-half-year-old Dutch warmbloods (Back *et al.*, 1995). Treadmill evaluations were performed at the trot before and after 70 days training under saddle or 70 days in pasture. The trained horses showed a reduction in hindlimb stance duration, which probably reflected an increase in strength allowing the necessary impulse to be generated during a shorter period of time. The hindlimbs showed less flexion and were maximally protracted earlier in the stride, and in the forelimbs the range of protraction and retraction decreased. Overall, the trained horses moved with greater impulse and showed a change in their balance in response to the demands of the rider that was reflected in the limb kinematics. The untrained horses, on the other hand, continued to trot in a more relaxed manner with a longer stride duration and a lower stride frequency.

Over a prolonged period of dressage training, horses learn to move with collection and self carriage. During trotting, for example, the hindlimbs provide more of the forward propulsive force as self carriage develops. At the same time, the forelimbs show a reduced propulsive force and an increased braking force. Consequently, the trained horse does not roll over the forelimbs; instead the forelimbs act to elevate the forehand and provide upward motion.

Effect of a rider

The presence of a rider affects both the kinematics and the ground reaction forces, with the changes being more pronounced in the forelimbs (Schamhardt *et al.*, 1991; Clayton *et al.*, 1999). Comparing horses trotting at the same speed in hand and with a rider, the peak vertical ground reaction force normalized to the mass of the system (horse or horse plus rider) is lower in both the forelimbs and the hindlimbs when horses are ridden. In

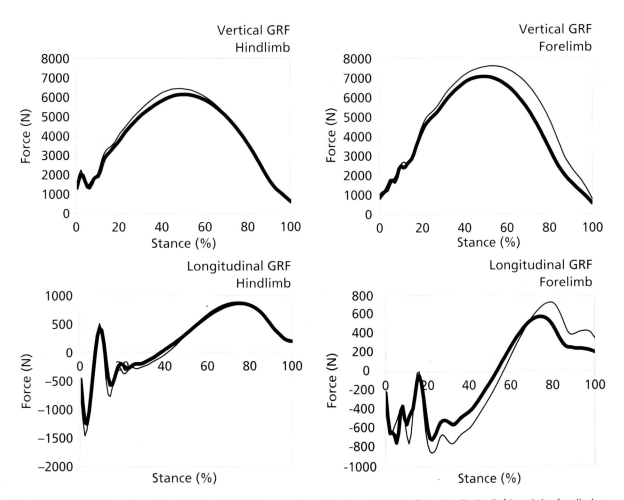

Fig. 8.2 Vertical (above) and longitudinal (below) ground reaction forces (GRFs) of the hindlimbs (left) and the forelimbs (right) for horses trotting at the same speed in hand (——) and with a rider (——).

the forelimbs the mass normalized propulsive force is higher in the terminal part of the stance phase in ridden horses (Fig. 8.2), and the fetlock joint is more extended between 50 and 70% stance. During walking, the effect of an experienced rider was almost identical to that of a sandbag of equal mass. During trotting, the posting motion of the rider gave rise to a left–right asymmetry in the ground reaction forces. However, the riders were able to shift part of the weight towards the hindlimbs (Schamhardt *et al.*, 1991).

A study performed by Schills *et al.* (1993) measured body segment angles and joint angles for riders of different levels of ability (beginning, intermediate, advanced) from a variety of equestrian disciplines (dressage, eventing, hunt seat, saddle seat, endurance, reining, western pleasure). Advanced riders positioned their trunk segment closer to the vertical, oriented the thigh and lower leg so they lay more underneath the body, and carried their upper arm further ahead of the trunk (Fig. 8.3). One of the consequences of this combination of actions was a more open angle at the hip joint.

GAIT ANALYSIS IN EQUESTRIAN SPORTS

Racing

Racing encompasses a broad spectrum of sports that occur over distances from as short as 200 m to greater than 160 km. The common denominator in all these sports is that the winner covers the set distance in the shortest time.

Quarter Horse racing

The Quarter Horse is the elite equine sprinter and was named from its ability to sprint over a distance of a quarter mile. The most important qualities of a sprinter are rapid acceleration and a high maximal speed. In sprinters, speed is more strongly influenced by stride frequency than stride length (Deuel & Lawrence, 1986). This is in contrast to galloping Thoroughbreds in which speed is altered primarily by changes in stride length (Ratzlaff *et al.*, 1985). Comparing Quarter Horses and Thoroughbreds galloping at 15 m/s, the stride length of the Quarter Horses is shorter by about 1.0–2.0 m (Deuel & Lawrence, 1986), with a correspondingly higher stride frequency. Values for the stride variables of 2-year-old Quarter Horse fillies galloping at a mean speed of 13.3 m/s are shown in Table 8.1.

Stride variables

There is no significant covariance between stride frequency and stride length in galloping Quarter Horses, so these variables are regarded as independent factors within the time domain and space domain (Deuel & Lawrence, 1986). As speed increases, stride frequency is increased by shortening the single support periods of the trailing hindlimb and leading forelimb, and the duration of the suspension. Linear regression analysis of the data predicts that at 14.9 m/s, overlap between the leading hindlimb and trailing forelimb approaches zero. Interestingly, at approximately this speed, two of four horses in the study showed strides with an extended suspension (i.e. a period of suspension between lift-off of the leading hindlimb and ground contact of the trailing

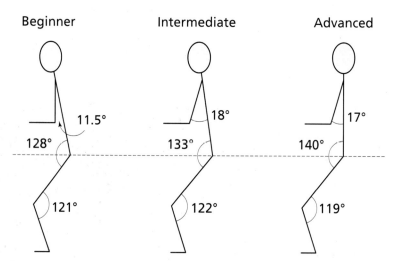

Fig. 8.3 Stick figures showing the angles of the arm, hip joint and knee joint of the beginner, intermediate and advanced riders at the sitting trot. (Reprinted from Schills *et al.*, 1993, ©Elsevier Science.)

forelimb) of 4.0 to 8.0 ms duration (Deuel & Lawrence, 1986). At a constant stride frequency, stride length is adjusted by increasing the distances between the trailing and leading forelimbs and between the leading forelimb and the trailing hindlimb. In Quarter Horse foals there is a significant correlation between stride length and mass (Leach & Cymbaluk, 1986). Small foals prefer to change speed by adjusting stride length, whereas foals with larger dimensions prefer to adjust their stride frequency.

Sidedness

Two-year-old Quarter Horse fillies show a leading limb preference; approximately twice as many strides were recorded on the right lead versus the left lead in spite of the horses being cued for the left and right leads an equal number of times. The horses either picked up the right lead during the transition or changed from the left to the right lead (Deuel & Lawrence, 1987a). Both speed and stride length were significantly longer on the left lead than the right lead, but stride frequency did not differ between the two leads. The trailing forelimb had a longer stance duration and a shorter period of overlap with the leading forelimb on the left lead, which was interpreted as a sign of an increased reliance on the right forelimb for support. The hindlimbs, however, did not show any linear or temporal asymmetries between the left and right leads.

Effect of urging

The effect of urging by the rider was studied by having the rider use a whip on the shoulder of the leading forelimb in rhythm with the stride. Use of the whip did not change the speed, but the horses maintained their speed with a reduced stride length and a higher stride frequency during urging. Also, the stance duration of the forelimbs was reduced (Deuel & Lawrence, 1987b).

Thoroughbred racing

Thoroughbreds race over short to middle distances. Most of the races are over distances in the range of one to two miles, though shorter and longer races do exist. Over the shorter distances, the requirements for acceleration and speed are similar to those for Quarter Horse racing, but as the distance increases stamina assumes more importance. In this breed high maximal speeds are achieved primarily as a result of having a long stride length (Leach *et al.*, 1987). Top class Thoroughbreds galloping at racing speed have had their stride lengths measured at 7.38 m for Secretariat and 6.66 m for Riva Ridge (Pratt & O'Connor, 1976). However, individual horses vary in terms of their preference to increase stride length or stride frequency as they approach top speed. In general, for Thoroughbreds galloping at sub-maximal speeds, stride length tends to show a decreased rate of increase whereas stride frequency tends to show an increased rate of increase (Yamanobe *et al.*, 1992). Stride lengths and stride frequencies for Thoroughbreds galloping at a range of speeds (Ishii *et al.*, 1989) are shown in Table 8.1

Stride variables

A study of part-Thoroughbred horses galloping on a variety of surfaces (sand, turf, woodchips, dirt) showed a linear relationship between stride length and speed, with stride length increasing from about 3.5 m at 6 m/s to around 7.5 m at 19 m/s. At the same time, stride duration decreased from 580 ms at 6 m/s to 440 ms at 19 m/s. The reduction in stride frequency was achieved through a large reduction in the swing phase from 200 ms to 100 ms, and a smaller reduction in the stance phase from 400 ms to 350 ms (Hellander *et al.*, 1983).

Stride length at the gallop comprises the sum of four inter-limb distances: the hind step, the diagonal step, the fore step and the suspension distance (Fig. 8.4). Alterations in stride length are associated with greater changes in the diagonal distance and the suspension distance than in the hind and fore steps (Ishii *et al.*, 1989). The suspension distance shows the greatest increase at moderate speeds but has a tendency to level off as maximal speed is approached, whereas the diagonal step tends to show an increasing rate of increase at higher speeds. Lengthening of the diagonal step is a consequence of an increased propulsive force from the hindlimbs. This may be associated with a higher forelimb braking force which, in turn, limits the suspension distance (Yamanobe *et al.*, 1992).

The temporal variables for the gallop stride include periods of single support when one limb only is in the stance phase, periods of overlap when two or more limbs are in the stance phase simultaneously and a suspension

Table 8.1 Mean values for stride variables of galloping Quarter Horses (QH) and Thoroughbreds (TB). Data for Quarter Horses are from Deuel and Lawrence (1986) and data for Thoroughbreds are from Ishii *et al.* (1989).

Speed (m/s)	Stride length (m)	Stride frequency (strides/s)	Breed
13.3	5.06	2.62	QH
6.6	3.63	1.82	TB
9.9	4.89	2.02	TB
13.8	6.18	2.23	TB
15.8	6.66	2.37	TB

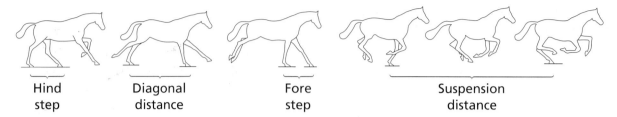

| Hind step | Diagonal distance | Fore step | Suspension distance |

Fig. 8.4 Inter-limb distances in the gallop. The sum of the inter-limb distances is the stride length.

phase when the horse is airborne. Duration of the suspension phase is highly correlated with stride duration. For Thoroughbreds galloping at 15 m/s, the suspension phase occupies 28% of stride duration (Leach *et al.*, 1987).

The stance phase durations of the four limbs differ significantly from each other, with the leading hindlimb and trailing forelimb having shorter stance durations than the contralateral limbs. Overlap is longest between the two hindlimbs, shortest between the two forelimbs, and of intermediate duration between the leading hind-trailing forelimb pair. As galloping speed increases there is a marked reduction in all the overlap durations, with overlap between the leading hind and trailing forelimbs decreasing linearly down to about 50 ms (Hellander *et al.*, 1983). Comparison between the extended canter of horses trained for dressage with horses trained for racing reveals that, at the same speed, there is no difference in stride length or stride frequency, but the racehorses had significantly shorter stance durations and overlap times (Clayton, 1993), which may be a consequence of race training. Following 8 weeks of high-intensity training on a treadmill, the stance duration of galloping Thoroughbreds was reduced by 8–20% (Corley & Goodship, 1994). These changes can be ascribed to greater muscular strength; the ability to generate higher ground reaction forces allows the necessary impulses to be created during a shorter stance phase, and the greater forces project the horse into a prolonged suspension phase. Race training also results in increases in stride duration and stride length (Leach *et al.*, 1987).

The advanced placements (time between footfalls) change in such a manner that, at faster galloping speeds, the hindlimbs act more in unison with each other while becoming more dissociated from the forelimbs. Thus the rhythm becomes more like a rabbit hop. As the advanced placement between the leading hind and the trailing forelimbs increases, the distance between placements of these limbs also increases. Dissociation of the actions of the hindlimbs and forelimbs causes a greater reliance on spinal flexion and extension. Thoroughbreds traveling at speeds greater than 13.5 m/s may show a short

extended suspension between lift off of the leading hindlimb and contact of the trailing forelimb. A third suspension, between lift off of the trailing forelimb and contact of the leading forelimb, has also been recorded occasionally. The percentage of Thoroughbreds showing multiple suspension phases increases with speed from 27% of horses at 15.5 m/s, to 50% at 17.0 m/s, and 70% at 19.5 m/s. The duration of these suspension phases also tends to increase with speed (Seder & Vickery, 1993).

Head and neck motion

The head and neck, which comprise approximately 10% of body weight, move in synchrony with the limbs. The neck is actively extended and lowered during the hindlimb stance phases with the head reaching its lowest point during the propulsive phase of the leading hindlimb (Bramble, 1984). This movement may counteract the tendency of the forequarters to rise as a result of the hindlimb propulsion (Pratt, 1983). Elevation of the head and neck begins as the trailing forelimb contacts the ground, continues through the forelimb stance phases and peaks at lift off of the leading forelimb.

Lead changes

Horses normally use a transverse gallop in which the leading limb is on the same side of the body for the fore and hind limb pairs. A lead change involves a reversal in the order of placement of the contralateral limb pairs, and Thoroughbreds normally change leads several times during a race. The most common strategy is to use the inside lead through the turns, and the opposite lead in the straightaways. Racehorses usually initiate the lead change with the forelimbs. During the forelimb swing phase the leading forelimb abbreviates the anterior part of its swing phase and is placed early to become the new trailing forelimb. The limb that was the trailing forelimb increases its swing phase duration substantially to become the new leading forelimb. The hindlimbs then change their lead in a similar manner during their next swing phase. For one stride (the stride in which the forelimb lead is changed) the sequence of limb placements follows a rotary sequence. Sometimes the hindlimb lead is not changed until several strides later, in which case the rotary sequence of limb placements is maintained during the intervening strides; this is also known as being disunited or on a crossed lead.

Acceleration

During acceleration, the initial increase in speed is due to a rapid increase in stride frequency accompanied by a relatively slow increase in stride length (Hiraga *et al.*, 1994). Stride frequency peaks within a few strides after leaving the starting gate, whereas stride length requires 25–30 strides to reach its maximal value. The diagonal distance increases relatively rapidly to reach maximal length within the first few strides. The airborne distance increases linearly after the first few strides until the 20th stride. The forelimb step length and the hindlimb step length tend to level off after the 20th stride. Hind step length is very short in the initial strides during which the horses use a half bound before establishing a leading limb for the hindlimb pair. The majority of horses use a rotary sequence of limb placements (crossed lead) during the initial acceleration before establishing the normal transverse sequence (Kai & Kubo, 1993; Hiraga *et al.*, 1994). Horses tend to hold their breath for 3–4 s immediately after leaving the starting gate after which they settle into a breathing rhythm that is synchronized with the stride cycle. The breath-holding follows inspiration (Kai & Kubo, 1993).

Ground reaction forces

The vertical ground reaction forces have been studied at racing speed in horses galloping round an 0.8 km track with well-banked turns and wearing instrumented shoes on all four feet (Ratzlaff *et al.*, 1987). On the straightaway the greatest vertical force was exerted by the leading forelimb, followed by the leading hindlimb, trailing hindlimb and trailing forelimb. On the banked turns, the greatest force was exerted on the leading forelimb, followed by the trailing forelimb, leading hindlimb and trailing hindlimb (Fig. 8.5). It is not surprising, therefore, that the majority of racing injuries occur in the leading limbs, especially the leading forelimb.

Fatigue

When racing Thoroughbreds become fatigued there is a decrement in performance shown by reductions in stride frequency and running speed. Stride length may increase or decrease depending on the horse. The absolute duration of both the stance and suspension phases of the stride increases, with suspension occupying a greater percentage of stride duration. Footfall of the leading hind is followed more closely by that of the trail-

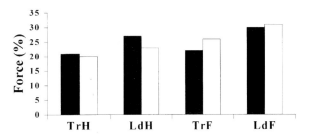

Fig. 8.5 Vertical ground reaction forces of Thoroughbreds galloping on a straightaway (dark shading) and through a turn (light shading). Forces are expressed as a percentage of the total force exerted on the four feet. TrH: trailing hindlimb; LdH: leading hindlimb; TrF: trailing forelimb; LdF: leading forelimb. (Data from Ratzlaff *et al.*, 1987.)

ing forelimb, and overlap between these two limbs increases during fatigue (Leach & Springings, 1979). Since the stride and respiratory cycles are synchronized in galloping horses, it has been suggested that the changes in limb coordination associated with fatigue may be related to the respiratory demands. By increasing the suspension phase, the duration of the inspiratory phase of the respiratory cycle is increased, which may be advantageous as the horse becomes fatigued (Leach & Springings, 1979).

Injury

Analysis of racetrack patrol videos (Ueda *et al.*, 1993) has shown that breakdown injuries often occur immediately after a lead change (47% cases), use of the whip (38% cases) or an oblique movement of the horse across the track (21% cases).

Training

An important consideration in Thoroughbred training is the need to stimulate skeletal adaptation without causing injury to the bones and joints. It has been suggested that the training regime should incorporate short sprints on a relatively frequent basis (every 3–6 days) to stimulate bone adaptation, especially with regard to the prevention of bucked shins (Moyer & Fisher, 1991). However, the distance of the sprints must be limited because horses that accumulate extensive distances at high speeds are more likely to suffer a fatal skeletal injury (Estberg *et al.*, 1995). Many complete fractures of the long bones are preceded by incomplete fractures (Stover *et al.*, 1992); indicating that they are a consequence of repeated limb trauma during training and racing.

Track surface

The material properties of the track surface affect both performance and lameness. On a harder surface there is a reduction in stride duration, whereas on a more compliant surface stride duration increases (Fredricson et al., 1983). This offers at least a partial explanation for the fact that faster race times are recorded on firmer track surfaces. However, there is a price to pay in terms of soundness. The incidence of lameness in Thoroughbreds that are in race training increases with the hardness of the track surface (Cheney et al., 1973). One of the factors that affects hardness is the composition and depth of the cushion. Hardness is reduced as the cushion gets deeper, but if the cushion depth is too deep (greater than 10 cm), the footing becomes insecure.

Standardbred racing

Racing Standardbreds are divided into two groups according to the gait they perform during racing. The tendency to trot, in which the diagonally opposite limb pairs move together, or to pace, in which the lateral pair of limbs move together, appears to be genetically determined. The offspring of pacers almost always pace, whereas about 20% of the offspring of trotters are pacers (Cothran et al., 1987).

Trotters

Stride variables

A good trotter should have a high maximal speed with a stride frequency in excess of 2.4 strides/s and a stride length greater than 5.45 m. It has been suggested that trotters achieve a high racing speed by selecting an optimal stride length then accelerating to the wire by increasing their stride frequency (Barrey et al., 1995).

Different studies vary in their findings regarding the relationship between speed, stride length and stride frequency. Barrey et al. (1995) found that both stride length and stride frequency increase linearly with speed, whereas Drevemo et al. (1980a) found speed to be moderately correlated with stride length but not correlated with stride duration. The latter study also found a close correlation between stride duration and swing duration. Swing time, which occupied about 75% stride, had much more effect on overall stride duration than stance time, which occupied only about 25% of stride. The treadmill study of Weeren et al. (1993) also found that stride length contributes more than stride frequency to an increase in speed, with the swing duration remaining constant at all speeds.

The temporal and linear stride variables of 30 Standardbreds trotting on a racetrack were studied using a camera car driven parallel to the horse as a pacemaker (Drevemo et al., 1980a). With the pacemaker car moving at 12 m/s, the actual speed of the individual strides varied

Table 8.2 Mean values for stride variables of Standardbred trotters and pacers. Data for trotters moving at 12.0 m/s are from Drevemo et al. (1980a,b) and at 14.2 m/s are from Barrey et al. (1995). Data for pacers are from Wilson et al. (1988b).

Speed (m/s)–gait	Stride length (m)	Stride duration (ms)	Suspension (ms)
12.0–trot	5.45	455.0	99.0
14.2–trot	5.65	396.8	N/A
11.5–pace	5.57	485.0	148.6
12.0–pace	5.57	465.9	141.2
13.1–pace	6.04	460.0	135.3
14.0–pace	6.28	448.4*	133.4

* In the original paper the stride duration is given as 499.4 ms, and the stride frequency is 2.23 strides/s. Apparently, the value for the stride duration is a typographical error.

from 11.3 to 12.4 m/s. The values of the stride variables are shown in Table 8.2. There was very little intra-individual variation (Drevemo et al., 1980b; Kobluk et al., 1989), indicating that each horse has a stable locomotion pattern that is repeated regularly with only minor deviations. The variation between individuals was two to three times greater than that within horses. Depending on the variable being studied, the coefficients of variation were of the order of 8–12%, though the variability within horses was about 60% less than that between horses.

Good trotters show a short stance phase duration, especially in the forelimbs (Bayer, 1973). The stance phase has been subdivided at the instant when the metacarpus is vertical in the forelimbs or when the hoof is vertically beneath the hip joint in the hindlimbs (Drevemo et al., 1980a). The early part was named the restraint phase and the later part was named the propulsion phase. Although the names suggest that these terms define functional phases of the stride, it should be noted that they are defined kinematically and so the implied functional relationship to the longitudinal ground reaction forces is an approximation only. The restraint phase accounts for the initial 40–45% stance, and is slightly longer in the hindlimbs than in the forelimbs. The propulsive phase is significantly longer in the right hind than in the other limbs, which has been interpreted as an indication of sidedness. The duration of the forelimb propulsive phase is negatively correlated with speed.

Diagonal dissociation is a term that encompasses the dissociation of the diagonal pair at contact with the ground (diagonal advanced placement) and at lift-off (diagonal advanced completion). Dissociation of the movements of the diagonal pair of limbs results in a short period of single support between the periods of bipedal support and periods of suspension. Duration of the diagonal dissociation is significantly longer at lift-off than at contact, with the forelimb acting in advance of the hindlimb both at contact and lift-off in the majority of horses. For a given diagonal, the duration of the dissociation at contact and lift-off are highly correlated. When the forelimb precedes the hindlimb, diagonal advanced placement is inversely correlated with the distance between the diagonal limb pair during bipedal support (diagonal length). When the hindlimb precedes the forelimb, the diagonal advanced placement is directly correlated with the diagonal distance (Drevemo et al., 1980b). About 25% of trotters showed highly significant differences between the left and right diagonal dissociations.

The mean duration of diagonal limb support at a speed of 12 m/s was 99 ms, with highly significant differences between the left and right diagonals in 4 out of 30 horses. Diagonal length, which is the distance between the diagonal limb pair during their stance phase, had a high coefficient of variation on the right diagonal, and the values for the left and right diagonals differed significantly in 5 out of 30 horses. The mean duration of the suspension phase was 99 ms, with 66% of the horses showing no significant difference between the left and right sides. The left and right suspensions were strongly correlated with the length and duration of the left and right hind steps, respectively. There was also a moderate correlation between suspension and stride duration (Drevemo et al., 1980b).

For Standardbreds trotting on a treadmill, the swing phase trajectories of the fore hooves are quite different from those of the hind hooves. The fore hooves are lifted higher but show less lateral deviation than the hind hooves in which the limbs swing wide to avoid interference. The hoof movements as seen in the frontal plane seem to be characteristic of the individual animal (Weeren et al., 1993).

Reproducibility of gait

The kinematic stride variables of trotting Standardbreds show good reproducibility in the short term during both overground (Drevemo et al., 1980c) and treadmill (Weeren et al., 1993) locomotion. A 5-month training period did not result in any significant changes in temporal parameters, but other aspects of the stride kinematics did change. In the forelimb there was more flexion of the elbow, more overextension of the carpus and a decrease in fetlock flexion after training. In the hindlimb there was an increase in overextension of the fetlock (Weeren et al., 1993). A longer training period of 3 years was associated with significant increases in stride length, stride duration and swing duration. The increase in stride duration resulted almost exclusively from the longer swing duration (Drevemo et al., 1980c).

Ground reaction forces

The peak vertical ground reaction force of a Standardbred trotting at a relatively slow speed of 8 m/s was 99% body weight and occurred around 50% stance. The braking longitudinal force had a maximal value of 6.4% body weight at 15% stance, while the propulsive component peaked at 75% stance with a value of 9.2% body weight. The forelimb longitudinal force changed from braking to propulsive at 40% stance (Quddus et al., 1978).

Sidedness

By definition the trot is a symmetrical gait, which implies that the movements of the left and right limbs are out of phase by 50%, with the left and right steps being equally spaced in time. In the 30 horses studied by Drevemo et al. (1980b), the kinematic variables for the entire group were symmetrical on the left and right sides. However, many individuals showed left–right asymmetries when trotting at high speeds, especially in the hindlimbs. Six of 30 horses had significant asymmetries between the fore steps, while 12 of 30 horses had significant asymmetries between the hind steps (Drevemo et al., 1980b). Some individuals had such marked asymmetries that, rather than trotting, they showed a transitional type of gait with a galloping motion of the hindlimbs. The asymmetries detected at racing speed by slow motion analysis are often not apparent during a clinical examination when the horse trots at a slower speed. Detection is important, though, because an asymmetrical gait is thought to be associated with poor performance (Dalin et al., 1985) and the development of locomotor pathology (Rooney, 1969).

Even 8-month-old Standardbreds that have not yet been trained show some differences between the kinematics of the left and right limbs (Drevemo et al., 1987). The fact that asymmetries are present at such a young age is strong evidence for congenital laterality or sidedness. Furthermore, when the same horses were re-evaluated at 18 months of age the differences between the left and right sides were even more pronounced in horses that had been trained, but not in those that were not trained in the interim.

An asymmetric appearance of the hindquarters has been associated with poor racing performance (Dalin et al., 1985). Five hundred Standardbreds in race training were evaluated for symmetry in the height of their tubera sacrale. The left tuber sacrale was lower than the right one in 9 horses, and the right tuber sacrale was lower than the left one in 30 horses. The asymmetric horses had significantly larger body size than the 461 horses that did not show asymmetry. The asymmetric horses had lower total earnings, a lower number of races per horse and less good racing records. It was concluded that horses in which the height of the tubera sacrale is asymmetrical are less likely to become successful racehorses.

Effect of track design

Lameness is a common problem in racing horses, and gait asymmetries that arise due to defects in the geometrical design of the racetrack were identified as a predisposing factor. Dalin *et al.* (1973) showed that when horses trot on a track with under-banked semi-circular turns the gait becomes asymmetrical at high speeds with the horses changing to a galloping motion in the hindlimbs. To overcome the tendency to slip sideways on the turns, the horse leans into the turns and places the feet sideways, using friction against the track surface to overcome the centrifugal force. The left limbs are adducted and placed on the ground closer to the horse's midline, which is associated with a lateral landing of the left hooves and medial deviation of the fetlock throughout the stance phase. Thermographic evaluation revealed that, after the horses performed at speed around inadequately banked turns, the left fore fetlock became warmer than the right one.

The traditional racetrack design of two straights joined by under-banked semi-circular turns is obviously not optimal for either performance or soundness of the horses. Fredricson *et al.* (1975) made suggestions for improving the geometric design of racetracks. They recommended the use of wide sweeping turns to reduce the horse's tendency to slide outwards and to facilitate adequate banking; on tighter turns the amount of banking required is so great that the surface material cannot be stabilized. Only the inner half of the track needs to be banked sufficiently for maximal speed; the middle and outer lanes can be less steeply banked to accommodate moderate and slow speed training. It has also been observed that gait asymmetries are most prevalent as the horse enters and leaves the turns. Therefore, the intercalation of a transitional curve between the true curve and the straight is highly recommended (Fredricson *et al.*, 1975).

Conformation of trotters

A study relating conformation to performance in Standardbred trotters (Magnusson, 1985) showed that traits associated with superior racing performance included height at the withers and large girth circumference around the point of the withers, which was indicative of prominent withers and a large area for attachment of the locomotor muscles. In contrast, girth circumference at the lowest point of the back had a negative correlation with performance. Outward rotation of the limb axes, which is typically regarded as a conforma-

tional fault, had a positive effect on racing ability. Conformational features that had a negative influence on performance included tied in at the knees and hocks, narrow hooves and greater width/circumference of the forelimbs. Overall it was concluded that the better performing horse was a lightweight, gracile type with tall withers, with open angles at the shoulder and stifle joints and normal-sized hooves.

Pacers

Stride variables

The pace is a symmetrical gait in which the lateral pair of limbs move more or less synchronously. Slow motion studies have shown that ground contact of the hind hoof precedes that of the front hoof (Crawford & Leach, 1984; Wilson *et al.*, 1988a), unlike the racing trot in which the front hoof usually precedes the hind hoof. At racing speed the dissociation is about 30 ms, which represents 7% of stride duration. With this amount of dissociation, the pace can be considered a four-beat gait.

The stride lengths and stride durations of Standardbreds pacing at a range of speeds between 11.5 and 14.0 m/s are shown in Table 8.2. Pacing speed increases primarily as a result of an increase in stride length with minimal change in stride frequency (Wilson *et al.*, 1988b). Lengthening of the stride is a result of covering a greater distance during the suspension phases, without much change in the distance between the lateral pair of limbs during their stance phases. Although the overall stride rate does not show much change with speed, overlap time is reduced and single support time is increased as a consequence of having longer diagonal advanced placements and diagonal advanced completions. These changes in timing create a distinctly four-beat gait. Perhaps horses that have higher stride frequencies do not have sufficient muscular strength to generate the large impulses needed to lengthen the strides during the short ground contact times that are associated with higher speeds. The best discriminators between speeds were stride length and overlap time, while the variables that limited pacing speed were stride rate and suspension time (Wilson *et al.*, 1988b).

At the end of a race, a pacer is moving at a speed close to 15 m/s. When horses with different levels of ability were classified according to their finishing placing, low-order finishers were found to have shorter distances between the lateral pair of limbs during their stance phase, whereas high-order finishers had a greater range of motion in the fore and hindlimbs. Comparing the last lap of a race with the preceding lap, speed and stride length were reduced during the last lap for low-order finishers but increased for high-order finishers. At the end of a race, an increase in the amount of overlap expressed as a percentage of the stride was a sign of fatigue.

Sidedness

Although the pace is generally described as a symmetrical gait, many pacers show temporal asymmetries between the left and right sides. Gait variables that show left–right asymmetries include stance duration, suspension, overlap, diagonal dissociation and single support (Crawford & Leach, 1984).

Conformation

Preliminary kinematic data of 2-year-old pacing fillies suggest that a long sloping scapula, substantial development of the brachiocephalicus, a long forearm and an elastic fetlock joint are associated with ergonomic efficiency (Sellett *et al.*, 1981).

Endurance racing

The primary requirement for an endurance horse is economy of movement, but the stride variables that contribute to energetic economy have not yet been evaluated. During a race an endurance horse takes many thousands of strides. Horses that maximize transfers of angular momentum between limb segments reduce their mechanical energy expenditure and so use less metabolic energy to cover a given distance.

Stride length has been shown to increase during the course of an 82 km endurance ride. Compared with prerace values, stride length at the walk increased to 115% at 41 km and 123% after 82 km. The length of the trot stride increased to 151% at 41 km and 149%

after 82 km compared with pre-race values (Lewczuk & Pfeffer, 1998). It was suggested that the increase in stride length was due to warming up during the course of the race.

Dressage

Since dressage competitions are judged subjectively, the esthetic quality of the gaits and the expressiveness of the movements are important factors in establishing the scores achieved in competition. The qualities of rhythm and relaxation are important at all levels of training and as the horse progresses to the more advanced levels, the amount of collection and self carriage must be developed to a higher degree. Collection describes a manner of moving in which the strides become shorter and more elevated, the cycle of hindlimb movement is well forward under the horse's body, and the vertebral column is rounded while the forehand is relatively elevated. Horses that are able to carry themselves in this manner are said to move in self carriage. As the horse becomes more collected, the range of pendular motion of the hindlimb is reduced (Holmström & Drevemo, 1997).

The Gaits

The gaits performed in competition are the walk, trot, canter, rein back, passage and piaffe. The walk, trot and canter each have several variations that differ in speed of progression. From slowest to fastest these are the collected, working, medium and extended gaits. Horses are supposed to maintain the same stride frequency (tempo) during the transitions between these gait types. In other words, they should change stride length independent of stride frequency.

The walk

The walk is a four-beat gait with a lateral footfall sequence: RH, RF, LH, LF. The footfalls should be evenly spaced in time, giving a regular, four-beat rhythm. The limb support sequences alternate between bipedal and tripedal supports (Fig. 8.6). The bipedal supports always consist of a forelimb and a hindlimb, which may be a diagonal or a lateral pair. The tripedal supports may be two hindlimbs and one forelimb or two forelimbs and one hindlimb.

The Fédération Equestre Internationale (FEI) recognizes four types of walk: collected, medium, extended and free. (There is no working walk.) The free walk, in which the horse is allowed freedom to stretch the neck, is only performed in lower levels of competition. The speed, tempo and stride length of the collected, medium and extended walks have been measured and compared

Summary

In racehorses, success is defined by the ability to maintain the highest average speed over the distance of the race. In sprinters, generation of high stride rates is of prime importance. Stride length assumes greater importance for horses racing over middle distances. Economy of movement and energy efficiency are prime considerations in endurance racing competitors. Research studies have focused on the trotting Standardbred for which considerable data are available describing stride kinematics and locomotor asymmetries. Studies have also been performed in pacing Standardbreds, Quarter Horses and Thoroughbreds. However, the sport of endurance racing has not been studied to any great extent.

Table 8.3 Mean values for stride kinematics for the collected, medium and extended walks in dressage horses. Data are from Clayton (1995, ©EVJ Ltd). Different superscripts indicate values that differ significantly, $p < 0.05$.

	Collected walk	Medium walk	Extended walk
Speed (m/s)	1.4[a]	1.7[b]	1.8[b]
Stride length (m)	1.57[a]	1.87[b]	1.93[b]
Stride frequency (strides/min)	52[a]	55[a,b]	56[b]
Lateral distance (cm)	158[a]	167[a]	166[a]
Tracking distance (cm)	-7[a]	19[b]	27[b]

(Table 8.3) in a group of national level FEI horses (Clayton, 1995).

Speed of the medium and extended walks is significantly faster than that of the collected walk. Compared with the collected walk, stride length is 23% longer and stride frequency is 8% longer in the extended walk, which agrees with Dušek et al. (1970) who found that increases in speed at all gaits up to a moderate gallop are caused mainly by increasing stride length. However, dressage horses did not fulfil the FEI requirement that the same stride frequency be maintained at all types of walk.

For dressage horses competing in the Seoul Olympics, the mean speed of the extended walk was 1.88 m/s, the stride length was 1.95 m and the stride duration was 1.03 s (Deuel & Park, 1990). These values are similar to the speed of 1.82 m/s achieved with a stride length of 1.93 m and a stride duration of 1.06 s reported by Clayton (1995) in horses of slightly lower caliber. On average, bipedal contact accounted for 61% of stride duration and tripedal contact for 39% of stride duration in the Olympic competitors (Deuel & Park, 1990).

Stride length in the walk can be considered as the sum of the lateral distance (distance between the hind hoof and the next placement of the ipsilateral fore hoof) plus the tracking distance (distance between the fore hoof and the next placement of the ipsilateral hind hoof). Changes in stride length at the walk are almost entirely due to adjustments in tracking distance (Table 8.3). Lengthening of the stride is accompanied by a wider arc of limb rotation during the stance phase. The angle between the cannon bone and the ground is more acute at ground contact and more obtuse at lift-off in the extended walk than in the collected walk, without any change in the carpal or tarsal angle at impact or at lift-off (Clayton, 1995).

Although dressage horses are required to maintain a regular, four-beat rhythm in the walk, only a minority of

horses achieve this (Clayton, 1995). When the rhythm becomes irregular, the horses show either lateral couplets (lateral or pacing rhythm), in which there is a shorter time between the lateral footfalls, or they show diagonal couplets (diagonal rhythm), in which there is a shorter time between the diagonal footfalls (Fig. 8.6). Clayton (1995) found that a majority of national level dressage horses showed lateral couplets, with the same footfall pattern being present in all types of walk. The average step durations measured for dressage finalists competing in the Seoul Olympics indicate that they moved with diagonal couplets (Deuel & Park, 1990).

In highly trained dressage horses, both the collected and extended walk strides have a longer stance duration in the hindlimbs than in the forelimbs (Clayton, 1995; Hodson et al., 1999), which is probably related to the fact that highly trained horses move in self carriage, which implies lightness of the forehand and a greater reliance on the hindlimbs for propulsion.

Half pirouette at the walk

The half pirouette in collected walk is a half circle in which the forelimbs move around the hindquarters. The inside hindlimb acts as a pivot point for the movement, but it continues to step in the rhythm of the walk strides.

In a study at the Atlanta Olympics (Hodson et al., 1999), the majority (8/11) horses completed the half pirouette in three strides; the remaining horses used four strides. This is consistent with the FEI rules, which stipulate three to four strides in a half pirouette. None of the horses maintained a regular four-beat rhythm in the walk pirouette. Instead, the footfall of the inside hindlimb occurred relatively early in the stride. Consequently, the time between footfalls of the outside fore and inside hind hooves was short, while the time between footfalls of the inside hind and inside fore hooves was long (Fig. 8.6). This indicates that, to compensate for the lack of forward movement, the horses become more reliant on the inside hindlimb to maintain their balance.

The trot

The trot is a two-beat gait in which the diagonal pairs of limbs move more or less synchronously, and the footfalls of the diagonal limb pairs are evenly spaced in time. The diagonal support phases are usually separated by periods of suspension, except in a very slow (jog) trot. Therefore, each stride has two diagonal support phases and two suspensions.

Slow motion analysis has shown a slight dissociation between ground contact and lift-off of the diagonal fore and hindlimbs. The interval between the fore and hind contacts is known as the diagonal advanced placement.

REGULAR

RHYTHM: **RH ------ RF ------ LH ------ LF ------ RH**

LATERAL

COUPLETS: **RH ---- RF -------- LH ---- LF -------- RH**

DIAGONAL

COUPLETS: **RH -------- RF ---- LH -------- LF ---- RH**

LEFT WALK

PIROUETTE: **RH ------ RF --- LH --------- LF ------ RH**

Time ⟶

Fig. 8.6 Temporal characteristics of a regular walk, a walk with lateral couplets, a walk with diagonal couplets and a half pirouette in walk.

The value is positive if the hindlimb contacts the ground before the forelimb, zero if the diagonal pair contact the ground simultaneously and negative if the hindlimb contacts the ground after the forelimb. Positive diagonal advanced placement (Fig. 8.7) is considered a desirable characteristic that is indicative of good balance (Holmström et al., 1995). It occurs in horses that travel with an elevated forehand, which is a characteristic of collection. However, a negative diagonal advanced placement does not preclude a horse from being successful in dressage. In the Seoul Olympics, 15% of the extended trot strides that were analyzed had a negative diagonal advanced placement (Deuel & Park, 1990).

Four types of trot are performed in competition: collected, working, medium and extended. Table 8.4 shows that speed and stride length differ significantly between each type of trot, and stride frequency is significantly slower in collected than extended trot (Clayton, 1994a). Deuel and Park (1990) have shown a positive relationship between speed and stride length and a negative relationship between speed and stride duration in a group of top level competitors. Interestingly, dressage horses that qualified for the individual medal finals in the Seoul Olympics tended to have higher speeds, longer stride lengths and higher stride frequencies in the extended trot than horses that failed to qualify (Deuel & Park, 1990).

Stride length at the trot depends on the diagonal distance (distance between the diagonal pair of limbs during their stance phase) and the tracking distance (distance between the fore hoof and the next contact of the ipsilateral hind hoof). Diagonal distance shows a

non-significant increase of 4.0 to 5.0 cm between working and medium trot, which is probably a consequence of the lengthening of the horse's frame. However, most of the lengthening of the stride is a result of greater over-tracking (46.0 cm increase from collected to extended trot), which represents the distance covered during the suspension. The best way to increase the over-tracking and, therefore, stride length is to prolong the suspension. This is achieved by pushing off with a higher vertical velocity. Suspension in the medium and extended trots is twice as long as that of the collected and working trots (Clayton, 1994a).

In the highest scoring dressage horses in the Seoul Olympics the speed of the extended trot was strongly influenced by stride length but not closely related to stride duration (Deuel & Park, 1990). This indicates greater reliance on changes in stride length rather than stride frequency in the elite dressage horses.

The speed of the extended trot (4.93 m/s) in the national level competitors recorded by Clayton (1994a) is similar to the speed recorded in Olympic competitors (4.98 m/s) by Deuel and Park (1990). However the Olympic competitors achieved this speed using a longer stride length (3.79 m versus 3.55 m) and a longer stride duration (0.763 s versus 0.722 s). This indicates that horses of a slightly lower caliber achieve the speed required in the extended trot using shorter, faster strides.

The stance durations of the forelimbs and hindlimbs do not differ from each other in any type of trot (Clayton, 1994a), but both the fore and hind stance durations are significantly shorter in the extended

Table 8.4 Mean values for stride kinematics of the collected, working, medium and extended trots in FEI level dressage horses. Data are from Clayton (1994a, © EVJ Ltd). Different superscripts indicate values that differ significantly, $p < 0.05$.

	Collected trot	Working trot	Medium trot	Extended trot
Speed (m/s)	3.20[a]	3.61[b]	4.47[c]	4.93[d]
Stride length (m)	2.50[a]	2.73[b]	3.26[c]	3.55[d]
Stride frequency (strides/min)	77[a]	79[a,b]	82[a,b]	83[b]
Diagonal distance (cm)	132[a]	132[a,b]	136[a,b]	137[b]
Tracking distance (cm)	7[a]	4[b]	27[c]	39[d]
Suspension (ms)	16[a]	17[a]	32[b]	37[b]

trot than in the collected trot. The angles of the cannon segment to the horizontal are significantly more acute at hoof contact and more obtuse at lift-off in the extended trot than in the collected trot (Clayton, 1994a). The hind cannon consistently has a more acute angle to the ground on its plantar side than the fore cannon throughout the stance phase. The difference ranges from about 10° at hoof contact to 20° at lift-off.

The passage

Like the trot, in passage and piaffe the diagonal limb pairs move more or less in synchrony. However, stride length and speed are significantly reduced from collected trot to passage and from passage to piaffe (Table 8.5). The stride frequency of passage and piaffe are the same as each other but significantly slower than that of collected trot (Clayton, 1997a).

Passage shows many similarities to the trot. It has two, well-defined suspensions in every stride, and a large positive diagonal advanced placement. The diagonal advanced placement tends to be even longer in the more successful competitors. During the swing phase the limbs are markedly elevated, and held momentarily in their most elevated position before being lowered to the ground (Fig 8.8). According to the FEI rules (Anon,

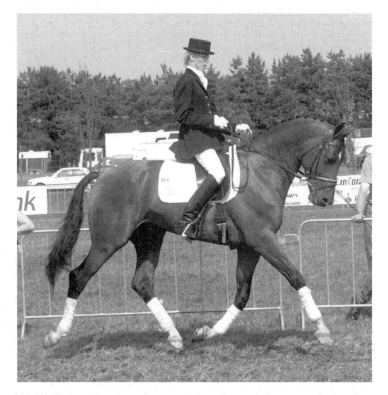

Fig. 8.7 Photograph of 'Cocktail Time' showing a large positive advanced placement during the trot (photo by Jacob Melissen, NL).

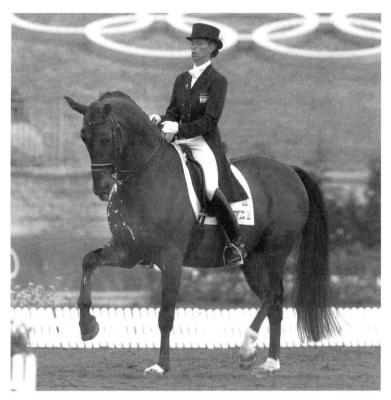

Fig. 8.8 Photograph of 'Bonfire' with gold medallist Anky van Grunsven performing the passage at the Olympic games, Sydney 2000 (photo by Jacob Melissen, NL).

1991) the toe of the fore hoof should be elevated to the middle of the contralateral cannon and the toe of the hind hoof should be raised slightly above the contralateral fetlock joint. None of the horses competing in the individual medal finals at the Barcelona Olympics achieved this amount of elevation in the forelimbs in passage (Argue, 1994).

The ground reaction forces in passage resemble those of the collected trot (Clayton, unpublished data). The forelimbs have a higher peak vertical force than the hindlimbs. The longitudinal GRF is almost entirely retarding in the forelimbs, and almost entirely propulsive in the hindlimbs. The forelimbs have the effect of elevating the forehand, while the hindlimbs provide forward and upward propulsion (Fig. 8.9).

The piaffe

Piaffe (or piaffer) is performed almost in place, so the stride length is very short (Table 8.5). The horses maintain their balance in the absence of forward movement by increasing the durations of the stance phases and the overlaps. There is always at least one hoof in contact with the ground, so piaffe has no suspension (airborne) phase. Therefore, piaffe is a stepping gait,

rather than a leaping gait, with a gradual transfer of body weight from one diagonal to the other. However, the amount of overlap between successive diagonal stance phases is shorter in the better-quality piaffe (Clayton, 1997a). As in passage, the limbs pause momentarily at their most elevated position in the swing phase (Fig 8.10). Each horse performs somewhat differently with its own individual coordination pattern and, although the mean value of the diagonal advanced

Table 8.5 Mean values for stride kinematics of the collected trot, passage and piaffe in dressage horses competing in the individual medal finals at the Barcelona Olympics. Data are from Clayton (1997a, EVJ Ltd). Different superscripts indicate values that differ significantly, $p < 0.05$.

	Collected trot	Passage	Piaffe
Speed (m/s)	3.3[a]	1.6[b]	0.2[c]
Stride length (m)	2.50[a]	1.75[b]	0.20[c]
Stride frequency (strides/min)	71[a]	55[b]	55[b]

placement for piaffe in a group of horses was negative (Argue, 1994; Holmström *et al.*, 1994), the best competitive horses have a positive diagonal advanced placement (Clayton, 1997a).

A unique feature of piaffe is the GRF profiles (Clayton, unpublished data). The vertical GRF has a small peak amplitude compared with the other diagonal gaits and the trace has a rather flattened profile during the long stance phase (Fig. 8.9). The longitudinal force is almost entirely propulsive in the forelimbs and almost entirely retarding in the hindlimbs (Fig. 8.9), which is the opposite of passage and collected trot.

The canter

The canter is the only asymmetrical gait of dressage horses. It has a transverse sequence of limb placements, so the leading fore and hindlimbs are on the same side of the body. Four types of canter are performed in dressage competitions: collected, working medium, and extended, which have significantly different speeds (Clayton, 1994b). The stride frequency is the same for the different types of canter, so changes in speed are accomplished by alterations in stride length (Table 8.6). Stride length increases as a result of a small increase in the distance between the two hindlimbs, a small increase in the distance between the two forelimbs, and a large increase in the distance covered during the suspension. The ability to generate a high vertical velocity at the start of the suspension allows the horse to stay airborne longer and to cover a greater distance during the suspension.

For horses competing in the individual medal final at the Seoul Olympic Games, the speed of the extended canter (7.03 m/s) was considerably faster than that recorded in slightly lower-caliber national level competitors (5.97 m/s). The difference was primarily a result of a longer stride length (4.15 m versus 3.47 m), which was combined with a slightly slower stride frequency (101 strides/min versus 105 strides/min) in the Olympic competitors. Higher overall competition scores have been recorded for horses with faster speeds and longer stride lengths in the extended canter. No upper limit was detected for optimal stride length (Deuel & Park, 1990). Higher scoring horses also showed shorter periods of

ground contact of the limbs, while increasing both the duration and distance covered during the suspension.

The rhythm of the stride differs between the collected and extended canters (Clayton, 1994b). In collected canter, the three footfalls are separated by relatively long intervals with a relatively short suspension. In extended canter the three footfalls are more closely grouped in time and the suspension is longer. The diagonal limb pair (leading hind and trailing fore) do not always make contact with the ground synchronously, though the dissociation is very small and usually only detectable with the aid of slow motion analysis. In the extended canter either the fore or hindlimb may contact the ground earlier (Deuel & Park, 1990; Clayton, 1994b).

The ground reaction forces at the canter (Merkens *et al.*, 1993) show marked differences between the trailing and leading limbs (Fig. 8.11). In collected canter the vertical ground reaction force is smallest in the trailing hindlimb (approximately equal to body weight) and largest in the trailing forelimb (1.5 times body weight). The vertical force in the leading hind and leading forelimbs was approximately 1.2 times body weight. With regard to the longitudinal ground reaction force, the trailing hindlimb is primarily propulsive; it acts to change the direction of movement of the center of mass from forward and downward to forward and horizontal. The leading hindlimb and trailing forelimb (diagonal pair) are principally responsible for supporting the body weight and supplying forward propulsion, with the trailing forelimb having a particularly large propulsive component. The leading forelimb raises the center of mass as the horse moves into the suspension by exerting large vertical and retarding forces. Therefore, it is the trailing limbs that produce most of the forward propulsion.

Lead changes at the canter

When a dressage horse performs a flying lead change, the leading hind and forelimbs change during the suspension phase. In high-level competitions, lead changes are performed in series at intervals of four, three, two or one strides. The characteristics of the canter strides during the two tempi (alternate stride) and one tempi

Table 8.6 Stride kinematics of the collected, working, medium and extended canters in FEI level dressage horses. Data are from Clayton (1994b, ©EVJ Ltd). Different superscripts indicate values that differ significantly, $p < 0.05$.

	Collected canter	Working canter	Medium canter	Extended canter
Speed (m/s)	3.27[a]	3.91[b]	4.90[c]	5.97[d]
Stride length (m)	2.00[a,b,c]	2.35[a,d,e]	2.94[b,d,f]	3.47[c,e,f]
Stride frequency (strides/min)	99[a]	99[a]	101[a]	105[a]
Suspension (ms)	0[a,b]	5[c,d]	54[a,c]	87[b,d]

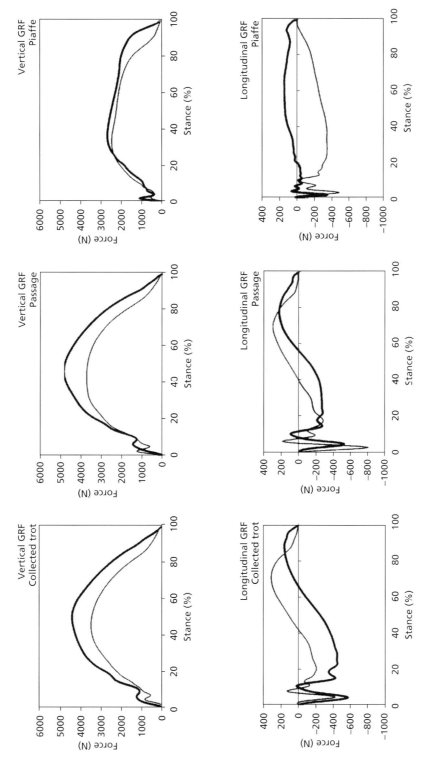

Fig. 8.9 Vertical (above) and longitudinal (below) ground reaction forces for collected trot (left), passage (center) and piaffe (right) for the forelimbs (———) and hindlimbs (———).

(every stride) lead changes are shown in Table 8.7 (Deuel & Park, 1990). During the lead changes, all four limbs have long stance durations and short swing durations, and there is a diagonal dissociation with contact of the leading hind hoof preceding that of the trailing fore hoof by 14.0–24.0 ms.

In the two tempi changes (Deuel & Park, 1990), the stride immediately preceding the change (pre-change stride) has a slower speed, shorter stride length and higher stride frequency than the stride following the change (post-change stride). The shorter stride length of the pre-change stride is a result of taking a shorter step between the two forelimbs and covering less distance during the suspension (Table 8.7). In pre-change strides ground contact of the trailing forelimb precedes that of the leading hindlimb, whereas in the post-change strides the sequence is reversed.

In the one tempi lead changes, the strides share characteristics of both the pre- and post-change strides in the two tempi changes (Table 8.7). The support sequence varies between horses, reflecting individual differences in technique, but the diagonal dissociation almost always involves placing the leading hindlimb before the trailing forelimb. There is a pronounced reliance on overlap between the two hindlimbs in the early part of the stride, which is similar to the post-change stride for the two tempi changes. Later in the stride there is a reliance on forelimb overlap. Higher competition scores are associated with a longer time in hindlimb support and a shorter time in forelimb support (Deuel & Park, 1990).

The canter pirouette

In the canter pirouette, horses are supposed to maintain the tempo and rhythm of the collected canter strides. However, a study of horses competing in the individual medal finals at the Barcelona Olympics showed that neither the tempo nor the rhythm of the collected canter strides was maintained in the canter pirouette. The tempo was significantly slower in the pirouette strides (68 strides/min) than in the collected canter strides (95 strides/min). The footfalls of the diagonal limb pair were dissociated in the pirouette strides, giving a distinct four-beat rhythm, in contrast to the three-beat rhythm of the canter strides. Also, there was no suspension between successive pirouette strides (Burns & Clayton, 1997).

The lack of forward movement in the pirouette makes it difficult for the horse to maintain its balance. The horse compensates by increasing the limb stance durations and the overlaps between limbs (Fig. 8.12). This was particularly obvious for the inside hindlimb, in which the stance duration was greatly prolonged as a means of maintaining the horse's balance in

the absence of forward movement (Burns & Clayton, 1997).

The capriole

Knezevic et al. (1987) used high-speed cinematography to describe the capriole in a Lipizzan stallion at the Spanish Riding School in Vienna. This is a movement in which the horse elevates the forehand, then leaps into the air and, at the culmination of the airborne phase, kicks backwards with the hindlimbs. At the culmination of the leap, the ventral rump contour was 158 cm above the ground. The hip, stifle and tarsal joints showed extreme extension when the hindlimbs were fully stretched behind the horse. Maximal extension of the fetlock and coffin joints occurred about 20 ms later.

Transitions

A study of transitions between the walk and trot classified the transitions into two types (Argue & Clayton, 1993a). Type 1 transitions are those in which all the limb support sequences are typical of the walk or trot. Type 2 transitions include intermediate steps between the two gaits in which the support sequences are not typical of either gait. Type 1 transitions are thought to be more desirable and should be rewarded by judges. The likelihood of performing a Type 1 transition may be influenced by the skill of the rider in giving the aids at the appropriate time in the stride.

For the transitions from walk to trot, in a Type 1 transition the horse springs from a diagonal support phase in the walk directly into the trot. Type 2 transitions are initiated from either a diagonal or a lateral

Table 8.7 Stride variables for the one tempi and two tempi lead changes. Data are from Deuel and Park (1990). TrH: trailing hindlimb; LdH: leading hindlimb; TrF: trailing forelimb; LdF: leading forelimb.

	One tempi stride	Two tempi stride before change	Two tempi stride after change
Speed (m/s)	3.36	3.65	3.95
Stride length (m)	2.08	2.21	2.44
Hind step			
TrH – LdH (m)	0.94	0.87	0.88
Diagonal step			
LdH – TrF (m)	0.97	0.97	0.93
Fore step			
TrF – LdF (m)	0.80	0.79	0.89
Suspension			
LdF – TrH (m)	−0.53	−0.47	−0.33
Stride frequency (strides/min)	97	99	97

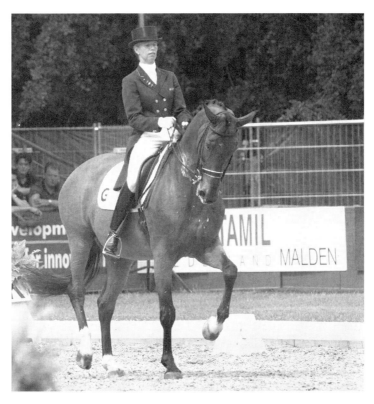

Fig. 8.10 Photograph of 'Bonfire' with Anky van Grunsven performing the piaffe at the Dutch dressage championships, Nijmegen 2000 (photo by Jacob Melissen, NL).

support phase in the walk. From a diagonal support phase, either the fore or hind hoof is raised, then the opposite diagonal pair is placed for a three-limb support. The original fore or hindlimb is lifted, and the horse springs from the remaining diagonal pair into the trot. In the transitions initiated from a lateral support phase, one limb is raised leaving a single supporting limb. The diagonal fore or hindlimb is then placed to give a diagonal support phase from which the horse springs into the trot. The ability to perform Type 1 transitions from walk to trot is significantly related to level of training; more highly trained horses perform a larger number of Type 1 walk–trot transitions (Argue & Clayton, 1993a).

Trot to walk transitions are initiated by placement of the second forelimb during a diagonal support phase at the trot. In Type 1 transitions, the horse then proceeds in the walk. In Type 2 transitions, the tripedal support phase is followed by lifting of the diagonal pair leaving a forelimb in single support. The diagonal hindlimb is then placed, and the horse continues in a normal walk sequence. The frequency of Type 1 transitions from trot to walk is significantly related to level of training, with the more highly trained horses showing a higher

percentage of Type 1 transitions (Argue & Clayton, 1993a).

Transitions between trot and canter are differentiated according to whether the horse initiates the canter from a forelimb or a hindlimb (Argue & Clayton, 1993b). Neither type of transition involves limb support sequences that are not typical of the trot or canter. A transition initiated by the forelimb starts with a diagonal support phase in trot. The opposite forelimb is then placed on the ground and it becomes the leading limb as the horse continues in a canter sequence. For the transitions initiated by a hindlimb, the forelimb is lifted during the diagonal support phase of the trot. The hindlimb that remains on the ground becomes the trailing hindlimb. The diagonal pair (leading hind–trailing forelimbs) are then placed on the ground and the horse continues in a canter sequence. The type of trot to canter transition is not related to the horse's level of training.

Two types of transitions were observed between canter and trot. In one type, the horse initiates the change by springing from the diagonal support phase of the canter to the opposite diagonal and then continues in the trot. The other type of transition is initiated from the leading

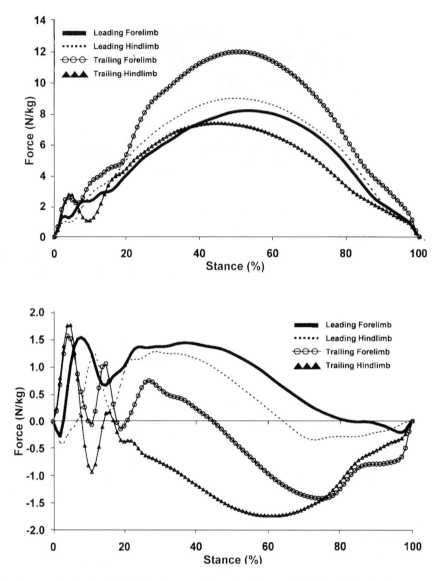

Fig. 8.11 Vertical (above) and longitudinal (below) ground reaction forces of the four limbs in the canter.

forelimb single support. Instead of proceeding into a suspension, the trailing hindlimb is placed on the ground to give a diagonal support phase, from which the horse springs into a suspension and continues in a trot sequence. The type of transition from canter to trot is not related to level of training (Argue & Clayton, 1993b).

Conformation of dressage horses

Elite dressage horses tend to have short necks, which perhaps reduces the leverage of the head and neck and so facilitates collection and self carriage. In the forelimb,

the scapula is sloping and the elbow joint has a large angle. A long humerus, a small hip angle and a long sloping femur are associated with high gait scores. The fore and hind phalanges tend to be long and upright (Holmström *et al.*, 1990).

Jumping

Jumping sports require the horse to raise its center of mass high enough for all of its body parts to clear the height and width of an obstacle. The jump is a form of extended suspension since it occurs between the stance

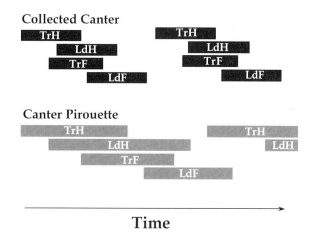

Fig. 8.12 Temporal characteristics of the collected canter strides and the canter pirouette strides. The shaded bars represent the stance phases of the limbs. TrH: trailing hindlimb; LdH: leading hindlimb; TrF: trailing forelimb; LdF: leading forelimb.

phases of the hindlimbs and the forelimbs, so it is most easily incorporated into the canter or gallop stride, though horses can also jump from the trot, walk or even the halt.

Summary

Dressage is a judged sport in which the quality of the horse's gaits (kinematics) and the horse's innate athleticism (balance, coordination) are important determinants of competitive success. There is a considerable body of research describing the performance of elite competitors in different gaits and movements, and studies of the mechanics of collection and self carriage are underway.

Terminology

Terminology for the strides during the approach and departure for horses jumping at a canter has been described (Clayton, 1989a). The stride in which the jump occurs is the jump stride; its components are the take off, jump suspension and landing. The take off comprises the stance phases of the two hindlimbs immediately preceding the jump. The jump suspension is the airborne phase from lift off of the last hind limb at take off to ground contact of the trailing forelimb at landing. The landing comprises the stance phases of the two forelimbs after the jump suspension. The strides preceding the jump stride are the approach strides and those fol-

lowing the jump stride are the departure strides. Both the approach and departure strides are numbered from the jump outwards (Fig. 8.13).

Jumping mechanics

The approach and take-off

The path of the horse's center of mass and the angular momentum of its body during the jump suspension are determined during the take off. After the jump suspension begins, these properties cannot be changed until the horse makes contact with an external object. Therefore, the approach and take off are extremely important in determining the outcome of the jump.

The positions of the limb placements on the take-off side do not differ between a vertical fence and an oxer, or between fences of different heights in the range of 1.10–1.40 m. One study showed that, in 92 of 96 trials, the limb placed closest to the fence on the take-off side was the leading forelimb in approach stride 1. In the remaining four trials, all of which were oxer fences, the limb placed closest to the fence was the leading hindlimb (Clayton & Barlow, 1989). Fewer knock downs occurred when there was a larger distance between the trailing forelimb in approach stride 1 and the base of the fence (Deuel & Park, 1991).

The timing and coordination of the limb movements during the approach, jump stride and departure are shown in Table 8.8. Approach stride 2 and the strides that precede it are fairly typical canter strides that have a three-beat rhythm with the head and neck elevated. The ability to maintain a high stride frequency during the approach is a characteristic of good jumpers (Barrey & Galloux, 1997).

Approach stride 1 is a short, quick stride; both the stride length and stride duration are significantly shorter than in approach stride 2. This stride has a distinctly four-beat rhythm with the leading hindlimb contacting the ground before the trailing forelimb. The neck is stretched forward and downward in preparation for take off. This action is similar to the 'gather' shown by human jumpers during the transition between the approach and take off. The objective of the gather is to lower the center of mass prior to the take-off foot contacting the ground. This avoids having to overcome a downward movement of the center of mass before driving the body into the air. It has even been suggested that the amount of lowering of the center of mass during the gather bears a direct relationship to the height jumped. The leading hindlimb has a very short stance duration in approach stride 1 and the horse's body does not roll forward over this limb as in a normal stride. The forelimbs are stretched forward at ground contact and, consequently, have a small angle between the palmar aspect of the metacarpus and the ground (Clayton & Barlow, 1991). The forelimbs initiate the upward movement of the forehand, converting forward movement into vertical movement. This involves reducing the horizontal speed, elevating the forehand and rotating the trunk segment into an appropriate position for take off. Because the forehand is already starting to move upwards, the leading forelimb is pulled off the ground relatively early, when it is more or less in a vertical position.

When a horse jumps a fence that is less than 1 m high, the center of mass is elevated only a small amount to allow clearance of the fence and, consequently, the forces required to jump a small fence are not much greater than those in a canter stride. For example, in jumping a fence 0.8 m high, the combined vertical

impulses of the fore and hindlimbs increases by only about 8% on the take-off side and 3% on the landing side. For fences higher than about 1.0 m, the need to elevate the center of mass increases progressively with the height of the fence, with a consequent increase in the vertical forces at take off and landing. A considerable increase in vertical forces has been recorded when the height of the fence was raised from 1.3 m to 1.5 m (Fig. 8.14) (Schamhardt *et al.*, 1993), and a vertical force of 3.85 times body weight has been measured in a horse jumping a vertical fence 1.53 m high (Preuschoft, 1989). Both forelimbs exert a large braking impulse that decelerates the forward movement. The trailing forelimb provides a little propulsion in the terminal part of its stance phase, but the leading forelimb provides a braking force only as a result of the early cessation of its stance phase (Schamhardt *et al.*, 1993). The braking action of the forelimbs causes a reduction in horizontal velocity (Clayton & Barlow, 1991) and an upward acceleration of the trunk segment (Barrey & Galloux, 1997). After the forelimbs leave the ground, the head and neck are raised, which helps to establish an advantageous position for optimal power production during the push off by the hindlimbs.

A short suspension intervenes between approach stride 1 and the jump stride. The jump stride is distinguished from the preceding and following strides by the inclusion of the jump suspension, which results in significant increases in stride length and stride duration. At take off the hindlimbs often contact the ground synchronously and at almost equal distances from the fence. Their functions are to provide upward and forward propulsion, and to reverse the direction of rotation of the trunk segment. Forward rotation of the trunk is necessary for the horse to leave the ground from the hindlimbs and land on the forelimbs. Both hindlimbs have relatively long stance durations, which allows the generation of large impulses. The two hindlimbs show

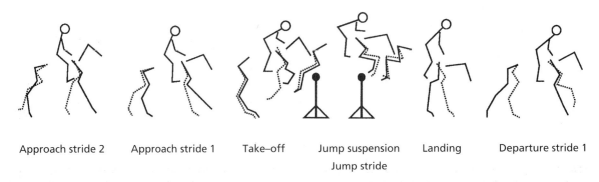

Approach stride 2   Approach stride 1   Take–off   Jump suspension   Landing   Departure stride 1

Jump stride

Fig. 8.13   Terminology for the strides preceding and following the jump.

Table 8.8 Stride characteristics of horses jumping a vertical fence 1.55 m high. Data from Clayton and Barlow (1991, © International Society of Biomechanics).

	Approach stride 1	Approach stride 2	Jump stride	Departure stride 1
Horizontal speed (m/s)	7.3	6.3	5.9	6.5
Stride length (m)	4.1	2.4	4.9	3.3
Stride frequency (str/min)	108	157	73	116
Stance TrH (ms)	157	145	197	147
Stance LdH (ms)	179	129	195	171
Stance TrF (ms)	149	188	140	174
Stance LdF (ms)	134	159	176	168

TrH: trailing hindlimb; LdH: Leading hindlimb; Tr F: trailing Forelimb; Ld F: Leading Forelimb

almost identical ground reaction force profiles. The vertical force rises to a plateau, with a peak amplitude around 130% body weight for a horse jumping a vertical fence 1.3 m high. The longitudinal forces are predominantly propulsive (Fig. 8.14).

Studies using an accelerometer attached to the thorax beneath the sternum have shown that the action of the hindlimbs produces a lower acceleration peak on the trunk segment than the push off by the forelimbs (Fig. 8.15). However, the inclination of the trunk axis during the hindlimb push off reduces the amplitude registered by the direction-sensitive accelerometer, so the acceleration due to the hindlimb action may be underestimated. The hindlimb acceleration peak at take off is significantly greater for fences with width (oxer – 1.48 g; water jump –1.74 g) than for those with height only (vertical

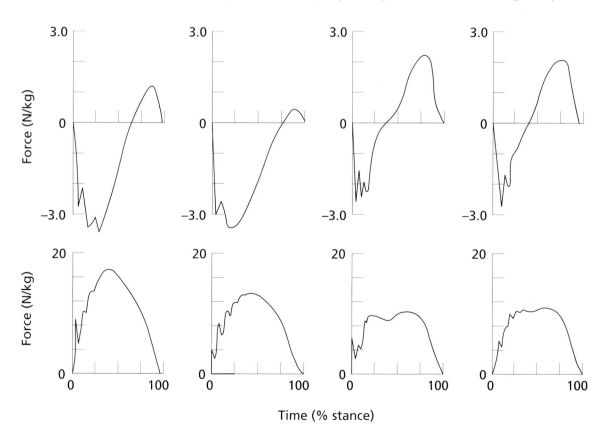

Fig. 8.14 Longitudinal (above) and vertical (below) ground reaction forces during the approach and take off for a horse jumping a vertical fence. The traces from left to right represent the trailing forelimb in approach stride 1, the leading forelimb in approach stride 1, the trailing hindlimb at take off and the leading hindlimb at take off.

−1.27 *g*) (Barrey & Galloux, 1997). This is because the flight path must be higher and longer when jumping a wider obstacle.

For elite show jumping horses jumping a vertical fence 1.50 m high during an international competition (Bogert *et al.*, 1994), a similar movement pattern was observed in all horses during take off. The duration of the take off phase averaged 221 ms. At the start of take-off the trunk was rotating backwards with an angular velocity of 150°/s. The direction of rotation changed almost linearly to 50°/s forward rotation at the start of the jump suspension. During this time the horizontal velocity initially decreased from 4.5 m/s at the start of take off to 3.6 m/s, then increased to 6.5 m/s at lift off. The vertical velocity, which was zero at the start of take off, reached a negative value of 1.0 m/s before increasing to 4.0 m/s at lift off. The initial downward movement of the trunk was a result of the total vertical GRF being less than body weight. The neck rotated downward throughout take off with an almost constant angular velocity.

The hip joint extended during the first 152 ms at take off, then maintained the same angle until leaving the ground. The stifle and hock joints initially flexed then extended with the transition from flexion to extension occurring earlier in the hock than the stifle. The fetlock showed two phases of dorsiflexion with a relatively constant angle in the period between. Maximal fetlock extension occurred late in the stance phase after which there was rapid flexion. The total power production by the hindlimbs was estimated to be 13 000 J, which represents an average power production of 59 000 W during the take-off phase. These findings indicate that most of the energy required to clear the fence is provided by the hindlimbs during take off (Bogert *et al.*, 1994).

Each horse has its own individual jumping technique that is repeatable from jump to jump. This produces a characteristic acceleration profile (Barrey & Galloux, 1997) and has a large effect on the ground reaction forces. Over a small fence, 0.8 m high, horses with good technique that fold their lower limbs during the jump suspension, had vertical and longitudinal force profiles that resembled those for a canter stride in shape and magnitude. However, a horse with poor jumping technique registered considerably higher forces both at take -off and landing (Schamhardt *et al.* 1993). The forces used by a poor jumper over a fence 0.8 m high were similar in magnitude to those used by a good jumper over a fence 1.3 m high. It might be expected from these results that horses with poor technique would show earlier signs of wear and tear injuries than horses with good technique. Poor jumpers, even when they clear a fence, tend to have a higher ratio between the acceleration provided during take off by the forelimbs and the hindlimbs. In other words, they are compensating for a weak acceleration impulse of the hindlimbs at take off by increasing the braking action of the forelimbs in approach stride 1 (Barrey & Galloux, 1997).

The jump suspension

The jump stride has a much longer stride length than the approach or departure strides due to the distance covered during the jump suspension. In one study the total distance jumped from take off to landing did not differ between a vertical fence and an oxer, but increased significantly with fence height (Clayton & Barlow, 1989). In a different study, the jump distance was longer over an oxer than a vertical fence, with the increase being approximately equal to the spread of the oxer (Deuel & Park, 1991).

After take off the motions of the body and limb segments are coordinated so that the angular velocity of the trunk remains almost constant throughout the jump suspension. All the segments act synergistically with the approximate contributions of the different segments to the angular momentum being 50% from the trunk, 25% from the hindlimbs, 2% from the head–neck and 5% from the forelimbs (Galloux & Barrey, 1997). The presence of the rider has virtually no effect on rotation of the horse's body.

As the horse passes over the top of the fence, the forelimbs generally have less clearance than the hindlimbs, and clearance by all limbs decreases with fence height (Jelen, 1976). Furthermore, a good horse paired with a good rider shows a smaller discrepancy between the height of the fence and the height of the limbs; in other words horses show less tendency to overjump with a good rider. Most jumping errors are a result of inappropriate aids from the rider (Lauk *et al.*, 1991). A study of trunk accelerations showed that 87% of jumping faults could be blamed on a forelimb error (Barrey & Galloux, 1997). More faults occur at vertical fences than at oxers or water jumps.

The landing and departure

During landing, the two forelimbs are separated by only a short distance. The metacarpal segment of the trailing forelimb is almost vertical when the hoof makes ground contact while the leading forelimb contacts the ground with a more acute angulation (Clayton & Barlow, 1991). The trailing hindlimb is usually placed between the previous placements of the two forelimbs, and this characteristic is associated with fewer jumping penalties (Deuel & Park, 1991). The leading hindlimb is placed further away from the fence than the forelimbs.

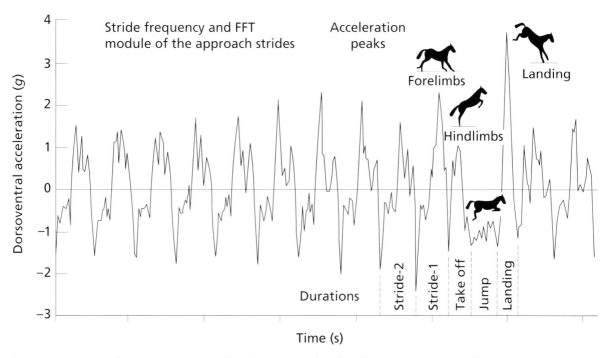

Fig. 8.15 Dorsoventral accelerometer recording of the approach, take off, jump suspension, landing and departure. FFT: Fast Fourier transformation (Reprinted from Barrey & Galloux, 1997, © EVJ Ltd.)

The placements of the leading forelimb and the leading hindlimb on the landing side are closer to the last element of an oxer than a vertical at all fence heights, and there is a trend toward landing further from the vertical than the oxer for the other limbs. The limb displacements from the fence on the landing side increase with fence height. Interestingly, the height of the fence has less effect on the later strides as the horse moves away from the fence (Clayton & Barlow, 1991). Therefore, the fewer the strides between fences in a combination, the more important it is to take into account the height and type of the in-going fence in determining the appropriate distance between fences.

During landing the trailing forelimb has a very short stance duration as the horse rapidly rolls forward onto the leading forelimb (Clayton & Barlow, 1991; Deuel & Park, 1991). Horses that have a longer time interval between contact of the two forelimbs are less likely to knock the fence down (Deuel & Park, 1991).

The trailing forelimb has the highest peak vertical forces both at take off and at landing (Fig. 8.16) (Schamhardt *et al.*, 1993), which may explain the fact that some horses have a preferred lead for take off and landing and habitually switch to this lead one or two strides before take off. These horses probably have either a subclinical lameness or a marked strength asymmetry between the left and right sides.

The forelimbs absorb the initial force of landing and this is reflected in the high peak amplitudes of the vertical forces, especially the trailing forelimb in which a vertical force peak of twice body weight has been recorded in a horse jumping a vertical fence 1.3 m high (Schamhardt *et al.*, 1993). This limb makes ground contact with an almost vertical orientation, which is not conducive to generating a braking force. Therefore, the longitudinal force is entirely propulsive for the trailing forelimb at landing, but for the leading forelimb the ground reaction force during landing is mostly braking with a smaller propulsive component in its terminal part (Merkens *et al.*, 1991; Schamhardt *et al.*, 1993). The actions of the trunk, hindlimbs and head and neck segments play a large role in reversing the direction of rotation of the horse's trunk which is necessary to allow the hindlimbs to contact the ground underneath the body mass.

In departure stride 1 the horse regains its balance and the hindlimbs re-establish forward movement by generating large propulsive longitudinal forces and impulses, especially in the trailing hindlimb (Schamhardt *et al.*, 1993). This stride has a four-beat rhythm (Fig. 8.13) with the leading hindlimb contacting the ground in advance of the trailing forelimb. The stride length is significantly shorter than

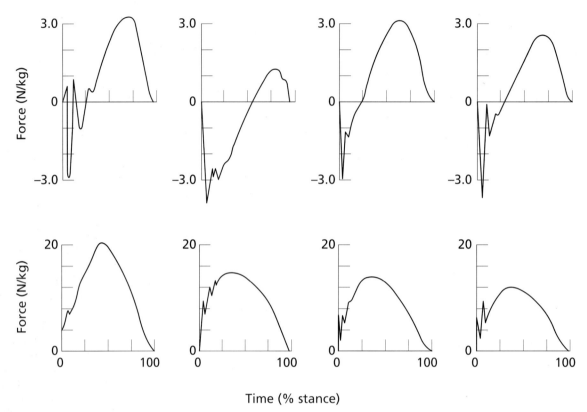

Fig. 8.16 Longitudinal (above) and vertical (below) ground reaction forces during the landing and departure for a horse jumping a vertical fence 1.3 m high. The traces from left to right represent the trailing forelimb at landing, the leading forelimb at landing, the trailing hindlimb in departure stride 1 and the leading hindlimb in departure stride 1.

in approach stride 2 (Clayton & Barlow, 1991), and the distance between the two hindlimb placements is particularly variable. Sometimes they are placed almost equidistant from the fence, other times they are widely separated. Fewer knock downs were recorded when the trailing hindlimb landed closer to the fence (Deuel & Park, 1991).

Water jump technique

A study performed during the Barcelona Olympics identified the factors that influence success in clearing a water jump. The vertical velocity and the angle of projection at take off were significantly greater, and the horizontal distance between the leading hindlimb and the center of mass at take off was significantly shorter, in horses that were successful in clearing the width of the water jump compared with those that failed to clear the entire width (Clayton *et al.*, 1995, 1996; Colborne *et al.*, 1995;). The horizontal velocity at take off did not influence success, nor did the height of the center of gravity at the start and end of the jump suspension. It was concluded that, to be a successful water jumper, a horse

must generate a large vertical velocity during the take off. Vertical velocity at the start of the jump suspension is highly correlated with the trunk angle at lift off and with the horizontal distance between the leading hind hoof and the horse's center of gravity at both the start and end of take off (Colborne *et al.*, 1995).

Conformation of jumping horses

The conformational trait that has been most consistently linked to successful jumping performance is height at the withers (Fabiani, 1973; Jelen, 1976; Langlois *et al.*, 1978). In addition to being tall, good jumpers are compact horses, built close to the ground and with width through the shoulders and hips (Langlois *et al.*, 1978). Body segment angles relative to the horizontal were large for the ilium and small for the femur, scapula and humerus. Elite show jumpers have larger hock angles than other horses (Holmström *et al.*, 1990). Jumping ability showed little change after 6 months of jumping training, indicating that innate ability is an important attribute if a horse is to be a good jumper (Fabiani, 1973).

Summary

Jumping horses require strength to raise the center of mass high enough to clear a large fence, together with exquisite coordination to allow all the body parts to clear the fence without over-jumping. The approach and take off determine the path of the center of gravity and the angular momentum of the body during the airborne phase. During the landing and departure, the balance and forward movement are re-established. Each horse has its own individual jumping technique that is repeatable from jump to jump.

Eventing

The sport of eventing was originally devised as a test of athleticism for cavalry horses, and the name 'the military' is still retained in some languages. Event horses perform three tests: dressage, speed and endurance and show jumping. Since dressage and show jumping are covered elsewhere in this chapter, this section will focus on studies that are specific to the sport of eventing, especially those describing performance in the speed and endurance phases, which include roads and tracks, steeplechase and cross country.

Dressage performance

In a study at the Barcelona Olympics, performance in the dressage phase was correlated with finishing place. Stride length and speed in the extended canter were positively related to points awarded by the judges for the canter. Horses that failed to complete the entire three day event had longer stride lengths and faster speeds in the extended canter during the dressage phase than horses that finished the competition (Deuel, 1995). The author suggested that characteristics of the extended canter that are highly rewarded by the judges have little relation to subsequent galloping and jumping performance, and qualities favored by dressage judges may even predict failure to finish the event.

Speed and endurance performance

Success in the speed and endurance phase is largely dependent on having a ground-covering stride. Recordings made during the steeplechase phase of the three day event at the Seoul Olympics (Deuel & Park, 1993) showed an average speed of 12.1 m/s with a stride length of 6.0 m and a stride frequency of 2.0 strides/s.

Superior performance in the entire competition was significantly associated with a faster speed and a longer stride length in the steeplechase phase. The score was optimized with a gallop stride frequency between 1.85 and 2.05 strides/s and a speed between 13.0 and 14.3 m/s. Up to 7 m there appeared to be no upper limit for optimal stride length.

In a study of the temporal and linear kinematics of horses jumping a steeplechase fence, 1.4 m high and 2.6 m wide at the base, during a young riders' competition (Leach & Ormrod, 1984), the average distance jumped was 5.2 m. The distances of the limbs from the base of the fence on the take-off side were: trailing forelimb 2.6 m, leading forelimb 2.1 m, trailing hindlimb 2.0 m and leading hindlimb 2.0 m. Unlike show jumpers, in which the trailing hindlimb is usually placed between the two forelimbs at take off, during steeplechasing both hindlimbs are placed closer to the fence than the leading forelimb. The forelimb stance durations were approximately 0.13 s, whereas the hindlimbs had longer stance durations of around 0.17 s. In a regression analysis the only temporal variable that was a significant predictor of the distance jumped was the overlap between the forelimb stance durations. The longer the forelimbs overlapped, the shorter the horizontal distance jumped. For the linear variables, the distance of the trailing forelimb from the base of the fence was positively related to the distance jumped. When this limb is further from the jump, the horse uses a flatter trajectory, which carries it farther across the fence.

Effect of added weight on jumping performance

In the past the competition rules stipulated that event horses had to carry a minimum weight of 75 kg (rider and tack), which represented anything from 10–17% of body weight depending on the weight of the horse. It was suggested that this imposed an unsafe burden on small horses. A study was performed (Clayton, 1997b) to compare the landing kinematics of small (maximum height 164 cm) event horses when carrying a 61 kg rider versus carrying the same rider plus an 18 kg weighted saddle pad. The test fence was a table fence with a sloping face that measured 1.1 m high, 1.9 m wide at the base and 1.3 m wide at the top. The results (Table 8.9) showed that with the extra weight the leading forelimb landed closer to the fence, which confirmed the riders' subjective impression that the horses were 'cutting down' during the landing. This was probably a result of failing to generate sufficient impulse during the take off to compensate for the extra weight.

During landing both the fetlock and carpal joints of the leading forelimb were significantly more extended

Summary

Event horses are versatile athletes. They must show relaxation and suppleness in the dressage phase; speed, strength, stamina and athleticism in the endurance phase; and suppleness and coordination in the show jumping phase. A long and energetically efficient galloping stride is an important quality in a potential eventer. More data are needed describing the techniques used to jump different types of cross country fences.

with the extra weight, which was a direct result of the greater force at landing. Since strain of the suspensory ligament and the superficial digital flexor tendon increase with extension of the fetlock, the extra weight may have put the horses at greater risk of suspensory desmitis or superficial digital flexor tendon strain. The stance duration of both hindlimbs increased in departure stride 1, which may have been indicative of the use of these limbs to restore the horses' balance by elevating the forehand which was burdened by the extra weight. As a result of these findings the minimum weight rule for event horses was abolished.

Cutting

Cutting horses perform almost independently of the rider; during the judging, points are lost if the rider cues the horse. The objective is to sort one calf from a herd and then to prevent it returning to the other calves. The sport evolved from the practical aspects of ranch work,

with the first competition taking place around the turn of the century. Since then, there has been increasing interest in cutting as a sport and it is currently one of the most rapidly growing equestrian sports. In competition the horse is judged for 2.5 minutes during which it usually cuts two or three calves.

Cutting is a high-intensity activity in which the horse must have quick reaction times and the ability to turn and accelerate in either direction in response to the unpredictable movements of the calf. Some horses are naturally more talented than others, and 'cow sense' is a highly prized trait. Genetic evaluation of over 3000 horses competing at the World Championship Futurities over a 9-year period yielded a heritability estimate of cutting ability of $19\% \pm 5\%$ (Ellersieck *et al.*, 1985).

The tactics used to keep the calf separate from the herd are similar to defensive play that blocks the progress of the offensive player in sports such as football. A study was performed to determine factors that differed between horses with different levels of ability (Clayton, 1989b). A group of cutting horses that were of similar ages, training histories and competitive opportunities, were divided into two groups according to their competitive winnings. The five horses in the 'average' group had won less than $35 000. The seven horses in the 'elite' group had won more than $35 000. The horses worked a mechanical flag rather than a live steer, which allowed the use of a standard test to ensure that all horses performed a similar series of turns and runs in each direction. The mechanical flag is a piece of heavy cloth measuring about 30 cm². All the horses had worked with the mechanical flag regularly and frequently during their careers.

Table 8.9 Temporal and linear kinematic variables for horses jumping a table fence with a 61 kg rider (rider weight) and with a 61 kg rider plus an 18 kg weighted saddle pad (added weight). Data are from Clayton (1997b, ©EVJ Ltd). TrF: trailing forelimb; LdF: leading forelimb; TrH: trailing hindlimb; LdH: leading hindlimb; D1: first departure stride.

	Rider weight	Added weight
Stance duration, TrF at landing (s)	0.18	0.18
Stance duration, LdF at landing (s)	0.21	0.21
Stance duration, TrH in stride D1 (s)	0.19*	0.20*
Stance duration, LdH in stride D1 (s)	0.21*	0.22*
Distance TrF to fence at landing (cm)	173.5	159.3
Distance LdF to fence at landing (cm)	240.4*	222.7*
Max carpal angle, TrF at landing (deg)	191.0	190.0
Max fetlock angle, TrF at landing (deg)	252.9	251.9
Max carpal angle, LdF at landing (deg)	190.7*	193.4*
Max fetlock angle, LdF at landing (deg)	247.4*	250.7*

* Values that differ significantly ($p < 0.05$).

Table 8.10 Comparison of elite and average cutting horses working a mechanical flag. Values are mean ± SD. Data are from Clayton (1989b).

	Elite horses	Average horses
Reaction time after flag starts moving (ms)	200 ± 66[*]	282 ± 74[*]
Time to stop after flag stops moving (ms)	386 ± 108[*]	492 ± 94[*]
Distance from flag at start of run (cm)	52 ± 23[*]	81 ± 32[*]
Maximal distance from flag during run (cm)	148 ± 28[*]	221 ± 23[*]
Distance from flag at end of run (cm)	55 ± 26[*]	78 ± 32[*]

[*] Values that differ significantly ($p < 0.05$).

Summary

Cutting is a high-intensity sport that requires great agility and an inherent 'cow sense'. Successful cutting horses have quick reaction times and an economical turning technique that allows them to follow the calf closely at all times.

Horses in the two groups differed significantly in several ways (Table 8.10). Elite horses had faster reaction times than average horses, which allowed them to respond more quickly when the flag began moving and to stop sooner after the flag stopped moving. The faster reaction times of the elite horses may have some value as a predictor of performance. As a result of their faster reaction times the elite horses were significantly closer to the flag throughout the run and were less likely to over-run the flag than the average horses. Other features of the performance were that elite horses leaned their shoulders in the direction of the turn before pushing off against the ground, which is a more effective method of turning. The average horses were more likely to move their hooves sideways as the first indication of turning, rather than leaning into the turn and pushing sideways. The elite horses also tended to turn using fewer strides than the average horses though this difference did not reach statistical significance.

REFERENCES

Anon (1991) *Rules for Dressage Events*, Switzerland: Fédération Equestre Internationale.

Argue, C.K. (1994) The kinematics of piaffe, passage and collected trot of dressage horses. *PhD thesis, University of Saskatchewan, Saskatoon.*

Argue, C.K. and Clayton, H.M. (1993a) A preliminary study of transitions between the walk and trot in dressage horses. *Acta Anat.* **146**: 179–182.

Argue, C.K. and Clayton, H.M. (1993b) A study of transitions between the trot and canter in dressage horses. *J. Equine Vet. Sci.* **13**: 171–174.

Back, W., Barneveld, A. Bruin, G., Schamhardt, H.C. and Hartman, W. (1994a) Kinematic detection of superior gait quality in young trotting warmbloods. *Vet. Quart.* **16** (Suppl 2): S91–96.

Back, W., Barneveld, H.C., Schamhardt, H.C., Bruin, G. and Hartman, W. (1994b) Longitudinal development of the kinematics of 4-, 10-, 18- and 26-month-old Dutch Warmblood horses. *Equine Vet. J.* **17** (Suppl.): 3–6.

Back, W., Hartman, W., Schamhardt, H.C., Bruin, G. and Barneveld, A. (1995) Kinematic response to a 70 day training period in trotting Warmbloods. *Equine Vet. J.* **18** (Suppl.): 127–135.

Barrey, E. and Galloux, P. (1997) Analysis of the equine jumping technique by accelerometry. *Equine Vet. J.* **23** (Suppl.): 45–49.

Barrey, E., Auvinet, B. and Courouce, A. (1995) Gait evaluation of race trotters using an accelerometric device. *Equine Vet. J.* **18** (Suppl.): 156–160.

Bayer, A. (1973) Bewegungsanalysen an Trabrennpferden mit Hilfe der Ungulographie. *Zbl. Vet. Med. A* **20** (Suppl.): 209–221.

Bodine-Rees, P. and Bone, J.P. (1976) Premotor reaction time component of biceps brachii, brachialis and brachioradialis muscles in varsity versus non-varsity women. *Biomechanics V-A*. Baltimore: University Park Press, pp. 96–101.

Bogert, A.J. van den, Jansen, M.O. and Deuel, N.R. (1994) Kinematics of the hind limb push-off in elite jumping horses. *Equine Vet. J.* **23** (Suppl.): 80–86.

Bramble, D.M. (1984) Locomotor-respiratory integration in running mammals. *Proc. Assoc. Equine Sports Med.* **4**: 42–53.

Burns, T.E. and Clayton, H.M. (1997) Comparison of the temporal kinematics of the canter pirouette and collected canter. *Equine Vet. J.* **23** (Suppl.): 58–61.

Cavagna, G.A., Heglund, N.C. and Taylor, C.R. (1977) Mechanical work in terrestrial locomotion: two basic mechanisms for minimizing energy expenditure. *Am. J. Physiol.* **233**: R243–R261.

Cheney, J.A., Shen, C.K. and Wheat, J.D. (1973) Relationship of racetrack surface to lameness in the Thoroughbred racehorse. *Am. J. Vet. Res.* **34**: 1285–1289.

Clayton, H.M. (1989a) Terminology for the description of equine jumping kinematics. *J. Equine Vet. Sci.* **9**: 341–348.

Clayton, H.M. (1989b) Kinematic analysis of cutting horses working a mechanical flag. *Am. J. Vet. Res.* **50**: 1418–1422.

Clayton, H.M. (1993) The extended canter: a comparison of some kinematic variables in horses trained for dressage and racing. *Acta Anat.* **146**: 183–187.

Clayton, H.M. (1994a) Comparison of the stride kinematics of the collected, working, medium and extended trot in horses. *Equine Vet. J.* **26**: 230–234.

Clayton, H.M. (1994b) Comparison of the collected, working, medium and extended canters. *Equine Vet. J.* **17** (Suppl.): 16–19.

Clayton, H.M. (1995) Comparison of the stride kinematics of the collected, medium, and extended walks in horses. *Am. J. Vet. Res.* **56**: 849–852.

Clayton, H.M. (1997a) Classification of collected trot, passage and piaffe using stance phase temporal variables. *Equine Vet. J.* **2** (Suppl.): 54–57.

Clayton, H.M. (1997b) Effect of added weight on landing kinematics of jumping horses. *Equine Vet. J.* **23** (Suppl.): 50–53.

Clayton, H.M. and Barlow, D.A. (1989) The effect of fence height and width on the limb placements of show jumping horses. *J. Equine. Vet. Sci.* **9**: 179–185.

Clayton, H.M. and Barlow, D.A. (1991) Stride characteristics of four Grand Prix jumping horses. *Equine Exerc. Physiol.* **3**: 51–157.

Clayton, H.M., Colborne, G.R. and Burns, T.E. (1995) Kinematics analysis of successful and unsuccessful attempts to clear a water jump. *Equine. Vet. J.* **18** (Suppl.): 166–169.

Clayton, H.M., Colborne, G.R., Lanovaz, J. and Burns, T.E. (1996) Linear kinematics of water jumping in Olympic show jumpers. *Pferdeheilkunde* **12**: 657–660.

Clayton, H.M., Lanovaz, J.L., Schamhardt, H.C., Willemen, M.A. and Colborne, G.R. (1998) Net joint moments and joint powers in the equine fore limb during the stance phase of the trot. *Equine. Vet. J.* **30** : 384–389.

Clayton, H.M., Lanovaz, J.L., Schamhardt, H.C. and Wessum, R. van (1999) Rider effects on ground reaction forces and fetlock kinematics at the trot. *Equine Vet. J.* **30** (Suppl.): 235–239.

Clayton, H.M., Hodson, E. and Lanovaz, J.L. (2000) The fore limb in walking horses. 2. Net joint moments and powers. *Equine Vet. J.* **32**: 295–300.

Colborne, G.R., Clayton, H.M. and Lanovaz, J.L. (1995) Factors that influence vertical velocity during take off over a water jump. *Equine Vet. J.* **18** (Suppl.): 138–140.

Corley, J.M. and Goodship, A.E. (1994) Treadmill training induced changes to some kinematic variables measured at the canter of Thoroughbred fillies. *Equine Vet. J.* **17** (Suppl.): 20–24.

Cothran, E.G., MacCluer, J.W., Weitkamp, L.R. and Bailey, E. (1987) Genetic differentiation associated with gait within American Standardbred horses. *Anim. Genetics* **18**: 285–296.

Crawford, W.H. and Leach, D.H. (1984) The effect of racetrack design on gait symmetry of the pacer. *Can. J. Comp. Med.* **48**: 374–380.

Dalin, G., Drevemo, S., Fredricson, I., Jonsson, K. and Nilsson, G. (1973) Ergonomic aspects of locomotor asymmetry in Standardbred horses trotting through turns. *Acta Vet. Scand.* **44** (Suppl.): 111–139.

Dalin, G., Magnusson, L.-E. and Thafvelin, B.C. (1985) Retrospective study of hindquarter asymmetry in Standardbred trotters and its correlation with performance. *Equine. Vet. J.* **17**: 292–296.

Deuel, N.R. (1995) Dressage canter kinematics and performances in an Olympic three-day event. *Proc. Eur. Assoc. Anim. Prod.* **46**: 341–344.

Deuel, N.R. and Lawrence, L.M. (1986) Gallop velocity and limb contact variables of Quarter Horses. *J. Equine Vet. Sci.* **6**: 143–147.

Deuel, N.R. and Lawrence, L.M. (1987a) Laterality in the gallop gait of horses. *J. Biomech.* **20**: 645–649.

Deuel, N.R. and Lawrence, L.M. (1987b) Effects of urging by the rider on equine gallop stride limb contacts. *Proc. Equine Nutr. Physiol.* **10**: 487–494.

Deuel, N.R. and Park, J. (1990) The gait patterns of Olympic dressage horses. *Int. J. Sport Biomech.* **6**: 198–226.

Deuel, N.R. and Park, J. (1991) Kinematic analysis of jumping sequences of Olympic show jumping horses. *Equine Exerc. Physiol.* **3**: 158–166.

Deuel, N.R. and Park, J. (1993) Gallop kinematics of Olympic three-day event horses. *Acta Anat.* **146**: 168–174.

Drevemo, S., Dalin, G., Fredricson, I. and Hjerten, G. (1980a) Equine locomotion. 1. The analysis of linear and temporal stride characteristics of trotting Standardbreds. *Equine Vet. J.* **12**: 60–65.

Drevemo, S., Fredricson, I., Dalin, G. and Bjorne, K. (1980b) Equine locomotion. 2. The analysis of coordination between limbs of trotting Standardbreds. *Equine Vet. J.* **12**: 66–70.

Drevemo, S., Dalin, G., Fredricson, I. and Bjorne, K. (1980c) Equine locomotion. 3. The reproductibility of gait in Standardbred trotters. *Equine Vet. J.* **12**: 71–73.

Drevemo, S., Fredricson, I., Hjerten, G. and McMiken, D. (1987) Early development of gait asymmetries in trotting Standardbred colts. *Equine Vet. J.* **19**: 189–191.

Dušek, J., Ehrlein, H.-J., Engelhardt, W.V. and Hornicke, H. (1970) Beziehungen zwischen Tritlange, Trittfrequenz und Geschwindigkeit bei Pferden. *A Tierzucht ZuchtBiol* **87**: 177–188.

Ellersieck, M.R., Lock, W.E., Vogt, G.W. *et al.* (1985) Genetic evaluation of cutting scores in horses. *J. Equine Vet. Sci.* **5**: 287–289.

Estberg, L., Stover, S., Gardner, I.A. *et al.* (1995) Several racing-career intensity characteristics are associated with racing-related fatal skeletal injury in California Thoroughbred racehorses. *Proc. Am. Assoc. Equine Practnr.* **41**: 82–83.

Fabiani, M. (1973) Proba wczesnej oceny zdolnosci koni do skokow. II Konie z Zakladow Treningowych w Kwidzynie i Bialym Borze. *Prace i Materiały Zootechniczne* **4**: 39–54.

Farley, C. and Taylor, R.C. (1991) A mechanical trigger for the trot-gallop transition in horses. *Science* **253**: 306–308.

Fredricson, I., Dalin, G., Drevemo, S. and Hjertén, G. (1975) A biotechnical approach to the geometric design of racetracks. *Equine Vet. J.* **7**: 91–96.

Fredricson, I., Hellander, J., Hjertén, G. *et al.* (1983) Gait-pattern stability in Thoroughbreds galloping on different track surfaces. *Svensk Veterinartidning* **35** (Suppl 3): 83–88.

Galloux, P. and Barrey, E. (1997) Components of the total kinetic moment in jumping horses. *Equine Vet. J.* **23** (Suppl.): 41–44.

Hellander, J., Fredricson, I., Hjertén, G., Drevemo, S. and Dalin, G. (1983) The galloping gait. I. Variable features at different speeds. *Svensk Veterinartidning* **35**: 75–82.

Hildebrand, M. (1962) Walking, running and jumping. *Int. Zoologist* **2**, 151–155.

Hiraga, A., Yamanobe, A. and Katsuyoshi, K. (1994) Relationships between stride length, stride frequency, step length and velocity at the start dash in a racehorse. *J. Equine Sci.* **5**: 127–130.

Hodson, E., Clayton, H.M. and Lanovaz, J.L. (1999) Temporal analysis of walk movements in the Grand Prix dressage test at the 1996 Olympic Games. *Appl. Anim. Behav. Sci.* **62**: 89–97.

Holmström, M. and Drevemo, S. (1997) Effects of trot quality and collection on the angular velocity in the hindlimbs of riding horses. *Equine Vet. J.* **2** (Suppl.): 62–65.

Holmström, M., Magnusson, L.E. and Philipsson, J. (1990) Variation in conformation of Swedish Warmblood horses and conformational characteristics of elite sport horses. *Equine Vet. J.* **22**: 186–193.

Holmström, M., Fredricson, I. and Drevemo, S. (1994) Biokinematic differences between riding horses judged as good and poor at the trot. *Equine Vet. J.* **17** (Suppl.): 51–56.

Holmström, M., Fredricson, I. and Drevemo, S. (1995) Biokinematic effects of collection on the trotting gaits in the elite dressage horse. *Equine Vet. J.* **27**: 281–287.

Hoyt, D.F. and Taylor, C.R. (1981) Gait and energetics of locomotion in horses. *Nature* **292**: 239–240.

Ishii, K., Amano, K. and Sakuraoka, H. (1989) Kinematic analysis of horse gaits. *Bull. Equine Res. Inst.* **26**: 1–9.

Jelen, B. (1976) Faktyczna I umowna wyokosc skokow koni przez przeszkody I niektore warunkujace ja czynniki. *Zootechniczna* **97**: 79–91.

Kai, M. and Kubo, K. (1993) Respiration pause and gait after the start dash in a horse. *Bull. Equine Res. Inst.* **30**: 26–29.

Knezevic, P.F. von, Kastner, J., Girtler, D. and Holzreiter, St (1987) Hochfrequenzkinematographische Messungen am Pferd in der Kapriole. *Dtsch tierartztl Wschr* **94**: 141–146.

Kobluk, C.N., Schnurr, D., Horney, F.D., Sumner-Smith, G., Willoughby, R.A. and DeKleer, V. (1989) Use of high-speed cinematography and computer generated gait diagrams for the study of equine hind limb kinematics. *Equine Vet. J.* **21**: 48–58.

Kroll, W. and Clarkson, P.M. (1977) Fractionated reflex time, resisted and unresisted fractionated reflex time under normal and fatigued conditions. In: Landers, D.M. & Christiana, R.W. (eds) *Psychology of Motor Behavior and Sport.* Champaign: Human Kinetic Publishers Inc., pp. 106–129.

Langlois, B., Froidevaux, J., Lamarche, L., *et al.* (1978) Analyse des liasons entre la morphologie et l'aptitude au galop au trot et au saut d'obstacles chez le cheval. *Ann. Genet. Sel. Anim.* **10**: 443–474.

Lauk, H.D., Auer, J. and Plocki, K.A. von (1991) Zum Problem "Barren" Uberblick, biomechanische Berechnungen und Verhaltungsbeobachtungen. *Pferdeheilkunde* **7**: 225–235.

Leach, D.H. and Cymbaluk, N. (1986) Relationships between stride length, stride frequency, velocity and morphometrics of foals. *Am. J. Vet. Res.* **47**: 2090–2097.

Leach, D.H. and Ormrod, K. (1984) The technique of jumping a steeplechase fence by competing event-horses. *Appl. Anim. Behav. Sci.* **12**: 15–24.

Leach, D.H. and Sprigings, E. (1979) Gait fatigue in the racing Thoroughbred. *J. Equine Med. Surg.* **3**: 436–443.

Leach, D.H., Sprigings, E.J. and Laverty, W.H. (1987) Multivariate statistical analysis of stride-timing measurements of nonfatigued racing Thoroughbreds. *Am. J. Vet. Res.* **48**: 880–888.

Lewczuk, D. and Pfeffer, M. (1998) Investigation on the horses' stride length during endurance race competition using video image analysis. In: *Conference on Equine Sports Medicine and Science.* The Netherlands: Wageningen Pers, pp. 249–250.

Magnusson, L.-E. (1985) Studies on the conformation and related traits of standardbred trotters in Sweden. *PhD thesis, Skara, Swedish University of Agricultural Sciences.*

Merkens, H.W., Schamhardt, H.C., Osch, G.J.V.M. van and Bogert, A.J. van den (1991) Ground reaction force analysis of Dutch Warmblood horses at canter and jumping. *Equine Exerc. Physiol.* **3**: 128–135.

Merkens, H.W., Schamhardt, H.C., Osch, G.J.V.M. van and Hartman, W. (1993) Ground reaction force patterns of Dutch Warmbloods at the canter. *Am. J. Vet. Res.* **54**: 670–674.

Moyer, W. and Fisher, J.R.S. (1991) Bucked shins: effects of differing track surfaces and proposed training regimens. *Proc. Am. Assoc. Equine. Practnr.* **37**: 541–547.

Normand, M.C., Lagasse, P.P., Rouillard, C.A. *et al.* (1982) Modifications occurring in motor programs during learning of a complex task in man. *Brain Res.* **241**: 87–93.

Persson, S.G.B., Essen-Gustavsson, B. and Lindholm, A. (1991) Energy profile and the locomotor pattern of trotting on an inclined treadmill. *Equine Exerc. Physiol.* **3**: 231–238.

Pratt, G.W. (1983) Remarks on gait analysis. *Equine Exerc. Physiol.* **2**: 245–262.

Pratt, G.W. and O'Connor, J.T. Jr. (1976) Force plate studies of equine biomechanics. *Am. J. Vet. Res.* **37**, 1251–1255.

Preuschoft, H. (1989) The external forces and internal stresses in the feet of dressage and jumping horses. *Z. Säugetierkunde* **54**: 172–190.

Quddus, M.A., Kingsbury, H.B. and Rooney, J.R. (1978) A force and motion study of the foreleg of a Standardbred trotter. *J. Equine Med. Surg.* **2**: 233–242.

Ratzlaff, M.H., Shindell, R.M. and White, K.K. (1985) The interrelationships of stride length and stride times to velocities of galloping horses. *J. Equine Vet. Sci.* **5**: 279–283.

Ratzlaff, M.H., Grant, B.D., Frame, J.M. and Hyde, M.L. (1987) Locomotor forces of galloping horses. *Equine Exerc. Physiol.* **2**: 574–586.

Rivero, J.-LL. and Clayton, H.M. (1996) The potential role of the muscle in kinematic characteristics. *Pferdeheilkunde* **12**: 635–640.

Roneus, N., Essen-Gustavsson, B., Johnston, C. and Persson, S. (1995) Lactate response to maximal exercise on the track: relation to muscle characteristics and kinematic variables. *Equine Vet. J.* **18** (Suppl.): 191–194.

Rooney, J.R. (1969) Lameness of the forelimb. In: *Biomechanics of Lameness in Horses.* Baltimore: Williams and Wilkins, 114–196.

Schamhardt, H.C., Merkens, H.W. and Osch, G.J.V.M. van (1991) Ground reaction force analysis of horse ridden at walk and trot. *Equine Exerc. Physiol.* **3**: 120–127.

Schamhardt, H.C., Merkens, H.W., Vogel, V. and Willekens, C. (1993) External loads on the limbs of jumping horses at take-off and landing. *Am. J. Vet. Res.* **54**: 675–680.

Schills, S.J., Greer, N.L., Stoner, L.J. and Kobluk, C.N. (1993) Kinematic analysis of the equestrian – walk, posting trot and sitting trot. *Hum. Movement Sci.* **12**: 693–712.

Seder, J.A. and Vickery, C.E. (1993) Double and triple fully airborne phases in the gaits of racing speed Thoroughbreds. *Abstr. Second Int. Workshop on Anim. Locom.*, pp. 59–60.

Sellett, L.C., Albert, W.W. and Groppel, J.L. (1981) Forelimb kinematics of the Standardbred pacing gait. *Proc. Equine Nutr. Physiol.*, pp. 210–215.

Stover, S.M., Johnson, B.J., Daft, B.M., *et al.* (1992) An association between complete and incomplete stress fractures of the humerus in racehorses. *Equine Vet. J.* **24**: 260–263.

Ueda, Y., Yoshida, K. and Oikawa, M. (1993) Analyses of race accident conditions through use of patrol video. *J. Equine Vet. Sci.* **13**: 707–710.

Viitsalo, J.T. and Komi, P.V. (1981) Interrelationships between electromyographic, mechanical, muscle structure and reflex time measurements. *Acta Physiol. Scand.* **111**: 97–103.

Weeren, P.R. van, Bogert, A.J. van den, Back, W., Bruin, G. and Barneveld, A. (1993) Kinematics of the Standardbred trotter measured at 6, 7, 8 and 9 m/s on a treadmill, before and after 5 months of prerace training. *Acta Anat.* **2–3**: 81–204.

Wilson, B.D., Neal, R.J., Howard, A. and Groenendyk, S. (1988a) The gait of pacers 1: kinematics of the racing stride. *Equine Vet. J.* **20**: 341–346.

Wilson, B.D., Neal, R.J., Howard, A. and Groenendyk, S. (1988b) The gait of pacers 2: factors influencing pacing speed. *Equine Vet. J.* **20**: 347–351.

Yamanobe, A., Hiraga, A. and Kubo, K. (1992) Relationships between stride frequency, stride length, step length and velocity with asymmetric gaits in the Thoroughbred horse. *Jap. J. Equine Sci.* **3**: 143–148.

9
Exercise Effects on the Skeletal Tissues

Allen E. Goodship and Helen L. Birch

INTRODUCTION

The horse has become one of the most successful animal athletes and is used at both amateur and professional levels in numerous types of sporting event. Its athletic capabilities have developed, through evolution, from the modern horse's ancestor: the small Hyracotherium (Eohippus). These creatures were only about the size of a fox terrier, with short legs and relatively long heads. They had three toes on the hindfeet and four on the forefeet, with digital pads (Fig. 9.1A). Since the first appearance of these animals some 50 million years ago in the Tertiary period evolution, predominantly on the North American continent, has led to the high-speed, long-legged ungulate equine species of modern times (Fig. 9.1B). This transformation has arisen due to environmental factors governing long-term changes in anatomical and physiological features, and also as a result of body systems and their inherent capacity for functional adaptation.

General adaptation during evolution, therefore, has resulted in considerable natural athletic potential. The morphological developments that have imparted advantage for high-speed locomotion include:

- elongated slender limbs, with muscles located proximally close to the center of mass
- controlled ranges of movement in the joints of the lower limb
- utilization of the collagenous components of the muscles to reduce energy requirements in posture and locomotion.

Additional energetic efficiency has been achieved by utilization of the elastic energy stored in the flexor tendons in the stance phase of locomotion; this conserved energy is then released in the take-off and swing phases of the gait cycle. Throughout equine development, there has also been a reduction in bone mass in the distal bones of the limb (an adaptation not without some risk). However this reduction in bone mass reduces the energy required for the changes in momentum that occur in cursorial locomotion with the oscillations of the limb (Currey, 1984). The different gaits also play a role in optimizing energetic efficiency in locomotion by minimizing oxygen uptake at particular speeds corresponding to the recognizable equine gaits. (Hoyt and Taylor 1981). The associated reduction in bone deformation that occurs at the trot/canter transition (Rubin & Lanyon, 1982), also reduces the risk of mechanical damage to the bony structures of the limb, at faster pace.

The systems of lever arms formed by the appendicular skeleton and its associated joints and muscles have also evolved for fast movement, the proximally located multipennate muscles acting on short levers such as the olecranon to effect rapid large arcs of movement of the lower

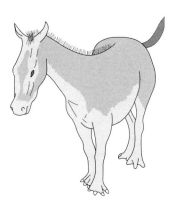

Fig. 9.1A An illustration of the primitive ancestor of the modern horse.

limb. In addition to the structural adaptations, physiological changes have resulted in increased athletic capacity of the evolving horse. Lactate tolerance, hemoglobin concentration, oxygen transport, heat exchange and muscle function all appear to be greater in the equine athlete than in its human counterpart (Wilson, 1991).

The ability of tissues, organs and systems to adapt to changes in functional demand enables individuals to be trained for enhanced athletic performance (within the limits of the performance potential of that individual and the suitability of the training regimen). It is the capacity for functional adaptation that allows the body systems to optimize structure and function for particular changes in conditions or demands throughout life. Different body systems respond to different types of input stimulus. The rate of change in these input conditions may also determine whether the system adapts or, alternatively, sustains damage, resulting in partial or total system failure. This chapter will focus on the skeletal tissues; however, the principles of adaptive response apply in general terms to all body tissues and systems.

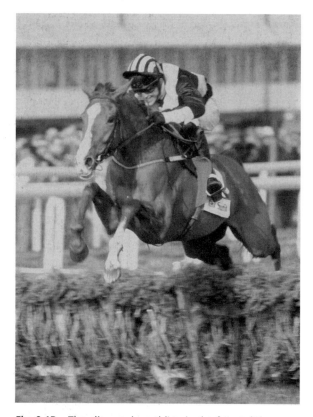

Fig. 9.1B The elite equine athlete in the form of the Thoroughbred racehorse.

Horses used for competitive events, whether at amateur or professional level, are by definition challenged to perform at a higher level than their wild counterparts. The ability to induce an increase in performance is a factor of both the inherent genetic potential of the individual horse and the ability of the trainer to utilize adaptive responses by applying an appropriate training regimen to maximize performance. Genetic potential can be increased by a combination of experience and science in selective breeding; however, it has been suggested that in the case of the racing Thoroughbred, due to gene pool limitations, the maximum improvement in 'genetic' performance has already been attained (Hill, 1988).

However, training methods and documentation of performance has to a large extent been based on tradition and experience. The lack of improvement in racing performance in terms of times to complete distances in classic races may be the result of the traditional approach to training together with differences in horse racing objectives compared with human racing objectives. In horse racing, national and world time performances are not the key goals: the objective is merely to win particular races. Notwithstanding possible differences in racing objectives, the developing science of equine sports medicine is in its infancy compared with the state of knowledge in the human field. Only when trainers are able to translate advances in scientific understanding into practical training methods will it become possible to assess any differences in performance or injury incidence compared with traditional training methods.

General responses to training

For most biological systems there is a capacity for adaptation to achieve an optimal state in the face of imposed conditions. The characteristics of the most effective stimuli to induce optimization may differ between systems and particular tissues. Therefore, it is important to understand these variations in stimulation and response for specific tissues, organs and systems when designing an effective conditioning and training protocol for specific athletic requirements. In general, training comprises the imposition of an increasing demand to elicit a progressive response and increased functional performance in the biological system being 'trained'. In essence the inherent capacity for functional adaptation is exploited in a controlled manner. The skill in training is to adjust the timing and extent of the input stimulus to achieve maximum increase in performance at the required time for athletic competition. An underestimate of the training input will not achieve maximum potential in performance, whereas an overestimate will exceed the capacity for functional adaptation and lead to over-training injuries with possible irreversible damage to tissues and systems.

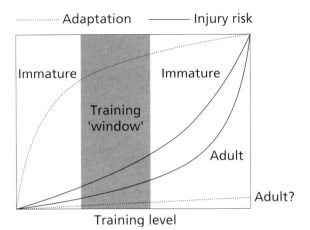

Fig. 9.2   A diagrammatic plot of training input as a function of gain in performance showing a 'safe zone' for maximizing training response; this safe zone will not be the same in terms of specific training input for different tissues.

The relationship between input stimulus and biological response is not linear. As the level and duration of training increases the respective gains in performance are reduced. The role of the scientific approach to training is to define in objective terms the specific responses of the different systems to defined training stimuli in order that the training protocol can lead to the attainment of the 'safe zone' (Fig. 9.2).

Tissue-specific responses to exercise are also seen in rehabilitation, where there is a need to both retrain tissues that may have undergone atrophy during the period in which an injury has been treated and also to condition the repair tissue formed as a consequence of injury. In the case of tendon injury, a controlled and monitored reintroduction of exercise will induce alignment of the collagen fibers formed during the repair process. This alignment occurs as a result of the tensile cyclical stresses sustained by the tendon.

In order to maximize the potential in all systems but also to avoid over-training or induced injury in any system, a training protocol must include a range of different specific stimuli. In terms of the skeletal system, the aim is to enhance the structural and material properties of each component to withstand the forces imposed during peak locomotor performance. Even within the skeletal system, the specific tissues respond to different types of stimulation. Our knowledge of the mechanisms controlling adaptation of skeletal tissues has increased markedly over the last decade and it is now possible to incorporate some scientific principles into training regimens for the equine athlete.

RESPONSE OF SPECIFIC SKELETAL TISSUES TO EXERCISE

Within the skeletal system the component tissues comprise bone, cartilage, tendon and ligament. There are, of course, subdivisions in which some of the extracellular matrices will have a specific composition at a specific site; for example, the composition of tendon differs between regions that are predominantly in axial tension, where the matrix is predominantly type I collagen, and regions where the tendon passes around a bone, where the matrix is fibrocartilage and contains a significant proportion of type II collagen. This chapter will not consider skeletal muscle since the morphology and functional characteristics are well documented in standard texts. In addition, the incidence of injury in equine athletes is greatest in the locomotor system and primarily affects the skeletal tissues outlined above (Rossdale *et al.*, 1985; Wilson *et al.*, 1996). The response of different component tissues and defined locomotor 'organs', such as synovial joints, is complex and not fully understood. Over the last decade the understanding of the underlying mechanisms that control the interactions between mechanical environment and skeletal tissue response has advanced significantly. Since different tissues respond to specific types of mechanical input, and entities such as joints consist of a number of different component tissues, it is impotant to understand the interaction of the adaptive changes in relation to the role of particular tissues within the structure. For instance, if training methods are used to increase bone mass and thus reduce fracture risk, the impact of increasing bone density on the shock-absorbing role of subchondral bone must also be considered. As will be discussed later, the increased stiffness of subchondral bone may be linked to detrimental effects on cartilage.

The effects of exercise, and thus information that might be applied to training protocols, will first be considered for each specific tissue. However, in application of the information to practical training methods, the conditioning of the *whole* animal has to be considered and appropriate compromises, as well as the potential for gains, addressed.

Bone

Bone, both as a tissue and an organ, responds to changes in imposed mechanical conditions. Indeed, the size and shape of component bones of the skeleton is determined not only by predetermined genetic factors but also by the exercise history and prevailing training input. The relationship between form and function in bone has

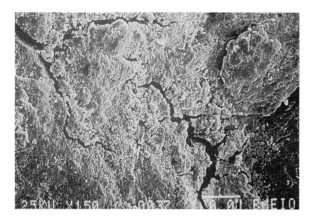

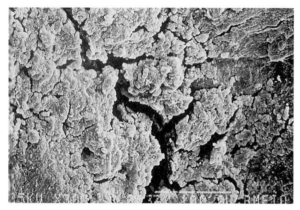

Fig. 9.3 A photomicograph of microcracking in bone; a fractel pattern of microcracks is seen in this process. (Tomlin *et al.*, 2000. © European Calcified Tissue Society)

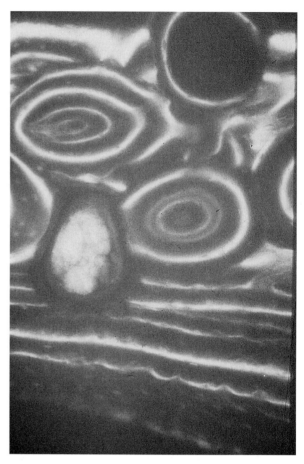

Fig. 9.4 A photomicrograph showing the porosity formed by osteoclastic resorption of damaged matrix and also formation of the secondary osteon. (With permission from WB Saunders: from Goodship *et al. Sciences Basic to Orthopaedics,* Hughes and McCarthy, (eds) 1998 .

been known for a long time, with the classic observations by Julius Wolff in the 1890s formulating the concepts that bone mass is related to the magnitude of prevailing mechanical forces and bone architecture reflects the distribution of these forces. For many bones these factors modulate the underlying genetically determined skeletal structure: hence the differences in 'bone stock' between individuals and breeds of horse. Since the horse in general and the equine athlete in particular have evolved for speed in locomotion, an unduly high mass of bone would increase energy requirements. There is thus a conflict between provision of an adequate 'safety factor' to avoid fracture with occasional overloads, and reducing bone mass for energetic efficiency but with fracture risk increasing during peak loading conditions. This conflict of requirements has resulted in a site-specific difference between functional loading conditions and bone mass. Thus the bones of the distal limb are less protected by in-built additional bone mass to allow for overload situations. Currey (1984) has related the incidence of bone fractures reported in the racehorse by Vaughan and

Mason (1975) to this biological strategy for energetic efficiency and shown that there is a greater incidence of fracture in the more distal bones of the limb. In addition, there appears to be a different damage limitation strategy in terms of avoiding catastrophic failure. Whereas in the majority of skeletal sites controlled increased loading results in adaptive hypertrophy, in the distal bones of the equine limb there appears to be a system of microcracking that may play a role in prevention of major crack propagation. This type of response has been observed in Thoroughbred horses subjected to controlled exercise conditions. Compared with horses given low-intensity exercise, those subjected to higher levels of exercise showed the presence of microcracks (Fig. 9.3) and these bones had significantly greater fracture toughness (Reilly *et al.*, 1997; Vashishth *et al.*, 1997).

In the circumstances just described, the exercise was imposed in a controlled manner. The adaptive response of bone requires a gradual increase in mechanical demand. If increased loading is imposed over too short a period at levels that are too great, then fatigue damage occurs. The presence of fatigue damage results in pain and reduced performance, lameness and even consequent gross fracture. This response is seen in ballet dancers, army recruits and racehorses.

Nunamaker *et al.* (1990, 1991) have given explanations for the site-specific accumulation of microdamage in the cortex of the cannon bone of horses in training. This condition, known as 'sore shins' or 'bucked shins', is a common exercise-related complication of training and is also seen in human athletes (Jones *et al.*, 1989). When a bone is subjected to a high number of loading cycles over a relatively short period of time the cells are unable to synthesize matrix fast enough to reduce the local tissue strains. Consequently, the yield strain of the material is exceeded and local matrix damage occurs. The local sites of damage may initiate a remodeling response, in which the bone-removing cells (osteoclasts) are activated and remove damaged matrix. This creates a local porosity within the bone cortex. The porosity is then filled in with circumferential layers of bone (lamellae) to form a secondary osteon (Fig. 9.4); thus, the damaged region of the bone will become remodelled with secondary osteonal bone. The secondary bone is a weaker material than primary bone. Therefore, some training methods that lead directly or indirectly to micro-damage, may induce a greater level of secondary remodeling of the skeleton. It has been shown that bone loaded to yield point will exhibit microcracking and this will lead to secondary osteon formation, even in species where such remodeling is normally minimal (Bentolila *et al.*, 1998). Provided that the training is progressed over an appropriate time course, the bone cell populations are able to increase matrix synthesis and deposition in a mechanically appropriate manner to model the structure and size of the bone and optimize the structure for the new functional requirements.

Current research is addressing the possibility of using blood markers both to monitor changes in bone during training and to identify individuals at risk of fracture. In a controlled exercise study over 1 year in 2-year-old Thoroughbreds, the effects of the exercise on two biochemical markers of bone formation were determined. These markers were the carboxy-terminal propeptide of type I collagen and the bone-specific alkaline phosphatase. In addition one potential marker of bone resorption, the pyridinoline cross-linked telopeptide domain of type I collagen, was also monitored. In both the low- and high-intensity exercised groups there was a significant reduction in marker lev-

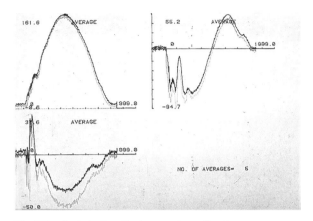

Fig. 9.5 A plot of vertical ground reaction force as a function of time showing the heel strike transient in the trotting pony.

els over the year – this is expected as a normal age-related change. However, it was encouraging that the pattern of reduction differed between groups in a way that indicated an increase in bone turnover in the high-intensity trained group (Price *et al.*, 1995). These results are encouraging as they indicate the potential to develop a non-invasive method of monitoring the effects of training on bone.

Basic research over the last two decades has provided evidence that the response of bone to increased loading can be elicited by very short periods of daily training (Rubin & Lanyon, 1984). Interestingly, the types of exercise that result in rapid and diverse loading of the bones are most potent in increasing bone mass. For example, in the human athlete, sports that involve weight bearing and high impact loading are more effective in increasing bone mass than non-weight bearing or low-impact activites (Fehling *et al.*, 1995; Heinonen *et al.*, 1995).

Different types of exercise can also affect specific sites of the skeleton. In human osteoporosis it has been shown that jumping exercises can increase bone mass in areas of the skeleton that are predilection sites for fracture, such as the neck of the femur in the hip and the vertebral bodies of the spine. Interestingly, a slight change in the way the jumps are performed causes the beneficial changes to be seen in the different parts of the skeleton (Bassey, personal communication). Again, only short periods of these osteogenic exercises are required; it is possibly that too long a period of exercise may result in a risk of fatigue damage.

There is some evidence that high-frequency transients are important in maintaining bone mass. These transients are seen in both man and horse and may be recorded at the time of heel strike (Fig. 9.5). In long-term space flight the reduction in gravity results in an

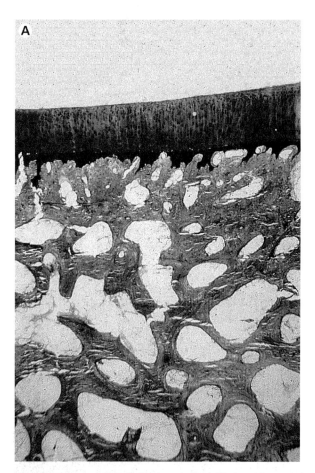 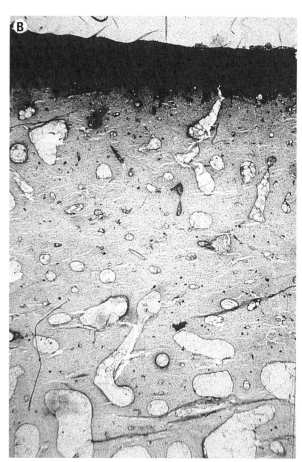

Fig. 9.6 The variation in thickness of calcified cartilage and underlying subchondral bone in the dorsal regions of the third carpal bone as a result of imposed exercise. (Reproduced with permission from Murray, RC. Does exercise cause adaptation or degeneration of the equine middle carpal joint? PhD thesis, University of Liege, 2000.)

absence of the heel strike transient. There is a generalized reduction in bone mass associated with long-term space flight but the distribution of bone loss varies, with the major losses occurring in the distal bones of the lower limb, particularly the calcaneus. In an experiment on the MIR space station a simulated heel strike transient was applied to one heel of an astronaut for around 10 minutes per day, and bone mass measured before and after the flight in both legs. The unstimulated limb showed a 5–7% reduction compared with pre-flight values; however, no significant loss of bone was detected in the stimulated limb (Goodship *et al.*, 1998). This suggests that very short periods of exercise that engenders high impact loading, such as trotting on a hard surface, will stimulate an increase in bone mass.

A very interesting recent finding by Qin *et al.* (1998) showed that bone formation can be stimulated by application of levels of bone deformation greatly below the levels that occur with locomotion, provided that

the cyclical loading is imposed with a very specific frequency. Very low levels of cyclical strain at around 30 cycles per second activate bone formation. Although this work is targeted at prevention and treatment of osteoporosis, there may be applications in the conditioning of bone in horses. For instance, use of this type of stimulus to initiate increased bone mass may reduce the incidence of fatigue fractures during the early phases of training.

The magnitude and rate of bone deformation increases with speed of locomotion. In the case of the horse, and other animals that can change gait, the gait transitions serve not only to optimize oxygen transport (Hoyt & Taylor, 1981) but also to limit strain magnitude in the limb bones (Rubin & Lanyon, 1982). Thus, it is likely that in the case of horses in which there is a natural or induced extension of a particular gait, such as occurs in trotting races, the training and performance of these animals results in high-magnitude strain levels in the limb bones. Consequently, horses subjected to high numbers of high-magnitude strain cycles, particularly over a short training period, are at risk of conditions such as bucked or sore shins.

As stated above, the changes in bone mass induced by osteogenic mechanical stimulation occur with only short periods of daily activity and are localized in those parts of the skeleton acting as the functional load paths. These regions of increased bone mass can indirectly affect other skeletal tissues. An example of this interaction is seen in the carpal joint. The bones of the carpal joint are short bones, characterized by an internal structure of cancellous bone supporting a thin overlying cortex and articular hyaline cartilage at the articular ends. Bones with this type of structure are usually loaded in near axial compression compared with the long bones, which have evolved a tubular form to resist the torsional and bending moments applied by muscles and locomotor forces.

The internal structure of the short bones comprises cancellous bone; although the rods and plates of bone in this architecture appear to be randomly arranged, this is not the case – they are in fact arranged strategically to provide maximum strength with minimum material. The prevailing loading conditions influence the geometrical arrangement and the size of the elements of cancellous bone. One of the functions of this type of bone, underlying an articular surface of a synovial joint, is to absorb shock or impact loads. This functional role of shock absorption acts to protect the overlying hyaline cartilage from damaging mechanical loads. It has been shown that adaptation of the subchondral bone can result in a decrease in the shock absorbing capacity. This is due to the increase in mass of the trabeculae increasing the bulk stiffness of the subchondral bone. The increased stiffness and reduced shock absorption causes the impact loads to damage the hyaline cartilage and contribute to degenerative joint disease (Radin *et al.*, 1973).

In response to exercise in the horse, it has been shown that the biological system attempts to preserve the integrity of the articular cartilage above the hypertrophied subchondral bone by increasing the thickness of the calcified layer while maintaining the thickness of the hyaline cartilage (Murray *et al.*, 1999) (Fig. 9.6). In two separate series of Thoroughbreds trained for both long periods of time (18 months) and short periods of time (4 months) the higher levels of exercise resulted in a site-specific adaptive hypertrophy in the radial and third metacarpal bones (Firth *et al.*, 1999). Although these horses were trained on a treadmill, similar adaptive responses were observed in a series of animals subjected to over-ground training in New Zealand. The effects of the increased level of exercise was to increase the bone mineral density in the dorsal regions of the radial and third carpal bones compared with the low-intensity exer-

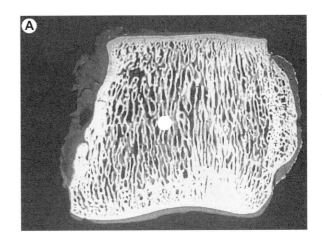

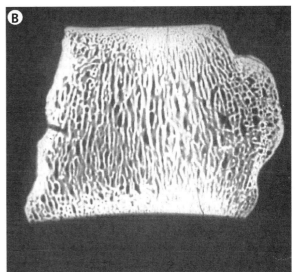

Fig. 9.7 Slab microradiographs of exercise and control carpal bones, showing localized intraosseous hypertrophy of the subchondral bone and underlying trabeculae in response to exercise. (From Firth *et al.* 1999, ©EVJ Ltd).

cised controls. Interestingly, the increased bone density of the trabecular bone in the dorsal location underlies the region of articular hyaline cartilage that is often found to be damaged on arthroscopic examination (Firth, personal communication). In addition the dramatic change in trabecular bone density between the palmar and dorsal regions of the two short bones is at the very plane in which slab or chip fractures occur in the third carpal bone (Fig. 9.7).

Only short periods of high-intensity physiological exercise are required to induce these changes in bone density. It could be argued that in most cases the management of the elite equine athlete is traditionally one of stable housing for the majority of the day interspersed with bouts of low-and high-intensity exercise. Thus, this traditional management system favors bone remodeling and, indeed, in terms of bony adaptation the levels and type of exercise used may increase the localized subchondral bone density in some joints such as the carpal joint and predispose the joint to degenerative joint disease. It is important, therefore, to balance the need to condition the bony skeleton to withstand the rigours of peak athletic performance with the potential for the adaptive response to become detrimental to the overall training goals. With increasing knowledge of the specific tissue responses, it should be possible to incorporate a scientific basis to the traditional approaches to training.

Cartilage

Mechanical effects on articular and physeal cartilage during growth

Hyaline cartilage forms the articular surface of the synovial joints of the limbs in the adult horse. The articular surface expands as the epiphysis grows by endochondral ossification of the spheriod physis, the secondary ossification center; longitudinal growth proceeds by ossification of the discoid physis. Mechanical forces influence the development of the bones not only by a direct action on bone cells but also indirectly by influences on the hyaline cartilage of these physes. There are complex interactions between the different growth centers and associated structures such as the periosteum. Changes in the levels of static and dynamic loads influence the rate of growth. Long bones with physes at both proximal and distal extremities can exhibit compensatory effects if there is a compromise of one physis. During growth, mechanical forces occur in the periosteum and it is well established, both experimentally and clinically, that sectioning of the periosteum can influence the curvature of the growing bone (Auer & Martens, 1982; Bertone *et al.*, 1985; Leitch, 1985). There are varying reports of the effects of exercise on the hyaline cartilage of these physes, in particular with reference to development of osteochondral defects.

Pathologies of the process of ossification, the osteochondroses (dyschondroplasias), can also be influenced by the mechanical environment and thus by the type and level of exercise given to developing animals. It has been shown recently that the incidence of osteochondroses, even in animals with a genetic predisposition, is influenced by exercise (Bruin & Creemers, 1994). Young horses subjected to high levels of exercise did not show as high an incidence of osteochondritis as the control group given lower levels of exercise.

In the young animal the spheroid physis provides not only an articular surface but also the capacity for growth and development of the epiphysis through the ossification of the growing hyaline cartilage precursor until, at skeletal maturity, the only cartilage present is the articular surface of the epiphysis. Hyaline cartilage is a connective tissue comprising cells and matrix and, as with all connective tissues, there is a complex interaction both between individual cells and between cells and their surrounding matrix. The morphology of cells differs within the thickness of the cartilage. The hyaline surface layer is separated from the underlying subchondral bone by a zone of calcified cartilage (Fig. 9.8).

In the neonate the articular cartilage across the entire joint surface has a very similar matrix composition. However, as the animal subjects the joints to weight-bearing and the forces of locomotion there is a topographical change in matrix composition within the joint. This has been shown in ovine (Little & Ghosh, 1997) and equine joints (Brama, 1999). The concept of a 'blank' joint at birth has been proposed by the group in Utrecht, suggesting that the composition of the matrix can be conditioned by the type and timing of imposed mechanical loading. This group also proposes the hypothesis that specific exercise in the early stages of postnatal development can influence the subsequent integrity of the articular surface.

Response of cartilage to exercise in the skeletally mature adult

It is known that there is a limited capacity for gross functional adaptation of articular cartilage to mechanical conditions in the adult; studies on young dogs have shown an adaptation to exercise as an increase in cartilage (Kiviranta *et al.*, 1988). A reduction in mechanical loading leads to a thinning of the cartilage. In addition,

CARTILAGE THICKNESS

- Total
  Exercised > control ($p < 0.0001$)

- Hyaline - no difference

- Calcified
  Exercised > control ($p < 0.0001$)
  Dorsal > palmar ($p < 0.003$)

Fig. 9.8 The thickness values of hyaline and calcified cartilage as function of exercise in the carpal bones of horses with high- and low-intensity exercise histories. (With permission from R.C. Murray, The Animal Health Trust, Newmarket.)

it has been demonstrated that reduced loading also results in fewer chondrocytes and a decrease in synthesis of matrix collagens type I and II (Pirttiniemi *et al.*, 1996), whereas increased exercise induces a complex array of responses. Recent research has shown that the osteochondral unit responds to the functional stimulus of exercise. Results showed an overall thickening of the cartilage, an increase in subchondral bone plate thickness and hypertrophy of the underlying subchondral bone. This spectrum of tissue changes associated with the joint is related to both the intensity and character of the exercise regimen. The increase in thickness of the cartilage resulted from an increase in thickness of the calcified layer, with the thickness of hyaline cartilage remaining constant compared with control group values; the subchondral bone also showed a dramatic response to exercise and was significantly thicker in exercised compared with non-exercised controls subjects. The changes observed in this study may indicate that topographical and exercise-related differences exist in the morphology and mechanical properties of carpal cartilage. Furthermore strenuous training may lead to deterioration of cartilage at sites with a high clinical incidence of lesions (Murray *et al.*, 1999) or predispose these sites to damage even after a period of recovery from the episode of high-intensity exercise (Little *et al.*, 1997).

Similar findings to the above were reported in dogs in which training had been initiated at the age of 15 weeks. The calcified and hyaline layers of the articular cartilage were increased in the running group compared with non-exercised controls. In addition, the running group were found to have a very marked increase in bone-forming surfaces (Oettmeier *et al.*, 1992). This study again emphasizes the need to appreciate the joint as an 'organ' in relation to adaptation to exercise. The volume and intensity of the exercise influence potential effects on the component tissues.

The increase in the thickness of the calcified cartilage might be interpreted as a mechanism to reduce the effect of high-impact loads transferred from the underlying bone to the susceptible hyaline cartilage at the articular surface by providing a stiffness gradient. Interestingly, there are reports of adaptive changes in human joints having different effects on the cartilage and associated subchondral mineralization zone. The thickness of the mineralization zone was related to local loading history and reflected loading patterns within the joint. A possible explanation for the difference in response between the mineralized zone and cartilage was given as a difference in response characteristics between osteocytes and chondrocytes or different site-specific loading conditions (Milz *et al.*, 1997).

One of the problems in determining the response of any tissue to functional changes in environment is being able to compare the different studies and extract common mechanisms that can then be applied to practical training programs. Many studies have been performed but on different species, with different types of exercise and at different stages of development. One classic study on long-term effects of exercise on cartilage in dogs showed no differences in structure or mechanical properties of cartilage between animals exercising and controls. The exercise group ran on a treadmill with 130% body weight loads for 75 minutes a day at 3 km/h 5 days a week over a period of 10 years, and the controls were allowed unrestricted cage activity (Newton *et al.*, 1997). However, another study looking at polarized light birefringence in relation to collagen organization found that there were changes in this aspect of cartilage morphology after 15 weeks of running 40 km per day, although collagen content and concentration of hydroxypyridinium cross-links were not significantly different (Arokoski *et al.*, 1996). These authors had also recognized site-dependent changes in glycosaminoglycan (GAG) content both within a joint and within the thickness of the cartilage. The findings were a depletion of GAG from the superficial zone in the high loaded areas of the joint as result of long-term exercise (Arokoski *et al.*, 1993).

Thus there is a range of responses reported in the literature, indicating the potential adaptive response of cartilage to mechanical loading both during development and after skeletal maturity. The concept of influencing the cartilage properties early in postnatal life to enhance resistance to injury in the adult is interesting and requires further research and validation. Conceptually it is attractive to provide a pattern of mechanical input during development of the skeletal system, resembling the demands that will be made during peak athletic performance as an adult. In fact, training from birth as a graded program would make more sense than traditional methods of superimposing a training program on a skeletal system that has developed under different functional demands.

The transition from functional adaptation to over-training injury is also difficult to define in terms of specific exercise levels; again there are suggestions in the literature that lack of exercise can be as detrimental as over-exercise. The difficulty is in determining what is 'just right.' However, once damaged, articular cartilage has only limited capacity for repair. Thus the relationship between defined local mechanical environment and tissue response is of critical importance in relation to maximizing performance and minimizing injury in the competition horse. However, certain sites, such as the dorsal margins of the radial and third carpal bones, are often associated with cartilage degeneration.

As a species the horse is prone to osteoarticular pathology. Although degenerative joint disease is also a common clinical problem in man, and the subject of extensive research, in terms of potential phamacological therapy to inhibit progression and effect a 'cure' for this devastating condition, little progress has been made. Therefore, it is important in conditioning both human and equine athletes to ensure that the type of training used to achieve high-performance goals does not result in immediate or subsequent cartilage and joint degeneration. Degenerative joint disease is a complex process with a multifactorial etiology; however, once initiated, many of the pathological processes are at present irreversible. Perhaps it is a paradox that the very nature of the mechanical stimulus that can be used to induce rapid bone formation also appears to be detrimental to the overlying hyaline articular cartilage.

The changes induced as a result of exercise in joints are related to the specific component tissues and the interactions of the consequences of these changes may be the underlying cause of the overall degenerative disease. For this reason it is important to consider the effects of exercise on the joint as an 'organ,' as proposed by Radin, and not as a group of independent tissues.

The data from studies reported above indicates that changes to the bony components occur very rapidly and that the exact type of stimulus that induces bone adaptation can, if continued, be detrimental to cartilage.

Since the repair capacity of cartilage is poor, it is important in training and competition of the equine athlete that the performance and risk factors – such as conformation, age, nutrition and training protocols – are geared to minimize any damage to the articular cartilage of synovial joints. Periods of immobilization of joint result in a type of disuse atrophy, in which the thickness of the articular cartilage is reduced. This aspect may also require more research in order to understand the optimal way in which normal thickness may be restored. Such information will be of use in designing rehabilitation protocols. The role of post-treatment manipulation in joint pathologies is well developed in human orthopedics, with protocols such as continuous passive motion being employed following joint surgery (Salter, 1981).

At a tissue level, there is evidence that both changes in static and dynamic loading conditions can elicit a response from chondrocytes in relation to the synthesis of matrix components. In living explants subjected to cyclical loading at frequencies greater than 0.1 Hz there is a dramatic increase in synthesis of cartilage oligomeric matrix protein (COMP) and fibronectin. The chondrocytes were found to be sensitive to both frequency and magnitude of mechanical stimulation. This work suggests that as a tissue, cartilage can remodel the matrix in response to specific mechanical loading condi-

tions (Wong *et al.*, 1999). Other *in vitro* studies on cartilage also indicate that the proteoglycan synthesis is modulated by both static and dynamic loading conditions (Steinmeyer & Knue, 1997). In other studies, exercise has been shown to influence decorin levels without an effect on GAG content (Visser *et al.*, 1998). These differences could be explained by a number of factors, such as the age when exercise is commenced, the volume and intensity of the specific training protocols and the duration of the training period. However, it does show the potential for conditioning joints by appropriate exercise regimens. There is a need to relate the scientific findings to practical training systems with appropriate monitoring to gain advantage in terms of reduced injury and improved performance for equine athletes.

Tendon and ligaments

General aspects of exercise and tendon injury

Perhaps another irony of equine exercise physiology and sports medicine is that understanding of the pathobiology of tendons and ligaments is poor yet the incidence of injury to the locomotor system in general is high (Rossdale *et al.*, 1985). A great proportion of locomotor injuries in equine atheletes involve the flexor tendons, accessory ligaments and the suspensory ligament. The injuries occur both in training and during athletic competition, resulting in significant wastage, with consequent financial and welfare implications. Recovery from tendon injury is protracted and incomplete; once injured, the tendon is permanently compromised to a greater or lesser extent. Treatments are numerous, indicating that no one approach is particularly effective. Rehabilitation is probably the most important component of the treatment regimen. Consequently, an appreciation of the mechanisms involved in the response of normal tendon to physical training could have implications for developing rehabilitation strategies in the management of tendon injuries. The extent of clinical pathological change can range from a minor disruption of a small number of fibrils to complete catastrophic rupture of the tendon. However, changes to the matrix at a molecular and ultrastructural level occur before a clinical injury is evident.

In most competition and race horses there is a high predisposition to injury in the superficial digital flexor tendon and, to some extent, the suspensory ligament of the forelimb. In addition to biomechanical predisposition resulting from individual conformation, external mechanical influences such as track surface contribute to injury risk. In some countries a change in track surface has led to a great increase in tendon injury, while reducing the incidence of bone fractures. Interestingly, the tendons of the hindlimbs are less frequently injured, although these were more often affected in draught horses pulling heavy loads. These observations provide further evidence that biomechanical factors are involved in the site-specific pathological changes, possibly as a result of a compromise in functional adaptation in these specific structures. In both the equine athlete and working horse, the flexor structures are afflicted rather than extensor tendons, yet there is scant data on the reasons for this apparent difference in biological response.

Recent work suggests that the role of the flexors in acting as elastic energy stores may predispose these particular tendons and ligaments to injury. One treatment of tendon injury of the flexor tendons was application of a graft using part of the lateral extensor tendon but there appears to be little scientific rationale for the development of this procedure. The characterization of cells within tendons and ligaments has not yet been well developed; however, there is now some evidence that the cells from different fibrous structures may respond to different types of stimulation with respect to both viability and matrix metabolism. The evidence will be presented and discussed later.

The methods used in training to condition tendons are for the most part based on a traditional empirical approach. Trainers often describe the effect of training as 'hardening' the tendons, yet these changes do not appear to be related to biological events within the tendon structure. Despite the extensive increase in the scientific understanding of training effects on muscle, and also the recent advances in elucidation of the factors that control functional adaptation of bone, the cellular and molecular

mechanisms involved in the adaptive response of tendon to increased mechanical demand are not well understood.

Lesions in the superficial digital flexor tendon (SDFT) of the horse are very similar to injuries seen in the human Achilles tendon, in the quadriceps tendons of jumping athletes and also the degenerative changes occurring in the rotator cuff of the shoulder. Thus, the horse may provide a natural model of tendon degeneration from which the underlying biological mechanisms and pathological processes of a number of tendon and ligament lesions, resulting from both exercise and aging, may be elucidated.

The response of tendons to training may also differ between specific tendons that have different biological functions (Birch *et al.*, 1997a). The incidence of injury being related to particular tendons suggests that the predisposition is associated with a specific function. The extensor tendons together with the deep digital flexor tendons (DDFT) have, in general, a low incidence of atraumatic failure in equine athletes, whereas the SDFT and suspensory ligament have a very high incidence of injury. Indeed, since the incidence of injury is based on clinically apparent lesions, and recent work has shown the presence of subclinical injury in a significant number of horses, the actual incidence of injury to these specific structures may be very much greater. The pattern of physiological loading in these tendons during the gait cycle may also add to the injury predisposition in the SDFT and suspensory ligament. *In vivo* force transducers have been used to show that levels of tensile force rise rapidly in the early part of the stance phase in both the superficial flexor tendon and suspensory ligament. The rise in force in the deep flexor tendon occurs more slowly and peaks at a lower level later in the stance phase (Fig. 9.9) (Platt *et al.*, 1994). The role of the tendons, as with other biological structures, is related to structural morphology. Thus with exercise, and particularly elite athletic performance, the different functional requirements will result in the need for changes in composition and structure of the tendons. It is this relationship and the mechanisms controlling it that are important in conditioning horses for peak performance while minimizing injury risk. A brief review of the functional morphology is appropriate to place the effects of exercise on tendon in context.

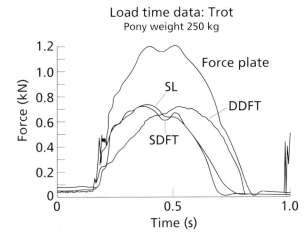

Fig. 9.9 A recording of tendon forces in the superficial (SDFT) and deep digital flexor tendon (DDFT) and suspensory ligament (SL) during locomotion. (From *Platt et al., 1994,* ©Elsevier Science Ltd.)

Functional morphology of tendons and ligaments in response to exercise

General functional characteristics

Tendons are the structures that link muscle to bone; this linkage spans one or more joints. Contraction of the muscle generates tensile forces, which are transmitted from the muscle to the bone by the fibrous framework of the muscle and its condensation into the tendon. These forces move one or more segments of the limb and the controlled and coordinated limb movements result in locomotion. The levels of force engendered in specific tendons, at particular times during locomotion, are dependent upon a large number of variables. Indirect effects of exercise such as muscle fatigue leading to uncoordinated movement can also result in excessive forces on some tendons where agonists and antagonists would normally operate in conjunction to stabilize joints.

Tendons are elastic and stretch to some extent. In specific tendons the elasticity of the tendon is utilized as a means of elastic energy storage to optimize the energetic efficiency of locomotion. The digital flexor tendons and the suspensory ligament fulfil such a role, which may contribute to the fact that these structures are a predilection site for injury. In order to maximize the level of energy stored, maximum deformation must occur in the tendon. Essentially the tendon acts in a manner analogous to the spring in a pogo stick. This energy saving role of tendons is also utilized in other species – perhaps the most evident is in the kangaroo, which is able to increase speed without an associated increased oxygen uptake (Morgan *et al.*, 1978), by utilizing the large Achilles tendons as springs.

Optimization for this role results in very low tensile failure safety margins compared with other less mass-critical regions of the skeletal system; consequently, at peak performance levels, functional strains are close to failure strains. Adaptive hypertrophy of these structures would compromise the compliance and optimization, representing a counterproductive mechanism.

Functional tensile strains in equine flexor tendons have been recorded *in vivo* using small implanted Hall effect transducers. Such studies suggest tensile strains of around 3% at the walk, 6–8% at the trot and 12–16% at the gallop (Stephens *et al.*, 1989). In the laboratory, tendons placed in materials test machines can be completely ruptured at around the 12–16% levels of tensile strain (Wilson, 1991). Thus, at peak locomotor performance, the flexor tendons are operating close to the level of gross tensile failure and it can be seen how narrow the safety margin is for elastic energy storage in these structures.

In laboratory testing, the plot of deformation as a function of applied load for collagenous tissues in general, and tendons in particular, shows a characteristic mechanical behavior (Fig. 9.10). At low levels of initial loading the structure extends considerably but as loading levels increase the incremental extension decreases to reach a linear relationship. The initial nonlinear part of the load/deformation plot is called the 'toe region' and is a result of a straightening of the 'crimp' in collagen fibrils. The limit of the toe region, in quantitative

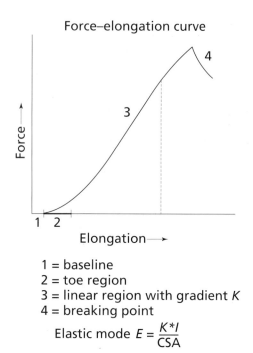

Force–elongation curve

1 = baseline
2 = toe region
3 = linear region with gradient *K*
4 = breaking point

Elastic mode $E = \dfrac{K*l}{CSA}$

Fig. 9.10 A plot of tensile loading of a tendon to failure, showing the 'toe' region of nonlinear deformation, the linear elastic region, yield followed by plastic deformation and failure.

terms, is determined by the crimp characteristics, such as wavelength and angle. These crimp characteristics may differ within the fascicles in different regions of the tendon; furthermore, changes may occur as a function of both exercise and natural aging. The subsequent linear region of the load deformation plot results predominantly from the material properties of the collagenous matrix. The gradient of this part of the load/deformation graph represents the tensile stiffness of the tendon.

If the structure is loaded beyond the elastic limit – to the yield point – an irreversible deformation occurs with an increased rate of extension; ultimately, tensile failure results. After yield and prior to structural failure the tendon will not return to the same zero point after loading, indicating plastic deformation and irreversible material damage.

Cyclical loading of the tendon, to a level not reaching yield, in a materials test machine over a period of time shows two phenomena that are relevant to the effects of exercise in the short term. First, as shown in Figure 9.11, there is a shift of the load/deformation plot to the right with each successive loading cycle until eventually a steady state is reached. This is known as 'preconditioning' and although it is a feature seen in laboratory testing of tendon it may have *in vivo* relevance in relation to 'warming up' prior to peak athletic performance. Secondly, as illustrated, the plot of loading followed by unloading of the tendon forms a loop, starting and finishing at the same point. The loop, termed hysteresis, is formed as a result of the elastic recoverability of the tendon being less than 100%. The area of the loop represents a loss of energy, largely in the form of heat, that occurs during stretch and release of the tendon.

The functional behaviour is related to the morphology of tendon and although tendons and ligaments have a rather uninteresting gross appearance they are in fact very complex structures. Tendon is formed of dense aligned fibrous connective tissue, which, as with all connective tissues, consists of *cells*, broadly termed tenocytes, and an extracellular *matrix*, comprising predominantly type I collagen. It is the collagen that imparts general tensile mechanical strength to the structure but the structural arrangements and chemical bonding of the collagen molecules influence the specific mechanical properties. The molecular composition and structural morphology of the matrix show differences between specific tendons and indeed regions along and within a particular tendon, which again relates to specific functional requirements. Interestingly, the strain at different levels of the superficial digital flexor tendon is uniform despite differences in cross-sectional area (Riemersna & Schamhardt, 1985). Changes in matrix composition, and associated functional properties, occur as a function of both age and exercise. The relationship between the morphology of the tendon and the functional performance applies to both the gross tendon and to the component structures, and may also be localized to specific regions within the overall structure.

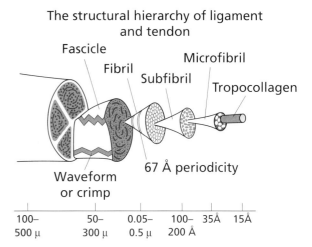

Fig. 9.12 A diagrammatic representation of the structural hierarchy of tendon (after Kastelic *et al.*, 1978, ©Harwood Academic).

General morphological features of tendon

Kastelic *et al.* (1978) described the complex structural hierarchy seen in tendons and ligaments (Fig. 9.12) in terms of the matrix morphology and arrangement. The fundamental molecular unit of tendon is tropocollagen. It is this protein that confers tensile strength and predominates in tendon matrix. The collagen molecules, or tropocollagen, are formed from three polypeptide chains wound together to form a right-handed superhelix. Five of these units are twisted to form the subfibril. Perhaps one of the most relevant structural components is the collagen fibril. When the fibril is viewed under the electron microscope a transverse banding can be seen with a 67 Å periodicity. The banding results from a quarter molecule stagger in the alignment of the component molecules of collagen.

The three-dimensional form of the collagen fibril is also relevant to changes that occur as a consequence of both exercise and aging. In the relaxed state and under low functional loads, the fibril shows a planar waveform or 'crimp'. This is well demonstrated using plane polarized light microscopy (Gathercole and Keller, 1991). This technique also allows measurement of both wavelength and angle of the crimp; these may vary between fibrils in different locations within the tendon. It is the crimp that causes the initial, nonlinear load/deformation behavior of the tendon.

Fibrils increase in diameter with age or maturation in tendons. In some other collagenous tissues, such as cornea and periodontal ligament, the initial small 40 nm diameter is maintained. However, in tendon, as the tissue matures, the initial unimodal diameter distribution changes, even in the newborn foal, to a bimodal

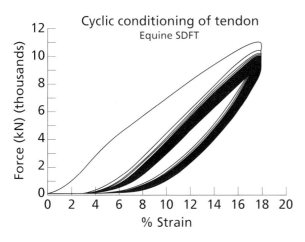

Fig. 9.11 Cyclical loading of a tendon within the elastic range, showing hysteresis due to energy loss and preconditioning to a steady state.

tissue distribution with larger diameter fibrils up to 150–200 nm appearing. The mean mass average diameter may differ between specific tendons and ligaments. The changes in fibril diameters, fibrillogenesis, may be influenced by the different GAGs present in the tendon matrix. These GAG chains may also change in level and type as a consequence of functional demand and age. Other non-collagenous proteins are also found in tendon matrix and have recently been implicated in possible mechanisms regulating adaptation.

The fibrils are grouped into fascicles surrounded by circumferentially arranged collagen fibers forming the inter-fascicular septa. The fascicles are polygonal and vary in size and shape when viewed in cross-section. The septal collagen is continuous with the tendon sheath surrounded by either a synovial sheath or the loose connective tissue of the paratenon. The cross-sectional area and shape of the tendon varies along its length. In areas where the tendon passes over and wraps around a bony prominence, the tissue is subjected to compressive forces. In these areas of compression the composition of the matrix differs from that in tensile regions. Compression leads to the formation of a fibrocartilaginous matrix with associated differences in molecular composition.

These levels of structure are influenced by both the type and level of functional demand and also by aging. The effects of exercise and athletic peak performance together with the influence of age-related changes can be considered first in terms of the entire structure and potential impact on functional performance, and secondly with respect to the effects of the constituent components of tendon.

Effects of short-term exercise

Preconditioning

The basic tropocollagen molecules are each formed from three polypeptide chains wound into a right-handed superhelix. The longitudinal arrangement of the molecules with a quarter stagger within the fibril results in a 67 nm banding appearance under the electron microscope. This packing arrangement is due to the interaction of hydrophilic and hydrophobic bonds between the collagen molecules. The factors controlling lateral packing of the molecules are not well understood. However, the effect of preconditioning of tendons, in which the load/deformation characteristics change in the initial period of cyclical loading, may be attributed to changes in collagen packing and water distribution. In laboratory testing of tendons using cyclical loading to strains below the yield point, initially, with each successive loading cycle, the load/deformation curve shifts to

the right. After a number of cycles the shift is no longer evident and the tendon reaches a steady state. The fact that the mechanical behavior of tendons changes during initial cyclical loading may well be important in the 'warming up' procedures prior to peak athletic performance. The effects of training on the preconditioning effects are not known; however, the role of preconditioning may be related to the risk of partial or gross failure of the tendon during peak performance. There is evidence that the modulus of the tendon is reduced once a steady state is reached (Grieshaber & Faust, 1992; Schatzmann et al., 1998).

Hyperthermia

The primary role of transmission of tensile forces from muscle to bone across one or more joints is supplemented, in the case of equine flexor tendons, by a postural role in supporting the metacarpophalangeal joint both in standing and locomotion. In addition these tendons play a role in the optimization of the energetic efficiency of locomotion. During high-speed locomotion the loading of the limb results in a hyperextension of the metacarpophalangeal joint, resulting in high tensile loads being imposed on the flexor tendons and suspensory ligament. At the gallop these structures are stretched almost to failure during the stance phase of the gait cycle, thus maximizing energy storage. This elastic energy is then released during the subsequent phase of the gait cycle. The energy storing role of the flexor tendons therefore contributes to improving the energetic efficiency of locomotion.

This additional role of the flexor tendons may compromise the normal process of functional adaptation in response to increased exercise, in terms of increased demand resulting in an increase in tissue mass. In order to maximize the energy storing capacity of the tendon, it must undergo maximal tensile strain.

Training for increased locomotor performance does not appear to have a consistent effect on all tendons and ligaments. During high-intensity exercise the cyclical loading of the superficial flexor tendon has been shown to induce an increase in temperature within the core of the tendon. This results from the elasticity of the tendon being less than 100% efficient, as shown by the area of hysteresis in the non-destructive load/deformation cycle. The area of the hysteresis represents energy loss; this energy is in the form of heat and lack of efficient conduction causes the localized elevation in core temperature. The internal tendon temperature rises to 45–47 °C during 7–10 minutes of peak performance. This level and duration of hyperthermia would normally result in cell death in fibroblasts from other sites, such as dermis (Wilson & Goodship, 1994). The temperature on the surface of the tendon showed a decrease during locomotion, resulting from proximity of the tendon to the overlying skin together with the cooling effect of the limb passing through the air.

Interestingly, clinical lesions of the superficial digital flexor tendon are also frequently seen as core lesions. Therefore, it was attractive to hypothesize that the site-specific hyperthermia resulted in cell death and the subsequent core degeneration. However, subsequent studies (Birch *et al.*, 1997b) indicate that tenocytes grown from the central core region of equine superficial digital flexor tendons are able to sustain temperatures that are lethal to fibroblasts from other sites such as the dermis of the skin. Furthermore, there is preliminary evidence that thermotolerance is an inherent property of these cells, evident in cells taken from mid-term fetal tendons, rather than an acquired resistance to metabolic stress (Gibbs *et al.*, 1995).

Although the tenocytes fom the central core of the SDFT can remain viable at high temperatures, it is possible that metabolic competence may be compromised, resulting in changes to the composition, structure and maintenance of the matrix in the core region. Further work is required to understand the biological significance of this site-specific temperature rise and the mechanisms controlling thermal tolerance in particular populations of tenocytes.

Longer-term changes in tendon resulting from exercise

Cross-sectional area

Various studies on horses and other species indicate tendon-specific differences in the response to exercise. An experimental study on the response of skeletal tissues to both an increase and decrease in exercise in rabbits and swine (Woo *et al.*, 1982) resulted in a significant change in both mass and material properties of tendons and ligaments. This and other studies suggest that periods of around four to six weeks of reduced functional input may induce changes to the material properties that can be irreversible (Woo *et al.*, 1987; Newton *et al.*, 1995). This suggests that the modern management of equine athletes, with relatively long periods spent in stables, and also the use of box rest in treating some tendon injuries, may not achieve an optimal level of conditioning or restoration of performance. In fact, under-exercising could result in a permanent impairment of the potential to enhance tendon properties. These findings may indicate support for early mobilization following injury and increased volume of exercise in training and they could be used in the development of scientifically based training and rehabilitation regimens.

The exercise studies in swine also showed a difference in response between the ligaments and the flexor and extensor tendons. The increase in exercise resulted in an increase in the properties and mass of the extensor tendons and ligaments but no significant increase in the flexor tendons. This finding was supported by our own observations on the effects of long-term exercise in Thoroughbred horses. One explanation for this differential response to increased exercise may be related to the fact that the extensor tendons do not act as energy storing tendons and are therefore able to exhibit an adaptive response in terms of an increase in cross-sectional area without risk of a consequent compromise in energy conservation. This type of adaptation was not seen in the flexor tendons. Similarly, in horses given controlled exercise for periods of up to 18 months, changes in cross-sectional area were not observed in the flexor tendons (Birch *et al.*, 1999).

Some studies, however, have reported an apparent increase in cross-sectional area of the SDFT in horses following increases levels of exercise (Gillis *et al.*, 1993). The level and type of exercise may be critical, since in the latter study two of the horses were reported to have shown clinical tendinitis. Thus it is possible that, in this study, the level of exercise for the particular horses was on the limit of functional adaptation and subclinical damage. In addition to the paucity of knowledge regarding adaptation of specific tendons to exercise, level and types of exercise that may contribute to damage rather than conditioning of tendons is also unknown.

This issue is further confused since some authors suggest that any increase in cross-sectional area of the superficial digital flexor tendon on ultrasound imaging is indicative of a pathological condition.

Fascicle/septal changes in response to exercise

The fascicles are separated by loose inter-fascicular fibrous tissue septa and are variable in cross-sectional shape and size. Gillis *et al.*, 1997 also reported an increase in the thickness of the inter-fascicular septa in horses that had been exercised. The factors controlling the size and number of fascicles have not been determined. Preliminary observations show the orientation of collagen fibers in the septa is circumferential around the fascicle and shows the presence of 'crimp' (Johns, 1998) (Fig. 9.13). Such a morphological arrangement would indicate a functional requirement to control fascicular transverse expansion and thickening could represent an internal adaptive change; alternatively, this thickening could also be interpreted as a repair response to overuse or subclinical injury.

The role of cells within the septal connective tissue may involve a paracrine control of the intra-fascicular tenocytes. Signaling peptides such as transforming growth factor (TGF) β have been shown to be localized in the septal tissues (Cauvin *et al.*, 1998). TGF β is

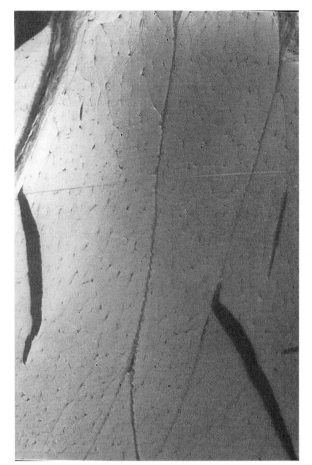

Fig. 9.13 A photomicrograph to show the circumferential orientation of collagen fibers around a tendon fascicle.

measure of cross-sectional area and by a more subjective evaluation of matrix integrity.

The apparent differences between these findings, in relation to the capacity of flexor tendons to undergo adaptive hypertrophy, might also result from the specific conditions of the exercise history and the type and age of the horses studied. Only by improving our understanding of the adaptive mechanisms of tendon can these differences be explained and new approaches developed for training and rehabilitation.

Effects of age and exercise on the crimp morphology of tendons
The morphological characteristics of the 'crimp' in the collagen fibril are related to the nonlinear region of the load/deformation curve. Thus the accumulated average of individual fiber characteristics will influence the mechanical behavior of the structure and its component parts. It could be speculated that the hyperthermia associated with exercise could affect cell metabolism and result in changes to matrix composition and structure. In terms of regional differences in crimp morphology, one study found no significant difference in crimp characteristics between peripheral and central regions in

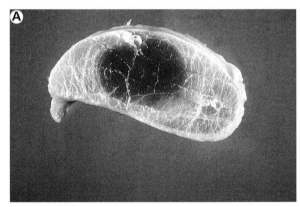

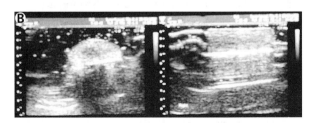

Fig. 9.14A A region of matrix damage seen in the central core of a superficial digital flexor tendon but not detected clinically. **B** A high-resolution ultrasound scan of the same tendon, showing a greater degree of anechogenicity in the damaged matrix.

involved in control of both proliferation and differentiation of cells, with known involvement in the development and repair of soft tissues (O'Kane & Fergusson, 1997).

In general, an adaptive response would result in an increase in tissue with normal if immature characteristics, whereas injury, and subsequent repair, is associated with a repair tissue, characterized by the collagen-type distribution and tissue architecture. Such subtle changes are difficult to detect by routine clinical examination. Modern imaging techniques such as ultrasonography, however, can now be used to assess the quality of the matrix in addition to detection of gross morphological abnormalities, but at a level that would not be detectable by normal manual clinical examination (Fig. 9.14). These techniques now have the potential to be used in conjunction with training and athletic performance to identify damage at an early stage, both from quantitative

Comparision of the stress–strain curves of central and peripheral fibers

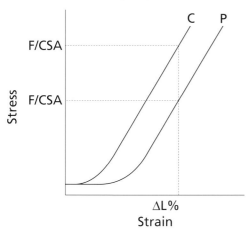

Fig. 9.15 A load/deformation plot of collagen fibers from central and peripheral regions of the superficial digital flexor tendon in an old horse, illustrating the effect of a lower toe limit strain on the greater increase in stress with extension experienced by the central fibers. (With permission from Wilmink *et al.,* 1992).

young horses. However, in older horses, particularly with some history of exercise, the crimp characteristics were significantly different between peripheral and central core regions. In the older horse, the changes in crimp length and angle resulted in a lower toe limit strain; thus for the same level of tensile strain the central fiber crimp would straighten before the crimp of the peripheral fibers. As levels of strain increase the stresses in the central fibers increase at a greater rate than in peripheral fibers (Fig. 9.15). The central fibers will then rupture at strains lower than those required to break the peripheral fibers (Wilmink *et al.,* 1992). This would provide one explanation for the frequent clinical finding of a partial tendon rupture with a central core lesion and also the typical acute pattern of central echogenicity seen with ultrasonographic imaging. Tensile tests to failure performed in the laboratory often also show an initial central core failure.

It is difficult to separate the effects of age and exercise on the site-related changes in crimp morphology. It could be argued that with both age and exercise the number of accumulated loading cycles increases. There is evidence that age-related changes occur with 'natural' levels of exercise in wild horses. A study on this topic showed a decrease in crimp angle in the central core of tendons from older horses. Interestingly, the crimp angle in peripheral fibrils did not change over the age range stud-

ied (Patterson-Kane *et al.,* 1997a). This again suggests a potential effect on tenocyte metabolism localized to the central core and may indicate the changes result more from accumulated effects of exercise rather than aging *per se.* However, in the controlled exercise study in young Thoroughbreds, although similar observations were made with respect to the reduction in crimp angle of fibers in the central core as a consequence of imposed exercise, the peripheral fibers showed a larger crimp angle than the corresponding fibers of the unexercised group. This observation requires further investigation but could be indicative of an exercise-related adaptation in the peripheral fibrils that would not be influenced by the potential hyperthermic influences occurring in the central core (Patterson-Kane *et al.,* 1998).

These findings may have implications for training methods, since it could be argued that training, and indeed athletic competition, was better carried out in younger rather than older horses. The monitoring of these central changes in crimp morphology *in vivo,* although desirable, is not yet possible. If the morphological changes in crimp are associated with other changes in matrix composition occurring with exercise, then the potential to develop markers may be greater.

Histological changes related to exercise and specific tendons
Degenerative lesions in tendons, particularly those with an energy storing role, are frequently seen in the central core. The level at which such lesions can be identified is to a large extent dependent up on the degree of degeneration. The gross appearance of abnormality observed as discoloration of the central area has been reported in the superficial digital flexor tendon of the horse (Wilson & Goodship, 1994) and in the human Achilles tendon (Kannus & Jozsa, 1991). Histologically, these lesions vary in level of abnormality from a minimal deviation from normal histological appearance of cells and matrix to well-defined areas of cell necrosis and matrix disruption (See Fig. 9.14A). The level of histologically observable damage might be expected to influence functional performance and may well be a result of exercise-induced damage. However, as yet, there is little evidence or data to link the levels and timing of functional input with these microscopic morphological features.

The cell populations found in the tendon are poorly described and understood. In histological sections of the superficial digital flexor tendon a number of different types of cell can be distinguished, based on the morphological appearance (Fig. 9.16). It is possible, however, that these differences could be a sectioning artifact. However, with vital staining and examination using real time confocal microscopy, the different cell populations

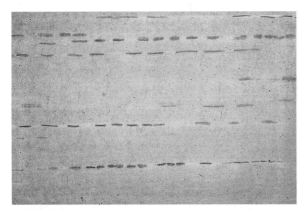

Fig. 9.16 A photomicrograph showing a longitudinal section of the superficial digital flexor tendon with morphologically distinct cell populations.

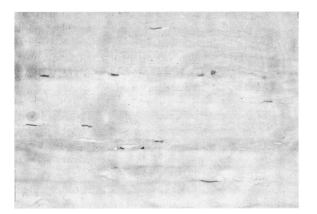

Fig. 9.17 A photomicrograph showing the histological appearance of tenocytes and matrix in a compression region of the superficial digital flexor tendon as it passes over the metacarpophalangeal joint.

can be verified. As yet the significance of these different populations has not been elucidated.

The distribution of cells and variation in terms of morphology are also different between specific tendons (Birch *et al.*, 1999). The superficial digital flexor tendon and the suspensory ligament have higher cellularity than the deep digital flexor tendon. The incidence of injury is far greater in the superficial flexor and suspensory ligament than in the deep flexor. Studies using intra-tendinous force transducers demonstrated a difference in the relationship between imposition of load and cell type and distribution during the stance phase of gait (Platt *et al.*, 1994). These differences may be related to the prevailing mechanical conditions in regions of tendon subjected to different mechanical conditions. The

histological appearance of the tensile regions differs from that in areas where the tendon wraps around bone, e.g. as in the metacarpophalangeal region of the superficial digital flexor tendon. In these areas tendon is subjected to compression forces and the constituent cells appear more like chondrocytes and are associated with a fibrocartilaginous extracellular matrix (Fig. 9.17). Although it has been established experimentally that the cell population responds to changes in mechanical conditions (Gillard *et al.*, 1979), the effects of different levels of exercise on these distinct regions of tendon are poorly understood.

Ultrastructural morphology – site and tendon-specific changes with age and exercise

The newly formed collagen fibrils are initially small in cross-sectional area, at around 40 nm, and increase in size as they mature, in some instances reaching 250 nm in diameter. Later, with old age, the fibril diameter

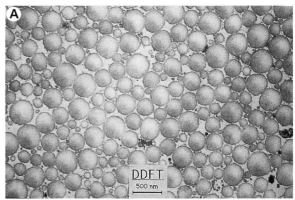

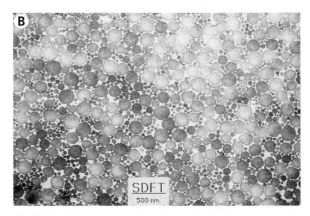

Fig. 9.18 An electron micrograph of transverse sections of (**A**) deep (DDFT) and (**B**) superficial (SDFT) digital flexor tendon to show the characteristic fibril profiles in each structure in the mature horse.

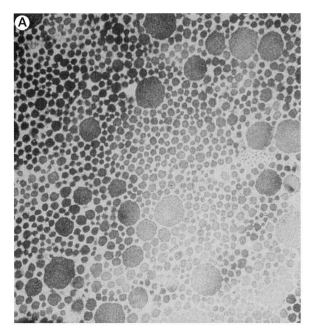

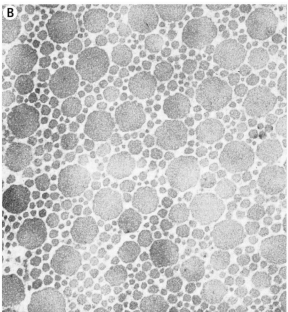

Fig. 9.19 (**A**) An electron micrograph of a transverse section of the central core region of the superficial digital flexor tendon of a 3-year-old Thoroughbred after 18 months of high-intensity training. This shows a predominance of small-diameter collagen fibrils with a mass average diameter of 105.9 nm. (**B**) a similar section from a control horse that had undergone low-intensity exercise only; here the more normal bimodal distribution of fibril diameters is seen, with a higher mass average diameter of 131.7 nm. (With permission from Patterson-Kane *et al.*, 1997b).

decreases. In the horse, a precocial animal showing advanced locomotor function at birth, the fibrils within the fascicle have a bimodal distribution of diameter size from birth. Altricial animals, such as the rat and man, in which locomotor function is poorly developed at birth, have tendons in which the fibrils are of small diameter throughout at birth; with development and commencement of locomotion, these species show an increase in diameters of some fibers giving an overall bimodal distribution. In all species there is an increase in mechanical strength with maturation and a decline in old age.

Several studies have investigated the effects of both exercise and the aging process on the distribution of collagen fibril diameters in flexor tendons. In addition to differences in fibril diameter profiles between specific tendons, there are also differences at the ultra-structural level between regions within an individual tendon.

The fibril profile may be related to the presence and distribution of GAGs. These molecules are present within the matrix and may regulate fibrillogenesis (Parry *et al.*, 1982). The functional interactions between mechanical role, cellular activity and regulation of matrix synthesis and maintenance are not yet understood.

During skeletal development the fibril diameter distributions change and there is also a maturation of the chemical cross-linking of the collagen. Both of these events result in an increase in tensile strength. There is also an initial change in the crimp morphology, discussed previously, in the early years of development. Interestingly the different levels of structure, replacement of immature cross-links, peaking of mass average fibril diameter, collagen fibril index and stabilization of crimp angle have all been shown to reach mature levels by two years of age in the Thoroughbred (Patterson-Kane *et al.*, 1997b).

The maturation of collagen fibrils in terms of diameter distributions does not result in a similar pattern in all tendons. The diameter profile differs between specific tendons; for example the superficial digital flexor tendon and the suspensory ligament show a relatively high proportion of small diameter fibrils in comparison to the deep digital flexor tendon (Fig. 9.18).

In response to exercise, particularly long-term exercise, there is a regional change in fibril diameter distribution within the superficial flexor tendon. The central core region exhibits an increase in the numbers of small-diameter collagen fibrils compared with the fibrils in the peripheral region and throughout the tendon of horses that have not undergone high intensity exercise (Fig. 9.19). Interestingly, in these studies there was no increase in cross-sectional area in these tendons, nor in collagen content or collagen-linked fluorescence (an indicator of age of collagen) (Birch *et al.*, 1997a). Thus it appears that long periods of exercise, even in 3-year-old horses, may disassemble the large-diameter collagen fibrils. This may represent accumulation of micro-damage prior to overt clinical injury; the mechanisms involved have yet to be determined but may result from increased levels of metalloproteinases. These preclinical degenerative changes could be related to a number of factors including the type, duration and intensity of exercise together with the age of the horse. The correlation between changes at this ultrastructural level and abnormalities detectable with modern high-resolution ultrasound imaging systems has not yet been established.

In a study using a shorter period of exercise (4 months), the regional differences in fibril diameter distribution were not seen. However, these horses were also 14 months younger than those examined after a long period of exercise. Thus it is not certain whether the difference in response was a result of a shorter period of exercise or sampling at a younger age. In addition, it has not yet been established that these ultrastructural changes are irreversible. It may be that following a reduction in exercise the small fibrils are able to reassemble into larger-diameter fibrils.

The development of tendon may be influenced by the imposed level of exercise. A study in Dutch Warmblood foals showed that the development of the superficial digital flexor tendon in terms of collagen fibril diameters was related to the type of exercise. Box rest was found to inhibit the development of tendon; however, inappropriate levels of exercise may damage the developing tendon. Interestingly, it was found that the delay in development resulting from box rest could be reversed by subsequent imposition of exercise. This may indicate that the effects of intense training could also be controlled by periods of different levels of exercise. Therefore it is important to determine the optimal levels of exercise for the early stages of postnatal development. It is also important to determine the windows of time during development when specific levels of exercise can be used to maximize the conditioning of tendon for the particular type of athletic performance to be undertaken in later life. Unfortunately, the nature of athletic competition, with participants working to their limits, means that injury is almost inevitable at some stage. However, a better understanding of the scientific principles underlying training should avoid unnecessary levels of injury, particularly during training, and thus improve welfare of the equine athlete.

Changes in molecular composition of tendon matrix resulting from exercise, aging and degeneration
As with many other tissues, water forms 60–70% of the wet weight of tendons and ligaments. The distribution of this water content may be involved in the preconditioning effects seen in the early cycles of loading and may be important in the warming-up process to reduce the risk of mechanically induced damage in subsequent high levels of loading associated with peak performance. In a controlled exercise study involving long-term exercise in 2 and 3-year-old Thoroughbreds, the water content of the extensor tendon was found to decrease with age. Training effects in the 3 year olds resulted in a decrease in water content; this provides additional evidence that exercise tends to accelerate age-related effects (Birch *et al.*, 1997).

The major component of the extracellular matrix dry weight is the protein collagen. Although there are around 13 different types of collagen, the type predominant in tendon is type I. Type II collagen, normally found as the predominant collagen of the matrix of articular cartilage, is also found in fibrocartilage present in the regions of tendons subjected to compressive forces as they wrap around bony prominences. There are also other collagens such as type III – normally accounting for 10% or less of the dry weight.

A number of non-collagenous proteins including the proteoglycans, decorin, biglycan, fibromodulin and cartilage oligomeric matrix protein (COMP) form a very small proportion of the dry weight, probably less than 1%. However, these molecules play a very significant role in controlling the composition and structure of the matrix with consequent effects on functional properties. Thus an understanding of the regulation of synthesis of these constituents may contribute to the development of more effective training and rehabilitation regimens and indeed lead towards the development of novel agents for the treatment of tendon injury.

The tensile strength of tendons results from cross-linking between overlapping collagen molecules. These cross-links increase as the collagen ages, changing from immature to mature cross-links. Another consequence of aging is the glycosylation of the collagen, making it possible to distinguish between newly formed and older collagen. In the study on the influence of long-term exercise in Thoroughbreds, the central core of the superficial digital flexor tendon in the exercised horses was found to contain an increase in small-diameter collagen fibrils; however there was no increase in collagen content or cross-sectional area. By determining the level of glycosylation, it was evident that the collagen was not newly formed but a degradation of the larger fibrils.

As with other tissues, the matrix of tendon and ligament is maintained by the cells and continuously degraded and renewed. Although figures of a half-life of 3–500 days are quoted (Nissen *et al.*, 1978) these are obtained from experimental data, often derived from studies on small rodents. The process and half-life of tendon matrix turnover in the horse in general, and for specific tendons in particular, have not been determined. It is possible that the effects of exercise on the composition of tendon matrix will be tendon specific since the effects of exercise on flexors and extensors has been shown to induce different responses in terms of mechanical properties. As with so many aspects of tendon pathophysiology, the mechanisms responsible for these changes are not understood. The effect of exercise on the formation of cross-links and turnover of matrix could be very significant in defining the optimal conditioning programs for tendon strength.

Recent work has shown that an interesting tendon matrix component, COMP, changes in response to age and tendon function. In the tensile regions of tendon the matrix levels rise from birth and peak at around 2 years of age, after which they decline. The effect of exercise on levels in the tensile region of the superficial flexor tendon was found to be an accelerated reduction, particularly in the central core region. Shorter-term exercise in younger horses did not result in significant changes. COMP levels in the compression region of the tendon also increase from birth but rise to reach a plateau at around 5–7 years of age (Smith *et al.*, 1999).

Interestingly, the GAG levels in the central core of the tendon is also affected by exercise, which reduces levels in the core of the superficial flexor and also in the suspensory ligament. In tendons that exhibited a discoloration of the central core, the GAG levels were increased. The factors that lead to an initial decrease and subsequent increase in this predilection site for injury are not yet understood. However, the link between these molecules and fibrillogenesis may be important in understanding the effects of both age and exercise on tendon structure and mechanical properties.

There is a need to apply more scientifically based approaches to training and performance assessments as the fundamental mechanisms become evident. Conventional arguments against athletic activity in young horses may be incorrect and, as with the protective effects of exercise on the development of osteochondral pathology, so too may exercise in younger horses lead to a reduced incidence of tendon injury.

Cell responses: changes with age and exercise; specific tendons
The cells are perhaps the most important component of connective tissues as they produce and maintain the extracellular matrix. This process involves the ability to condition the matrix to changes in functional demand and to initiate and effect repair to microscopic and gross injury. Although cells in tendons are often referred to as fibroblasts or tenocytes, there is increasing evidence that there are distinct subpopulations which may differ both between and within tendons and ligaments. There is

also evidence that cells in different locations may play specific roles in the response to mechanical and biological stimulation. Cells present in the inter-fascicular septa have been shown to play a role in the synthesis of growth factors that may influence the metabolic activity of the fibrillar tenocytes (Cauvin *et al.*, 1998). The fibrillar tenocytes themselves are varied in morphological appearance and in distribution as a function of specific tendon and age.

As yet, the identification and specific characterization of these cells has not been elucidated fully. There is evidence that fibroblasts differ in response to metabolic stress. The cells from the central core region of the superficial digital flexor tendon are resistant to the localized hyperthermia that occurs during high-speed locomotion (Birch *et al.*, 1997b); fibroblasts from other regions such as the dermis showed poor tolerance to hyperthermia. Preliminary data suggest that this is not a conditioned response resulting from repeated exposure to metabolic stress but an inherent characteristic that can be demonstrated in cells grown from embryonic tendons (Gibbs *et al.*, 1995)

On histological section there are differences in the morphology and distribution of tenocytes in different specific tendons. However, little is known about the factors that relate to the presence of particular cells within specific tendons in terms of their functional roles. There is evidence that tenocytes respond to mechanical stimulation in cell culture. Studies have shown that tenocytes can synthesize small peptides that may regulate both proliferation of cells and synthesis of extracellular matrix components (Banes *et al.*, 1999a).

As with other connective tissues there is some morphological evidence of cell-to-cell interaction in the form of gap junctions between cell processes (McNeilly *et al.*, 1996). The cells within tendon exhibit cytoplasmic processes and these form junctions between cells. The pattern is similar to that seen with osteocytes in bone; mechanical loading of bone results in an increase in the number of gap junctions. The effects of loading of tendons, in terms of specific cellular responses, have not yet been determined. However, the cells are likely to be responsive to mechanical signals *in vivo*, and this may play a role in maintaining matrix integrity. There is some evidence from *ex vivo* studies that gap junctions may play a role in regulating the response of tenocytes to mechanical stimulation (Banes *et al.*, 1999b).

Although specific cellular responses have not been elucidated, it is known that the metabolic activity of tenocytes can be modified by changing the mechanical environment. Cells in the tension regions of a tendon express messages for and synthesize type I collagen, whereas cells in regions of tendon that wrap around bone produce type II collagen and other matrix components typical of the fibrocartilaginous matrix seen in these areas of compression. An interesting study by Gillard *et al.* (1979) demonstrated the potential for tendon cells to respond to changes in the normal mechanical environment. The compression region of a deep digital flexor tendon was released to remove the compressive forces and introduce tensile forces; this resulted in a change in the molecular composition of the matrix from fibrocartilaginous to fibrous type I collagen.

Other non-collagenous components of tendon matrix are also synthesized in response to changes in the mechanical environment and in response to aging. One such component is COMP. In the superficial flexor tendon, COMP levels overall increase up to 1 year of age and decline to minimal levels by 2 years of age. However, in the compressive region of the tendon the levels increase to a plateau and are maintained throughout life. The levels of COMP in the tensile regions are further reduced by increased levels of exercise. Although the significance of this matrix component is not fully understood, it may play a role in the ability of the tendon to undergo functional adaptation. In older horses the reduction in COMP must be related to other molecular and structural changes that are now known to occur as a result of long periods of exercise (Smith *et al.*, 1999). The role of COMP also needs to be evaluated in the non-energy storing tendons, such as the extensors, which do show evidence of functional adaptation.

Interestingly, the tenocytes from tendons in older horses can be grown in culture and, when stimulated by TGF β, these cells produce COMP (Smith *et al.*, personal communication). Thus the effects of aging and possibly exercise may involve a suppression of signaling molecules, rather than an age-related inability of the tenocytes to synthesize these non-collagenous proteins. This may indicate potential to develop therapeutic agents to stimulate a response from tenocytes.

CONCLUSION

The whole area of the effects of exercise in relation to both conditioning and rehabilitation of the equine athlete, and the assessment of performance potential subsequent to injury, requires much more investigation. From the scientific evidence it is apparent that the training requirements to condition the individual components of the skeletal system are different. Indeed, conditioning of the whole animal also requires consideration of other vital elements, such as the cardiovascular and respiratory systems, and the integration of these separate conditioning programs with each other. Specific inputs can be characterized for the different component tissues.

Despite scientific advances, training methods remain essentially empirical and the value of extensive research has still to be audited effectively in the commercial arena of equine athletic competition. There is also a need to provide a scientific basis for a complete program of treatment and rehabilitation, including physiotherapy, osteopathy and many of the currently popular paraveterinary disciplines. The position of 'team physiotherapist' is one common to many human athletic activities but relatively less common in association with equine athletes. Perhaps the links between science, training and performance that seem to have occurred in human sports medicine are now beginning to be considered for the equine athlete?

REFERENCES

Arokoski, J., Kiviranta, I., Jurvelin, J., Tammi, M. and Helminen, H.J. (1993) Long-distance running causes site-dependent decrease of cartilage glycosaminoglycan content in the knee joints of beagle dogs. *Arthritis Rheum.* **36**(10): 1451–1459.

Arokoski, J.P., Hyttinen, M.M., Lapvetelainen, T. *et al.* (1996) Decreased birefringence of the superficial zone collagen network in the canine knee (stifle) articular cartilage after long distance running training, detected by quantitative polarised light microscopy. *Ann. Rheum. Dis.* **55**(4):253–264.

Auer, J.A. and Martens, R.J. (1982) Periosteal transection and periosteal stripping for correction of angular limb deformities in foals. *Am. J. Vet. Res.* **43**(9): 1530–1534.

Banes, A.J., Horesovsky, G., Larson, C. *et al.* (1999a) Mechanical load stimulates expression of novel genes *in vivo* in avian flexor tendon cells. *Osteoarthritis Cartilage* **7**(1): 141–153.

Banes, A.J., Weinhold, P., Yang, X. *et al.* (1999b) Gap junctions regulate responses of tendon cells *ex vivo* to mechanical bading. *Clin. Orthop.* **367**(Suppl): 356–370.

Bentolila, V., Boyce, T.M., Fyhrie, D.P., Drumb, R., Skerry, T.M. and Schaffler, M.B. (1998) Intracortical remodeling in adult rat long bones after fatigue loading. *Bone* **23**(3): 275–281.

Bertone, A.L., Park, R.D. and Turner, A.S. (1985) Periosteal transection and stripping for treatment of angular limb deformities in foals: radiographic observations. *J. Am. Vet. Med. Assoc.* **187**(2): 153–156.

Birch, H.L., Wilson, A.M. and Goodship, A.E. (1997a) Physical training induces alterations in tendon matrix composition which are structure specific. *Proc. Brit. Orthopaed. Res. Soc.*, Cardiff.

Birch, H.L., Wilson, A.M. and Goodship, A.E. (1997b) The effect of exercise-induced localised hyperthermia on tendon cell survival. *J. Exp. Biol.* **200**(Pt 11): 1703–1708.

Birch, H.L., Bailey, J.V., Bailey, A.J. and Goodship, A.E. (1999) Age-related changes to the molecular and cellular components of equine flexor tendons. *Equine Vet. J.* **31**(5): 391–396.

Birch, H.L., McLaughlin, L., Smith, R.K.W. and Goodship, A.E. (1999) Treadmill exercise induced tendon hypertrophy: assessment of tendons with different mechanical functions. *Equine Vet. J. Suppl.* **30**, 222–226.

Brama, P. (1999) Dynamics of equine cartilage. *PhD thesis, University of Utrecht, Netherlands.*

Bruin, G. and Creemers, J. (1994) Het voorkomen van osteochondrose. *Praktijkanderzoek Paardenhoverij Maart,* pp 15–17

Cauvin, E.R., Smith, R.K., May, S.A., and Ferguson, M.W.J. (1998) Immunohistochemical localisation of TGF-b in equine tendons. A study in age-related changes in TGF-b expression. *Proc. British Connective Tissue Soc. Cardiff.* In: *Int. J. Exp. Pathol.* **79**: A23.

Currey, J.D. (1984) *Mechanical Adaptations of Bone.* Princeton Press.

Fehling, P.C., Alekel, L., Clasey, J., Rector, A. and Stillman, R.J. (1995) A comparison of bone mineral densities among female athletes in impact loading and active loading sports. *Bone* **17**(3): 205–210.

Firth, E.C., Delahunt, J., Wichtel, J.W., Birch, H.L. and Goodship, A.E. (1999) Galloping exercise induces regional changes in bone density within the third and radial carpal bones of Thoroughbred horses. *Equine Vet. J.* **31**(2): 111–115.

Gathercole, L.J. and Keller, A. (1991) Crimp morphology in the fibre-forming collagens. *Matrix* **11**, 214–234.

Gibbs J., Birch, H.L., and Goodship, A.E. (1995) An investigation into the thermal sensitivity of equine fetal tendon fibroblasts. *Proc. Brit. Orthopaed. Res. Soc.* Dundee

Gillard, G.C., Reilly, H.C., Bell-Booth, P.G. and Flint, M.H. (1979) The influence of mechanical forces on the glycosaminoglycan content of the rabbit flexor digitorum profundus tendon. *Connect Tissue Res.* **7**(1): 37–46.

Gillis, C.L., Meagher, D.M., Pool, R.R. *et al.* (1993) Ultrasonographically detected changes in equine superficial digital flexor tendons during the first months of race training. *Am. J. Vet. Res.* **54**(11): 1797–1802.

Gillis C. Pool R.R., Meagher D.M., Stover S.M., Reiser K, Willits N (1997) Effect of maturation and aging on the histomorphometric and biochemical characteristics of equine superficial digital flexor tendon. *Am J Vet Res.* **58**: 425–30

Goodship, A.E., Cunningham, J.L., Oganov, V., Darling, J., Miles, A.W. and Owen, G.W. (1998) Bone loss during long term space flight is prevented by the application of a short term impulsive mechanical stimulus. *Acta Astronautica* **43**(3–6): 65–76.

Grieshaber, F.A. and Faust, U. (1992) Mechanical characteristics of biological soft tissue *Biomed. Tech. (Berl.)* **37**(12): 278–286.

Heinonen, A., Oja, P., Kannus, P. *et al.* (1995) Bone mineral density in female athletes representing sports with different loading characteristics of the skeleton. *Bone* **17**(3): 197–203.

Hill, W.G. (1988) Why aren't horses faster? *Nature* **332**(6166): 678.

Hoyt, D.F. and Taylor, C.R. (1981) Gait and energetics of locomotion in horses. Nature **292**: 239–240.

Jones, B.H., Harris, J.M., Vinh, T.N. and Rubin, C. (1989) Exercise-induced stress fractures and stress reactions of bone: epidemiology, etiology, and classification. *Exerc. Sport Sci. Rev.* **17**: 379–422.

Johns, P (1998) The effect of exercise on the cross-sectional area of fasciles in the equine superficial digital flexor tendon. *BSc Dissertation,* University College London.

Kannus, P. and Jozsa, L. (1991) Histopathological changes preceding spontaneous rupture of a tendon. A controlled study of 891 patients. *J. Bone Joint Surg.* [*Am*] **73**, 1507–1525.

Kastelic, J., Galeski, A. and Baer, E. (1978) The multicomposite structure of tendon. *Connect. Tissue Res.* **6**(1): 11–23.

Kiviranta, I., Tammi, M., Jurvelin, J., Saamanen, A.M. and Helminen, H.J. (1988) Moderate running exercise augments glycosaminoglycans and thickness of articular cartilage in the knee joint of young beagle dogs. *J. Orthop. Res.* **6**(2): 188–195.

Leitch, M. (1985) Musculoskeletal disorders in neonatal foals. *Vet. Clin. North Am.: Equine Pract.* **1**(1): 189–207.

Little, C.B. and Ghosh, P. (1997) Variation in proteoglycan metabolism by articular chondrocytes in different joint regions is determined by post-natal mechanical loading. *Osteoarth. Cart.* **5**(1): 49–62.

Little, C.B., Ghosh, P. and Rose, R. (1997) The effect of strenuous versus moderate exercise on the metabolism of proteoglycans in articular cartilage from different weight-bearing regions of the equine third carpal bone. *Osteoarth. Cart.* **5**(3): 161–72.

McNeilly, C.M., Banes, A.J., Benjamin, M. and Ralphs, J.R. (1996) Tendon cells *in vivo* form a three dimensional network of cell processes linked by gap junctions *J. Anat.* **189**(3): 593–600.

Milz, S., Eckstein, F. and Putz, R. (1997) Thickness distribution of the subchondral mineralization zone of the trochlear notch and its correlation with the cartilage thickness: an expression of functional adaptation to mechanical stress acting on the humeroulnar joint? *Anat. Rec.* **248**(2): 189–197.

Morgan, D.L., Proske, U. and Warren, D. (1978) Measurements of muscle stiffness and the mechanism of elastic storage of energy in hopping kangaroos. *J. Physiol. (Lond.)* **282**: 253–261.

Murray, R.C., Zhu, C.F., Goodship, A.E., Lakhani, K.H., Agrawal, C.M. and Athanasiou, K.A. (1999) Exercise affects the mechanical properties and histological appearance of equine articular cartilage. *Orthop. Res.* **17**(5): 725–731.

Newton P.O., Woo SL-Y, Mackenna D.A., Akeson WH (1995) Immobilisation of the knee alters the mechanical and ultra-strucutral properties of the rabbit anterior cruciate ligament *J. Orthop Res.* **13** 191–200

Newton, P.M., Mow, V.C., Garnder, T.R., Buckwalter, J.A. and Albright, J.P. (1997) The effect of lifelong exercise on canine articular cartilage. *Am. J. Sports Med.* **25**(3): 282–287.

Nissen R, Cardinale GJ, Udenfriend S Increased turnover of arterial collagen in hypertensive rats. Proc Natl Acad Sci USA 1978 **75**: 451–3

Nunamaker, D.M., Butterweck, D.M. and Provost, M.T. (1990) Fatigue fractures in thoroughbred racehorses: relationships with age, peak bone strain, and training. *J. Orthop. Res.* **8**(4): 604–611.

Nunamaker, D.M., Butterweck, D.M. and Black, J. (1991) In vitro comparison of Thoroughbred and Standardbred racehorses with regard to local fatigue failure of the third metacarpal bone. *Am. J. Vet. Res.* **52**(1): 97–100.

Oettmeier, R., Arokoski, J., Roth, A.J., Helminen, H.J., Tammi, M. and Abendroth, K. (1992) Quantitative study of articular cartilage and subchondral bone remodeling in the knee joint of dogs after strenuous running training. *J. Bone Miner. Res.* **7**(Suppl. 2): S419–424.

O'Kane, S. and Ferguson, M.W. (1997) Transforming growth factor beta s and wound heading. *Int. J. Biochem. Cell Biol.* **29**(1): 63–78.

Patterson-Kane J.C., Firth E.C., Goodship A.E., Parry D.A. (1997a) Age-related differences in collagen crimp patterns in the superficial digitalflexor tendon core region of untrained horses. *Aust. Vet. J.* **75**: 39–44.

Patterson-Kane, J.C., Parry, D.A.D., Birch, H.L. et al. (1997b) An age-related study of morphology and crosslink composition of collagen fibrils in the digital flexor tendons of young Thoroughbred horses. *Connective Tissue Res.* **36,** 253–260.

Patterson-Kane, J.C. Wilson, A.M., Firth, E.C. *et al.* (1998) Exercise-related alterations in crimp morphology in the central regions of superficial digital flexor tendons from young thoroughbreds: a controlled study. *Equine Vet. J.* **30,** 61–64.

Parry, D.A., Flint, M.H., Gillard, G.C. and Craig, A.S. (1982) A role for glycosaminoglycans in the development of coellagen fibrils. *FEBS left* 149(1): 1–7.

Pirttiniemi, P., Kantomaa, T., Salo, L. and Tuominen, M. (1996) Effect of reduced articular function on deposition of type I and type II collagens in the mandibular condylar cartilage of the rat. *Arch. Oral Biol.* 41(1): 127–131.

Platt, D., Wilson, A.M., Timbs, A., Wright, I.M., and Goodship, A.E. (1994) Novel force transducer for measurement of tendon force in vivo. *J. Biomech.* 27(12): 1489–1493.

Price, J.S., Jackson, B., Eastell, R. *et al.* (1995) The response of the skeleton to physical training; a biochemical study in horses. *Bone* 17(3): 221–227.

Qin, Y.X., Rubin, C.T. and McLeod, K.J. (1998) Nonlinear dependence of loading intensity and cycle number in the maintenance of bone mass and morphology. *J. Orthop. Res.* 16(4): 482–489.

Radin, E.L., Parker, H.G., Pugh, J.W., Steinberg, R.S., Paul, I.L. and Rose, R.M. (1973) Response of joints to impact loading. 3. Relationship between trabecular microfractures and cartilage degeneration. *J. Biomech.* 6(1): 51–57.

Reilly, G.C., Currey, J.D. and Goodship, A.E. (1997) Exercise of young thoroughbred horses increases impact strength of the third metacarpal bone. *J. Orthop. Res.* 15(6): 862–868.

Riemersma, D.J. and Schamhardt, H.C. (1985) In vitro mechanical properties of tendons in relation to cross-sectional area and collagen content. *Res. Vet. Sci.* 39(3): 263–70.

Rossdale, P.D., Hopes, R, Digby, N.J. and Offord, K. (1985) Epidemiological study of wastage among racehorses 1982 and 1983. *Vet. Rec.* 116(3): 66–69.

Rubin, C.T. and Lanyon, L.E. (1982) Limb mechanics as a function of speed and gait: a study of functional strains in the radius and tibia of horse and dog. *J. Exp. Biol.* 101: 187–211.

Salter, R.B. (1981) Royal College Lecture: Prevention of arthritis through preservation of cartilage. *J. Can. Assoc. Radiol.* 32(1): 5–7.

Schatzmann, L., Brunner, P. and Staubli, H.U. (1998) Effect of cyclic preconditioning on the tensile properties of human quadriceps tendons and patellar ligaments. *Knee Surg. Sports Traumatol. Arthrosc.* 6(Suppl. 1): S56–61.

Smith, R.K.W., Williams, L., Birch, H.L., van Weeren, R. and Goodship, A.E. (1999) Should equine athletes commence training during skeletal development? Changes in tendon matrix associated with, development, ageing, function and exercise *Equine Vet. J.* (Suppl. 30): 201–209.

Steinmeyer, J. and Knue, S. (1997) The proteoglycan metabolism of mature bovine articular cartilage explants superimposed to continuously applied cyclic mechanical loading. *Biochem. Biophys. Res. Commun.* 240(1): 216–221.

Stephens, P.R., Nunamaker, D.M. and Butterweck, D.M. (1989) Application of a Hall-effect transducer for measurement of tendon strains in horses. *Am. J. Vet. Res.* 50(7): 1089–1095.

Tomlin, J.L. Lawes, T.J., Blunn, G.W., Goodship, A.E. and Muir, P. (2000) Fractographic examination of racing greyhound central (navicular) tarsal bone failure surfaces using scanning electron Microscopy. *Calcif. Tissue Int.* 67, 260–266.

Vashishth, D., Behiri, J.C. and Bonfield, W. (1997) Crack growth resistance in cortical bone: concept of microcrack toughening. *J. Biomech.* 30(8): 763–769.

Vaughan, L.C. and Mason, B.J.E. (1975) *A Clinico-pathological Study of Racing Accidents in Horses. A report of a study on equine fatal accidents on racecourses financed by the Horserace BettingLevy Board.* Dorking: Adlard and Sons Ltd, Bartholomew Press.

Visser, N.A., de Koning, M.H., Lammi, M.J., Hakkinen, A., Tammi, M. and van Kampen, G.P. (1998) Increase of decorin content in articular cartilage following running. *Connect. Tissue Res.* 37(3–4): 295–302.

Webbon, P.M. (1977) A post mortem study of equine digital flexor tendons. *Equine Vet. J.,* **9,** 61–67.

Wilmink J, Wilson A.M., Goodship A.E. Functional significance of the morphology and micromechanicm of collagen fibres in relation to partial rupture of the superficial digital flexor tendon in racehorses. *Res. Vet. Sci.* 1992; **53:** 354–9

Wilson, A.M. (1991) The effect of exercise intensity on the biochemistry, morphology and mechanical properties of tendon. *PhD thesis,* University of Bristol, UK.

Wilson, A.M. and Goodship, A.E. Exercise-induced hyperthermia as a possible mechanism for tendon degeneration. *J Biomech* 1994; **27 :** 899–905.

Wilson, J.H., Robinson, R.A., Jensen, R.C. and McArdle, C.J. (1996) Equine soft tissue injuries associated with racing. Descriptive statistics from American racetracks. In: Rantanen, N.W. and Hauser, M.L. (eds) *The Equine Athlete: Tendon, Ligament and Soft Tissue Injuries.* Matthew, R. Rantanen Design.

Wong, M., Siegrist, M. and Cao X (1999) Cyclic compression of articular cartilage explants is associated with progressive consolidation and altered expression pattern of extracellular matrix proteins. *Matrix Biol.* 18(4): 391–399.

Woo, S.L.Y., Gomez, M.A., Sites, T.J., Newton, P.O. Orlando, C.A and Akeson, W.H. (1987) The biomechanical and morphological changes in the medial collateral ligament of the rabbit after immobilization and remobilization. *J. Bone Joint Surg.,* **69A,** 1200–1211.

Woo, S.L., Gomez, M.A., Woo, Y.K. and Akeson, W.H. (1982) Mechanical properties of tendons and ligaments. II. The relationships of immobilization and exercise on tissue remodeling. *Biorheology* 19(3): 397–408.

10
Gait Adaptation in Lameness

H.H. Florian Buchner

INTRODUCTION

Horses are kept as domestic animals due to their outstanding locomotor skills, which have been employed for military use, transportation and sports. Perfect athletic performance, of course, needs a sound locomotor system. Maintenance of soundness and detection of lameness are of prime importance for horse owners. The ability to study the gait of horses and assess the small deviations associated with locomotor problems is limited by the physiological ability of the human eye. Therefore, locomotion research in horses started very early with studies of the gait of lame horses. As early as 1899, Muybridge published series of photographic plates of both sound and lame horses in his fascinating book *Animals in Motion*. These nice studies were the start of modern kinematic research on lameness in horses, which is and will continue to be a central theme of equine locomotion analysis (Leach & Crawford, 1983).

Definitions

Lameness is not a disease but a symptom of a locomotor disturbance. Generally, lameness can be defined as an alteration of the normal gait due to a functional or structural disorder in the locomotor system (Wittmann, 1931; Knezevic *et al.*, 1982; West, 1984; Stashak, 1987; Wyn-Jones, 1988; Speirs, 1994; Wilson & Keegan, 1995). A detailed description of the locomotion pattern is a central part of each lameness examination. The goal is to localize the cause of the lameness and to make a diagnosis that is as specific as possible as a basis for veterinary therapy.

Classification of lameness

In a clinical setting various classifications of lameness are used to differentiate various pathological gait patterns. Such classifications provide only a rough framework and a real lameness cannot always be fitted into a single category. Nevertheless, placing a lameness in one of the categories is a first step for the clinician in reaching a diagnosis. Locomotion analysis, on the other hand, should provide specific details of the various lamenesses as well as fundamental relations and principles. These can be used to understand the different types of lameness and to provide the scientific basis for interpreting the observations made during lameness examinations. Figure 10.1 shows the traditional classifications for lameness. The cause of the lameness is most often pain in one or more limbs. Sometimes diseases of peripheral nerves, blood vessels or muscles cause specific lamenesses and occasionally purely mechanical restrictions can be found. The type of lameness describes the phase of the stride when the disturbance is visible. A supporting limb lameness is caused by pain during the stance phase, while swinging limb lameness is caused by problems during the swing phase. Pure swinging limb lamenesses are extremely rare and are most often a component of mixed lameness with features of both supporting and swinging limb lameness. The third classification describes the site of the lameness as a fore or a hindlimb lameness or as a bilateral lameness, when both fore or hindlimbs are affected.

If a specific structure can be proven as the origin of lameness and a specific diagnosis established, locomotion analysis techniques can be used to define the associated locomotor patterns. A special situation is represented by induced lamenesses, which have been used in several clinical studies for evaluations of diagnostic

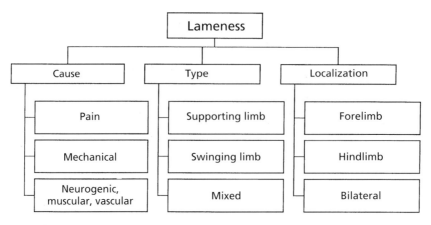

Fig. 10.1 Classification of lameness.

or therapeutic regimes. Lameness models have been reported to induce hoof lameness (Merkens & Schamhardt, 1988a; Foreman & Lawrence, 1991), arthritis of the carpal joint (Auer & Butter 1986; Firth *et al.*, 1987; Peloso *et al.*, 1993) and tendonitis (Silver *et al.*, 1983; Williams *et al.*, 1984). The ability to induce a more or less transient lameness in groups of sound horses offers an important and reliable method to study the locomotor pattern in horses with specific, well-defined lamenesses in a controlled manner that minimizes individual variations.

Locomotion research can provide information regarding several aspects of equine locomotion. This chapter will describe the results of locomotion research in the area of lameness during the past century from different viewpoints and with different objectives.

1. First, the kinematics that are specific to different types of lameness will be described. This will provide a more complete insight into the gait adaptations and how horses deal with and compensate for pain in a limb. The findings are of fundamental importance for the orthopedic specialist.
2. The effectiveness of the locomotor adaptations in terms of load reduction in the painful limb and load redistribution will be evaluated using kinetic methods. The connection of kinetic and kinematic findings allows an analysis of the mechanisms by which a horse manages a lameness.
3. The patterns of some well-defined lamenesses will be presented and analyzed to determine their specific signs, which will serve as a diagnostic database.
4. The possible use of locomotion analysis techniques in clinical settings, such as the documentation of diagnostic or therapeutic regimes or the diagnosis of insidious lamenesses, will then be described and discussed with all the pros and cons of these methods.

5. Finally, the effects of several frequently used diagnostic or therapeutic aids will be evaluated. In these studies locomotion analysis technology is used to evaluate the proposed effects and to support or reject their use based on scientific fundamentals.

KINEMATICS OF LAMENESS

The judgment of an observer as to whether a horse is lame or not is based on a comparison of the gait or details of the locomotion pattern with a sound reference. Such a reference for an objective determination of a lameness can be found using three different approaches:

1. A comparison with the 'normal' locomotion pattern in the population, which is based on the experience of the clinician. This requires a sufficient number of observations in sound horses to establish a standard and to eliminate the problem of individuality. This 'standard horse', however, may not be the best method for kinematic assessments due to the small differences caused by lameness compared with the wide inter-individual variation in sound horses.
2. A comparison using the horse's own pattern as an individual control. Since the sound pattern of the individual is usually unknown during lameness examinations, diagnostic nerve blocks serve as a tool to restore kinematics that are close to the sound pattern during a clinical evaluation. In a research setting similar comparisons are possible using lameness models, where the sound locomotion pattern of each horse before lameness induction serves as an individual control and minute deviations due to lameness can be easily differentiated from the small intra-individual variations.

3. An assessment of the movements of the left and right sides of the body in terms of locomotor symmetry or asymmetry within an individual horse. This approach allows an immediate comparison of affected and unaffected limbs independent of individual characteristics.

Using one of these three methods, several general characteristics of supporting limb lameness and swinging limb lameness have been described.

Supporting limb lameness

Lameness that results from the efforts of the horse to avoid pain during the stance phase is defined as supporting limb lameness and often originates in ailments of the hoof or the distal limb. These ailments cause pain during loading and the horses try to minimize the pain by changes in various aspects of the locomotor pattern, which can be classified into four categories: the temporal stride pattern, the movement of the hoof, the angular pattern of the limb joints and head and trunk movements.

Temporal stride pattern

Many studies (Hugelshofer, 1982; Clayton, 1986b; Girtler, 1988a, 1988b 1988c; Dohne, 1991; Tietje, 1992; Buchner et al., 1995a; Keegan et al., 1997) have tried to find relationships between lameness and the timing of the limb placements, described as stride variables. However, these studies did not find typical changes or asymmetry patterns. This is in contradiction to subjective impressions, where some observers describe that a shortening of the loading phase of the lame limb seems to be a typical sign for a supporting limb lameness (Wittmann, 1931; Ratzlaff et al., 1982; Hajer et al., 1988). Nevertheless, some general temporal patterns can be seen if the lameness is moderate or severe. Slight or 'subclinical' lamenesses, on the other hand, do not show significant temporal deviations from the sound stride pattern (Buchner et al., 1995a).

Generally, lame horses tend to move with a slower velocity. This is of utmost importance for the interpretation of the stride pattern in lame horses, because all stride variables are heavily dependent on velocity (Dusek et al., 1970; Leach & Cymbaluk, 1986; Leach & Drevemo, 1991). Comparisons of different assessments, for example before and after diagnostic anesthesias, are valid only if recorded at the same velocity or using statistical correction methods (Kübber et al., 1994). Horses reduce their velocity by decreasing stride duration, stride length and all the dependent variables, such as stance duration or contralateral advanced placement. On the other hand, when horses are forced to maintain a constant velocity on the treadmill, variable results regarding stride duration and stride length in lame horses have been

Table 10.1 Mean and standard deviation of stride variables in 11 horses evaluated when sound and with two degrees of induced forelimb lameness in the hoof at the trot (3.5 m/s).

Variable	Lameness degree		
	0	1	2
Stride duration (ms)	715 (36)	707 (42)	693 (53)[c]
Stance duration (ms)			
Lame forelimb	312 (17)	313 (15)	318 (16)
Sound forelimb	307 (16)	306 (15)	312 (15)[c]
Ipsilateral hindlimb	291 (20)	287 (25)	290 (22)
Diagonal hindlimb	291 (17)	284 (20)[a]	285 (19)[c]
Relative stance duration (%)			
Lame forelimb	43.7 (2.4)	44.3 (2.4)	46.0 (2.8)[bc]
Sound forelimb	43.0 (2.4)	43.4 (2.8)	45.3 (3.4)[bc]
Ipsilateral hindlimb	40.7 (3.1)	40.7 (3.7)	42.0 (3.8)[bc]
Diagonal hindlimb	40.7 (2.9)	40.3 (3.3)	41.3 (3.2)
Advanced placement (ms)			
Lame diagonal	0 (18)	–9 (19)[a]	–16 (26)[c]
Sound diagonal	3 (22)	–2 (24)	–10 (24)[bc]
Lame → sound forelimb	360 (20)	358 (26)	341 (28)[bc]
Sound → lame forelimb	355 (18)	350 (19)	352 (28)
Ipsi. → diag. hindlimb	358 (19)	357 (20)	359 (21)
Diag. → ipsi. hindlimb	357 (18)	351 (24)	335 (36)[bc]
Suspension (ms)			
Lame diagonal	36 (24)	35 (26)	14 (29)[bc]
Sound diagonal	39 (20)	38 (20)	32 (27)

Significant differences between the values of a variable for different lameness degrees are indicated by superscripts. [a]: degree 0 versus 1; [b]: degree 1 versus 2; [c]: degree 0 versus 2. Diagonal advanced placement is positive when the hindlimb precedes the forelimb and vice versa.
(Reprinted with permission from Buchner, H.H.F., Savelberg, H.H.C.M., Schamhardt, H.C. and Barneveld, A. (1995) Temporal stride patterns in horses with experimentally induced fore or hind limb lameness. *Equine Vet. J.* **18**(Suppl.): 161–165.)

reported (Buchner et al., 1995a; Pollhammer-Zeilinger, 1996; Keegan et al., 1997). When showing different degrees of hoof lameness, provoked by the screw model of Merkens and Schamhardt (1988a), horses maintained the velocity by taking shorter, but quicker, strides than in the sound condition (Table 10.1) (Buchner et al., 1995a; Galisteo et al., 1997). However, in horses suffering from navicular disease no consistent changes in stride duration and stride length were found between the lame pattern and the sound pattern after diagnostic anesthesia (Pollhammer-Zeilinger, 1996; Keegan et al., 1997).

Generally, a consistent feature in all studies is a shortening of the swing duration in lame horses compared to the same horses without lameness (Hugelshofer, 1982; Dohne, 1991; Tietje, 1992; Buchner et al., 1995a; Keegan et al., 1997). In other words, horses lengthen the stance phase duration rather than shortening it to diminish the pain. This is in contradiction to the opinions that shortened stance durations are indicative of supporting limb lameness (Ratzlaff et al., 1982; Clayton, 1986a). Furthermore, there is no difference in stance duration between the lame and the sound limb (Girtler, 1988c; Tietje, 1992; Buchner et al., 1995a). The horses maintain their symmetry; both limbs are kept on the ground longer with increasing lameness, while both swing durations decrease. This does not contradict the findings of differences in stance durations between left and right limbs in some particular horses. Absolute symmetry is nearly impossible in nature and significant left/right differences as a sign of handedness or leggedness are found in various breeds (Meij & Meij, 1980; Deuel & Lawrence, 1987; Drevemo et al., 1987). Asymmetry in stance duration is therefore not a sign of a supporting limb lameness, but a typical individual characteristic.

In forelimb lamenesses a real asymmetry due to lameness can be found in the suspension phase at the trot (Table 10.1) (Clayton, 1986a; Buchner et al., 1995a). The suspension phase following the lame diagonal stance phase, which means the time when none of the limbs is on the ground after the stance phase of the lame forelimb and diagonal hindlimb, is significantly shortened in lame horses. This is a sign of reduced propulsion during the stance phase of the lame limb. The suspension following the sound diagonal, on the other hand, is unchanged. This asymmetry can only be seen in forelimb lameness, not in hindlimb lameness. During hindlimb lameness, generally the same temporal pattern is found in most stride variables, and the duration of the suspension phase does not change. Horses with hindlimb lameness keep this variable constant and perfectly symmetrical.

The asymmetric suspension phase in forelimb lameness has some implications for the coordination of the placements of the different limbs. The duration of the step from the lame to the sound forelimb is shorter than the contralateral step or than the step duration without lameness (Table 10.1) as a result of the clearly shortened suspension between the lame and sound diagonals.

An interesting pattern is seen in the diagonal advanced placement. As already mentioned, during forelimb lameness, the stance phases of the forelimbs tend to increase, with the fore hooves being placed earlier and lifted later. This results in an earlier placement of the forelimbs in relation to the diagonal hindlimbs. Sound horses place their diagonal limb pairs almost synchronously or even place the hindlimbs earlier than the fore-

Summary

Horses with supporting limb lameness tend to have longer stance durations in their forelimbs, but provide less propulsion during the stance phase of the lame limb, so that the following suspension phase is reduced. This is an important method of reducing the peak loads on the limbs, which will be discussed in detail below.

limbs (positive diagonal advanced placement). The latter sequence may be indicative of superior gait quality in dressage horses (Holmström et al., 1994). Lameness reverses this pattern. Similarly, horses on a treadmill show this earlier forelimb placement, perhaps due to a need for longer ground contact, possibly as a sign of a remaining insecurity even after a long period of habituation to the treadmill (Buchner et al., 1994).

Hoof movement

Hoof movement can be visualized as the hoof trajectory during the stride. Figure 10.2 shows the trajectory of a fore hoof on a treadmill seen from the right side. The stance phase is characterized by a constant vertical position on the treadmill belt during the horizontal movement from right to left in the figure. After lift off, the flight arc of the hoof shows the elevation during the swing phase and ends with the hoof landing at the start of the next stance phase.

Different features can be seen in this figure showing typical changes in the hoof trajectory due to various degrees of forelimb lameness. The maximal height of the hoof during protraction of the limb is said to be lower during both supporting limb lameness and swinging limb lameness (Stashak, 1987). In supporting limb lameness, a lower flight arc might reduce pain on impact. In swinging limb lameness, difficulties in flexing the joints may cause a lowering of the flight arc. However, this could not be confirmed in recordings of horses suffering from navicular disease. Several authors investigated this lameness for characteristic patterns, but did not find consistent changes in maximal hoof height (Ratzlaff & Grant, 1986; Pollhammer-Zeilinger, 1996; Keegan et al., 1997). In experimentally induced forehoof lameness (Buchner et al., 1996a) as well as in patients with forelimb lamenesses (Girtler et al., 1987) a higher flight arc was found in the sound forelimb and an unchanged height in the lame limb (Fig. 10.2). During hindlimb lameness, a lower flight arc was found in the lame limb, while the sound limb had an unchanged flight arc (Buchner et al., 1996a). Both patterns give the same impression: the hoof of the lame side is lower than the contralateral hoof.

Changes in the pro- and retraction of the limbs of lame horses are visible at the walk. Retraction of the forelimbs is slightly reduced during forelimb lameness. For the interpretation of this pattern a comparison with the changes in hindlimb movement during hindlimb lameness is interesting. Lame hindlimbs show a reduction in protraction rather than retraction. Perhaps the position of the limb relative to the body center of mass influences this feature. During walking, vertical ground reaction forces of the forelimbs reach peak values in the second half of the stance phase, when the limb is retracted, which brings it closer to the body center of mass. On the other hand, the position of the hindlimbs relative to the body center of mass causes peak loading in the first half of the stance phase (Merkens *et al.*, 1986). The changes in pro- or retraction, which are more obvious during walking than trotting, might reduce the total load on the lame limb by shortening the period of high load.

The changes in the temporal stride pattern also have implications for the linear stride variables. The distances between hoof placements of sound and lame limbs and vice versa, which are called the step lengths, might give information about the cause of the lameness. A shortening of the step length from the lame to the sound limb is said to be typical for a supporting limb lameness (Wittmann, 1931; Stashak, 1987). Horses with sesamoiditis (Clayton, 1986b) and hoof lameness (Buchner *et al.*, 1996) showed this feature. This shortening corresponds with the temporal variables in terms of the shorter

Summary

The hoof flight arc does not change much in the lame limb, while hoof landing pattern might depend more on individual characteristics. The reduced swing duration leads to a shorter step length from lame to sound limb but a slightly higher flight arc in the sound limb.

advanced placement between lame and sound forelimbs as well as the clearly shortened suspension phase following the lame diagonal. The linear stride variables offer further proof of reduced propulsion during the stance phase of the painful limb.

Few studies have described specific changes in the hoof landing pattern due to lameness. Toe first or heel first might give information about the localization of the pain, in the heel or toe region (Ratzlaff & Grant, 1986; Stashak, 1987; Clayton, 1988; Tietje, 1992; Wilson & Keegan, 1995). Measurements of induced hoof lameness, caused by pressure-inducing screws on the sole, did not influence the hoof landing angle (Buchner *et al.*, 1996a), which may have been due to the position of the screws being in the middle, between toe and heel. Differences in the hoof position and motion just before landing were described by Knezevic *et al.* (1982) for a horse with carpal lameness. Changes in limb movement during the swing phase may also cause changes in the hoof landing pattern. However, a lack of quantitative data precludes making precise conclusions at

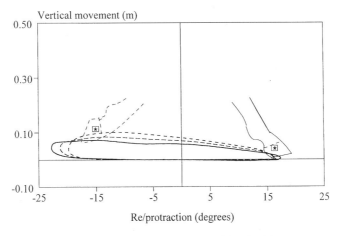

Fig. 10.2 Hoof trajectory of a lame forelimb during different degrees of forelimb lameness.
(—) lameness degree 0 (sound); (- - -) lameness degree 1; (– – –) lameness degree 2. (Reprinted with permission from Buchner, H.H.F., Savelberg, H.H.C.M., Schamhardt, H.C. and Barneveld, A. (1996) Limb movement adaptations in horses with experimentally induced fore or hind limb lameness. *Equine Vet. J.* **28**: 63–70.)

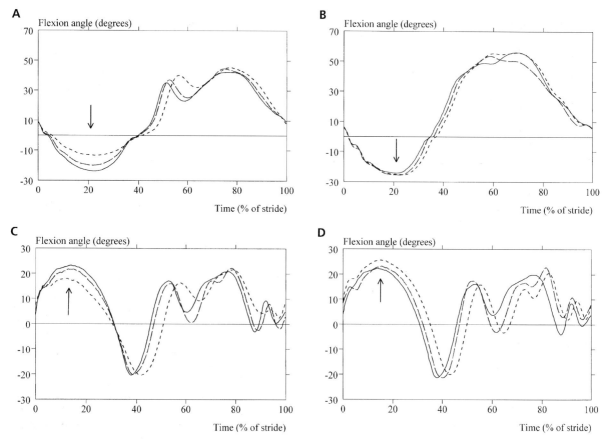

Fig. 10.3 Joint angle pattern of the fetlock (**A**) and coffin (**C**) joints of a lame forelimb, and the fetlock (**B**) and coffin (**D**) joints of the contralateral sound forelimb during different degrees of forelimb lameness. (———) lameness degree 0 (sound); (— — —) lameness degree 1; (- - -) lameness degree 2. (Reprinted with permission from: Buchner, H.H.F., *et al.* (1996) Limb movement adaptations in horses with experimentally induced fore or hind limb lameness. *Equine Vet. J.* **28**: 63–70.)

this time. To differentiate between individual landing patterns and specific lameness patterns, it will be necessary to perform studies with a number of horses that have a similar diagnosis or the same induced lameness.

Limb movement and joint angle patterns

The joint movement patterns of the equine limbs are important indicators of both physiologic locomotor capacity (Back *et al.*, 1994; Holmström *et al.*, 1994) and disturbances of the gait due to lameness (Adrian *et al.*, 1977; Ratzlaff & Grant, 1986; Back *et al.*, 1993; Peloso *et al.*, 1993; Buchner *et al.*, 1996a; Keegan *et al.*, 1997). The amount of hyperextension of the fetlock joint and flexion of the carpal and tarsal joints correlated very well with subjective judgments of gait quality in the areas of suppleness and strength (Back *et al.*, 1994). In lame horses, the proximal (shoulder, carpus, stifle, tarsus) and

distal (fetlock, coffin) joints reflect different aspects of limb motion and show different changes due to lameness.

During supporting limb lameness the horse tries to reduce the load on the painful limb. The amount of loading can be measured directly using a force plate, and it can be assessed indirectly from the distal joint patterns during the stance phase. At the trot, the fetlock joint shows increasing hyperextension until the moment of maximal loading in the middle of the stance phase (Fig. 10.3A). The hyperextension then decreases gradually until the end of the stance phase. The fetlock joint angle during the stance phase is determined by and resembles the pattern of the vertical ground reaction force as measured in sound horses with a force plate (Riemersma *et al.*, 1988) or a force shoe (Ratzlaff *et al.*, 1993). This relationship is valid also in lame horses, when changes in the fetlock and coffin joint patterns correspond to a decrease in the vertical ground reaction

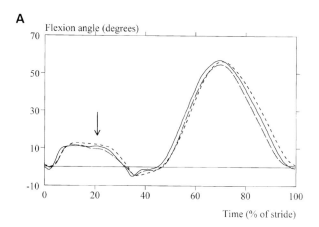

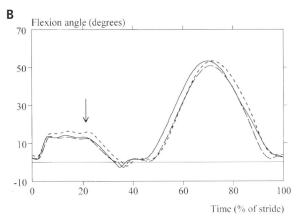

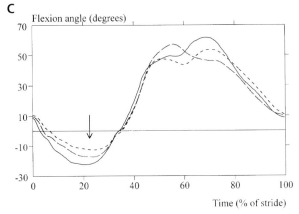

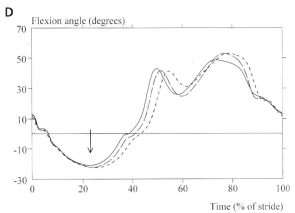

Table 10.2 Joint angle variables of the forelimbs of 11 horses at the trot when sound and with two degrees of induced forelimb lameness at the trot (3.5 m/s).

Variable	Limb	Lameness degree		
		0	1	2
Maximal carpal flexion	Lame	80.3 (7.7)	81.1 (6.3)	79.4 (5.2)
	Sound	79.8 (10.4)	80.1 (10.0)	78.3 (11.2)
Maximal fetlock hyperextension	Lame	−19.1 (4.0)	−17.0 (4.1)[a]	−11.5 (5.2)[bc]
	Sound	−20.0 (3.7)	−21.2 (3.4)[a]	−21.9 (3.9)[c]
Maximal coffin flexion	Lame	23.6 (3.3)	22.8 (3.5)	20.4 (3.4)[bc]
	Sound	23.5 (4.0)	24.6 (4.1)	27.3 (3.5)[bc]

Data are presented as mean (SD), and are expressed in degrees. Significant differences ($p < 0.05$) between different lameness degrees are indicated by superscripts.[a]: degree 0 versus 1; [b]: degree 1 versus 2; [c]: degree 0 versus 2. (Reprinted with permission from: Buchner, H.H.F., Savelberg, H.H.C.M., Schamhardt, H.C. and Barneveld, A. (1996). Limb movement adaptations in horses with experimentally induced fore or hind limb lameness. *Equine Vet. J.* **28**: 63–70.)

Fig. 10.4 Joint angle pattern of the tarsal (**A**) and fetlock (**B**) and fetlock (**C**) joints of a lame hindlimb and tarsal (**D**) joints of the contralateral sound hindlimb during different degrees of hindlimb lameness. (——) lameness degree 0 (sound); (— — —) lameness degree 1; (- - -) lameness degree 2. (Reprinted with permission from Buchner, H.H.F., *et al.* (1996) Limb movement adaptations in horses with experimentally induced fore or hind limb lameness. *Equine Vet. J.* **28**: 63–70.)

force in the lame limb and a compensatory increase in the contralateral sound limb (Merkens & Schamhardt, 1988b).

During supporting limb lameness, both the fetlock and coffin joint patterns change distinctly with increasing lameness (Table 10.2). In the lame limb, fetlock hyperextension at the middle of the stance phase is reduced with each degree of lameness (Fig. 10.3A). In contrast, fetlock hyperextension in the contralateral sound limb shows increased maximal values (Fig. 10.3B). This asymmetry indicates a compensation of the reduced loading of the lame limb by the contralateral

Summary

The proximal joint pattern shows the efforts of the horse to smooth limb loading, while the distal joint pattern reflects an absolute decrease in loading of the lame limb. This decrease in limb loading cannot be achieved by changing the limb movement pattern. It is the result of adaptations in head and trunk movements.

sound limb. Similarly, coffin joint flexion is reduced, but the effects are a little less obvious and occur earlier in the stride cycle (Fig. 10.3C,D). Based on this strong correlation, the fetlock joint pattern can be used as indicator of a supporting limb lameness or the supporting limb component of a mixed lameness (Back *et al.*, 1993). However, the range of fetlock joint motion proved to be less sensitive in detecting slight lamenesses (Peloso *et al.*, 1993), probably due to the higher variability in swing phase flexion. Therefore, maximal fetlock hyperextension during stance, which resembles the clinical assessment of fetlock sinking, is a sensitive measure of a supporting limb lameness. The asymmetric pattern of lame and contralateral sound limbs can be used as a symmetry variable for lameness quantifications.

In contrast to the distal joints, the proximal joints play a more active role in lameness management. The shoulder and tarsus normally flex as the limbs are loaded, but movements of these joints are more dependent on muscular control than the fetlock joint, where passive support by the interosseus (suspensory) ligament is the most significant factor. In contrast to the distal joints, flexion of the proximal joints during loading of the limbs is increased rather than reduced in the lame limb. In the shoulder joint of the lame forelimb this increase is rather small, but tarsal flexion changes more distinctly, which may indicate an increased functioning of a shock absorbing mechanism (Fig. 10.4A–D) (Hjertén *et al.*, 1994; Back *et al.*, 1995b). These increases in shoulder and tarsal joint flexion during the stance phase of the lame limb are not due to increased loading. They are the result of a more gentle braking of the flexion by the extensor muscles. Consequently, loading of the lame limb with the body weight occurs more gradually, and this reduces the peak forces in the hoof. This finding corresponds with the changes in the ground reaction force pattern in lame horses: there is a marked decrease in the first peak of the vertical ground reaction force in a lame limb at the walk, while the forces at mid stance are slightly higher (Merkens & Schamhardt, 1988a). This increased damping is expressed more in the hindlimb than the forelimb; this is thought to be related to the

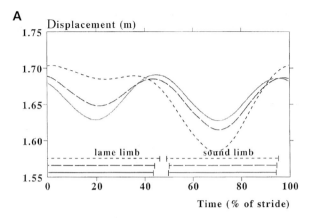

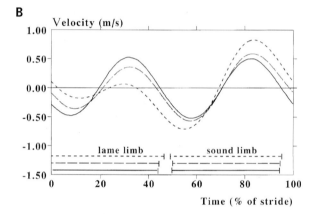

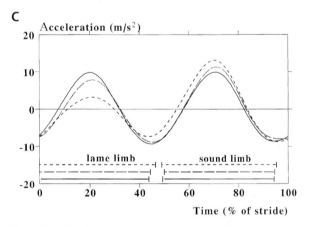

Fig. 10.5 Head movement pattern during different degrees of forelimb lameness. **A**: vertical displacement; **B**: vertical velocity; **C**: vertical acceleration. The horizontal bars indicate the stance phases of the limbs.
(——) lameness degree 0 (sound); (— — —) lameness degree 1; (- - -) lameness degree 2. (Reprinted with permission from Buchner, H.H.F., *et al.* (1996) Head and trunk movement adaptations in horses with experimentally induced fore or hind limb lameness. *Equine Vet. J.* **28**: 71–76.)

considerably greater range of motion in the tarsal/stifle joint complex compared with the shoulder/elbow joint complex (Back *et al.*, 1995a, b).

Head and trunk movement

The simplest, most sensitive, and most frequently used indicator for the clinical diagnosis of lameness is the characteristic vertical movement of the horse's head and trunk (Stashak, 1987; Wyn-Jones, 1988). A more or less asymmetric pattern of head movement is the starting point for each student to diagnose a forelimb lameness and, similarly, croup or hip movement is used to diagnose a hindlimb lameness. Sound horses at a trot show a perfect sinusoidal pattern for all midline body locations including the head, withers and croup (Girtler & Floss, 1984; Buchner *et al.*, 1996b). During one stride, two symmetric waves can be seen (Fig. 10.5A), which occur almost synchronously in all three body parts. The height of these structures falls from the beginning of the diagonal stance phase, reaching the lowest position at mid stance, then rising to their highest level at or shortly after the end of the stance phase. During the suspension phase, the body starts to fall again into the next diagonal limb stance phase. These sinusoidal cycles are repeated twice in each stride. The derivatives of this vertical movement, vertical velocity and vertical acceleration of the head or withers, show similar sinusoidal patterns, but shifted by 12.5% per derivative to the left (Fig. 10.5B,C). Vertical velocity reaches minimal values shortly after the beginning of the stance phase and maximal values shortly before the end of stance. Acceleration is maximal in the middle of the stance phase and minimal during the suspension phase, when it falls to its minimum value which is equal to gravitational acceleration.

During lameness, characteristic changes in the patterns of all these body segments occur. The most obvious of these is the vertical head movement pattern (Girtler & Floss, 1984; Peloso *et al.*, 1993; Buchner *et al.*, 1996b; Keegan *et al.*, 1997). The lowering and lifting of the head during the stance phase of the lame limb decreases, with a compensatory increase in both movements during the stance phase of the contralateral sound forelimb (Fig. 10.5). These changes are proportional to the degree of lameness and in severe lameness the first wave may not be visible. The sinusoidal pattern with two cycles per stride then changes to show a single cycle during each stride (Girtler & Floss, 1984). Vertical velocity of the head changes in accordance with the vertical movement. Both minimal and maximal vertical velocity during the lame stance phase decrease. During the sound stance phase both values increase, which also results in a more positive velocity of the head at the start of the subsequent lame stance phase. This means that, at impact,

the head shows less downward movement with increasing lameness. During severe forelimb lameness, the head may even be lifted slightly at the instant of impact of the lame limb. Finally, vertical acceleration of the head also changes from a symmetrical pattern to an asymmetrical pattern (Fig. 10.5C).

For a quantitative analysis of the lameness, the acceleration values are even more useful than the head movement pattern, since vertical acceleration is less sensitive to changes in absolute head height. Furthermore, changes in the acceleration peaks quite accurately represent changes in the vertical forces acting on the limbs, since forces (F) are determined by the mass (m) of a body and its vertical acceleration (a): $F = ma$. Therefore, reduced vertical acceleration of the head and trunk during the stance phase of the lame limb results in a lower vertical force, or less loading of the lame limb.

During forelimb lameness the withers and croup show the same vertical movement pattern as the head, but the oscillations are less pronounced (Buchner *et al.*, 1996b). Nevertheless, there is a large decrease in the vertical acceleration depending on the degree of lameness. Due to the mass of the trunk, which accounts for about 65% of total body mass (Buchner *et al.*, 1997), this causes a highly significant decrease in limb loading.

The locomotion patterns of the head, withers and croup during hindlimb lameness are similar to those of a forelimb lameness, but show some distinctive characteristics. The os sacrum, which lies on the midline, shows a perfectly sinusoidal up and down motion in sound horses. During lameness, it shows less lowering and lifting during the stance phase of the lame limb, which is exactly the same as the motion of the withers during forelimb lameness (Buchner *et al.*, 1996b). The tuber coxae, however, which is more laterally placed, has an asymmetric locomotion pattern even in sound horses (Buchner *et al.*, 1993). The amplitude of motion, which is measured as the distance between lowest and highest positions of the tuber coxae, is smaller during the stance phase of the ipsilateral hindlimb than during the contralateral stance phase (Fig. 10.6A). Rotation of the croup around the sagittal axis through the hip joint causes different displacements in the ipsilateral and contralateral tuber coxae. The sum of the rotational movement and the vertical translational movement of the whole trunk causes this typical asymmetric pattern even in sound horses.

In hindlimb lameness, the asymmetry on the lame side of the body increases. This means that vertical motion of the left tuber coxae during left hindlimb lameness is diminished or absent during the left hindlimb stance phase (Fig. 10.6B) and increased during the right hindlimb stance phase (May & Wyn-Jones, 1987; Buchner *et al.*, 1996b). The larger motion amplitudes of the tuber coxae compared with midline os sacrum are

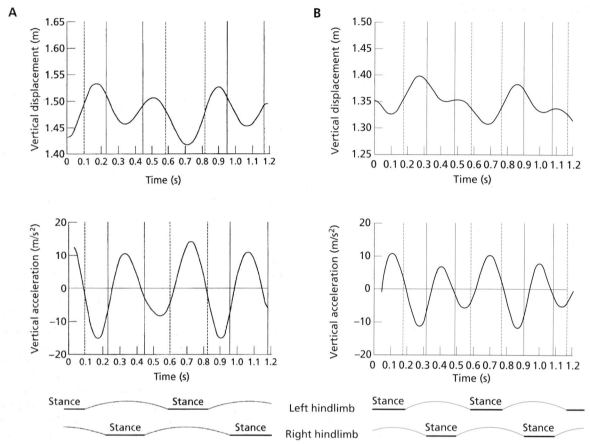

Fig. 10.6 (A) Vertical displacement and vertical acceleration of the right tuber coxae in a sound horse (**A**) and in a horse with a moderate lameness of the right hindlimb (**B**) at the trot. The horizontal bars indicate the stance phases of the hindlimbs. (Redrawn with permission from Buchner, F., Kastner, J., Girtler, D. and Knezevic, P.F. (1993) Quantification of hind limb lameness in the horse. *Acta Anat.* **146**: 196–199. Reproduced with permission from S. Karger AG, Basel.)

more easily detected by many people, but the pattern of the os sacrum is similar to head and withers movement and is, therefore, easier to describe. Movement of the withers during hindlimb lameness is similar to, but less pronounced, than os sacrum movement. Head movement, on the other hand, shows a different pattern in fore and hindlimb lameness. While the head movements

Summary

Based on a knowledge of these principles and the interactions between trunk and head movement patterns, the observer can quantify the lameness and differentiate between fore and hindlimb lameness. The use of these kinematic lameness quantification methods will be discussed later in the chapter.

are unchanged or even increased during the stance phase of the lame hindlimb, the displacement amplitude of the head decreases during the stance phase of the sound hindlimb. Therefore, the head drops during stance of the lame diagonal in moderate to severe hindlimb lameness. This is to allow the horse to reduce some of the load on the lame hindlimb (this will be discussed in more detail below). Dropping of the head as a compensating mechanism for a hindlimb lameness mimics the head movements in a supporting limb lameness of the ipsilateral forelimb and, consequently, is described as false forelimb lameness (Uhlir *et al.*, 1997) or sagittal lameness. A false lameness can be differentiated from a real or true forelimb lameness by diagnostic anesthesia. Positive diagnostic anesthesia in the lame hindlimb reduces the sagittal forelimb lameness too. True forelimb lameness, on the other hand, will not be changed by the hindlimb anesthesia.

Swinging limb and mixed lameness

Pure swinging limb lameness, i.e. lameness that causes changes during the swing phase without problems during the stance phase, is extremely rare. The two major reasons for a pure swinging limb lameness are a mechanical problem, such as an advanced ankylosis of a limb joint, or a neural problem such as paresis of the radial nerve. Adrian *et al.* (1977) published goniograms of a 9-year-old stallion with an osseous ankylosis of the metacarpophalangeal joint. Flexion testing in this limb did not cause pain, but the limb showed hardly any flexion or extension during the entire stride. The author has observed a similar locomotion pattern in horses with ankylosis of the stifle or talocrural joint. In all cases, the affected limb could support the body without pain, but also without any flexion or extension during the stride.

Much more common and of clinical significance are the mixed lamenesses, where pain or pain reactions are obvious during both stance and swing phases. Typical examples are shoulder and carpal lameness or stifle and tarsal lameness. The most extensive information is available for carpal lameness. Several clinical studies in patients (Ratzlaff *et al.*, 1982; Ratzlaff & Grant, 1986; Clayton, 1987a) as well as studies using lameness models (Morris & Seeherman, 1987; Back *et al.*, 1993; Peloso *et al.*, 1993) investigated the locomotion pattern of horses with carpal joint problems. In these studies the various symptoms can be differentiated into signs that are typical of a supporting limb lameness and other signs that are typical of swing phase problems. The temporal variables do not show a consistent pattern in the different studies. Clayton (1986a, 1987a,b) studied three horses, suffering from a shoulder, carpal and tarsal problems. She found in all three cases shorter stance phase durations in the lame limb compared with the sound limb. Ratzlaff *et al.* (1982), focusing on carpal lameness, found variable results regarding stance duration and suggested that a shortened stance duration occurred with a predominance of the supporting limb lameness component, while a lengthened stance duration indicated a predominance of the swinging limb lameness. Of course, the variability of the patient histories, even in horses suffering from carpal lameness, preclude making general conclusions.

Three studies provoked carpal lameness using toxins (Back *et al.*, 1993), antibiotics (Peloso *et al.*, 1993) or surgical manipulation (Morris & Seeherman, 1987). If trotting velocity was checked to be constant, no significant changes were found in the stance phase duration between the sound and lame limbs, or between the same limb before and after lameness induction (Morris & Seeherman, 1987; Peloso *et al.*, 1993). Obviously, individual left/right differences play a major role compared with the influence of a mixed lameness. In most cases, a

high degree of symmetry is maintained and the right/left differences in temporal variables do not help to diagnose a specific lameness.

The characteristics of the caudal and cranial phases of the stride might be a useful criterion to distinguish between swinging and supporting limb lameness (Wittmann, 1931; Hajer *et al.*, 1988). In swinging limb lameness the cranial phase is said to be shorter in the lame limb due to pain during the swing phase and its effect on protraction. Indeed, Clayton (1986a, 1987b) found shorter cranial phases in shoulder and tarsal lameness, but in a horse with carpal lameness (Clayton 1987a) both phases were equal. Therefore, reduction of the cranial phase is indicative of some swing phase problems, but lack of such a reduction does not exclude a swinging limb lameness.

Equivocal results were found regarding the joint angle pattern in horses with mixed lameness. Looking at the different limb joints, a very clear differentiation between swing phase and stance phase problems can be made. During the swing phase, flexion of the affected joint (carpal, tarsal, fetlock) was decreased in all studies (Fig. 10.7A). The restriction can be seen in both the maximal flexion and the total range of motion. The limb gives the impression of moving stiffly with a lower flight arc of the hoof. This is most obvious during carpal lameness (Back *et al.*, 1993), but is also found in tarsal (Clayton, 1987b) and shoulder lameness (Clayton, 1986a). This feature is clearly different from a supporting limb lameness, where the carpal joint angle during the swing phase was unchanged, and the tarsal joint angle was even increased (Buchner *et al.*, 1996a). Therefore, the presence and degree of left/right differences in flexion of a carpal or tarsal joint seem to be useful indicators for the swinging limb component of a mixed lameness, as Back *et al.* (1993) proposed. The decreased flexion of a painful joint results from the horse's efforts to avoid painful positions. This effort can be detected even earlier in the stride cycle at the start of the swing phase; when flexion of the carpus begins, the angular velocity of this joint is reduced (Ratzlaff *et al.*, 1982).

The characteristics of the supporting limb lameness component of the mixed lameness have already been described. In general, all variables typical for a supporting limb lameness can also be seen in mixed lamenesses (Clayton, 1986a; Peloso *et al.*, 1993). The most significant features is that fetlock hyperextension in the lame limb is reduced as sign of less loading, which is achieved by reduced head displacement. The contributions of the supporting and swinging limb lameness components are quite variable depending on the individual condition.

Figure 10.7 shows the carpal and fetlock joint patterns in a pony with induced carpal lameness, a typical example of a mixed lameness. The combined angle-angle graph of

A

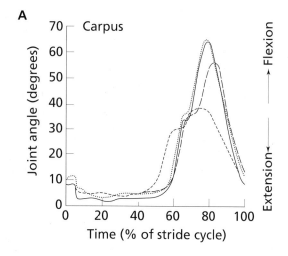

B

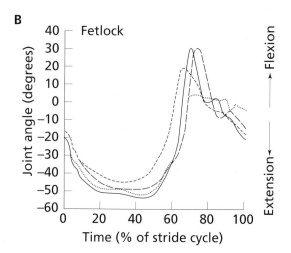

C

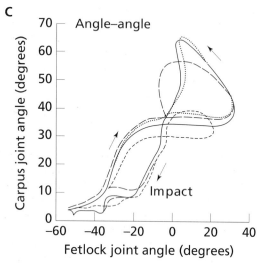

Fig. 10.7 Joint angle patterns of carpal and fetlock joints of one pony at the walk during different degrees of induced carpal lameness, and angle-angle diagram of fetlock and carpal joints. (——) sound; (— — —) severe lameness; (- - -) moderate lameness; (·······) sound. (Reprinted with permission from Back, W., Barneveld, A., Weeren, P.R. van and Bogert, A.J. van den (1993) Kinematic gait analysis in equine carpal lameness. *Acta Anat.* **146**: 86–89. ©Karger, Basel)

both joints illustrates the changes during various lameness degrees very clearly. Fetlock hyperextension and carpal flexion give useful information about both aspects of the lameness, but not necessarily about its location. Though the proximal limb joints are more at risk for swinging limb lameness, distal limb problems more often show supporting limb lameness. The coupling of different joints, such as the tarsal and stifle joints, impedes the ability to localize the disease. Furthermore, slow protraction due to joint pain causes similar decreases in the range of joint motion in the coupled joint regardless of whether the pain is in this joint or the neighboring joint.

Bilateral lameness

A special situation, and a more challenging task for a veterinarian, is the presence of a bilateral lameness. A number of orthopedic diseases, such as navicular disease, distal

limb arthrosis and bone spavin, may be present in both limbs to a more or less similar extent. The presence and degree of bilateral problems are often difficult to assess, because of the lack of the typical asymmetric pattern associated with unilateral lameness (Seeherman, 1991). The locomotion of horses suffering from bilateral lameness has been described as stiff, short or shuffling (Stashak, 1987). Such characteristics are difficult to distinguish from the normal locomotor pattern of the individual horse, which is usually unknown to the veterinarian. In this situation, local diagnostic anesthesia is used to detect locomotor asymmetries by eliminating pain in one limb and thus facilitating the detection of pain in the contralateral limb. However, a study of the effects of local anesthesia in sound horses showed changes in the locomotion pattern, perhaps due to the changed proprioception in the anesthetized limb (Kübber *et al.*, 1994). Therefore, in mild cases it is difficult to decide whether a change in locomotion pattern is due to bilateral lameness, or just to the lost sensitivity in one limb.

Quantitative locomotion analysis in bilaterally lame horses suffers from the same problems as the clinical assessment. If the horse does not show left-to-right asymmetries and if there are no individual control data for the horse when it was sound, it is impossible to make a diagnosis of lameness (Hugelshofer, 1982). The use of a bilateral hoof lameness model showed some gait adaptations that allowed the horses to reduce their discomfort, even when the usual transfer of weight to the contralateral limb was impossible (Buchner *et al.*, 1995b). The adaptations were similar to those seen in unilateral supporting limb lameness. With regard to the temporal variables, stride duration was reduced, while relative stance duration increased. The most distinct change in temporal coordination, however, was in the diagonal advanced placement. During slight bilateral lameness, horses placed their forelimbs earlier than the hindlimbs compared with the sound situation. Again, this variable proved to be a reliable indicator for unilateral or bilateral locomotor problems.

A second variable that is indicative of bilateral pain is fetlock hyperextension, which was reduced equally in both forelimbs during an induced bilateral lameness. By changing the temporal stride pattern and slightly reducing the vertical displacement of the trunk, the horse achieved the same amount of load reduction (and pain relief) as seen in unilateral lameness.

THE MECHANISMS OF EQUINE LAMENESS MANAGEMENT

If horses feel pain in a limb when moving, they adjust their locomotion pattern to diminish the pain, which causes the visible signs of lameness. The various kinematic changes described in the previous sections are components of the overall effort to achieve pain reduction. In a supporting limb lameness, pain reduction means reducing the load on the affected limb. The success of the efforts of the load-reducing strategy can be assessed by measuring the ground reaction forces (GRFs) using a force plate (Gingerich *et al.*, 1979; Morris & Seeherman, 1987; Merkens & Schamhardt, 1988a, 1988b), force shoes (Hugelshofer, 1982; Dohne, 1991) or the EGA-system (Tietje, 1992). A synchronous view of kinetic and kinematic findings provides a more complete picture of how horses manage a lameness and gives a better understanding of the mechanisms that redistribute the load away from the lame limb without serious overloading of the sound limbs.

Load reduction in the lame limb

As lameness increases, horses show progressive reductions in their vertical and longitudinal deceleration forces. These differences can be seen in the GRF tracings at the walk (Merkens & Schamhardt, 1988a) as well as at the trot (Morris & Seeherman, 1987; Clayton *et al.*, 2000a). At the walk the peak vertical force decreases, while the GRF pattern becomes smoother: the dip

Summary

Horses manage and relieve the pain in bilateral lameness even when the typical asymmetric, contralateral compensation is not possible. Diagnosis of bilateral lamenesses remains difficult, especially in mild cases. Repeated measurements using diagnostic anesthesia or by screening the horses over longer periods can monitor fetlock joint angle and diagonal advanced placement to detect mild gait deficits.

between the two vertical force peaks diminishes in mild lameness and disappears in moderate lameness (Fig. 10.8) (Merkens & Schamhardt, 1988a). At the trot the single force peak is decreased in amplitude in lame horses (Morris & Seeherman, 1987; Clayton *et al.*, 2000a). The degree of unloading is, of course, dependent on the degree of lameness, but there are no absolute data calibrating the lameness degree with GRF data. A mean decrease of 11.5% in the vertical load due to an easily observable carpal lameness has been reported by Morris and Seeherman (1987). Tietje found mean load differences of about 1000 N or 15% between groups of 50 sound horses and 60 lame horses. These load reductions correspond to only moderate lameness at the trot. Clayton *et al.* (2000a) recorded horses with induced tendinitis of the superficial flexor tendon and found 27% less peak vertical force compared with the control recording. However, these horses, showing moderate to severe lameness also reduced their running velocity by 10% which contributes to the overall load reduction. If lameness is more severe, the load is reduced progressively to zero load in a non-weight-bearing lameness. In lame horses, the fetlock joint angle–time diagram (Back *et al.*, 1993; Buchner *et al.*, 1996a) resembles the vertical force pattern shown by Merkens and Schamhardt (1988a) or Morris and Seeherman (1987). The reduction of the fetlock hyperextension of about 8° in a grade 2 lameness might be quite comparable to the reduction of peak vertical force by about 10% that was reported in horses with an easily observable lameness by Morris and Seeherman (1987). Similarly, Clayton *et al.* (2000a) found a decrease in fetlock hyperextension of 10° corresponding to the decrease in the peak vertical GRF of 27%.

Based on the kinematic analyses, the reduced loading in a lame forelimb can be explained by two major mechanisms: smoother loading of the lame limb and decreased vertical movement of the head and trunk. The loading is smoothed by small adjustments in several aspects of limb timing. The swing duration of the forelimbs is reduced, while the relative stance duration is increased by 2.3% of the stride duration. The longer ground contact distributes the effort required to lift the body over a longer period. Furthermore, the earlier placement of the lame forelimb allows it to accept the body load at a time when the trunk is at a higher point in its sinusoidal motion cycle and has a relatively low downward velocity. This reduces the effort required to lift the body, as discussed in the second mechanism below. Additionally, braking of the descending body is

smoothed by slightly more flexion of the shoulder joint.

The second mechanism to reduce peak load involves the vertical displacement of the body. During the stance phase of the lame limb, the head and neck and, to a lesser extent, the trunk are not lowered as normal. Keeping the body at a more constant height needs less maximal vertical acceleration and results in a decreased peak vertical force in the lame limb. Additionally, horses

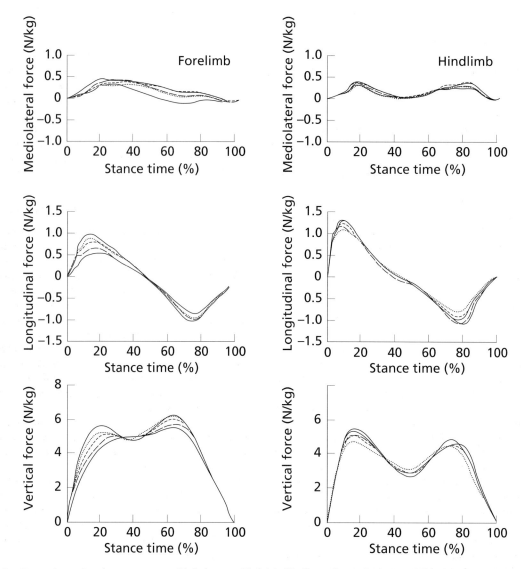

Fig. 10.8 Ground reaction force patterns of left fore and left hindlimbs at the walk during different degrees of left forelimb lameness. The forces are expressed in N/kg body mass during a standardized stance time.
(——) control session; (– – –) only lame at the trot; (— — —) mild lameness at the walk; (——) moderate lameness at the walk; (·········) digital nerve block. (Reprinted with permission from Merkens, H.W. and Schamhardt, H.C. (1988a) Evaluation of equine locomotion during different degrees of experimentally induced lameness. I. Lameness model and quantification of ground reaction force patterns of the limbs. *Equine Vet. J.* **6** (Suppl.): 99–106.)

adjust their head and neck movement to control the load distribution in all limbs. Since the head and neck are heavy, representing about 10% of total body mass (Buchner *et al.*, 1997), and they have a long lever arm relative to the body center of mass, their position has a relatively large effect in loading or unloading the forelimbs. This influence of head and neck movement has been evaluated using an inverse dynamics model (Vorstenbosch *et al.*, 1997). The dynamic forces acting on the trunk and then on the limbs were calculated from the kinematics of head and neck, their inertial properties and the geometric properties. Differences of only 10 cm in vertical amplitude of the head during the stance phases of lame and sound limbs caused differences in the vertical force of nearly 500 N and differences of about 230 Nm in the sagittal torque acting on the trunk. Therefore, the head is an effective tool for redistributing the load from the painful limb to the other limbs.

These dynamic influences of the head and neck movements should not be confused with the relatively small static influences on the position of the body center of mass (BCM) due to different head positions. If the head and neck move caudally by 10 cm, the BCM shifts caudally by only 1 cm. For a 500 kg horse, assuming a distance of 100 cm between fore and hindlimbs, this means a transfer of only 50 N from fore to hindlimb. Therefore, the dynamic influences of the asymmetric head and neck movement in lame horses have about 10 times more effect than the static component.

Redistribution of the load

The reduction of the peak load in the lame limb is not accompanied by equivalent increases of peak loads in the sound limbs. This remarkable fact has been observed both in kinematic studies that evaluated the fetlock joint pattern of all limbs and in kinetic studies of the vertical loads on all four limbs. The explanation lies in the characteristic head and trunk movements. Using the maximal hyperextension of the fetlock joint as a load indicator, at the trot a decrease of 7.6° in the lame limb was accompanied by an increase of only 1.9° in the contralateral forelimb, no change in the diagonal hindlimb and a 2.6° decrease in the ipsilateral hindlimb (Buchner *et al.*, 1996a). The same relationships were found by Morris and Seeherman (1987), Tietje (1992) and by model calculations (Vorstenbosch *et al.*, 1997). The reduction of maximal head acceleration during the lame diagonal stance phase reduces the load on the lame forelimb, but increases the load on the diagonal hindlimb due to a reduced torque at the neck–trunk connection. At the same time, reduced acceleration of the whole trunk adds to the reduction of loading of the lame forelimb, but counteracts and equalizes the torque effects of the head on the diagonal

Summary

Summing up all details, the body receives less vertical impulse during the stance phase of the lame limb, despite the small prolongation of the stance duration. This smaller vertical impulse leads to a distinct reduction in the duration of the subsequent suspension phase and the contralateral limb has to cope with a higher vertical impulse associated with the descending trunk and head.

hindlimb. During the sound diagonal stance phase, the trunk acceleration hardly changes. Increased head movements, however, slightly increase the loading of the contralateral forelimb and decrease that of the ipsilateral hindlimb.

So, if the reduction of the peak load in the lame limb is not compensated by the other limbs, where does the load go? Two phenomena are involved in answering this question:

1. A redistribution within the lame limb
2. A decrease of total load during the whole stride cycle.

The changes in limb timing smooth the loading of the lamb limb which enables the horse to reduce the peak load more than either the total load or the impulse. The difference has been quantified for a carpal lameness model by Morris and Seeherman (1987) whose results showed 11.5% reduction in peak force, but only 8.4% reduction in time integrated force (impulse) in the lame limb. In severe induced tendinitis, a decrease of 27% in peak vertical force corresponded to 15% reduction in the vertical impulse (Clayton *et al.*, 2000a) (Fig. 10.9). The same principle works in the contralateral limb but in the opposite direction. A small increase in peak load and a longer stance phase lead to a greater increase in total load. For their carpal lameness model Morris and Seeherman (1987) showed that while the peak vertical force in the contralateral limb hardly changed, the time integrated force (impulse) increased by 4.7%. The overall changes were a decrease of 13.7 G msec in the lame forelimb, an increase of 7.7 G msec in the contralateral limb, an increase of 2 G msec in the diagonal hindlimb and a decrease of 6.5 G msec in the ipsilateral hindlimb. Overall, the total vertical impulse decreased by 10.5 G msec per stride.

The remaining difference in impulses between lame and sound limbs can be explained by the second phenomenon, the reduction of the total load. This has already been suggested by Morris and Seeherman (1987) and is now confirmed by the results of our study. When forced to keep a constant velocity on the treadmill, the horses increase their stride frequency by reducing the duration of the swing phase. In this way the horses reduce the load within one stride by distributing it over a larger number of strides.

These results show that a lameness in one limb will not necessarily increase the risk of damaging the contralateral limb or the other sound limbs. If high peak forces are responsible for compensatory injuries, the mechanisms described above enable a maximal decrease of peak force in the lame limb together with a minimal increase in the sound limbs.

Special mechanisms in hindlimb lameness

In general, similar mechanisms to those described for forelimb lamenesses are found in trotting horses suffering from a hindlimb lameness. Limb timing and joint patterns differ only slightly from forelimb lamenesses, but larger differences are found in trunk and head movements.

Asymmetry in the vertical acceleration of the trunk during hindlimb lameness is similar to forelimb lameness, with the asymmetry in the hind quarters being enhanced by longitudinal rotational movements in the vertebral spine. These allow a significant reduction of loading in the lame hindlimb, which is reflected by 7.3° less hyperextension of the fetlock joint during a grade 2 lameness. To a certain extent, this is a substitute for the head movements during forelimb lameness. The head movements during hindlimb lameness are small and play only a

minor role in lameness management. However, they may be confusing to the observer, as a small asymmetry during moderate hindlimb lameness seems to simulate lameness in the ipsilateral forelimb, which is described as false lameness by Uhlir *et al.* (1997). However, the asymmetry in head rotation is contrary to the movements of the withers and as a result forelimb loading is almost unchanged compared with the sound situation. In the hindlimbs the same head asymmetry enhances the load redistribution from the lame to the contralateral limb, but is less effective than during forelimb lamenesses.

Limb timing is influenced much less by hindlimb lameness. Stride frequency increases as in forelimb lameness, but the increase in relative stance duration is small and both diagonal advanced placement and suspension phases do not change at all (Buchner *et al.*, 1995a). There are two possible explanations for this temporal stability. First, load damping may be more effective in the hindlimbs as a result of greater tarsal flexion during loading of the lame limb. Secondly, a lower percentage of the body weight is carried by the hindlimbs (46.8%) compared with the forelimbs (53.2%) (Merkens *et al.*, 1993), which may facilitate the management of a supporting limb lameness.

SPECIFIC LAMENESSES

The most ambitious aim in the use of locomotion analysis for the diagnosis of lameness in horses is the exact localization of the ailment within a limb, thus making the diagnosis of a specific disease (Leach & Crawford, 1983; Clayton, 1986a). A precondition for such a specific diagnosis is a database that includes kinematic patterns of various specific diseases, based on sufficient measurements to eliminate the variation due to individual locomotion patterns. Recordings have been made in individual horses with specific ailments, and studies have been performed in groups of horses with equal, induced lamenesses. Analysis of the results of these studies presented two major problems that impede formulation of a definition of characteristic lameness patterns in specific lameness:

(a) *The individual locomotion pattern.* Several studies found a high level of reproducible individuality in the locomotion pattern of horses (Drevemo *et al.*, 1980; van Weeren *et al.*, 1993), seen as a low intra-individual variation compared to the high inter-individual variation. The low intra-individual variation allows for repeated, reliable assessments of the locomotion pattern after diagnostic or therapeutic manipulations. The accurate measurement techniques enable the detection of

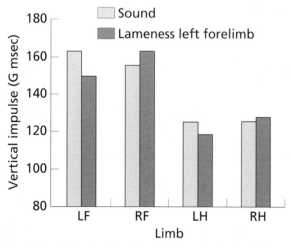

Fig. 10.9 Redistribution of vertical impulse from the lame forelimb to the other limbs during induced superficial digital flexor tendinitis in one forelimb. (Data from Clayton, H.M., Schamhardt, H.C., Willemen, M.A., Lanovaz, J.L. and Colborne, G.R. (2000a) Kinematics and ground reaction forces in horses with superficial digital flexor tendinitis. *Am. J. Vet. Res.* **61**, 191–196. ©American Veterinary Medical Association.)

really small, but significant differences due to the various lamenesses. However, these differences are often smaller than differences between horses due to their individual locomotion patterns.

(b) *The wide variety of orthopedic diseases.* Many horses suffer from more than one disease. Even horses suffering from very similar diseases or syndromes, such as navicular disease or carpal lameness, show a variety of orthopedic and radiological findings. In two studies analysing seven horses with carpal lameness, seven different diagnoses were reported (Ratzlaff *et al.*, 1982; Clayton, 1986a). Navicular disease seems to be more uniform, but additional ailments can occur. In the thorough study of Girtler (1988a, 1988b, 1988c) six out of seven horses with navicular disease had additional problems, such as arthrosis, tendinitis, sesamoiditis or bone spavin. This problem might have existed, though it was not described, in other studies of horses with navicular disease by Pollhammer-Zeilinger (1996), Hütter (1997) and Keegan *et al.* (1997). Therefore, it is difficult to use horses with naturally occurring lameness to extract specific patterns for a specific ailment. General conclusions can be drawn only by analysis of a large number of horses suffering from more or less the same disease; then, general symptoms have to be separated from specific symptoms. Large numbers of horses have been studied for only a few diseases and in these diseases the general symptoms dominate over specific details.

Navicular disease

There are five studies reporting kinematic data from horses with navicular disease (Ratzlaff & Grant, 1986; Girtler, 1988a, 1988b, 1988c;, Pollhammer-Zeilinger, 1996; Keegan *et al.*, 1997; Hütter, 1997). Comparing their results with those from other lameness studies, the same general characteristics as described for supporting limb lameness can be found. There is a tendency to longer stance durations, but this feature is not shown by all horses (Pollhammer-Zeilinger, 1996). Fetlock joint hyperextension is reduced and vertical head movement, which depends on the degree of asymmetry of the pathologic process, shows its characteristic asymmetric pattern. Even hoof landing, as described by Ratzlaff and Grant (1986), does not show a consistent pattern in all horses (Hütter, 1997). Keegan found also a reduced maximal flexion in the carpal joint during the swing phase, which he explained as a general symptom of a reduced loading followed by a less energetic protraction of the limb. Therefore, no really specific kinematic

patterns for navicular disease could be found to differentiate navicular disease from other supporting limb lamenesses.

Carpal lameness

Carpal lameness is the most intensively studied orthopedic syndrome using locomotion analysis techniques. Both patient studies (Ratzlaff *et al.*, 1982; Clayton, 1987a) as well as studies of induced, uniform carpal lameness (Auer *et al.*, 1980; Morris & Seeherman, 1987; Back *et al.*, 1993; Peloso *et al.*, 1993) serve as a database for a detailed analysis. As in navicular disease, there are reliable general signs of lameness, including reduced fetlock hyperextension and a head movement pattern that are indicative of the supporting limb lameness component. Reduced carpal flexion is a consistent sign of the swinging limb lameness component. Ratzlaff *et al.* (1982) also described changes in the angular velocity as a good indicator to differentiate swinging and supporting limb lameness. Clayton (1987a) described a specific detail in the vertical movement pattern of the carpal region in a horse with a fracture of the third carpal bone. This involved lowering of the lame limb at lift off and during the early swing phase. This pattern is visible also in the horse recorded by Ratzlaff and Grant (1986) as well as in one horse of Girtler (1988b). Another horse in Girtler's Study (1988b) that was suffering from tendinitis showed the same carpal pattern, which might point to a common phenomenon of pain during maximal extension of the carpal joint and the wish to flex and unload the lame limb as early as possible.

Tendinitis

An integrated study of the kinematics and GRFs before and after the induction of superficial digital flexor (SDF) tendinitis in one forelimb (Clayton *et al.*, 2000a) showed that the peak vertical GRF was significantly lower in the lame limb, and this was associated with less flexion of the coffin joint and less extension of the fetlock joint in the lame limb compared with the compensating limb. Carpal joint kinematics did not change. At the lame evaluation the compensating limb had a more protracted orientation throughout its stance phase, though its total range of limb rotation from ground contact to lift off did not change. This facilitated a smooth transfer of body weight from the lame to the compensating limb without the need to raise the body mass into a suspension. In association with its more protracted orientation, the compensating limb had a higher braking longitudinal force and impulse than the lame limb, while the propulsive components of the longitudinal ground reaction force did not differ between limbs. The center of pressure began to move rapidly toward the toe relatively early in the stance phase in the lame limb, which was interpreted as a consequence of the lower GRFs in the lame limb. The lame limb also showed significant reductions in the peak values for the net joint moments on the palmar aspect of the fetlock, carpal and elbow joints, which are the joints crossed by the SDF musculotendinous unit. The total mechanical energy absorbed was significantly lower at every joint in the lame limb compared with the compensating limb (Clayton *et al.*, 2000b).

In the early stance phase, oscillations in the longitudinal force peaks correspond approximately with changes in the vertical loading pattern of the limb, and it has been suggested (Dow *et al.*, 1991) that changes in the slope of the vertical ground reaction force during these periods correspond to a reduced rate of loading of the fetlock as this joint reaches its full extension. Unfortunately, findings from the lame and compensating limbs were not differentiated by Dow *et al.* (1991), but all horses whose values for the vertical force slope for one or both limbs were outside the 95% confidence limits of the population under study had an SDF injury. Clinical lameness was only apparent when the deviation of the vertical force slope was outside the 99% confidence limits of the population. Clayton *et al.* (2000a) also found a significant difference in the slope of the vertical ground reaction force that was indicative of a greatly reduced loading rate in the lame limb and a more rapid loading rate in the compensating limb. It coincided with a divergence between the angles of the coffin and fetlock in the two limbs as a consequence of the differences in loading. However, the large variations in the force curves between and within horses is likely to preclude their use as a diagnostic tool.

Peculiar lamenesses

There are some rare orthopedic diseases in which the locomotion pattern is so unique that it will be recognized by everybody who has seen it previously. Two of these specific lamenesses have been described kinematically in detail.

Stringhalt

This extraordinary locomotion pattern can be seen in horses often without a known underlying cause, which leads to the diagnosis of idiopathic stringhalt. Girtler (1988c) presented the flight arc and temporal data of such a patient. The hoof was lifted to a maximum height of nearly 60 cm instead of the normal height of 15 to 20 cm, with the peak of the flight arc being reached quite late during the swing phase and the hoof then being lowered nearly vertically to the ground (Fig. 10.10). In the affected limb, the stance phase was reduced and the swing phase was lengthened, whereas the sound limb showed the opposite changes. Step duration from the

Summary

Different lamenesses show patterns that allow for a reliable classification into supporting or swinging limb lameness, but more specific characteristics have not yet been found. Furthermore, it is not clear whether the detection of specific kinematic patterns for each orthopedic disease is only a matter of further research and intelligent analysis methods, such as artificial neural networks, or if specific patterns do not exist. Perhaps horses react in a uniform way to pain in a limb, due to the limited degree of freedom in their locomotion patterns. If that is the case, there may be only general signs that serve as indicators for classification as a supporting or a swinging limb lameness. Therefore, specific lameness diagnosis is still a very difficult topic that may never be resolved.

sound to the lame limb was longer than the contralateral step. This strange locomotion pattern is much more obvious at the walk than at the trot, and is seen even at very slow velocities.

Fibrotic myopathy

Like stringhalt, the typical locomotion pattern of fibrotic myopathy is more obvious at the walk than at the trot. Fibrosis of torn muscle fibers of the semitendinosus muscle impedes protraction of the hindlimb at its most cranial position, when the muscle is maximally stretched. At the walk, the hind hoof jerks backward and downward just before landing instead of a smooth forward movement till impact (Fig. 10.11). Clayton (1988) analyzed a typical example of a horse with this ailment and described some kinematic details for the trot. The flight arc stopped its forward movement at 84% of the swing phase and the hoof contacted the ground toe first, after being lowered almost vertically rather than being retracted prior to contact. Consequently, the diagonal distance was shorter for the affected diagonal limb pair. These differences were found even at the trot, in which the characteristics are less obvious than at the walk, which normally shows more hindlimb protraction than the slow trot (Buchner *et al.*, 1996a).

CLINICAL USE OF LOCOMOTION ANALYSIS

Accurate and objective assessments of locomotor disturbances using locomotion analysis techniques provide the

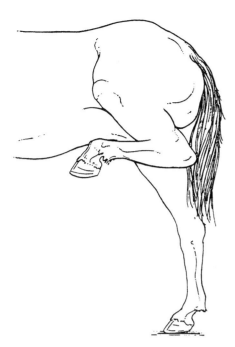

Fig. 10.10 Typical high elevation of the hindlimb during the swing phase in a horse at the walk suffering from stringhalt.

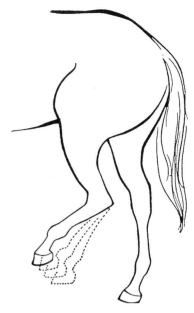

Fig. 10.11 Typical movement pattern of a hindlimb in a horse at the walk suffering from fibrotic myopathy of the semitendinosus muscle. The foot jerks backward and downward just before landing. (Reprinted from Stashak, T.S. (1987) Fibrotic and ossifying myopathy. In: Stashak, T.S. (ed.), *Adams' Lameness in Horses,* 4th edn. Philadelphia: Lea & Febiger, p. 731.)

veterinarian with valuable tools for advanced diagnostics in a clinical setting. Both qualitative and quantitative methods can be used to assess lameness objectively, to augment diagnostic procedures or to verify therapeutic effects. Qualitative assessments use slow motion video-recordings to detect changes in hoof motion and landing as well as locomotor asymmetries (Seeherman, 1991, 1992). The big advantage of qualitative gait analysis is the low technical effort and the simplicity of interpretation of the slow motion video images by veterinarian and horse owner. The same criteria are assessed as during a standard orthopedic examination, but with a higher temporal resolution and with as many replays as necessary.

Quantitative assessments need more sophisticated methods and can measure all kinematic or kinetic details described in the previous sections. For clinical applications, however, the need for a rapid turnaround time usually restricts the analysis to localization of the lame limb and quantification of the lameness degree. Several methods and variables are available to define symmetry indices for lameness quantification (Table 10.3). These indices have to meet several criteria to be of practical, diagnostic value. First, they must be sufficiently sensitive to lameness to ensure that even small disturbances in the locomotion pattern are reflected by distinct changes in the symmetry index. Secondly, an index value should be indicative of a certain degree of lameness, and the inter-

individual variation in this variable should be smaller than the differences between lameness degrees. Thirdly, the variable should be easy to measure and interpret. These criteria can be fulfilled by variables derived from both kinetic and kinematic analyses.

Kinematic lameness indicators

The typical asymmetric pattern of head, withers or croup movements in lame horses enables their use for the calculation of symmetry indices to quantify lameness that are similar to the traditional, subjective assessments by the veterinarian. Kastner (1989) first used the vertical accelerations of the head to calculate a symmetry index named HAAS: Head Acceleration ASymmetry. He used the following equation:

$$HAAS = \frac{LAA - RAA}{BAA}$$

HAAS: **H**ead **A**cceleration **AS**ymmetry
LAA: **L**eft vertical head **A**cceleration **A**mplitude
RAA: **R**ight vertical head **A**cceleration **A**mplitude
BAA: **B**igger vertical head **A**cceleration **A**mplitude

The HAAS index is zero in sound horses with symmetric head movements during the left and right forelimb stance phases. The index tends to −1 if the left limb is lame and it tends to +1 if the right limb is lame. This simple equation has also been applied to locations other than the head, giving rise to WAAS (Withers Acceleration ASymmetry) (Kübber et al., 1994) or SAAS (Sacral Acceleration ASymmetry) (Uhlir et al., 1997). Similarly, using slightly different calculation methods, the hip acceleration can be recorded and analyzed (Buchner et al., 1993) or the vertical displacements in both hips can be compared (May & Wyn-Jones, 1987). These symmetry indices perform very well and fulfill all the criteria for clinical application.

More sophisticated calculation methods were used by Peham et al. (1996) to reduce the influence of unsteady head movements. After processing the data using a system-matched filter, the symmetry of the vertical head movement pattern was analyzed by determination of the Fourier series. The symmetry of the horse's movements can then be calculated by comparing the values of the Fourier coefficients and presenting the data as a symmetry percentage (Table 10.3) (Peham et al., 1995).

A different kinematic method was reported by Pourcelot et al. (1997). They applied an intercorrelation method to analyze the contralateral symmetry of both the vertical joint motion and the joint angle changes during one stride. The results of these calculations are presented as kinematic indices for the comparison of each pair of markers or limb joints, or as an averaged fore or hindlimb index. In contrast to the HAAS, these symmetry indices have the value 1 in perfectly sound and symmetric horses and tend to zero in severe lameness.

Accelerometer

Acceleration can be calculated by double differentiation of the displacement of a point, or it can be measured directly using an accelerometer. Conversely, acceleration data can be integrated to calculate velocity or displacement. Barrey et al. (1994) used accelerometers fixed to the sternum of horses to record the horizontal and vertical movements of the trunk. In addition to providing performance indices, this method can be used to assess both symmetry between successive half strides and regularity between successive strides by calculating the autocorrelation function of the acceleration signal. This allows the detection of lame horses as those showing symmetry values lower than 95%, with 100% as the result in perfectly symmetrically moving horses (Barrey & Debrosse, 1996).

An accelerometer mounted to the horse's head has been used to detect head motion asymmetries by Weishaupt et al. (1993). They recorded the vertical head acceleration directly and quantified the improvement of the gait in a lame horse due to analgesics and local anesthetics, in a similar manner to Kastner (1989).

Both accelerometric methods have the advantage of needing little instrumentation and of offering results in a short time using automated data analysis software.

Force plates, force shoes, EGA system

Pratt and O'Connor (1978) introduced the force plate in equine locomotion research. The vertical and horizontal force tracings allow a clinically appropriate analysis of limb loading and have often been used to satisfy the urgent need for objective assessments of orthopedic therapies. Gingerich et al. (1979) measured the different

Table 10.3 Symmetry indices using kinematic or kinetic variables.				
Author	Index	Variables	Method	Soundness value
Morris & Seeherman (1987)	L/R ratio	Ground reaction forces, impulses, timing	Quotient	1
Merkens et al. (1988)	H(orse)INDEX	Ground reaction forces, impulses, timing	Quotient, factors	1
Kastner (1989)	HAAS	Head vertical acceleration	Quotient	0
Buchner et al. (1993)	HAQ	Hip vertical acceleration	Quotient	1.28
Kübber et al. (1994)	WAAS	Withers vertical acceleration	Quotient	0
Peham et al. (1996)	Symmetry	Vertical head movement	Fourier analysis	100%
Buchner et al. (1996b)	Various indices	Head, withers, sacrum, tuber coxae, vertical displacement, maximal acceleration, vertical acceleration amplitude	Quotient	1
Uhlir et al. (1997)	SAAS	Sacral vertical acceleration	Quotient	0
Pourcelot et al. (1997)	Symmetry indices, forelimb, hindlimb index	Joint displacement, joint angles	Intercorrelation	1

loadings of the limbs due to various forms of carpal lame-nesses and the effect of hyaluronic acid as a therapeutic agent. Similarly, Goodship *et al.* (1983) evaluated differ-ent therapeutic regimes for tendinitis and Morris and Seeherman (1987) evaluated induced carpal lameness. Merkens *et al.* (1988) and Merkens and Schamhardt (1988a, 1988b) tried to establish a clinically oriented assessment system based on the bilateral symmetry of fore and hindlimbs. Both amplitude and temporal variables were used to define various symmetry indices that were combined into a single H(orse)INDEX (Table 10.3). Furthermore, graphical displays of the vertical and hori-zontal forces can be presented that allow a quick qualita-tive assessment of the presence of asymmetries by the veterinarian (Fig. 10.12) (Merkens *et al.*, 1988).

The major advantage of force plate analysis is that it does not require any instrumentation on the horse, so there are minimal problems for the horse and its owner. Furthermore, the results are very accurate and reliable. A disadvantage is the large number of trials needed to get enough data when using a small force plate; this requires some time and patience for all concerned. With larger force plates, however, fewer trials are needed due to the higher percentage of successful trials.

A special application of the force plate as a diagnostic instrument has been described by Aviad (1988), who used the stability of the force versus time signal of horses standing with the lame limb on a force plate to assess the weight-bearing stability and improvement due to therapy.

Clayton *et al.* (1999) have used the force plate to detect postural sway in standing horses as an indicator of neurological disease. In human subjects, certain neuro-logical diseases are associated with an increase in post-ural sway, which may be exacerbated by the application of a blindfold to remove visual proprioception. In horses, postural sway is assessed by having the horses stand with both fore or both hind feet on the force plate, without and with a blindfold. The movements of the cen-ter of pressure are monitored over a period of time. Variables that are measured include the radius and velocity of the movements of the center of pressure, and the craniocaudal and mediolateral range of motion. The findings are plotted graphically as a stabilogram (Fig. 10.13). Increases in the measured variables have been detected in horses with various neurological diseases including cervical vertebral stenosis (wobblers), equine protozoal myelitis and vestibular disease.

Besides force plate studies, two other kinetic devices have been used for the analysis of equine lameness: force shoes and the EGA system. Force shoes measure GRFs in special measuring devices integrated into a horse shoe. Different types of force shoes using piezoelectric trans-ducers (Ratzlaff *et al.*, 1990) or strain gauges (Roepstorff & Drevemo, 1993) have been designed. Problems in the

design of force shoes include the delicate nature of the instrumentation and the considerable weight of the shoes (Hugelshofer, 1982; Dohne, 1991), which impedes their use in a clinical situation. However, the technology is improving, and a clinically useful force shoe may even-tually be developed.

Auer and Butler (1986) first described the Kaegi sys-tem as a tool for assessing limb loading patterns in lame horses. The system, later improved and described as the EGA system (Huskamp *et al.*, 1990; Tietje, 1992), meas-ures vertical forces in a number of sensors, which are integrated into a special floor. This system needs no instrumentation on the horse and offers data describing the loading of each limb as well as temporal stride vari-ables. Despite the simplicity of use, the high cost of the EGA system prevented the widespread adoption of its use.

Artificial neural networks

A nice computational method to assess the results of locomotion analysis, and to detect asymmetry or lame-ness, is the use of artificial neural networks (ANNs). ANNs are computer programs that use similar methods to the human brain to recognize characteristic patterns in the kinematic or kinetic variables. As with human learning experiences, neural networks need to be trained with input data and the corresponding output message. For example, the ANN might be given input data describing the joint angle values or symmetry indices of the head and sacrum, together with the corresponding output message that there is a grade 2 lameness in the left forelimb. After several training cycles, the networks can use different, new input data to arrive at a conclusion describing the corresponding, unknown output information.

There have been two studies in which kinematic data from groups of lame horses were used as input data for an ANN: Schobesberger (1996) used data from 175 horses with a variety of different orthopedic diseases, and Loon *et al.* (1995) used the results of the lameness study of Buchner *et al.* (1995a, 1996a, 1996b). Both authors were able to detect the lame limb and to assess the lameness degree with probabilities between 75 and 85%. However, both concluded that the quality and the reliability depended on using a sufficiently high number of training data. Schobesberger estimated the necessary amount of input data for a correct diagnosis in 90% of the cases to be about 6600 input values, and to reach 95% probability of a correct diagnosis, 13 200 input val-ues were required. The fact that ANNs require such a large amount of kinematic input data to be adequately trained is likely to restrict their clinical use for lameness diagnosis in the near future.

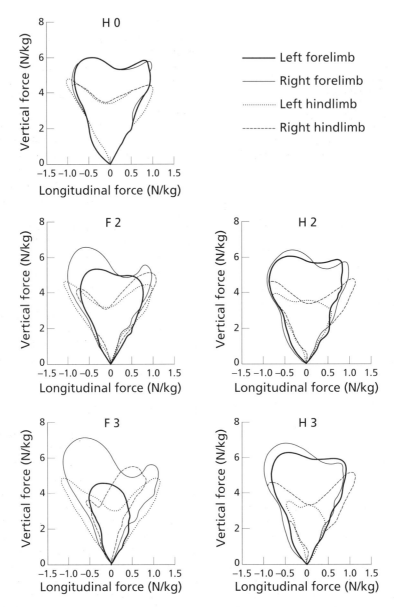

Fig. 10.12 Vertical-longitudinal force curves (vector– dynamograms) of all limbs of one horse during sound control session (H0), moderate left forelimb lameness (F2), severe left forelimb lameness (F3), mild left hindlimb lameness (H2) and moderate left hindlimb lameness (H3). (Reprinted with permission from Merkens, H.W. and Schamhardt, H.C. (1988b) Evaluation of equine locomotion during different degrees of experimentally induced lameness. II. Distribution of ground reaction force patterns or the concurrently loaded limbs. *Equine Vet. J.* **6** (Suppl.): 107–112.)

BIOMECHANICAL STUDIES OF DIAGNOSTIC, THERAPEUTIC OR PREVENTIVE AIDS IN EQUINE ORTHOPEDICS

A number of biomechanical studies have used kinematic or kinetic techniques to evaluate the use of diagnostic or therapeutic procedures or tools in equine orthopedics. Some of these procedures or tools are frequently used, but their effects are often small and difficult to quantify. Knowledge regarding the effects of these methods has been based primarily on experience or logical assumptions, but not on objectively determined results. Such quantitative studies have been performed on the effect

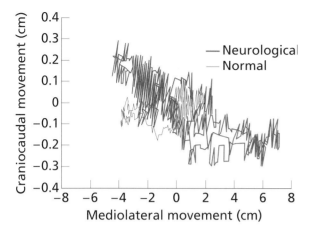

Fig. 10.13 Stabilogram showing craniocaudal and mediolateral movements of the center of pressure of the two forelimbs in a normal horse (dark line) and a horse with vestibular disease (light line). Measurements were made over a period of 10 seconds at a sampling frequency of 2000 Hz.

of flexion tests, the influence of diagnostic nerve blocks on sound horses, the benefit of bandages, the effects of desmotomy of the accessory ligament of the deep digital flexor tendon and the value of various orthopedic shoeing techniques. The biomechanical aspects of shoeing are described in chapter 6 and will not be considered here.

Flexion tests

A flexion test is a standard procedure during equine lameness examinations. The objective is to test if pain in a certain region and a worsening of a lameness can be provoked by prolonged flexion of the regional joints. Typical examples of flexion tests are digital flexion, carpal flexion and hock flexion (spavin) tests. Two factors have a significant influence on the outcome of a flexion test: the force applied and the duration of force application. Keg *et al.* (1997a) analyzed the forces used by a group of clinicians using a force transducer, the 'flex-o-meter' (Fig. 10.14). They found a considerable inter-individual variation between different clinicians of about 20% of the mean force. Furthermore, there was a significant sex difference in mean force: female examiners used a mean force of 114 N compared with 144 N in male examiners. The intra-individual variation, which is the variation within repeated flexion tests by the same person, was smaller, only about 12%. Therefore, to achieve a high repeatability, it is necessary to be consistent in performing the flexion tests. The same person should perform flexion tests in both limbs of the

same horse to allow for a correct interpretation, and it is not possible to equate the results found by different examiners.

The second variable, the duration of the forced joint flexion, is also very important. Two studies analysed the influence of changing flexion force and duration on the outcome of the test in sound horses (Keg *et al.*, 1997b; Verschooten & Verbeeck, 1997). Both studies found dramatic increases in the number of positive flexion tests by increasing the time of flexion to 3 or 5 minutes. This factor was more important than the force, in which an increase of 25% resulted in only one additional horse out of eight becoming lame (Keg *et al.*, 1997b). Increasing the force from 100 N to 150 N caused only about 6% more positive results in the flexion tests (Verschooten & Verbeeck, 1997). Both studies stressed the importance of standardizing the flexion tests in regard to force and duration, and both concluded that 60 seconds is an adequate duration for the flexion test. For the applied force, Keg *et al.* (1997b) suggested 150 N, while Verschooten and Verbeeck (1997) preferred only 100 N. More important, however, is the principle of using the same person to apply all the flexion tests within one horse to achieve the necessary consistency in the applied force.

Diagnostic anesthesia

The effects of diagnostic nerve blocks on the gait of lame horses has often been described (Girtler *et al.*, 1987; Merkens & Schamhardt, 1988a, 1988b; Keg *et al.*, 1992, 1994, 1996a; Keegan *et al.*, 1997) and can easily be quantified. More ambiguous results are reported concerning the effect of diagnostic anesthesias on the gait of sound horses. This information is important for differentiating sound horses from those with slight bilateral lameness. Bilaterally lame horses do not show any asymmetries in their gait patterns, but diagnostic nerve blocks of one affected limb cause a visible lameness of the contralateral limb. This is the only way to prove a bilateral orthopedic problem. This diagnostic procedure, however, is based on the assumption that diagnostic blocks in sound horses do not affect their locomotor pattern or, at least, have a different effect than in bilaterally lame horses. Several investigators tested this assumption using different methods. All the studies of diagnostic anesthesia in sound horses found slight gait changes, but they differed in quality and quantity. Kübber *et al.* (1994) and Drevemo *et al.* (1999) found some kinematic changes that were indicative of a slight increase in weight-bearing on the anesthetized limb. Kübber *et al.* (1994) reported increased asymmetry in the symmetry variables of head and withers after the nerve block in 9 of 12 sound horses, while Drevemo *et al.*

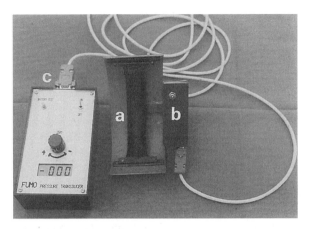

Fig. 10.14 Flex-o-meter. a: polyvinylchloride plate with rubber tube as inner lining; b: electronic manometer; c: charge amplifier.

(1999) found an increased range in the joint angle pattern of the fetlock joint. The changes were very small and some were very close to the border of statistical significance. Looking at the loading of the limbs using a force plate, however, Keg *et al.* (1996b) could not find differences in the vertical load before and after local nerve blocks. Only one variable, the time of change from a decelerative to an accelerative horizontal force, changed significantly. This indicates a change in the proprioceptive information and a consequent slight change in the locomotion pattern of the horses. This change in proprioception was also proposed by Kübber *et al.* (1994) and Drevemo *et al.* (1999) and leads to the conclusion that sound horses do indeed show small changes in their gait pattern after a local nerve block. However, these changes are very small. There might however be a gray zone, in which it is impossible to differentiate between the response to desensitization of the limbs in horses with a slight or subclinical, bilateral lameness from the reactions of sound horses.

Bandages

Bandages on the limbs of horses are a widely used tool and serve several different functions. There are the important medical uses in wound management or immobilization, and the therapeutic uses for applying pressure, cold, heat, water or various medical agents (Stashak, 1987). Another important use of bandages is to afford protection against injuries of the distal limbs due to interfering, over-reaching, hitting a fence or any other cause of skin trauma (Dyson, 1994). The most controversial use of bandages is to prevent tendon strains or joint injuries associated with loading during

locomotion. The distal limbs are often bandaged to prevent or support tendinitis or arthritis of the fetlock joint. There are some studies, however, which disprove this protective function or even indicate possible adverse effects of bandages for this purpose. The effects of bandages can be evaluated directly using invasive methods, such as strain gauges implanted into the tendons, or indirectly, using non-invasive, kinematic methods. Keegan *et al.* (1992) implanted strain gauges into the suspensory ligaments of nine horses. They compared ligamentous strain while standing and walking with two types of casts and four types of supportive bandaging materials, as well as different bandaging techniques. The results clearly showed that significant support can be expected only for the full cast and the dorsal fetlock splint. There was no effect of any bandage on suspensory ligament strain.

Kobluk *et al.* (1990) applied the close relationship between fetlock joint angle and suspensory ligament strain to evaluate the supporting capacities of bandages. They measured the kinematics of galloping horses that had been wrapped with different types of support bandages. Some horses showed slightly decreased fetlock hyperextension with bandages, but others showed no decrease or even had increased fetlock joint angles. In general, there was no proof for a protective effect of supporting bandages on fetlock joint angle or tendon strain during loading of the limbs. There might be a physical restriction of the amount of flexion during the swing phase, but this is unlikely to prevent injuries associated with limb loading.

On the other hand, bandages cause pressure on the limb, with the amount of pressure being dependent on the type of bandage and the speed of locomotion. Morlock *et al.* (1994) quantified the pressures on the metacarpal skin using a small pressure-sensitive mat. They measured local peak pressures up to $14.4\,N/cm^2$ at the gallop and maximal total forces up to $235\,N$ under the bandage. They concluded that even when no kinematic effect can be seen, the pressure under the bandage might impede blood flow in the distal limb, which could be counterproductive in terms of protection and performance of the horse. Furthermore, if bandages were applied tightly enough to support the tendons during locomotion, the forces applied to the limb at different locations under the bandage, for example the metacarpal skin, are likely to cause problems that would outweigh any positive effects at the tendons or fetlock joint.

Desmotomy

The effectiveness of various pharmaceuticals for the therapy of lameness has been quantified in terms of changes in the lameness degree or loading of the limbs. A study of the therapeutic effects of desmotomy of the accessory ligament of the deep digital flexor tendon (also known as the distal check ligament, DCL) took this a step further and used inverse dynamic analysis to assess the consequences of this procedure for the digital joints and tendons (Buchner *et al.*, 1996c; Becker *et al.*, 1998a). Desmotomy of the DCL is usually performed in young, growing horses suffering from flexural deformity of the distal interphalangeal joint (McIlwraith & Fessler, 1978). Recently, desmotomy of the DCL has also been proposed as a possible therapy for DCL desmitis, using a similar rationale to desmotomy of the accessory ligament of the superficial digital flexor tendon to treat an SDF tendinitis (Becker *et al.*, 1998a). In a long-term study all clinical, ultrasonographical, histological and biomechanical aspects of the desmotomy were assessed to evaluate the advantages or disadvantages of the desmotomy for treating chronic desmitis of the the DCL. A combination of kinetic, kinematic and radiologic techniques were used to study the function of the DCL for normal locomotion and to follow the changes in joint moments, tendon forces and limb kinematics at intervals of 10 days and 6 months after DCL desmotomy in sound horses.

Ten days after desmotomy the horses had no visible lameness or changes in limb loading, but alterations in the locomotion pattern were clearly indicative of the loss of biomechanical function of the DCL (Buchner *et al.*, 1996c). During the whole stance phase a caudad shift of the point of force application at the hoof (center of pressure) reduced the moment arm of the GRF and, consequently, the net joint moment at the coffin joint. Despite the loss of DCL function, the joint motion pattern at the beginning and in the middle of the stance phase was not changed. An increase in function of the SDFT compensated for the loss of the DCL, so the fetlock joint angle was unchanged during maximal vertical loading at midstance. At the end of the stance phase, it was primarily the deep digital flexor tendon (DDFT), rather than the SDFT, that took over the function of the deficient DCL (Fig. 10.15). However, the DDFT could not fully compensate the DCL function. Consequently, some kinematic changes occurred in the later part of the stance phase: the fetlock joint remained hyperextended for a longer time before flexing rapidly at the end of the stance phase, whereas the carpal joint started to flex earlier in the stride cycle. The increased loading of SDFT and DDFT was found to be within the normal range of loading at the walk and the trot. Therefore, it was concluded that there is no risk of damage to the compensating tendons after DCL desmotomy, provided locomotion is controlled during the recovery period.

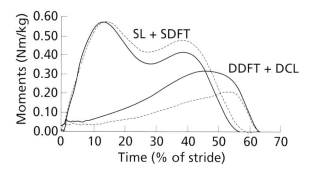

Fig. 10.15 Tendon moments at the fetlock joint of suspensory ligament and superficial digital flexor tendon (SL + SDFT), and deep digital flexor tendon and its distal check ligament (DDFT + DCL), averaged over six horses at the walk before and after desmotomy of the DCL. (——) before desmotomy; (– – –) after desmotomy. (Reprinted with permission from: Buchner, H.H.F., Savelberg, H.H.C.M. and Becker, C.K. (1996c) Load redistribution after desmotomy of the accessory ligament of the deep digital flexor tendon in adult horses. *Vet. Quart.* **18** (S2): S70–74.)

These experimental findings nicely confirmed most of the details that had been predicted by a model analysis of Bogert *et al.* (1989). By using a computer model to simulate the loss of the DCL, the increase in the DDFT force, as well as the change in the position of the point of force application, were predicted correctly, but the increase in the force of the suspensory ligament (SL) was overestimated. Obviously, the SDFT could compensate for the DCL desmotomy by maintaining the normal midstance angle of the fetlock joint so that SL loading was unchanged.

Six months after the desmotomy, the function of the DCL was partly restored by scar tissue formation, which restored 80% of the original tensile strength of the DCL, while its length had increased by 1 cm (Becker *et al.*, 1998b). This healing process restored its biomechanical function to a certain extent and reduced the typical locomotor changes seen 10 days after the desmotomy. However, most of the locomotor changes persisted, especially the caudad shift of the point of force application, and it was assumed that healing would continue for a longer period of time.

In conclusion this study documented the biomechanical changes due to DCL desmotomy and quantified the consequences for the net joint moments and the loading of the tendons. Even 6 months after desmotomy, healing was still in progress and DCL function was not fully restored. These experimental and model studies of DCL function show the potency of non-invasive methods for assessing the biomechanical effects of therapeutic procedures on the internal forces in limb joints and tendons. Similar studies have been performed to assess the effects of various types of orthopedic shoes and to enable an objective assessment of the benefit of these therapeutic measures for the health of the horse.

REFERENCES

Adrian, M., Grant, B., Ratzlaff, M. *et al.* (1977) Electrogoniometric analysis of equine metacarpophalangeal joint lameness. *Am. J. Vet. Res.* **38**: 431–435.

Auer, J. and Butler, K.D. (1986) An introduction to the Kaegi equine gait analysis system in the horse. *J.A.V.M.A.* 209–226.

Auer, J.A., Fackelman, G.E., Gingerich, D.A. and Fetter, A.W. (1980) Effect of hyaluronic acid in naturally occurring and experimentally induced osteoarthritis. *Am. J. Vet. Res.* **41**: 568–574.

Aviad, A.D. (1988) The use of the standing force plate as a quantitative measure of equine lameness. *J. Equine Vet. Sci.* **8**: 460–462.

Back, W., Barneveld, A., Weeren, P.R. van and Bogert, A.J. van den (1993) Kinematic gait analysis in equine carpal lameness. *Acta Anat.* **146**(Suppl.): 86–89.

Back, W., Barneveld, A., Bruin, G. *et al.* (1994) Kinematic detection of superior gait quality in young trotting warmbloods. *Vet. Quart.* **16**: 91–96.

Back, W., Schamhardt, H.C., Savelberg, H.H.C.M. *et al.* (1995a) How the horses move: 1. Significance of graphical representations of equine forelimb kinematics. *Equine Vet. J.* **27**: 31–38.

Back, W., Schamhardt, H.C., Savelberg, H.H.C.M. *et al.* (1995b) How the horses move: 2. Significance of graphical representations of equine hind limb kinematics. *Equine Vet. J.* **27**: 39–45.

Barrey, E. and Debrosse, F. (1996) Lameness detection using an accelerometric device. *Pferdeheilkunde* **12**: 617–622.

Barrey, E., Hermelin, M., Vaudelin, J.L. *et al.* (1994) Utilisation of an accelerometric device in equine gait analysis. *Equine Vet. J.* **17**(Suppl.): 7–12.

Becker, C.K., Savelberg, H.H.C.M., Buchner, H.H.F. and Barneveld, A. (1998a) Long-term consequences of experimental desmotomy of the accessory ligament of the deep digital flexor tendon in adult horses. *Am. J. Vet. Res.* **59**(3): 347–351.

Becker, C.K., Savelberg, H.H.C.M., Buchner, H.H.F. and Barneveld, A. (1998b) Effects of experimental desmotomy on material properties, histomorphology and ultrasonographic features of the accessory ligament of the deep digital flexor tendon in clinically normal horses. *Am. J. Vet. Res.* **59**(3): 352–358.

Bogert, A.J., van den, Sauren, A.A.H.J. and Hartman, W. (1988) Computer simulation of the equine hindlimb during locomotion. *Biol. Sport.* **5**(Suppl. 1): 131–143.

Bogert, A.J. van den, Schamhardt, H.C., Sauren, A.A.H.J. and Hartman, W. (1989) Computer simulation of equine locomotion and its application to the study of force distribution in the limbs. In: Bogert, A.J., van den (1989) Computer simulation of locomotion in the horse. *PhD thesis, Utrecht University*, pp. 111–136.

Buchner, H.H.F., Kastner, J., Girtler, D. and Knezevic, P.F. (1993) Quantification of hind limb lameness in the horse. *Acta Anat.* **146**: 196–199.

Buchner, H.H.F., Savelberg, H.H.C.M., Schamhardt, H.C. *et al.* (1994) Kinematics of treadmill versus overground locomotion in horses. *Vet. Quart.* **16**(Suppl. 2): 87–90.

Buchner, H.H.F., Savelberg, H.H.C.M., Schamhardt, H.C. and Barneveld, A. (1995a) Temporal stride patterns in horses with experimentally induced fore or hind limb lameness. *Equine Vet. J.* **18**(Suppl.): 161–165.

Buchner, H.H.F., Savelberg, H.H.C.M., Schamhardt, H.C. and Barneveld, A. (1995b) Bilateral lameness in horses – a kinematic study. *Vet. Quart.* **17**: 103–105.

Buchner, H.H.F., Savelberg, H.H.C.M., Schamhardt, H.C. and Barneveld, A. (1996a) Limb movement adaptations in horses with experimentally induced fore or hind limb lameness. *Equine Vet. J.* **28**: 63–70.

Buchner, H.H.F., Savelberg, H.H.C.M., Schamhardt, H.C. and Barneveld, A. (1996b) Head and trunk movement adaptations in horses with experimentally induced fore or hind limb lameness. *Equine Vet. J.* **28**: 71–76.

Buchner, H.H.F., Savelberg, H.H.C.M. and Becker, C.K. (1996c) Load redistribution after desmotomy of the accessory ligament of the deep digital flexor tendon in adult horses. *Vet. Quart.* **18**: S70–74.

Buchner, H.H.F., Savelberg, H.H.C.M., Schamhardt, H.C. and Barneveld, A. (1997) Inertial properties in Dutch Warmblood horses. *J. Biomech.* **30**: 653–658.

Clayton, H.M. (1986a) Cinematographic analysis of the gait of lame horses. *J. Equine Vet. Sci.* **6**: 70–78.

Clayton, H.M. (1986b) Cinematographic analysis of the gait of lame horses II: chronic sesamoiditis. *J. Equine Vet. Sci.* **6**: 310–320.

Clayton, H.M. (1987a) Cinematographic analysis of the gait of lame horses III: fracture of the third carpal bone. *J. Equine Vet. Sci.* **7**: 130–135.

Clayton, H.M. (1987b) Cinematographic analysis of the gait of lame horses IV: degenerative joint disease of the distal intertarsal joint. *J. Equine. Vet. Sci.* **7**: 274–278.

Clayton, H.M. (1988) Cinematographic analysis of the gait of lame horses V: fibrotic myopathy. *J. Equine Vet. Sci.* **8**: 297–301.

Clayton, H.M., Schott, H.C., Littlefield, L and Lanovaz, J.L. (1999) Center of pressure analysis in normal and neurological horses. *J. Vet. Internal Med.* **13**: 241 (abstract).

Clayton, H.M. Schamhardt, H.C., Willemen, M.A., Lanovaz, J.L. and Colborne, G.R. (2000a) Kinematics and ground reaction forces in horses with superficial digital flexor tendinitis. *Am. J. Vet. Res.* **61**, 191–196.

Clayton, H.M., Schamhardt, H.C., Willemen, M.A., Lanovaz, J.L. and Colborne, G.R. (2000b) Net joint moments and joint powers in horses with superficial digital flexor tendinitis. *Am. J. Vet. Res.* **61**, 197–201.

Deuel, N.R. and Lawrence, L.M. (1987) Laterality in the gallop gait of horses. *J. Biomech.* **20**: 645–649.

Dohne, W. (1991) Biokinetische Untersuchungen am Huf des Pferdes mittels eines Kraftme β schuhes. *Dissertation, Hannover.*

Dow, S.M., Leendertz, J.A., Silver, C.A. and Goodship, A.E. (1991) Identification of subclinical tendon injury from ground reaction force analysis. *Equine. Vet. J.* **23**: 266–272.

Drevemo, S., Dalin, G., Fredricson, I. and Björne, K. (1980) Equine locomotion: 3. The reproducibility of gait in standardbred trotters. *Equine Vet. J.* **12**: 71–73.

Drevemo, S., Fredricson, I., Hjertén, G. and McMiken, D. (1987) Early development of gait asymmetries in trotting standardbred colts. *Equine Vet. J.* **19**: 189–191.

Drevemo, S., Johnston, C., Roepstorff, L. and Gustas, P. (1999) Nerve block and intra-articular anaesthesia of the forelimb in the sound horse. *Equine Vet. J.* (Suppl.) **30**: 266–269.

Dusek, J., Ehrlein, H.J., Engelhardt, W.V. and Hörnicke, H. (1970) Beziehungen zwischen Trittlänge, Trittfrequenz und Geschwindigkeit bei Pferden. *Zeitschr. Tierzüchtung und Züchtingsbiologie* **87**: 177–88.

Dyson, S.J. (1994) Training the event horse. In: Hodgson, D.R. and Rose, R.J. (eds.), *The Athletic Horse*. Philadelphia: W.B. Saunders, pp. 419–428.

Firth, E.C., Wensing, T. and Seuren, F. (1987) An induced synovitis disease model in ponies. *Cornell Vet.* **77**: 107–118.

Foreman, J.H. and Lawrence, L.M. (1991) Lameness and heart rate elevation in the exercising horse. *J. Equine Vet. Sci.* **11**: 353–356.

Galisteo, A.M., Cano, M.R., Morales, J.L. *et al.* (1997) Kinematics in horses at the trot before and after an induced forelimb supporting lameness. *Equine Vet. J.* **23**(Suppl.): 97–101.

Gingerich, D.A., Auer, J.A. and Fackelman, G.E. (1979) Force plate studies on the effect of exogeneous hyaluronic acid on joint function in equine arthritis. *J. Vet. Pharmacol. Therap.* **2**: 291–298.

Girtler, D. (1988a) Untersuchungen über die Dauer des Bewegungszyklus – Stützbeinphase, Hangbeinphase, Phasenverschiebung – bei lahmen und bewegungsgestörten Pferden im Schritt und Trab sowie kinetische Beurteilungen zu deren Bewegungsmuster. *Wien Tierärztl Mschr* **5**: 217–231.

Girtler, D. (1988b) Untersuchungen über die Dauer des Bewegungszyklus – Stützbeinphase, Hangbeinphase, Phasenverschiebung – bei lahmen und bewegungsgestörten Pferden im Schritt und Trab sowie kinetische Beurteilungen zu deren Bewegungsmuster. *Wien Tierärztl Mschr* **5**: 225–270.

Girtler, D. (1988c) Untersuchungen über die Dauer des Bewegungszyklus – Stützbeinphase, Hangbeinphase, Phasenverschiebung – bei lahmen und bewegungsgestörten Pferden im Schritt und Trab sowie kinetische Beurteilungen zu deren Bewegungsmuster. *Wien Tierärztl Mschr* **5**: 310–324.

Girtler, D. and Floss, F.N. (1984) Zur Bewegung gesunder und bewegungsgestörter Pferde. In: Knezevic, P.F. (ed.), *Orthopädie bei Huf-und Klauentieren*. Hannover: Schlütersche, pp. 132–139.

Girtler, D., Kastner, J. and Holzreiter, S. (1987) Die Bewegung eines stützbeinlahmen Pferdes vor und nach diagnostischen Leitungsanästhesien dargestellt in Weg-Zeit-Diagrammen. *Wien Tierärztl Mschr* **4**: 13–142.

Goodship, A.E., Brown, P.N., Mac Fie, H.J.H. *et al.* (1983) A quantitative force plate assessment of equine locomotor performance. In: Snow, D.H., Persson, S.G.B., Rose, R.J. (eds) *Equine Exercise Physiology*. Cambridge: Granta, pp. 263–270.

Hajer, R., Hendrikse, J., Rutgers, J.E. *et al.* (1988) Het klinisch onderzoek bij grote huisdieren. Utrecht: Wetenschappelijke Uitgeverij Bunge, pp. 178–214.

Hjertén, G., Drevemo, S. and Eriksson, L.E. (1994) Shortening of the hind limb in the horse during the stance phase. *Equine Vet. J.* **17**(Suppl.): 48–50.

Holmström, M., Fredricson, I. and Drevemo, S. (1994) Biokinematic differences between riding horses judged as good and poor at the trot. *Equine Vet. J.* **17**(Suppl.): 51–56.

Hugelshofer, J. (1982) Vergleichende Kraft und Belastungszeit Messung an den Vorderhufen von gesunden und an Podotrochlose erkrankten Pferden Vet. Med. *Diss., Giessen.*

Huskamp, B., Tietje, S., Novak, M. and Stadtbäumer, G. (1990) Fussungs – und Bewegungsmuster gesunder und strahlbeinlahmer Pferde – gemessen mit dem Equine Gait Analysis System (EGA-system). *Pferdeheilkunde* **6**: 231–236.

Hütter, H. (1997) Aussagekraft der Winkeländerung der Zehengelenke von podotrochlosekranken Pferden. *Dissertation Veterinärmedizinische, Universität Wien.*

Kastner, J. (1989) Bewegungsmessung auf dem Weg zur klinischen Methode. *Österreich Hochschulzeitung* **9**: 15–16.

Keegan, K.G., Baker, G.J., Boero, M.J. *et al.* (1992) Evaluation of support bandaging during measurements of proximal sesamoidean ligament strain in horses by use of a mercury strain gauge. *Am. J. Vet. Res.* **53**: 1203–1208.

Keegan, K.G., Wilson, D.J., Wilson, D.A. *et al.* (1997) Effects of anesthesia of the palmar digital nerves on kinematic gait analysis in horses with and without navicular disease. *Am. J. Vet. Res.* **58**: 218–223.

Keg, P.R., Belt, A.J.M. van den, Merkens, H.W. *et al.* (1992) The effect of regional nerve blocks on the lameness caused by collagenase-induced tendonitis in the midmetacarpal region of the horse: a study using gait analysis, and ultrasonography to determine tendon healing. *J. Vet. Med. Assn.* **39**: 349–364.

Keg, P.R., Barneveld, A., Schamhardt, H.C. and van den Belt, A.J.M. (1994) Clinical and force plate evaluation of the effect of a high plantar nerve block in lameness caused by induced mid-metatarsal tendinitis. *Vet. Quart.* **16**: S70–75.

Keg, P.R., Schamhardt, H.C., Weeren, P.R. van and Barneveld, A. (1996a) The effect of high palmar nerve block on lameness provoked by collagenase induced desmitis of the lateral branch of the suspensory ligament. *Vet. Quart.* **18**: S103–105.

Keg, P.R., Schamhardt, H.C., Weeren, P.R. van and Barneveld, A. (1996b) The effect of diagnostic regional nerve blocks in the forelimb on the locomotion of clinically sound horses. *Vet. Quart.* **18**: S106–109.

Keg, P.R., Weeren, P.R. van, Schamhardt, H.C. and Barneveld, A. (1997a) Variations in the force applied to flexion tests of the distal limb of horses. *Vet. Rec.* **141**: 435–438.

Keg, P.R., Weeren, P.R. van, Back, W. and Barneveld, A. (1997b) Influence of the force applied and its period of application on the outcome of the flexion test of the distal forelimb of the horse. *Vet. Rec.* **141**: 463–466.

Kobluk, C.N., Martinez del Campo, L., Harvey-Fulton, K.A. *et al.* (1990) A kinematic investigation of the effect of a cohesive elastic bandage on the gait of the exercising Thoroughbred racehorse. *Proc. Am. Assoc. Equine Pratnr.*, Lexington, pp. 135–148.

Knezevic, P.F. (1982) Untersuchung auf Bewegungsstörung und /oder Lahmheit. In: Dietz, O. and Wiesner, E. (eds) *Handbuch der Pferdekrankheiten für Wissenschaft und Praxis.* Basel: S. Karger, pp. 40–53.

Knezevic, P.F., Floss, F.N. and Girtler, D. (1982) Erste klinische Ergebnisse rechnergestützter kinematographischer Bewegungsanalyse beim Pferd. *Proc. 14th Conf. Europ. Soc. Vet. Surg.*, Istanbul, pp. 89–94.

Kübber, P., Kastner, J., Girtler, D. and Knezevic, P.F. (1994) Erkenntnisse über den Einfluss der tiefen Palmaranästhesie auf das Gangbild des lahmheitsfreien Pferdes mit Hilfe einer kinematischen Meßmethode. *Pferdeheilkunde* **1**: 11–21.

Leach, D.H. and Crawford, W.H. (1983) Guidelines for the future of equine locomotion research. *Equine Vet. J.* **15**: 103–110.

Leach, D.H. and Cymbaluk, N.F. (1986) Relationship between stride length, stride frequency, velocity and morphometrics of foals. *Am. J. Vet. Res.* **47**: 2090–2097.

Leach, D.H. and Drevemo, S. (1991) Velocity-dependent changes in stride frequency and length of trotters on a treadmill. *Equine Exerc. Physiol.* **3**: 136–140.

Loon, J.P.A.M. van, Savelberg, H.H.C.M., Buchner, H.H.F. and Schamhardt, H.C. (1995) Lameness diagnosis in horses using artificial neural networks. *ESMAC Conference*, Enschede, p. 43

May, S.A. and Wyn-Jones, G. (1987) Identification of hindlimb lameness. *Equine Vet. J.* **19**: 185–188.

McIlwraith, C.W. and Fessler, J. (1978) Evaluation of inferior check ligament desmotomy for treatment of aquired flexor tendon contracture in the horse. *J. Am. Vet. Assoc.* **294**: 293.

Meij, H.S. and Meij, J.C.P. (1980) Functional asymmetry in the motor system of the horse. *South African J. Science* **76**: 552–556.

Merkens, H.W. and Schamhardt, H.C. (1988a) Evaluation of equine locomotion during different degrees of experimentally induced lameness. I. Lameness model and quantification of ground reaction force patterns of the limbs. *Equine Vet. J.* **6**(Suppl.): 99–106.

Merkens, H.W. and Schamhardt, H.C. (1988b) Evaluation of equine locomotion during different degrees of experimentally induced lameness. II. Distribution of ground reaction force patterns on the concurrently loaded limbs. *Equine Vet. J.* **6**(Suppl.): 107–112.

Merkens, H.W., Schamhardt, H.C., Hartman, W. and Kersjes, A.W. (1986) Ground reaction force patterns of Dutch Warmblood horses at normal walk. *Equine Vet. J.* **18**: 207–214.

Merkens, H.W., Schamhardt, H.C., Hartman, W. and Kersjes, A.W. (1988) The use of H(orse) INDEX: A method of analysing the ground reaction force patterns of lame and normal gaited horses at the walk. *Equine Vet. J.* **20**: 29–36.

Merkens, H.W., Schamhardt, H.C., Osch van, G.J.V.M. and Bogert, A.J. van den (1993) Ground reaction force patterns of Dutch warmblood horses at normal trot. *Equine Vet. J.* **25**: 134–137.

Morlock, M.M., Kobluk, C.N., Jones, J.H. *et al.* (1994) Influence of bandage material on pressure distribution under the bandage on the distal forelimb of the galloping horse. *Gait & Posture* **2**: 253–260.

Morris, E.A. and Seeherman, H.J. (1987) Redistribution of ground reaction forces in experimentally induced equine carpal lameness. *Equine Exerc. Physiol.* **2**: 553–563.

Muybridge, E. (1899) *Animals in Motion*. Republished (1957) Brown, L.S. (ed.), New York: Dover publications.

Peham, C., Scheidl, M. and Girtler, D. (1995) Definition eines Lahmheitsmaßes mit Hilfe der Spektralanalyse. In: Knezevic, P.F. (ed.) *Orthopädie bei Huf-und Klauentieren*. Stuttgart: Schattauer, pp. 412–423.

Peham, C., Scheidl, M. and Licka, T. (1996) A method of signal processing in motion analysis of the trotting horse. *J. Biomech.* **29**: 1111–1114.

Peloso, J.G., Stick, J.A., Soutas-Little, R.W. *et al.* (1993) Computer-assisted three dimensional gait analysis of amphotericin-induced carpal lameness in horses. *Am. J. Vet. Res.* **54**: 1535–1543.

Pollhammer-Zeilinger, S. (1996) Messung des Bewegungsmusters podotrochlosekranker Pferde auf dem Laufband mit Hilfe eines High Speed Videosystems. *Dissertation, Wien.*

Pourcelot, P., Degueurce, C., Audigié, F. *et al.* (1997) Kinematic analysis of the locomotion symmetry of sound horses at a slow trot. *Equine Vet. J.* **23**(Suppl.): 93–96.

Pratt, G.W. and O'Connor, J.T. (1978) A relationship between gait and breakdown in the horse. *Am. J. Vet. Res.* **39**: 249–253.

Ratzlaff, M.H., Grant, B.D. and Adrian, M. (1982) Quantitative evaluation of equine carpal lameness. *J. Equine Vet. Sci.* **2**: 78–88.

Ratzlaff, M., Hyde, M.L., Grant, B. *et al.* (1990) Measurements of vertical forces and temporal components of the strides of horses using instrumented shoes. *J. Equine Vet. Sci.* **10**: 23–35.

Ratzlaff, M.H. and Grant, B.D. (1986) The use of electrogoniometry and cinematography in the diagnosis and evaluation of forelimb lameness. *Proc. Am. Assoc. Equine Pract.* **31**: pp. 183–198.

Ratzlaff, M.H., Wilson, P.D., Hyde, M.L. *et al.* (1993) Relationships between locomotor forces, hoof position and joint motion during the support phase of the stride of galloping horses. *Acta Anat.* **146**: 200–204.

Riemersma, D.J., Schamhardt, H.C., Hartman, W. and Lammertink, J.L.M.A. (1988) Kinetics and kinematics of the equine hind limb: in vivo tendon loads and force plate measurements in ponies. *Am. J. Vet. Res.* **49**: 1344–1352.

Roepstorff, L. and Drevemo, S. (1993) Concept of a force-measuring horse shoe. *Acta Anat.* **146**: 114–119.

Schobesberger, H. (1996) Einsatz eines neuronalen Netzes bei der Lahmheitsuntersuchung von Pferden im Trab. *Dissertation, Wien.*

Seeherman, H.J. (1991) The use of high-speed treadmills for lameness and hoof balance evaluations in the horse. *Vet. Clin. N. Amer.: Equine Pract.* **7**: 271–309.

Seeherman, H.J. (1992) Gait analysis. In: Robinson, N.E. (ed.), *Current Therapy in Equine Medicine 3*. Philadelphia: W.B. Saunders, pp. 786–790.

Silver, C.A., Brown, P.N. and Goodship, A.E. (1983) Biomechanical assessment of locomotor performance in the horse. *Equine Vet. J.* **1**(Suppl.): 23–35.

Speirs, V.C. (1994) Lameness: approaches to therapy and rehabilitation. In: Hodgson, D.R. and Rose, R.J. (eds.) *The Athletic Horse*. Philadelphia: W.B. Saunders, pp. 343–70.

Stashak, T.S. (1987) Diagnosis of lameness. In: Stashak, T.S. (eds.) *Adams' Lameness in Horses*, 4th edn. Philadelphia: Lea & Febiger, pp. 100–156, 731, 840–877.

Tietje, S. (1992) Das EGA-System (Equine Gait analysis) – eine Möglichkeit zur Bewegungsanalyse und Lahmheitsuntersuchung beim Pferd. *Dissertation, München.*

Uhlir, C., Licka, T., Kübber, P. *et al.* (1997) Compensatory movements of horses with a stance phase lameness. *Equine Vet. J.* **23**(Suppl.): 102–105.

Verschooten, F. and Verbeeck, J. (1997) Flexion test of the metacarpophalangeal and interphalangeal joints and flexion angle of the metacarpophalangeal joint in sound horses. *Equine Vet. J.* **29**: 50–54.

Vorstenbosch, M.A.T.M., Buchner, H.H.F., Savelberg, H.H.C.M. *et al.* (1997) Modelling study of compensatory head movements in lame horses. *Am. J. Vet. Res.* **58**: 713–718.

Weeren, P.R., van, Bogert, A.J. van den, Back, W. *et al.* (1993) Kinematics of the standardbred trotter measured at 6, 7, 8 and 9 m/s on a treadmill, before and after 5 months of prerace training. *Acta Anat.* **146**: 154–161.

Weishaupt, M.A., Schatzmann, U. and Straub, R. (1993) Quantifizierung der Stützbeinlahmheit mit Hilfe akzelerometrischer Messungen am Kopf des Pferdes. *Pferdeheilkunde* **9**: 375–377.

West, G.P. (1984) *Black's Veterinary Dictionary*. London: A & C Black, pp. 442–444.

Williams, I.F., McGullagh, K.G., Goodship, A.E. and Silver, I.A. (1984) Studies on the pathogenesis of equine tendonitis following collagenase injury. *Res. Vet. Sci.* **36**: 326–338.

Wilson, D.A. and Keegan, K.G. (1995) Pathophysiology and diagnosis of musculoskeletal disease. In: Kobluk, C.N., Ames, T.R. and Geor, R.J. (eds.), *The Horse, Diseases & Clinical Management*. Philadelphia: W.B. Saunders, pp. 607–658.

Wittmann F. (1931) Die Untersuchung auf Lahmheit. In: Wittmann F. *Chirurgische Diagnostik des Pferdes.* Stuttgart: Ferdinand Enke Verlag, pp. 140–149.

Wyn-Jones, G. (1988) The diagnosis of the causes of lameness. In: *Equine Lameness.* Oxford: Blackwell Scientific Publications, pp. 1–22.

11
The Effects of Conformation

Mikael Holmström

INTRODUCTION

For as long as the horse has been used by man, conformation has been regarded as an important indicator of performance and soundness. In accordance with the variety of uses, many different types and breeds of horses have evolved, ranging from heavy draught horses to light, refined and racehorses. The result is that a huge number of breeds exist today, each with its own specific conformational characteristics. However the conformational traits are not always related to performance and soundness. This chapter will focus on conformational characteristics that, subjectively or objectively evaluated, are considered important for the performance and soundness of the sport horse.

THE STUDY OF EQUINE CONFORMATION

History and tradition

Much has been written about the conformation of the horse during the past 200 years, but very little is based on research. This does not mean that the work is of less interest. It is thought-provoking that many of the relationships between conformation and performance described by Bourgelat (1750) and Magne (1866) correspond well with the results from recent research. They stressed the importance of the hindquarter conformation. Horses with hindlimbs placed well underneath themselves were found suitable for dressage work, whereas those with hindlimbs camped out behind were likely to show good speed. Another early author, Hörman (1837), wrote that a long and forwardly sloping femur facilitates lifting of the hindlimb and the horse's ability to step under itself. Ehrengranat (1818) maintained that a sloping shoulder, long radius, short fore cannon and a flat croup are desir-able for good movement. According to Schmidt (1928), a small hock angle means that, although the horse will be able to step under itself easily, it will not be able to carry weight on the hind quarters due to decreased strength in the hock. Thus, he regarded a normal hock angle as advantageous for the function of the hindlimbs. Most authors of handbooks on conformation evaluation believe that a large hock angle leads to rigid and incorrect hindlimb movements as well as an increased strain on the hindlimb joints (Wrangel 1911–1913; Forsell, 1927; Anon, 1940; Bengtsson, 1983). Much of these horsemen's knowledge is still in practice but parts of it seem to have been forgotten in recent years.

In Sweden, the results from research based on both subjective evaluation and quantitative analysis has confirmed some and rejected other aspects of these old relationships. Some of the 'forgotten' relationships have also been rediscovered. Even though objective methods for conformation evaluation will probably play a more important role in the future, traditional subjective evaluation will always be important. It must be kept in mind that there are aspects of the conformation that cannot be measured by objective methods.

Subjective evaluation

Traditional subjective evaluation of conformation is currently performed in many different ways. Almost every country has its own protocol. Furthermore, many breeds have their own specific regulations that instruct the judges how to judge according to the standards of the breed. A problem with traditional evaluation is that subjective evaluations of conformation vary greatly between judges, although some morphological characteristics are assessed more consistently than others (van Vleck & Albrechtsen, 1965; Grundler, 1980; Magnusson, 1985a). It

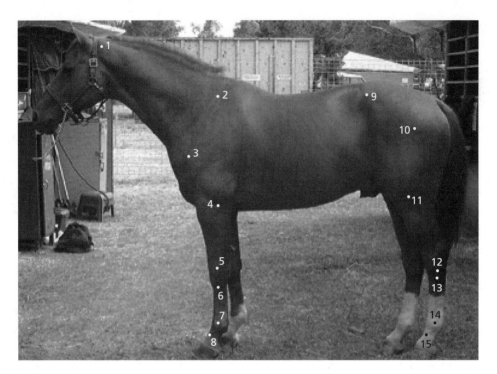

Fig. 11.1 Standard position and reference points.
Head and forelimbs **1:** The cranial end of the wing of the atlas; **2:** the proximal end of the spine of the scapula; **3:** the posterior part of the greater tubercle of the humerus; **4:** the transition between the proximal and middle thirds of the lateral collateral ligament of the elbow joint; **5:** the lateral tuberosity of the distal end of the radius; **6:** the space between the fourth carpal and the third and fourth metacarpal bones; **7:** the proximal attachment of the lateral collateral ligament of the fetlock joint to the distal end of the third metacarpal bone; **8:** the proximal attachment of the lateral collateral ligament of the pastern joint to the distal end of the first phalanx.
Hindlimbs **9:** the proximal end of the lateral angle of the ileum; **10:** the center of the anterior part of the greater trochanter of the femur; **11:** the proximal attachment of the lateral collateral ligament of the stifle joint to the femur; **12:** the attachment of the long lateral ligament of the hock joint to the plantar border of the calcaneus bone; **13:** the space between the forth tarsal and the third and fourth metatarsal bones; **14:** the proximal attachment of the lateral collateral ligament of the fetlock joint to the distal end of the third metatarsal bone; **15:** the proximal attachment of the lateral collateral ligament of the pastern joint to the distal end of the first phalanx.

is obvious that the reliability of the evaluation is dependent on the skill and experience of the individual judge.

The importance of the traditional conformation evaluation also varies between breeds. In race horses and Standardbred trotters, racing performance is the main parameter when selecting individuals for breeding. In riding horses intended for dressage and jumping, the selection is mainly based on conformation and performance tests carried out at 3–4 years of age. Since riding horses perform in competition much later in life than race horses, it is desirable to have a method for prediction of breeding value in young stallions and mares that do not have any performance record. Because the selection of stallions in most countries is stepwise, and performance tests are only applied to those that reach

minimum conformation standards, it is very important that conformation evaluation is based on correct criteria.

Quantitative analyses

Quantitative methods for measuring conformation can be used for an objective evaluation. Several studies have been carried out, especially on riding horses. The results do often show a great deal of conformity, but in most cases it is impossible to directly compare such parameters as angle measurements from different studies, due to differences in methods of measurement.

Quantitative conformational analysis, as a complement to the traditional evaluation, has been proven to

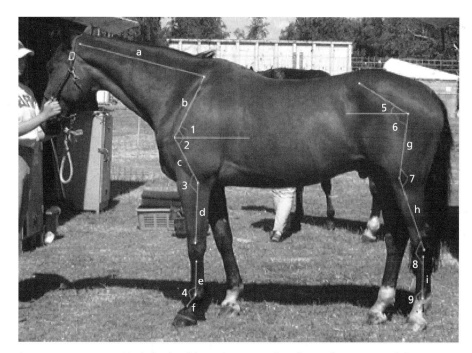

Fig. 11.2   Length measurements   a: Neck; **b:** shoulder; **c:** humerus; **d:** radius; **e:** fore cannon; **f:** fore pastern; **g:** femur; **h:** tibia; **i:** hind cannon; **j:** hind pastern.
Angle measurements   1: Shoulder inclination; **2:** shoulder joint; **3:** elbow joint; **4:** fore fetlock joint; **5:** pelvis inclination; **6:** femur inclination; **7:** stifle joint; **8:** hock joint; **9:** hind fetlock joint.

increase the accuracy in the prediction of performance potential in young riding horses (Holmström & Philipsson, 1993). However, applying this knowledge in practice, i.e. in breeding evaluation programs, talent scouting, etc., has been very difficult. Much of the resistance to quantitative analysis is due to the deeply rooted tradition of subjective evaluations in the horse industry, combined with a lack of familiarity with the new methods. In addition, there are some shortcomings in the method itself. Obtaining quantitative measurements has, until recently, been a slow procedure – too slow to be incorporated into stallion tests and other similar events. New computerized methods have now been developed that will speed up the process and make it possible to measure many horses in a short time.

In Sweden a method is used that was originally developed by Magnusson (1985a) for a study on Standardbred trotters. It is based on reference points marked on the horse with small paper dots glued to the skin (Fig. 11.1). When the technique was first used, all measurements were registered 'by hand' from a picture projected on a wall using a simple measuring band and a protractor. The measurements were transferred to the computer via punch cards. Now, however, the whole procedure is computerized. A picture of the horse is digit-

ized from a regular camcorder or a digital camera into a laptop computer. The measurements are registered by clicking with the mouse on the white markers. The computer then calculates all length and angle measurements (Fig. 11.2). The whole procedure takes about 10 minutes.

CONFORMATION, PERFORMANCE AND SOUNDNESS

Searching for talented young sport horses involves evaluation of many different qualities. Temperament, movement and jumping ability are of course the most important in riding horses, but the significance of conformation must not be neglected. Furthermore, dressage riders seek 'good looking' horses, with conformation that facilitates good movements, soundness and, above all, the ability to show a high level of collection. The competition results of Grand Prix horses are certainly dependent on the skill of their riders and trainers, but their conformation and movement must have the basic qualities that create the necessary conditions for successful training of the horse. Resistance from the horse is often interpreted as poor temperament but might just as well be due to pain or lack of ability to carry

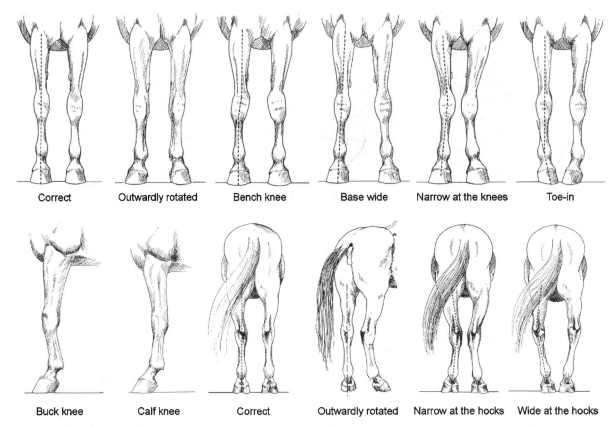

Correct	Outwardly rotated	Bench knee	Base wide	Narrow at the knees	Toe-in
Buck knee	Calf knee	Correct	Outwardly rotated	Narrow at the hocks	Wide at the hocks

Fig. 11.3 Deviations of limb and toe axes in the fore and hindlimbs.

weight on the hindlimbs caused by inappropriate conformation and/or movement. Potential world class Grand Prix dressage horses are difficult to find because many promising young horses with excellent gaits fail to learn passage, piaffe and other collected movements, resulting in years of wasted training. The ability to collect and work in balance is also very important in a jumping horse.

Conformation is also important in the selection of most other performance horses. However, a successful use of conformation as an indicator of performance requires good knowledge of the relationships between conformation and performance, as well as a reliable method for its evaluation. In most cases a subjective evaluation is not sufficient. Many important variables are almost impossible to judge correctly without objective measurements.

This chapter will focus on objective measurements and subjective conformational characteristics that are important for the function of sport horses. For those who have a specific interest in the characteristics of a specific breed, that information can be obtained from the respective breeding organization.

Deviations of limb and toe axis

One important part of the subjective evaluation is to describe deviations of limb and toe axes, if any. The most common deviations are described in Figure 11.3. Deviations from the straight (normal) limb and toe axes have traditionally been considered as a considerable weakness. However, not all deviations from what has been the desired conformation should be judged as abnormal, according to two Swedish studies. About 80% of all Warmblood riding horses and Standardbred trotters had outwardly rotated hindlimbs (Magnusson & Thafvelin, 1985a; Holmström *et al.*, 1990). The frequency of this 'faulty conformation' is so high that it must be regarded as normal. Boldt (1978) maintains in his dressage handbook that outwardly rotated hindlimbs facilitate exercises such as half-pass and shoulder-in. In this context, it is important to distinguish between hindlimb rotation and toe-out conformation as well as between rotated hindlimbs and hindlimbs that are narrow at the hocks (cow hocked). Confusion between these characteristics should be avoided, especially as the rotated hindlimb conformation should be considered normal. To judge

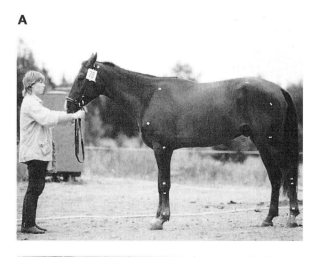

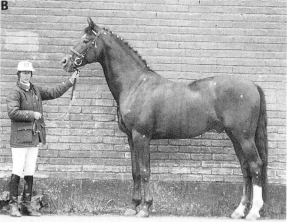

Fig. 11.4 Horses with low set neck **(A)** and well set neck **(B)**.

ance, bench kneed horses have been reported to have a higher frequency of splints on the medial side of the third metacarpal bone (Adams, 1970; Davidson, 1970; Nordin, 1980).

The frequency of toe-in and/or bench knee conformation, as well as of most other deviations, was the same among the elite dressage horses and show jumpers as in a group of riding school horses (Table 11.1). This indicates that mild to moderate deviations from the 'normal' limb conformation do not impair either soundness or performance in riding horses. However, it is important to emphasize that, even though mild and moderate deviations can be accepted, severe deviations of any type should be considered as a major weakness.

According to Adams (1974), calf knee (back at the knee) conformation may predispose to lameness, whereas buck knee (over at the knee) conformation is less serious. This is probably true for race horses that overextend the carpal joint considerably during mid stance phase. It is also likely to be true for jumpers and other horses moving at speed, but the effect on soundness in dressage horses might not be so important.

Head, neck and body

Many of the criteria that are used to describe the head, neck and body are very difficult or impossible to analyze objectively. Such criteria are type, the setting of the neck, the shape of the withers, the 'harmony' of the horse, etc. They have to be evaluated subjectively. Other characteristics, such as length of the neck and body or height at the withers, can be objectively measured.

It is obvious that there are significant relationships between head, neck and body characteristics and performance, which are reflected in the difference between, for example, a slow, heavy draught horse and a fast, elegant race horse. Thus, differences between breeds have, to a large extent, originated from different demands upon the horses. However, within a certain breed it is much more difficult to correctly describe and evaluate the relatively subtle differences, and this difficulty has been associated with a rather great variation between judges (van Vleck & Albrechtsen, 1965; Grundler, 1980; Magnusson, 1985a). Long experience, a deep understanding of the influence of conformation on performance and, when appropriate, inclusion of objective measurements can minimize these discrepancies. Figure 11.4 shows two horses, one with a low set neck and the other with a well set neck.

In handbooks on evaluation of the conformation of sport horses, some characteristics are described more consistently. A long and well set neck are considered important for most kinds of performances (Wrangel, 1911–1913; Forsell, 1927; Anon, 1940; Boldt, 1978; Bengtsson, 1983) and a long well developed withers is

this aspect of conformation, the observer should stand behind the point of the hock rather than behind the tail of the horse. The latter position makes it impossible to see if the rotated hindlimb is also narrow at the hocks.

Bench kneed conformation in the forelimbs together with a toe-in conformation is a very common type of deviation in riding horses, while outwardly rotated forelimbs are seldom seen in adult riding horses (Holmström *et al.*, 1990). According to Magnusson and Thafvelin (1985a) the converse is the case in Standardbred trotters. This difference may partly be explained by the fact that trotters are narrower through the chest than the riding horses, even after adjustment for different height at the withers. As in the hindlimbs, there is often confusion between outwardly rotated forelimbs and a toe-out conformation. Even though bench knee conformation in a riding horse does not have any documented negative effects on the long-term perform-

Table 11.1 Frequencies (percent) of subjectively scored deviations of limb and toe axes in different groups of riding horses. (Data are from Holmström et al., 1990. ©EVJ Ltd.)

Characteristic	[Mild]				[Moderate]				[Severe]				[Total]			
	1	2	3	4	1	2	3	4	1	2	3	4	1	2	3	4
Forelimbs																
Front view																
Outwardly rotated	3.0	7.1	3.0	3.7	–	3.6	–	0.6	–	–	–	–	3.0	10.7	3.0	4.3
Bench knee	48.4	32.5	53.0	48.4	6.1	21.4	11.0	11.8	–	–	–	–	54.5	53.6	64.0	60.2
Base wide	–	–	–	–	–	–	1.0	0.6	–	–	–	–	–	–	1.0	0.6
Narrow at knees	9.1	21.4	10.0	11.8	–	–	–	–	–	–	–	–	9.1	21.4	10.0	11.8
Toe-in	39.4	25.7	37.0	37.2	9.1	10.7	7.0	8.1	–	–	3.0	1.9	48.5	46.4	47.0	47.2
Side view																
Buck knee	18.2	35.7	6.0	13.8	3.0	10.7	2.0	3.7	6.1	–	–	1.2	27.3	46.4	8.0	18.7
Calf knee	9.1	7.1	21.0	16.2	3.0	–	3.0	2.5	–	–	–	–	12.1	7.1	24.0	18.7
Hindlimbs																
Rear view																
Outwardly rotated	84.9	82.1	67.0	73.3	3.0	3.6	7.0	5.6	–	–	–	–	87.9	85.7	74.0	78.9
Narrow at the hocks	–	7.1	10.0	7.4	–	–	–	–	–	–	–	–	–	7.1	10.0	7.4
Wide at the hocks	–	14.3	3.0	4.4	–	–	1.0	0.6	–	–	–	–	–	14.3	4.0	5.0
Toe-out	–	0	1.0	0.6	–	–	–	–	–	–	–	–	–	–	1.0	0.6
Side view																
Camped under	–	7.1	4.0	3.7	–	–	1.0	0.6	–	–	–	–	–	7.0	5.0	4.3

1: Elite dressage horses (n = 33); 2: elite show jumpers (n = 28); 3: riding school horses (n = 100); 4: total (n = 161).

Table 11.3 Significant conformational differences between horses treated for recurrent lameness and other insured horses.

Variable	Lame horses Mean (s.d.)	Sound horses Mean (s.d.)
Height at the withers	165.4 (4.2)	163.5 (3.6)*
Femur inclination	86.7 (1.7)	85.4 (2.3)**
Hind fetlock joint angle	156.6 (6.2)	153.8 (6.4)*

*: $P < 0.05$; **: $P < 0.01$; ***: $P < 0.001$.

said to be important for horses that are working under saddle. Results from objective studies show that elite show jumpers have significantly longer necks than elite dressage horses or 'normal' horses (Holmström, unpublished data) (Table 11.2). Other studies showed significantly shorter necks in elite dressage horses than in other riding horses but there was no significant correlation between the length of the neck and gaits under saddle in 4-year-old riding horses (Holmström et al., 1990; Holmström & Philipsson, 1993).

Overall, these findings indicate that a long neck might be an advantage for jumping horses, which is probably because it makes it easier for the horse to maintain balance over the fence. In dressage horses the length of the neck seems to be of less importance: the setting of the neck is probably more important than its length. It is generally agreed among riders and trainers of riding horses that a low set neck makes it very difficult to work the horse in a proper frame. However, there are no data supporting this statement, mainly because of the difficulties of objectively measuring the setting of the neck.

The setting of the head to the neck is also of importance. A wide throat latch has always been considered important in race horses, trotters and quarter horses because it is said to facilitate breathing. In dressage horses a wide distance between the wing of the atlas (first cervical vertebra) and the posterior ridge of the mandible has been considered important by riders. In a study of differences between elite dressage horses, elite jumping horses and 'normal' horses it was found that both the dressage horses and the jumpers had significantly greater width in this area than other horses (Holmström, unpublished data). A possible explanation is that a small distance might cause problems, like pain or a mechanical resistance, at higher levels of collection when the horse is required to perform a maximal flexion at the poll.

Height at the withers has been linked to jumping performance in several studies (Neisser, 1976; Langlois et al., 1978). Müller and Schwark (1979) found that show jumpers were taller at the withers than dressage horses.

Even though there is a positive correlation between height at the withers and jumping performance up to a certain limit (around 172 cm), it must be remembered that there is a great variation among elite show jumpers. The range of the height at the withers was between 158 cm and 178 cm in a study of the World Cup finalists in 1997 (Holmström, unpublished data).

It is generally agreed that height at the withers is not related to stride length in different gaits (von Wagener, 1934; Krüger, 1957; Dušek et al., 1970; Dušek, 1974). However, Holmström & Philipsson (1993) found positive correlations between height at the withers and subjective scores for the canter in 4-year-old riding horses. Elite dressage horses have not been found to be larger than other riding horses. In Standardbred trotters many authors have found a positive correlation between height at the withers and performance (Bantoiu, 1922; Richter, 1953; Magnusson, 1985d), while a negative correlation between height at the withers and soundness was found by Magnusson (1985c). In a study of relationships between conformation and soundness in insured riding horses in Sweden, horses with recurrent lameness problems were significantly taller at the withers than the sound horses (Table 11.3) (Holmström, unpublished data).

Swedish Warmblood riding horses (Holmström et al., 1990) and Hannovarian stallions (Dušek, 1974) have a long body form, i.e. the length of the body is greater than the height at the withers. Oldenburg and East Friesian breeds have also been shown to have this body form (Degen, 1953; Weferling, 1964). Müller and Schwark (1979), on the other hand, measured 687 horses competing in dressage, show jumping and three-day events and found them to have a rather short body form. The horses had about the same height at the withers as Swedish Warmbloods but it was not clear how the body length was measured. Neisser (1976) and Schwark et al. (1977) found negative correlations between body length and performance in show jumping. The influence of body length on performance is therefore still somewhat unclear and further studies are needed in different types of sport horses.

Magnusson (1985c) found that Standardbred trotters with a short back had fewer problems with back pain then those with a long back. On the other hand, horses with short backs showed more scalping problems. This confirms the statement that a short back is a strong back but predisposes to interference, such as over-reaching, forging and scalping (Pritchard, 1965; Nordin, 1980). Several authors have claimed that there is an increased stress to the distal parts of the limbs in horses with toe-out and toe-in conformation (Churchill, 1962; Rooney, 1968; Beeman, 1973; Magnusson, 1985c). This can often be noticed as synovial distensions of the fetlock and the coffin joints, as well as swelling of the distal metacarpal growth plate.

Table 11.2 Comparison of adjusted means for length and angle measurements between elite dressage horses (n = 40), elite show jumpers (n = 51), 4 year olds tested at Quality Events (n = 217) and horses with back problems or recurrent lameness problems (n = 52). Differences in sex, and, for the stifle angle, differences in femur inclination, have been taken into consideration.

Variable	Quality Events 1996	Dressage	Jumping	Injured
Length measurements (cm)				
Neck	70.51[a]	71.55[ab]	74.02[c]	72.87[bc]
Scapula	40.07[a]	42.00[c]	40.51[a]	41.00[ab]
Humerus	32.10[a]	33.07[b]	32.14[a]	32.01[a]
Radius	37.15[a]	37.64[b]	37.69[a]	37.58[ab]
Fore cannon	20.92[a]	21.56[b]	21.37[b]	21.14[ab]
Fore pastern	9.12[a]	9.52[b]	9.51[b]	9.16[a]
Femur	40.24[a]	41.20[b]	40.36[a]	40.09[a]
Tibia	48.52[a]	49.14[ab]	49.74[b]	49.40[ab]
Hind cannon	26.83[a]	27.36[b]	26.68[a]	26.55[ab]
Hind pastern	8.74[a]	9.01[ab]	9.34[b]	9.07[ab]
Angle measurements (degrees)				
Shoulder inclination	64.5[a]	66.3[a]	67.0[b]	66.5[b]
Shoulder joint	126.3[a]	124.5[b]	126.2[a]	126.0[a]
Elbow joint	152.4[a]	148.5[b]	151.1[a]	150.7[a]
Fore fetlock joint	148.7[a]	149.9[ab]	151.3[b]	148.2[a]
Pelvis inclination	31.0[a]	27.5[b]	28.2[b]	31.0[a]
Femur inclination	85.4[a]	84.7[b]	84.5[b]	87.8[c]
Stifle joint	154.1[a]	155.6[b]	154.0[a]	153.4[a]
Hock joint	159.4[a]	160.4[a]	159.2[a]	157.0[b]
Hind fetlock joint	154.6[a]	153.4[a]	155.7[a]	156.1[a]

Values with different superscripts differ significantly from each other.

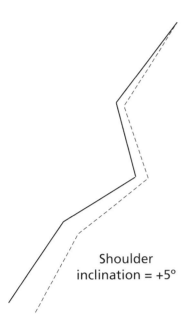

Shoulder
inclination = +5°

Fig. 11.5 Possible effect of different shoulder conformationon forelimb orientation at the beginning of the swing phase retraction: 5⁰ difference in shoulder inclination and all other angles unchanged.

Forelimbs

A long and sloping shoulder has always been considered as advantageous for the movements of the forelimbs (Ehrengranat, 1818). Sellet *et al.* (1981) suggested that a long sloping scapula was associated with ergonomic efficiency in 2-year-old pacing fillies. In a study of conformational characteristics of elite dressage horses and show jumpers, both groups had significantly more sloping shoulders (Holmström *et al.*, 1990). There was also a significant correlation between high gait scores and a sloping shoulder in 4-year-old riding horses (Holmström *et al.*, 1993). In a recent study (Table 11.2), the opposite result was found (Holmström, unpublished data). The slope of the shoulder, objectively measured, does not seem to be directly connected to elite performance in riding horses. Henninges (1933), however, found a positive correlation between a sloping shoulder and stride length in walk. Theoretically, a more sloping shoulder might facilitate the forward and upward movement of the forelimbs during the last part of the swing phase in trot (Fig. 11.5).

Subjectively, it is very difficult to correctly estimate the real slope of the shoulder. The problem is that in some horses there is a considerable discrepancy between the external outline of the shoulder and the real inclination (Fig. 11.6A,B). To be able to judge the slope of the shoulder correctly, it is necessary to palpate the position of the scapula. On the other hand there is one important aspect of the shoulder that might have been underestimated. A seemingly long and sloping shoulder in combination with a long and well-developed withers will place the rider more to the rear on the horse, resulting in better balance. As a result of the better balance, the horse will be able to move its forelimbs more freely, and reach higher and more forward. Thus, the effect of a 'subjectively' sloping shoulder on the forelimb movements might be more important than the real or 'objective' slope.

Of the forelimb conformational details, the length of the humerus showed the strongest correlation to good gaits in 4-year-old riding horses (Table 11.4) (Holmström *et al.*, 1993; Holmström, unpublished data). Elite dressage horses have been shown to have a significantly longer humerus than both show jumpers and 'nor-

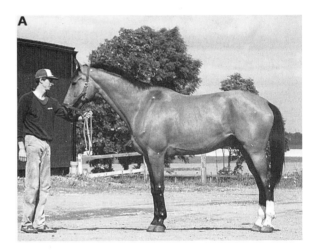

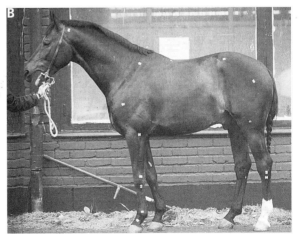

Fig. 11.6 A,B Horses with different slopes of the shoulders and scapula. Note the discrepancy between the real slope and the outer contour in B.

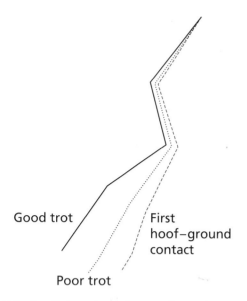

Fig. 11.7 Forelimb angles at the most forward position of the limb.

mal' horses (Table 11.2). In older literature, the importance of a long radius and a short fore cannon is often stressed (Ehrengranat, 1818; Schmidt, 1928; Wrangel, 1911–1913) but the length of the humerus is never mentioned.

In the subjective judging procedure good forelimb movements are often described in terms of 'freedom of the shoulders.' The analyses of high-speed films have shown that 'freedom of the shoulders' is not an adequate expression. The difference in forelimb movements between good and poor horses has very little to do with the movements of the shoulder or the shoulder joint. The most significant differences between good and poor forelimb movements were found in the elbow and carpal joints, with the elbow being more important (Holmström *et al.*, 1994). At the most forward position of the forelimb, the elbow joint was flexed ~30° more in the horses with good forelimb movements compared to those with poor movement. Consequently, the fore hoof was lifted higher above the ground and reached more forward. The effect of the greater flexion in the elbow and carpal joints is shown in Fig. 11.7. The significance of the elbow joint flexion for the forelimb movements explains why a correlation was found between the length of the humerus and gait score in the conformational studies: a long humerus gives a long triceps muscle that may facilitate a larger range of elbow movements. The humerus is significantly shorter in which less knee action in the forelimbs is preferred, or in which the forelimb movements have no influence on performance (Holmström, unpublished data). According to Sellet *et*

al. (1981) a long forearm is important in pacing Standardbreds.

The fore pastern has been shown to be significantly longer in elite dressage and jumping horses than in other riding horses, while the inclination to the horizontal plane showed no differences (Holmström, 1990). Horses with short, upright fore pasterns are considered to be prone to injuries, as are those with long sloping pasterns. (Adams, 1974). Magnusson (1985c) found more swellings of the superficial flexor tendon in horses with upright pasterns. The short upright pastern will probably also have a negative effect on the movements due to there being less elasticity. Ergonomic efficiency in pacing horses has shown to be correlated to an elastic fetlock joint (Sellet *et al.*, 1981).

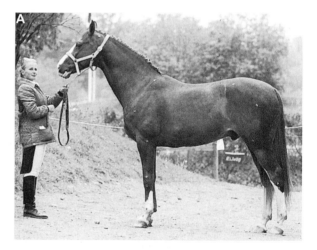

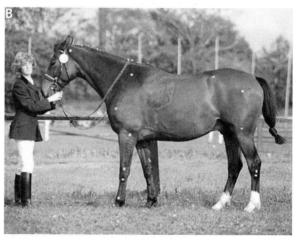

Fig. 11.8 Horse with large discrepancy between the slopes of the pelvis and the croup (**A**), compared to a horse with rather good correspondence between pelvis and croup (**B**).

Table 11.4 Results from multiple regression analyses of the effects of conformation measurements and scores on gaits under saddle and jumping ability, 1984 and 1996. Partial regression coefficients for variables that showed either significant correlation to the performance traits or significant differences between elite and 'normal' horses were calculated. Effects of sex and event (site) were included in the model.

Variable	Gaits under saddle		Jumping ability	
	1984	1996	1984	1996
Objective measurements				
Humerus length	0.16***	0.12**	0.10**	−0.13
Pelvis inclination	−0.04*	−0.005	−0.005	0.03
Femur inclination	−0.21***	−0.13***	−0.08**	0
Stifle angle	0.04*	−0.006	0.09	−0.04
Hock angle			0.01	0.11*
Subjective scores				
Type	0.11		−0.04	0.02
Head, neck and body	0.12		0.11	0.18
Extremities	−0.08		0.02	−0.28
Walk	0.38***		0.25***	0.05
Trot	0.19**		0.45***	0.11
Coeff. of determination, R2 (%)				
Conformation score	26.12		25.13	0
Objective measurements	24.76	13.32	13.32	1.31
Score + measurements	24.76	42.24	42.61	0.42

*: $P < 0.05$; **: $P < 0.01$; ***: $P < 0.001$

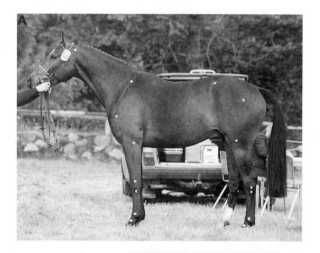

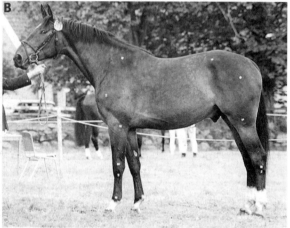

Fig. 11.9 Comparison of horses with a forward sloping femur (**A**) and a vertical femur (**B**). Note the effect on the overall placing of the hindlimb.

Hindlimbs

The importance of the hindlimbs for sport horse performance is obvious. The hind quarters constitute the 'engine' of the horse that, depending on the type of performance, should lift the horse over a fence, push it forward at a high speed or over long distances or, as in dressage horses, carry a lot of weight. Both horsemanship handbooks and many scientific studies indicate that good conformation of the hindlimbs is essential for good performance and soundness.

A small angle of the pelvis to the horizontal plane has been reported to have a positive effect on performance in dressage and jumping horses. In a recent study, elite dressage and jumping horses had significantly flatter pelvises than 'normal' riding horses (Table 11.2). The same results were found in a similar study in 1988 (Holmström et al.,

1990). Holmström et al. (1993) also found a positive correlation between the slope of the pelvis and scores for the walk at 4-year-old tests for riding horses. Ehrengranat (1818) states that a flat croup is desirable for good movements. However, there is not always a good correspondence between the slope of the croup and pelvis. Many horses have a flat croup combined with a steep pelvis (Fig. 11.8). This must be taken into consideration when evaluating conformation subjectively. In analyses of high-speed films it has been found that dressage horses classified as good movers had a larger rotation of the pelvis during the stride than those classified as poor movers (Holmström et al., 1994). Pelvic rotation is one of the biomechanical parameters that contributes to elastic gaits in good dressage horses, while a non-rotating pelvis results in short and inelastic gaits. A flat pelvic conformation facilitates pelvic rotation. Rotation of the pelvis during the stride is more pronounced in passage than in the other paces, and the degree of change in the pelvic movement pattern from trot in hand to passage is approximately the same in all horses, irrespective of the initial pattern (Holmström et al., 1995a,b). Pelvic rotation in the trot might be a determinant of passage performance. Thus, it is important to evaluate pelvis slope correctly in riding horses.

In Standardbred trotters a steeply sloping pelvis has been reported to be related to synovial distention in the femoropatellar joint and the medial synovial sac of the stifle joint, and also to have a negative effect on the soundness of the hock joints (Magnusson, 1985c). On the other hand, a flat pelvis is significantly correlated with pain on palpation of the croup muscles. The length of the pelvis has been reported to have a positive correlation to jumping ability (Langlois et al., 1974) and to stride length in the walk (Kronacher & Ogrizek, 1931).

Probably the most important individual conformational detail for most sport horses is the femur. A long and forwardly sloping femur places the hindlimb more under the horse, which allows the horse to keep its balance more easily and carry more weight on the hindlimbs, since the hindlimb position is closer to the center of gravity. In a study of Brandenburg horses, Kronacher & Ogrizek (1931) showed a positive correlation between stride length in walk and the length of the pelvis and femur. The slope of the femur has been reported by many authors to be related to performance. Langlois et al. (1978) showed that good jumping performance was significantly correlated to a forwardly sloping femur, i.e. a small angle of the femur to the horizontal plane (Fig. 11.9). In 4-year-old riding horses the forward sloping femur has been shown to have the strongest correlation to gait quality of all studied variables (Holmström et al., 1993). In a recent study both elite dressage and jumping horses had significantly more

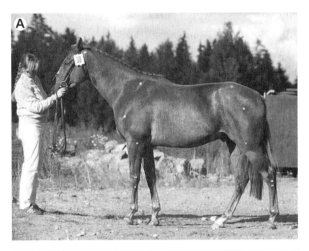

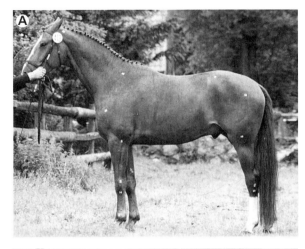

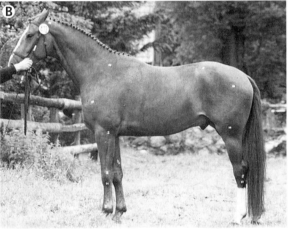

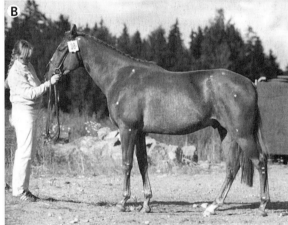

Fig. 11.10 Horses with small hock joint angle (**A**) and large hock joint angle (**B**).

Fig. 11.11 Horses with good (**A**) and poor (**B**) hindlimb conformation.

forward sloping femurs than 'normal' horses (Table 11.2). More than 150 years ago this correlation was stated by Hörman (1837). Other authors claimed that horses intended for dressage work should be well camped under (Bourgelat, 1750; Magne, 1866), which is very much the result of a forward sloping femur.

A forwardly sloping femur has also been shown to have a positive effect on soundness. In a study of riding horses with recurrent lameness and back problems attending one of the major horse clinics in Sweden, the femur was significantly more vertical than in 'normal' horses and elite horses (Table 11.2). Going through insurance company records of riding horses that were measured at quality events as 4 year olds, horses with recorded recurrent lameness and back problems had a significantly more vertical femur than the sound horses (Table 11.3) (Holmström, unpublished data).

In riding horses, the stifle angle should not be too small. Elite dressage horses have been shown to have a significantly straighter stifle angle than elite show jumpers and 'normal' horses (Table 11.2). A small stifle angle results in a lot of strain to the quadriceps femoris muscle, i.e. the muscle that extends the stifle. The quadriceps femoris probably is the most strained group of muscles when a horse works in collected gaits. If the muscles cannot 'lock' the stifle in an extended position when maximum load is put on the hindlimbs, the horse must transfer weight to its forelimbs and it is then no longer working in balance. In Standardbred trotters a positive correlation has been found between stifle angle and performance (Magnusson, 1985d).

Comparing the hock angles of elite dressage and jumping horses with 'normal' horses (Fig. 11.10), it has been found that the dressage horses in general had larger hock angles or, more correctly, there were no sickle hocked dressage horses (Holmström *et al.*, 1990). However, it could not be proved that the gaits improved with larger hock angles (Holmström *et al.*, 1993). A more recent study failed to show any differences in the hock angle between elite horses and others, mainly because the mean hock angle in the 'normal' horses had increased from 155.4° to 159.4°, which was almost the same as in the elite horses (Table 11.2). Horses with lameness and back problems had significantly smaller hock angles than sound horses (Table 11.2).

Magnusson (1985c) found that small hock angles (sickle hocks) were related to more synovial distentions in the stifle and hock joints as well as to more curbs. This has also been reported by several other authors (Smythe, 1963; Pritchard, 1965; Davidson, 1970; Beeman, 1973; Adams, 1974). Rooney (1968) and Hickman (1977) had the opinion that sickle hocked horses more often get bone spavin. Icelandic Toelter horses show a significant correlation between small hock angles and bone spavin (Eksell *et al.*, 1998). All these findings confirm what was said by Schmidt (1928), that a horse with a small hock angle will be able to step underneath itself but will not be able to carry weight on the hindlimbs due to decreased resistance and strength in the hock.

Studies using high-speed films have shown that in good dressage horses there is a considerable compression of the hock joint (~15°) during the mid-stance phase in trot and even greater compression in passage and piaffe (Holmström *et al.*, 1995a). In jumping horses and race horses, the compression is larger than in dressage horses. It is concluded that sickle hocked horses, or horses with small hock joint angles, should be avoided.

The slope of the hind pastern is, to some extent, influenced by the rest of the hindlimb conformation. A straight hock is significantly correlated to a more sloping pastern (Magnusson, 1985b). Riding horses with soundness problems had a significantly steeper pastern. This might be an effect of a smaller hock angle in these horses; however, the difference in hock angle was not statistically significantly (Table 11.3) (Holmström, unpublished data).

Generally, the hindlimb conformation should be regarded as one unit when evaluated. There are many different combinations of angles that result in a 'good hindlimb conformation', but it is generally characterized by a somewhat flat pelvis, a forwardly sloping femur, a normal to straight stifle and a normal to straight hock (Fig. 11.11). If the horse is weak in one part this can be compensated by strength somewhere else. The overall result is a strong hindlimb that can endure stress, carry weight and store elastic strain energy. Thus, looking at one characteristic at a time is not sufficient. All aspects of hindlimb conformation must be taken into account. This makes it more difficult to do an accurate evaluation

subjectively, and that is why inclusion of objective measurements has proven to improve the accuracy of the evaluation (Holmström *et al.*, 1993).

Preliminary studies on riding ponies, race horses and Icelandic Toelter horses indicate that the most favorable conformation for each type of performance is almost the same as that described above in sport horses. The differences found are variations on the same theme (Holmström, unpublished data). These variations are nevertheless important to investigate, and further studies will be carried out in the future.

REFERENCES

Adams, O.R. (1974) *Lameness in Horses*, 3rd edn. Philadelphia: Lea and Febiger, pp. 1–32.

Anon (1940) *Riding Instructions for the Swedish Army*.

Beeman, G.M. (1973) Correlations of defects in conformation to pathology in the horse. *Proc. 19th Ann. Meetg. Am. Assoc. Equine Pract.*, Atlanta, Georgia, pp. 177–197.

Bengtsson (1983) *ABC om hästar*, 7th edn. [In Swedish] Stockholm: LT:s Förlag.

Boldt, H. (1978) In: Haberbeck, H. and Haberbeck, H.-R. (eds) *Das Dressurpherd*. Verlagsgesellschaft GmbH: Lage-Lippe, pp. 60–71.

Bourgelat, C. (1750) *Elémens d'Hippiatique au Nouveaux Principes sur la Connaissance et sur la Médicine de Chevaux*. T. 1, Lyon.

Churchill, E.A. (1962) Predisposing factors to lameness in Standardbreds. *Proc. 8th Ann. Meetg. Am. Assoc. Equine Pract.*, Chicago, Illinois, pp. 191–194.

Davidson, A.H. (1970) Some relationships of conformation to lameness and the evaluation of the potential. *Proc. 16th Ann. Meetg. Am. Assoc. Equine Pract.*, Montreal, Quebec, pp. 399–404.

Degen, K. (1953) Variationsstatistische Körpermassuntersuchungen an 500 Oldenburger Zuchtstuten. *Dissertation, Hannover*.

Dušek, J. (1974) Beitrag zum Problem der Beziehung zwischen der Höhe des Pherdes und der Bewegungsmechanik bei den Hannoveranerhengsten. *Bayer. Landw. Jb.* **52**: 209–213.

Dušek, J., Ehrlein, H.-J., v Engelhardt, W. and Hörnicke, H. (1970) Beziehungen zwischen trittlänge, Trittfrekvenz und Geschwindigkeit bei Pferden. *Z. Tierzücht. ZüchtBiol.* **87**: 177–188.

Ehrengranat, A. (1818) *Om hästens rörelser i deras samband med ridkonsten*. [In Swedish] Lund.

Eksell, P., Axelsson, M., Broström, H., Ronéus, B., Häggström, J. and Carlsten, J. (1998) Prevalence and risk factors of bone spavin in icelandic horses in Sweden: a radiographic field study. *Acta Vet. Scand.* **39**: 339–348.

Forsell, G. (1927) *Om hästen, dess anatomiska byggnad, ytterlära, vård och sjukdomar*. [In Swedish] Stockholm: Hugo Gerbers Förlag, pp. 34–51.

Grundler, C. (1980) Aussagewert Verschiedener Hilfsmerkmale zur Beurteilung des Zücht – und Gebrauchswertes von Warmblutpferden. *Dissertation, München*.

Henninges, H.E. (1933) Untersuchungen über den Einfluss der Körpermasse und Gliedmassenvinkel auf die Leistungsschrittlänge bei Pommerschen Warmblutstuten. *Dissertation, Berlin*.

Hickman, J. (1977) *Farriery*. London: J.A. Allen & Co. Ltd.

Holmström, M. and Philipsson, J. (1993) Relationship between conformation, performance and health in 4-year old Swedish Warmblood Riding Horses. *Livestock Prod. Sci.* **33**: 293–312.

Holmström, M., Magnusson, L.-E. and Philipsson, J. (1990) Variation in conformation of Swedish Warmblood horses and conformational characteristics of elite sport horses. *Equine Vet. J.* **22**: 186–193.

Holmström, M., Fredricson, I. and Drevemo, S. (1994) Biokinematic differences between riding horses judged as good and poor at the trot. *Equine Vet. J.* **17**(Suppl.): 51–56.

Holmström, M., Fredricson, I. and Drevemo, S. (1995a) Biokinematic effects of collection in the elite dressage trot. *Equine Vet. J.* **27**: 281–287.

Holmström, M., Fredricson, I. and Drevemo, S. (1995b) Variation in angular pattern adaptation from trot in hand to passage and piaffe in the Grand Prix dressage horse. *Equine Vet. J.* **18**(Suppl.): 132–137.

Hörman, J. (1837) *Hästens exteriör. Hästen både naturhistoriskt och tekniskt betraktad.* [In Swedish] Skara, pp. 39–122.

Kronacher, C. and Ogrizek, A. (1931) Exteriur und Leistungsfähigkeit des Pferdes und besondere Berücksichtigung der Gliedmassenvinklung und Schrittlängenverhältnisse. *Z. Tierzücht. ZüchtBiol.* **23**: 183–228.

Krüger, L. (1957) Die estimmung der Arbeitsfähigkeit bei Pferd und Rind durch leistungsprüfungen, Physiologische und Psychologische. Messweret und durch die Exteriurbeurteilung. *Z. Tierzüct. ZüchtBiol.* **69**: 289–320; **70**: 1–20.

Langlois, B., Froideveaux, J., Lamarche, L., Legault, P., Tassencourt, L. and Theret, M. (1978) Analyse de liaisons centre la morphologie et l'aptitude au galop, au trot et au saut d'obstacle chez le cheval. *Ann. Génét. Sél. Anim.* **10**: 443–474.

Magne, J.L. (1866) *Valet af hästar eller beskrivning av alla de kännetecken som utvisa hästars brukbarhet till olika behov.* [In Swedish]. Stockholm, pp. 38–93.

Magnusson, L.-E. (1985a) Studies on the conformation and related traits of Standardbred trotters in Sweden. I. An objective method for measuring the equine conformation. *Thesis, SLU, Skara.*

Magnusson, L.-E. (1985b) Studies on the conformation and related traits of Standardbred trotters in Sweden. II. The variation in conformation of the Standardbred trotter. *Thesis, SLU, Skara.*

Magnusson, L.-E. (1985c) Studies on the conformation and related traits of Standardbred trotters in Sweden. IV. Relationship between conformation and soundness in 4-year old Standardbred trotters. *Thesis, SLU, Skara.*

Magnusson, L.-E. (1985d) Studies on the conformation and related traits of Standardbred trotters in Sweden. V. Relationship between conformation and performance in 4-year old Standardbred trotters. *Thesis, SLU, Skara.*

Müller, J. and Schwark, H.J. (1979) Merkmalsvarians und Genetische Bedingtkeit von im Turniersport Erfassten Leistungsmerkmalen. Züchterische Weiterentwicklung der Sportpferderassen. *Vorträge de III Int. Wissenschaftliches Symp.*, Leipzig, pp. 45–52.

Neisser, E. (1976) Korrelative Zusammenhänge Zwischen Phänotyp und Leistung beim Sportpferd. *Arch. Tierzücht.* **19**: 51–60.

Nordin, S. (1980) Sören Nordins Travskola. [In Swedish]. *Trav och galoppronden 49.*

Pritchard, C.C. (1965) Relationship between conformation and lamemess in the equine foot. *Auburn Vet.* **22**: 11–26; 29.

Rooney, J.R. (1968) Biomechanics of the equine lameness. *Cornell Vet.* **58**(Suppl.): 49–58.

Schmidt, P. (1928) *Handbok i hästbedömning.* [In Swedish]. Uppsala, Stockholm: Almquist and Wiksell.

Schwark, H.J., Schreiber, K. and Sasse, L. (1977) Merkmalskorrelationen bei Sportpferden. Paper presented at: *28th Annual Meetg. Europ. Assoc. Anim. Prod.*, Brussels, H1.05, pp. 1–7.

Sellet, L.C., Albert, W.W. and Groppel, J.L. (1981) Forelimb kinematics of the Standardbred pacing gait. *Proc. Equine Nutr. Physiol.*, pp. 210–215.

Smythe, R.H. (1963) *Horses in Action.* London: Country Life Ltd.

van Vleck, L.D. and Albrechtsen, R. (1965) Differences between appraisers in the New York type appraisal program. *J. Dairy Sci.* **48**: 61–64.

Weferling, C.G. (1964) Körpermessungen bei Oldenburgischen und Ostfriesischen Warmblutstuten. *Dissertation, Hannover.*

von Wagener, H. (1934) *Untersuchungen an Spitzenpferden des Spring - und Schulstalles der Kavallerieschule Hannover.* Hannover: Scharper Verlag.

Wrangel, C.G. (1911–1913) *Handbok för hästvänner.* [In Swedish] Facsimile-uppl. Bröd. Ekstrand Tryckeri AB, Lund, 1981, pp. 336–455.

12

Hereditary Aspects of the Locomotor System

Albert Barneveld and P. Rene van Weeren

INTRODUCTION

In the science of genetics three important eras can be discerned. The first started soon after the domestication of the first species. At that time man started interfering with the animals' gene pools by developing breeding programs that were purely empirically based and that were prompted by the observation that various traits had a genetic background. The second era started with the publications of Mendel in the 1860s, or rather perhaps with the rediscovery of his work in 1900 by de Vries in Amsterdam, Correns in Germany and Tschermak in Vienna. The Mendelian laws introduced the gene concept, while Galton and Pearson laid the basis for the science of biometric genetics, which developed rapidly in the 20th century, making fast progress possible in the genetic improvement of various breeds of animals and plants. The third era is based in the discovery of the molecular structure of DNA by Watson and Crick in 1953, but did not actually start before the 1980s, when the revolutionary surge of molecular genetics took place. Progress in this area has been breathtakingly fast and developments still occur at an ever increasing rate. The localization and identification of specific genes has been made possible by molecular genetic techniques and several (mainly single gene-based) genetic diseases have already been elucidated. It is to be expected that the science of molecular genetics will further expand in the (near) future, shedding light on a large number of polygenic traits and disorders and offering more and more possibilities in both an investigational sense and in the field of genetic manipulation.

In relation to the equine locomotor system, genetics are important at three levels. First, as a determinant of athletic capacity. In this respect there is a relation with conformation and a strong interaction with other performance-determining characteristics that are not related to the musculoskeletal system, such as the capacity of the circulatory and respiratory system and the character of the horse. A second level at which genetics may have an important influence on locomotor capacity is the determination of the susceptibility of musculoskeletal tissues for injury. Thirdly, there are a number of genetically determined disorders that may directly influence locomotor performance.

In this chapter a short overview is given of the historical role of horse breeding with respect to locomotor performance, both in the pre-Mendelian era and during the 20th century when breeding became, to a certain extent, more science than the art it was in earlier days. Some attention is paid to a number of disorders of the locomotor system that have a genetic background and the chapter concludes with a brief summary of recent developments in equine genetics and the implications they may have in the future for equine locomotion performance.

THE PRE-MENDELIAN ERA

The relation between conformation and gait and the fact that variation in many conformational traits is for a large part inherited has formed the basis for the selection of performance horses for millennia and still to a large extent forms this basis in many breeds of horses today. As early as the 4th century BC the great Greek hippologist Xenophon gave detailed descriptions of the conformational characteristics of a good performance horse. He made comments on the quality of the horn, the slope of the pastern, the robustness of the metacarpal and metatarsal bones and the desired joint angles in fore and hindlimbs. According to Xenophon a well-developed hind quarter is the best sign that a horse will move fast and smoothly; this statement shows his knowledge that propulsion comes from the hindlimbs. This insight is also evidenced by the statement that a short, strong lumbar region is preferred to a long back (*cited by* Schauder, 1923). From Xenophon onwards all great hippologists to some degree stress the same conformational characteristics as desirable traits. This applies to the great Arab horsemen from the early Middle Ages, like Akhi Hizam al-Furusiyah wa al-Khayl who published on the conformation of horses in AD 860 (Dunlop & Williams, 1996), and also to the famous European *ecuyers* from the 17th and 18th centuries such as William Cavendysh (1674) and Jacques de Solleysel (1733). Natural selection in different biotopes and selection by man for different purposes resulted in various horse breeds, ranging from the small and sturdy Shetland pony, that on average stands not more than 11 hands, to the Shire, 'the great horse of the Middle Ages,' that had to carry the heavily armored knights of those days. The Shire may be more than 17 hands high and may weigh more than 2000 lbs.

All breeds descend from the same common ancestor, a Przewalski-like horse that stood about 13 hands. It took ages to develop these breeds and selection was based in most cases on both conformation and performance. In some breeds, performance became the most important selection criterion; this applies to the Thoroughbred, the famous racing breed that was founded on the gene pool of three arab stallions that were imported to England in the early 18th century: The Darley Arabian, The Godolphin Barb and The Beyerley Turk. In the breeding of racing Thoroughbreds, speed was practically the only criterion for selection. Later, Trotters and Pacers were bred along similar lines.

FROM EMPIRICISM TO SCIENCE

Performance

In horse breeding selection always has been based on conformational characteristics, and the evaluation of gait. These traits can be scored in a semi-quantitative way, but some degree of subjectivity remains. This is in contrast to many commercially used farm animals where traits such as milk production, growth rate, fat thickness and food conversion can easily be measured and used as a basis for breeding programs. There is no doubt that gait, and even more so the complex concept of performance, are polygenic traits that can also be heavily influenced by environmental factors.

Performance can arbitrarily be divided into three areas: working, riding and racing (Hintz, 1980). With respect to working, pulling has been considered by various authors. Estimations of heritability range from from 0.12 ± 0.14 (Lonka, 1946) to 0.58 ± 0.20 (Varo, 1947) with a mean estimated heritability over several reports of 0.25 (Hintz, 1980). Cutting performance or 'cow sense' has received little attention so far. Ellersieck *et al.* (1985) estimated heritability at 0.19 ± 0.05. With respect to riding performance, estimates vary as widely as from 0.00 ± 0.12 for log of total earnings and log of average annual earnings for three-day eventing (Bade *et al.*, 1975b) to 0.71 ± 0.41 for points for jumping (Bade *et al.*, 1975a). Mean values for log earnings from jumping, three-day eventing and dressage are 0.18, 0.19 and 0.17, respectively (Hintz, 1980).

Most efforts have been made to investigate the heritability of racing performance. In the 1930s Harry H. Laughlin tried to find 'the laws by which nature governs the transmission of racing capacity from one generation of Thoroughbred horses to another.' He quantified performance by first calculating a formula (the so-called '*Standard Mean Seconds per Furlong*,' St.M.S.F.) that determined a standard mean time, taking into account the variables of age, weight to be carried and distance. The quality of performance for an individual horse could now be calculated by dividing the St.M.S.F. by the actual mean seconds per furlong of that horse (Laughlin, 1934a, 1934b). Though innovative, his method has not been widely applied.

Although racing performance is seemingly easy to quantify using parameters such as number of races won, best time and (total) earnings, many factors complicate this procedure. For instance, many methods use the ranking in a certain athletic event. However, although high ranking in a certain event may be synonymous with good performance for a given individual horse, this does not necessarily give information about the genetic value of this individual for the population, as much depends on the level of the event in which the individual took part. Nowadays, transformations of earnings are used in most cases (Ricard, 1998). Heritability estimates for the different variables cover a wide range. Field and Cunningham (1976) came to an exceptionally high heritability for timeform rating of 0.93 ± 0.13 using the offspring-sire regression approach. However, Langlois (1975) found a heritability of 0.30 when considering log of annual earnings, using the same method. Tables 12.1 and 12.2 summarize the heritability estimations of racing performance for Thoroughbreds and Trotters as given by Hintz (1980).

Conformation

The heritability of conformational characteristics has been estimated by various authors. Dušek (1970) used

Table 12.1 Average estimates of heritability for a number of performance criteria in Thoroughbred race horses, calculated by weighting the estimate by number of offspring used to obtain estimate. (Adapted from Hintz, 1980. ©American Society of Animal Science.)

Criterion	Weighted average estimate	Range
Performance rates	0.55	0.36–0.68
Log of earnings	0.49	0.38–0.60
Handicap weights	0.49	0.24–0.61
Best handicap weight	0.33	–
Best time	0.23	0.13–0.34
Time	0.15	0.06–0.29
Earnings	0.09	0.03–0.14

Table 12.2 Average estimates of heritability for a number of performance criteria in Trotters, calculated by weighting the estimate by number of offspring used to obtain estimate. (Adapted from Hintz, 1980. ©American Society of Animal Science.)

Criterion	Weighted average estimate	Range
Log of earnings	0.41	–
Time	0.34	0.04–0.48
Best time	0.25	0.12–0.36
Earnings	0.20	0.00–0.26

the 0–5 scale (from 'good' to 'bad') by which horses from the Trakehner Studbook were judged to calculate heritability coefficients. The h^2-value for 'swing' was of an intermediate level (0.42), the value for 'regularity of the gait' rather low (0.24). Other parameters that were measured on this scale were 'conformation', 'type' and 'total impression.' Although parameters like these can be scored on a semi-quantitative scale, they are so broad and susceptible to individual variation in judgment that the resulting h^2-values are of questionable value.

The Royal Dutch Warmblood Studbook introduced a system for the linear scoring of conformational traits and gait at the end of the 1980s. This system, together with the assessment of some health-related items, is one of the pillars of the Dutch selection system for stallions and their progeny (Barneveld, 1996). In this system a large number of conformation traits are scored on a 0–40 scale in which a population mean of 20 is assumed. The rather fine scale and the use of more specific characteristics (such as slope of the shoulder, length of the back, slope of the pastern, etc.), makes a better estimation of heritability possible. In general, heritability was found to

be rather low for these traits, ranging from 0.09 (slope of the pastern) to 0.26 (length of the neck and position of the croup) (Koenen *et al.*, 1995). Heritability coefficients for gait characteristics varied between 0.15 and 0.20. Also in other studbooks linear scoring systems have been successfully introduced (van Bergen & van Arendonk, 1993; Samoré *et al.*, 1997).

Some of these conformational characteristics are correlated with performance. A long, sloping shoulder is positively correlated with dressage results (Holmström *et al.*, 1990, 1994). A long and strongly muscled croup is positively related to show jumping performance (Langlois *et al.*, 1978). However, the vast majority of conformational traits that are scored using the linear system do not directly correlate with performance. This fact, together with the low to moderate heritability estimates for conformation (Preisinger *et al.*, 1991; von Butler-Wemken *et al.*, 1992), indicate that conformation results should be considered of minor importance in a direct selection for performance (Koenen *et al.*, 1995).

This is different when the test results of (potential) breeding stock are considered. When evaluating the system of stationary performance testing (SPT) of stallions in the Dutch Warmblood population by comparing SPT results of the sires with competition results of the offspring, Huizinga *et al.*, (1991) came to an estimated genetic correlation of 0.84 for show jumping and 0.83 for dressage. Though there is some bias due to selection and the subjectivity of scoring, they concluded that selection on SPT of stallions before entering breeding service is an effective tool to breed for competitive performance.

INHERITED DISORDERS OF THE LOCOMOTOR SYSTEM

A discrimination should be made between inherited conformational traits that may predispose to lameness or other aberrations of the locomotor system and genetically determined disorders of the musculoskeletal system that will affect performance. Stashak (1987a) describes conformation of the horse as 'the key to its method of progression.' He then elaborates on a number of faulty conformations that may predispose to various pathologic conditions of the musculoskeletal system: for instance a toe-out conformation results in a greater likelihood of limb interference and plaiting; a palmar deviation of the carpal joints ('calf knees') may predispose to slab fractures of the carpal bones; and the commonly seen cow hocked conformation may lead to bone spavin. Apart from these conformation-related disorders, there are direct genetically determined aberrations of the musculoskeletal system which are much rarer than conformational imperfections. Some of these have been known for a long time to have a genetic background. The mechanism of others has only recently been elucidated using modern molecular genetic techniques.

Single gene disorders of the locomotor system

Many monogenic anomalies in the horse have been described, a minority of which are related to the locomotor system (Galizzi Vecchiotti Antaldi, 1980a,b). Most of these disorders are inherited as autosomal recessive genes. Björck *et al.* (1973) described progressive congenital cerebellar ataxia in the Gotland pony breed as being inherited as an autosomal recessive gene with full penetrance. In Arabs a clinically similar condition described by Gerber *et al.* (1995) caused almost total hypoplasia or atrophy of the Purkinje cell layer. A lethal form of arthrogryposis associated with polydactylia in the Norwegian Fjord horse was described by Nes *et al.* (1982) as a new autosomal recessive mutation. Valberg *et al.* (1996) gave evidence for a familial basis for polysaccharide storage myopathy and associated exertional rhabdomyolysis in Quarter Horse-related breeds, the pattern of inheritance of which resembled an autosomal recessive disorder. Hermans (1970) described ulnar and tibial malformation (persistence) in the Shetland pony with associated locomotor problems.

Some disorders are inherited as dominant traits. An example that has been known for centuries in both animals and man is hereditary multiple exostoses. In the horse the condition is generally inherited as a single autosomal dominant gene (Gardner *et al.*, 1975; Shupe *et al.*, 1979), though some report that, as in man, three genes are involved, two autosomal and one X-linked (Monteiro & Barata, 1980).

Hyperkalemic periodic paralysis (HYPP) in Quarter Horses is a rather novel autosomal dominant disorder with a variable penetrance that has been extensively studied in recent years, not in the least because the disease is homologous to *adynamica episodica hereditaria* or Gamstorp's disease in man (Pickar *et al.*, 1991). It has been shown that HYPP in the Quarter Horse population can be traced back to a single stallion (Bowling *et al.*, 1996). Indications exist that the inherited predisposition for the disease has a positive genetic correlation with muscular appearance. This could mean that the HYPP rate has increased as a result of selection for more muscular appearance (Naylor, 1994). Cloning of the horse cDNA by cross-species PCR and subsequent sequencing revealed, as in man, that a defect in the sodium channel α-subunit gene was responsible for the condition (Rudolph *et al.*, 1992).

Polygenic disorders of the musculoskeletal system

Osteochondrosis (OC) can be defined as a disturbance of the process of endochondral ossification as this occurs in the growing individual. Of the group of so-called developmental orthopedic diseases it is by far the most common (McIlwraith, 1986). Epidemiological data suggest that the disorder is present in many breeds of horses in 10–25% of the population (Jeffcott, 1997). The exact pathogenesis of the disease is still unclear and subject to investigation (Jeffcott, 1991; Jeffcott & Henson, 1998). However, there is universal agreement that the disease is multifactorial (Hurtig & Pool, 1996) and that genetics play a role. Therefore, like many diseases and performance characteristics the phenotypic expression of OC is influenced by the environment plus a genetic component consisting of many genes in the genome (Gerber & Bailey, 1995).

From population studies that were mainly conducted in Trotters in the Scandinavian countries, it became clear that the disease was more prevalent in the offspring of certain stallions than of others (Hoppe & Philipsson, 1985; Philipsson, 1996), though these sires did not necessarily show signs of the condition themselves (Schougaard *et al.*, 1990). Heritability estimates for OC in the talocrural joint have been given at 0.24–0.27 by Philipsson *et al.* (1993), at a corresponding 0.26 by Schougaard *et al.* (1990), but at 0.52 by Grøndahl and Dolvik (1993) in their study on Norwegian Trotters. Winter *et al.* (1996) came to a very low heritability of 0.07 for the condition, but they used a pre-selected population, namely horses sold at auction. A recent overview is given by Philipsson *et al.* (1998). For the other frequently affected joint, the stifle, no such figures have been reported.

Recently, van Weeren and Barneveld (1999) showed that osteochondrosis is a very dynamic process in which lesions develop, but may also regress spontaneously. They also demonstrated the presence of osteochondrotic lesions in many joints other than the commonly affected hock and stifle. These findings shed a different light on this condition and put the question of whether there is a genetic difference between animals that show the condition at 3 years of age and animals that have shown the condition since foals, but in which the lesions subsequently regressed spontaneously. In addition to this, when considering the stifle joint, they found significant difference in the prevalence of the condition in foals that were the offspring of OC-free parents compared with foals whose parents were suffering from the condition in the same joint. This was not the case with respect to osetochondrotic lesions in the hock joint and might be an indication of a different genetic background in these two joints (van Weeren *et al.*, 1999).

Other frequently encountered lameness-causing disorders of the locomotor system that are not developmental in origin, but are more of a degenerative nature, include navicular disease, sesamoiditis, osteoarthritis of the fetlock joint and bone spavin.

Navicular disease, a degenerative disorder of the podotrochlea including the navicular bone, the navicular bursa, the distal sesamoid impar ligament, the collateral sesamoid ligament and the distal part of the deep digital flexor tendon, has been known as an important cause of lameness for ages (Youatt, 1836). An inherited basis for the disease has been suggested (Numans & van de Watering, 1973). Using a radiological classification of the navicular bone as a measure for the disease, Bos *et al.* (1986) found variation between daughter groups consisting of 3-year-old mares from different sires, supporting the theory that navicular disease has, to a certain extent, a genetic basis. However, they also concluded that the results of the radiological evaluation of the sires did not have predictive value for the progeny. In a large study that included 590 female offspring from 30 sires, the heritability of the radiographic classification of the navicular bone was estimated as 0.26–0.34 (van der Veen *et al.*, 1994). At the Heinz Gerber International Workshop on Genetics and Disease in the Horse that was held in Interlaken in 1995, D. Stornetta from Berne also presented evidence for a hereditary basis for navicular disease. He found a significant difference in the blind radiological evaluation (lateral and tangential views and Oxspring view) in the offspring of two Freiberger stallions (Rossdale, 1995).

Hermans *et al.* (1987) investigated the genetic background of congenital luxation of the patella in Shetland ponies. Németh (1974) demonstrated a phenotypic correlation between navicular disease and sesamoiditis. For sesamoiditis a relatively low heritability of 0.11–0.17 has been estimated (Barneveld, 1996). For osteoarthritis or degenerative joint disease of the fetlock joint, which can also be graded using a radiological scale, heritability was found to be comparable (0.13–0.26; Barneveld, 1996).

Bone spavin is commonly associated with poor conformation in which sickle hocks and cow hocks are predisposing factors (Stashak, 1987b). It is therefore not surprising that the disease to a certain extent is thought to have a genetic basis. Barneveld (1983) studied 168 3- and 4-year-old Warmblood offspring of 11 stallions and concluded that bone spavin indeed had a hereditary basis and was related to the conformation of the hindlimb. In the study by van der Veen *et al.* (1994) bone spavin was found to have a heritability of 0.20–0.35.

'Wobbler disease' is a pathological disorder of the spinal cord rather than of the locomotor system. However, as it produces ataxia the condition may severely affect locomotor performance. An early report on Wobbler disease stated that the syndrome was familial (Dimock, 1950). However, this could not be confirmed in a later large-scale retrospective study (Falco *et al.*, 1976), nor in a prospective study in which clinically and radiographically confirmed 'wobbler' mares and stallions were mated (Wagner *et al.*, 1985). In the latter study the high incidence of a number of developmental orthopedic diseases (OC, physitis, contracted tendons) was remarkable.

ACTUAL AND FUTURE DEVELOPMENTS IN MOLECULAR GENETICS

Thanks to the development of various molecular genetic techniques the knowledge of the genome in many species has increased rapidly. In recent years genetic maps have been published for, among others, man, mouse, cattle, pigs, sheep and chicken. A first draft of the complete human map is now available. In this 'genetic boom' the knowledge of equine genetics has lagged behind. Harrison (1998) gives three reasons for this. First, the traditionality of the horse industry, which resents scientific input into breeding schemes. Secondly, the fact that funding of research has been more directed towards veterinary items, neglecting genetic research. Thirdly, due to the cost of maintaining horses, the long generation interval and the long time it takes before a performance variable can be assessed, traditional crossing experiments have been limited.

In spite of having a late start, equine genetics have become a primary focus of interest. In 1995 an international workshop on genetics and diseases in the horse was held in Interlaken, Switzerland. Various general genetic topics and a large number of inherited disorders were discussed (Rossdale, 1995). Later that year the First International Equine Gene Mapping Workshop was organized in Lexington, Kentucky. Seventy-one delegates from 21 countries decided to develop a genome map of the horse within 3–5 years (Marti & Binns 1998). From then on the number of publications on equine gene mapping has steadily increased.

The first physical mapping of an equine gene (the gene complex for α-globin), using the technique of fluorescence *in situ* hybridization (FISH), was reported in 1993 by Oakenfull *et al.* In early 1997 the physical location of six genes was known (Breen *et al.*, 1997). At present, the number of microsatellites characterized in the horse is rapidly increasing (Marti & Binns, 1998; Marti *et al.*, 1998). Godard *et al.* (1998) produced a bacterial artificial chromosome (BAC) library of 40 000 clones of 100 kb on average characterized by PCR screening of approximately 130 microsatellite sequences and exogenic gene sequences retrieved from databases. Lindgren *et al.* (1998) published the first linkage map of the horse genome by segregation analysis of 140 genetic markers within 8 half-sib families. The marker set was calculated to cover at least 50% of the genome.

There is no doubt that the application of modern molecular genetic techniques to equine genetics will continue. This might result in the unraveling and complete understanding of certain monogenic disorders, which has already happened with respect to lethal white foal syndrome. This hereditary defect, that is homologous to Hirschsprung disease in man, was shown to be the result of a single TC AG dinucleotide mutation in the endothelin-B receptor gene which changed isoleucine to lysine at position 118 of the receptor protein. In the heterozygous horse this mutation produces the overo phenotype. In the homozygous individual it causes agangliosis of the bowel and is lethal (Metallinos *et al.*, 1998; Yang *et al.*, 1998). However, the production of a reliable horse genome linkage map and of large numbers of genetic markers is more interesting for the unraveling of polygenic traits. These may include the susceptibility to a number of more complex diseases (e.g. OC, navicular disease, bone spavin), the biochemical quality of the various tissues that make up the equine musculoskeletal system which determines the resistance to injury, or the genetic basis of performance characteristics. Though environmental factors play an important role in at least two of these areas, genetic markers will be used in the near future as guidelines for horse breeding, giving this ancient art a more scientific basis.

It has been estimated that the first horses were domesticated in about 3000 BC (Dunlop & Williams, 1996). Having just entered the third Christian millennium, or the sixth millennium in the history of the domestication of the horse, it may be anticipated that, thanks to the developments in molecular genetics, horse breeding will have a fundamentally different basis in the millennium to come than in the preceding 5000 years.

REFERENCES

Bade, B., Glodek, P. and Schormann, H. (1975a) Die Entwicklung von Selektionskriterien für die Reitpferdezucht. I. Genetische Parameter für Kriterien der Eigenleistungsprüfung von Junghengsten auf Station. *Züchtungsk.* **47**: 67–77.

Bade, B., Glodek, P. and Schormann, H. (1975b) Die Entwicklung von Selektionskriterien für die Reitpferdezucht. II. Genetische Parameter für Kriterien der Nachkommenprüfung von Hengsten im Feld. *Züchtungsk.* **47**: 154–163.

Barneveld, A. (1983) Spat bij het paard. *PhD thesis, Utrecht University*.

Barneveld, A. (1996) The role of breeding in sports performance and health with special emphasis on lameness prevention. *Pferdeheilk.* **12**: 689–692.

Björck, G., Everz, K.E., Hansen, H.-J. and Henricson, B. (1973) Congenital cerebellar ataxia in the Gotland pony breed. *Zbl. Vet. Med. A.* **20**: 341–354.

Bos, H., van der Meij, G.J.W. and Dik, K.J. (1986) Heredity of navicular disease. *Vet. Quart.* **8**: 68–72.

Bowling, A.T., Byrns, G. and Spiers, S. (1996) Evidence for a single pedigree source of the hyperkalemic periodic paralysis susceptibility gene in Quarter Horses. *Anim. Gen.* **27**: 279–281.

Breen, M., Lindgren, G., Binns, M.M. *et al.* (1997) Genetical and physical assignments of equine microsatellites – first integration of anchored markers in horse genome mapping. *Mamm. Gen.* **8**: 267–273.

Cavendysh, G. (1674) *Méthode nouvelle et invention extraordinaire de dresser les chevaux et les travailler selon la nature.* Londres: Tho. Milbourne.

De Solleysel, J. (1733) *Le parfait maréschal, qui enseigne a connoistre la beauté, la bonté et les défauts des chevaux,* 2ième partie. Paris: Pierre-Jean Mariette.

Dimock, W.W. (1950) 'Wobbles' – An hereditary disease in horses. *J. Hered.* **41**: 319–323.

Dunlop, R.H. and Williams, D.J. (eds) (1996) *Veterinary Medicine. An illustrated history.* St. Louis: Mosby.

Dušek, J. (1970) Zur Heritabilität des Körperbaus und des Ganges bei Pferden. *Z. Tierz. Zücht.-biol.* **87**: 14–29.

Ellersieck, M.R., Lock, W.E., Vogt, D.W. and Aippersbach, R. (1985) Genetic evaluation of cutting scores in horses. *J. Equine Vet. Sci.* **5**: 287–289.

Falco, M.J., Whitwell, K. and Palmer, A.C. (1976) An investigation into the genetics of 'wobbler disease' in Thoroughbred horses in Britain. *Equine Vet. J.* **8**: 165–169.

Field, J.K. and Cunningham, E.P. (1976) A further study of the inheritance of racing performance in Thoroughbred horses. *J. Hered.* **67**: 247–248.

Galizzi Vecchiotti Antaldi, G. (1980a) Eredità patologica nel cavallo. I. *Riv. Zootec. Vet.* **9**: 53–61.

Galizzi Vecchiotti Antaldi, G. (1980b) Eredità patologica nel cavallo. II. *Riv. Zootec. Vet.* **9**: 123–132.

Gardner, E.J., Shupe, J.C., Leone, N.C. and Olson, A.E. (1975) Hereditary multiple exostosis. A comparative genetic evaluation in man and horses. *J. Hered.* **66**: 318–322.

Gerber, V and Bailey, E. (1995) Genetics and disease in the horse. *Equine Vet. J.* **27**: 400–401.

Gerber, H. Gaillard, C.L., Fatzer, R. *et al.* (1995) Cerebellär Abiotrophie bei Vollblutaraber-Fohlen. *Pferdeheilk.* **11**: 423–431.

Godard, S., Schibler, L., Oustry, A., Cribiu, E.P. and Guérin, G. (1998) Construction of a horse BAC library and cytogenetical assignment of 20 type I and type II markers. *Mamm. Gen.* **9**: 633–637.

Grøndahl, A.M. and Dolvik, N.I. (1993) Heritability estimation of osteochondrosis in the tibiotarsal joint and of bony fragments in the palmar/plantar portion of the metacarpo- and metatarsophalangeal joints of horses. *J. Am. Vet. Med. Assoc.* **203**: 101–104.

Harrison, S.P. (1998) Progress in the molecular genetics of the horse. *Equine Vet. J.* **30**: 1–2.

Hermans, W.A. (1970) A hereditary anomaly in Shetland ponies. *Neth. J. Vet. Sci.* **3**: 55–63.

Hermans, W.A., Kersjes, A.W., van der Mey, G.J.W. and Dik, K.J. (1987) Investigations into the heredity of congenital lateral patellar (sub)luxation in the Shetland pony. *Vet. Quart.* **9**: 1–8.

Hintz, R.L. (1980) Genetics of performance in the horse. *J. Anim. Sci.* **51**: 582–594.

Holmström, M., Magnusson, L.E. and Philipsson, J. (1990) Variation in conformation of Swedish warmblood horses and conformational characteristics of élite sport horses. *Equine Vet. J.* **22**: 186–193.

Holmström, M., Fredricson, I. and Drevemo, S. (1994) Biokinematic differences between riding horses with good and poor trot. *Equine Vet. J.* **17** (Suppl.): 51–56.

Hoppe, F. and Philipsson, J. (1985) A genetic study of osteochondrosis dissecans in Swedish horses. *Equine Pract.* **7**: 7–15.

Huizinga, H.A., van der Werf, J.H.J., Korver, S. and van der Meij, G.J.W. (1991) Stationary performance testing of stallions from the Dutch Warmblood riding horse population. 1. Estimated genetic parameters of scored traits and the genetic relation with dressage and jumping competition from offspring of breeding stallions. *Livest. Prod. Sci.* **27**: 231–244.

Hurtig, M.B. and Pool, P.R. (1996) Pathogenesis of equine osteochondrosis. In: McIlwraith, C.W. and Trotter, G.W. (eds) *Joint Disease in the Horse.* Philadelphia: Saunders, pp. 335–358.

Jeffcott, L.B. (1991) Osteochondrosis in the horse – searching for the key to pathogenesis. *Equine Vet. J.* **13**: 331–338.

Jeffcott, L.B. (1997) Osteochondrosis in horses. *In Practice* **19**: 64–71.

Jeffcott, L.B. and Henson, F.M.D. (1998) Studies on growth cartilage in the horse and their application to aethiopathogenesis of dyschondroplasia (osteochondrosis). *Vet. J.* **156**: 177–192.

Koenen, E.P.C., van Veldhuizen, A.E. and Brascamp, E.W. (1995) Genetic parameters of linear scored conformation traits and their relation to dressage and show-jumping performance in the Dutch Warmblood riding horse population. *Livest. Prod. Sci.* **43**: 85–94.

Langlois, B. (1975) Analyse statistique et génétique des gains de *pur sang anglais* de trois ans dans les courses plates françaises. *Ann. Génét. Sél. Anim.* **7**: 387–408.

Langlois, B., Froidevaux, J., Lamarche, L. *et al.* (1978) Analyse des liaisons entre la morphologie et l'aptitude au galop, au trot et au saut d'obstacles chez le cheval. *Ann. Génét. Sél. Anim.* **10**: 443–474.

Laughlin, H.H. (1934a) Racing capacity in the Thoroughbred horse. Part 1. The measure of racing capacity. *The Sci. Monthly* **38**: 210–222.

Laughlin, H.H. (1934b) Racing capacity in the Thoroughbred horse. Part 2. The inheritance of racing capacity. *The Sci. Monthly* **38**: 310–321.

Lindgren, G., Sandberg, K., Persson, H. *et al.* (1998) A primary male autosomal linkage map of the horse genome. *Genome Res.* **8**: 951–966.

Lonka, T. (1946) The evaluation of the pulling ability of horses. *Valt. Maatalousk. Julk.* **126**: 45–50.

McIlwraith, C.W. (1986) Incidence of developmental joint problems. In: McIlwraith, C.W. (ed) *AQHA Developmental Orthopedic Disease Symposium*, Amarillo, AQHA, pp. 15–20.

Marti, E. and Binns, M. (1998) Horse genome mapping: a new era in horse genetics? *Equine Vet. J.* **30**: 13–17.

Marti, E., Breen, M., Fischer, P., Swinburne, J. and Binns, M.M. (1998) Six new cosmid derived and physically mapped equine dinucleotide repeat microsatellites. *Anim. Gen.* **29**: 236–238.

Metallinos, D.L., Bowling, A.T. and Rine, J. (1998) A missense mutation in the endothelin-B receptor gene is associated with Lethal White Foal Syndrome: an equine version of Hirschsprung Disease. *Mamm. Genome* **9**: 426–431.

Monteiro, J. and Barata, G. (1980) Exostoses no cavalo. Estudo da sua hereditariedade. *Rev. Port. Ciênc. Vet.* **75**: 31–39.

Naylor, J.M. (1994) Equine hyperkalemic periodic paralysis: review and implications. *Can. Vet. J.* **35**: 279–285.

Németh, F. (1974) De sesambeenskreupelheid bij het paard. *PhD thesis, Utrecht University.*

Nes, N., Løno, O.M. and Bjerkås, I. (1982) Hereditary lethal arthrogryposis ('muscle contracture') in horses. *Nord. Vet. Med.* **34**: 425–430.

Numans, S.R. and van de Watering, C.C. (1973) Navicular disease: podotrochleitis chronica aseptica, podotrochleosis. *Equine Vet. J.* **5**: 1–7.

Oakenfull, E.A., Buckle, V.J. and Clegg, J.B. (1993) Localization of the horse *(Equus caballus)* α-globin gene complex to chromosome 13 by fluorescense in situ hybridization. *Cytogenet. Cell. Genet.* **62**: 136–138.

Philipsson, J. (1996) Pathogenesis of osteochondrosis – genetic implications. In: McIlwraith, C.W. and Trotter, G.W. (eds) *Joint Disease in the Horse.* Philadelphia: Saunders, pp. 359–362.

Philipsson, J., Andréasson, E., Sandgren, B., Dalin, G. and Carlsten, J. (1993) Osteochondrosis in the tarsocrural joint and osteochondral fragments in the fetlock joints in Standardbred trotters. II. Heritability. *Equine Vet. J.* **16** (Suppl.): 38–41.

Philipsson, J., Brendow, E., Dalin, G. and Wallin, L. (1998) Genetic aspects of diseases and lesions in horses. *Proc. World Congr. Genet. Appl. to Livest. Prod.* **6**: 408–415.

Pickar, J.G., Spier, S.J., Snyder, R.J. and Carlsen, A.C. (1991) Altered ion permeability in skeletal muscle from horses with hyperkalemic periodic paralysis. *Am. J. Physiol.* **260**: C926–C933.

Preisinger, R., Wilkens, J. and Kalm, E. (1991) Estimation for conformation traits for foals and their practical implications. *Livest. Prod. Sci.* **29**: 77–86.

Ricard, A. (1998) Developments in the genetic evaluation of performance traits in horses. *Proc. World Congr. Genet. Appl. to Livest. Prod.* **6**: 388–395.

Rossdale, P.D. (1995) Genetics and disease in the horse: Heinz Gerber International Workshop. *Equine Vet. J.* **27**: 411–415.

Rudolph J.A., Spier, S.J., Byrns, G. and Hoffman, E.P. (1992) Linkage of hyperkalaemic periodic paralysis in Quarter Horses to the horse adult skeletal muscle sodium channel gene. *Anim. Gen.* **23**: 241–250.

Samoré, A.B., Pagnacco, G., Miglior, F. (1997) Genetic parameters and breeding values for linear type traits in the Haflinger horse. *Livest. Prod. Sci.* **52**: 105–111.

Schauder, W. (1923) Historisch-kritische Studie über die Bewegungslehre des Pferdes. (1. Teil) *Berl. Tierärztl. Wschr.* **39**: 123–126.

Schougaard, H., Falk Rønne, J. and Philipsson, J. (1990) A radiographic study of tibiotarsal osteochondrosis in a selected population of trotting horses in Denmark and its possible genetic significance. *Equine Vet. J.* **22**: 288–289.

Shupe, L., Leone, N.C., Olson, A.E. and Gardner, E.J. (1979) Hereditary multiple exostoses: clinicopathologic features of a comparative study in horses and man. *Am. J. Vet. Res.* **40**: 751–757.

Stashak, T.S. (1987a) The relationship between conformation and lameness. In: Stashak, T.S. (ed) *Adams' Lameness in Horses*, 4th edn. Philadelphia: Lea and Febiger, pp. 71–99.

Stashak, T.S. (1987b) Bone spavin (osteoarthritis or degenerative joint disease of the distal tarsal joints). In: Stashak, T.S. (ed) *Adams' Lameness in Horses*, 4th edn. Philadelphia: Lea and Febiger, p. 695.

Valberg, S.J., Geyer, C., Sorum, S.A. and Cardinet, III G.H. (1996) Familial basis of exertional rhabdomyolysis in Quarter Horse related breeds. *Am. J. Vet. Res.* **57**: 286–290.

van Bergen, H.M.J.M. and van Arendonk, J.A.M. (1993) Genetic parameters for linear type traits in Shetland ponies. *Livest. Prod. Sci.* **36**: 273–284.

van der Veen, G., Kingmans, J., van Veldhuizen, A.E. *et al.* (1994) The frequency and heritability of navicular disease, sesamoidosis, fetlock joint arthrosis, bone spavin, osteochondrosis of the hock: a radiographic progeny study. *Zeist, Koninklijk Warmbloed Paardenstamboek Nederland, 47 pp.*

van Weeren, P.R. and Barneveld, A. (1999) The effect of exercise on the distribution and manifestation of osteochondrotic lesions in the Warmblood foal. *Equine Vet. J.* **31** (Suppl.): 16–25.

van Weeren, P.R., Sloet van Oldruitenborgh-Oosterbaan, M.M. and Barneveld, A. (1999) The influence of birth weight, rate of weight gain and final achieved height and sex on the development of osteochondrosis in a population of genetically predisposed warmblood foals. *Equine Vet. J.* **31** (Suppl.): 26–30.

Varo, M. (1947) The development of the Finnish horses' pulling power. *Maataloust. Aikakausk.* **19**: 69–82.

von Butler-Wemken, I., Duda, J. and Kaiser, M. (1992) Genetische Analysen für Exterieurgesamtbeurteilungen und Beziehungen zu Körpermaßen bei Trakehner Stuten. *Züchtungsk.* **64**: 92–100.

Wagner, P.C., Grant, B.D., Watrous, B.J., Appell, L.H., and Blythe, L.L. (1985) A study of the heritability of cervical malformation in horses. *Proc. Am. Assoc. Equine Pract.* **31**: 43–50.

Winter, D., Bruns, E., Glodek, P. and Hertsch, B. (1996) Genetische Disposition von Gliedmaßenerkrankungen beim Reitpferd. *Züchtungsk.* **68**: 92–108.

Yang, G.C., Croaker, D., Zhang, A.L., Manglick, P., Cartmill, T. and Cass, D. (1998) A dinucleotide mutation in the endothelin-B receptor gene is associated with lethal white foal disease (LWFS); a horse variant of Hirschsprung disease (HSCR). *Hum. Mol. Gen.* **7**: 1047–1052.

Youatt, W. (1836) Animal pathology. *The Veterinarian* **9**: 362–368.

13

Mechanical Analysis of Locomotion

Liduin S. Meershoek and Anton J. van den Bogert

INTRODUCTION

Visual examination of equine gait has been the main clinical tool for diagnosis of lameness in horses during the past two or three millennia. Similarly, trainers and breeders routinely examine gait visually in order to predict sport performance. Recent developments in gait measurement techniques (Clayton, 1996) have made it possible to perform gait analysis in a quantitative manner, which results in better reproducibility, improved temporal and spatial resolution, and is less dependent on the experience and judgment of the clinician or trainer. The separate analysis of either movements or forces, *kinematics* or *kinetics* respectively, can enhance our understanding equine gait. However, an even more powerful method is to analyze movements and forces simultaneously using Newton's laws of *dynamics*.

Kinematic variables, such as limb trajectories, joint angles and angular velocities, have been used frequently in the past two decades to quantify equine gait (e.g. van Weeren *et al.*, 1993). These variables contain essentially the same information that is presented to the eye of a clinician, the only difference being the quantitative nature of the information and the increased spatio-temporal resolution. This resolution is important, because equine gait is very reproducible and small or fast changes in movement, invisible to the human eye, are relevant. Until now, however, automated kinematic gait analysis has not resulted in a better ability to quantify and characterize lameness, as compared to visual examination by an experienced clinician (Back *et al.*, 1993). However, some success has been reported in prediction of performance using gait analysis (Deuel & Park, 1993; Back *et al.*, 1995).

A different type of gait information is obtained by using *kinetic* variables. Kinetic variables are variables related to forces. Internal kinetic variables such as tendon forces (Riemersma *et al.*, 1996) and bone strain (Hartman *et al.*, 1984; Biewener *et al.*, 1988) have been measured in horses. These measurements are, however, invasive and limited to research applications. For routine gait evaluation, the only non-invasive kinetic measuring device is the force platform, which measures forces between hoof and ground. After initial work by Pratt and O'Connor (1976), clinical applications were explored (Merkens & Schamhardt, 1988; Dow *et al.*, 1991). These studies have shown that although force plate signals do not always provide enough information for full diagnostics, they are useful to quantify lameness and to indicate the affected limb.

Isaac Newton (England, 1642–1727) formulated the basic laws of *dynamics*, establishing a relationship between force, mass and translational movement: $F = m \cdot a$. Leonhard Euler (Germany, 1707–1783) further developed these laws to describe rotation of rigid bodies, whereas Joseph Louis Lagrange (France/Italy, 1736–1813) formulated equations for linked multibody systems which are the basis of modern robotics. The laws of dynamics have proved useful to predict motion resulting from known forces (*forward dynamics*), or to estimate the forces that were the cause of an observed motion (*inverse dynamics*). Since Elftman introduced the inverse dynamics analysis in biomechanics (1939) it has been applied successfully in human movement research. Examples can be found in orthopedics (Andriacchi, 1993), in motor control (Winter & Eng, 1995) and in sport (Yeadon & Challis, 1994). It provides an opportunity for interpretation of gait that is not possible with kinematic or kinetic measurements alone. This opportunity has also been explored for basic questions on equine gait (Bartel *et al.*, 1978; Schryver *et al.*, 1978; Clayton *et al.*, 1998).

Inverse dynamic analysis treats the locomotor system as a system of linked rigid segments, with hypothetical torque (or moment) motors at each joint representing the action of muscles. The analysis combines kinematic and force platform data to derive these joint moments throughout the movement cycle (Fig. 13.1). The methods have been well established in

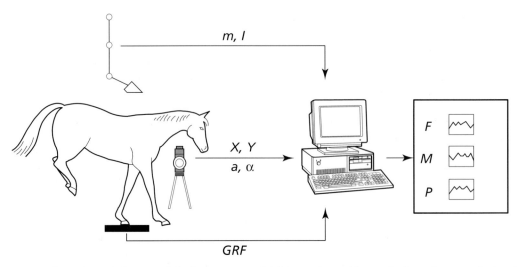

Fig. 13.1 Inverse dynamic analysis uses a linked segment model, kinematics and force platform data to calculate joint moments, forces and powers. (See text for details.)

the literature, both in two dimensions (Winter, 1990) and in three dimensions (Vaughan, 1984; van den Bogert, 1994). Software to perform inverse dynamic analysis on any user-specified locomotor system, allowing for horses as well as humans, is available from the major manufacturers of gait analysis equipment.

The moment at the center of rotation of a joint is directly related to the combination of muscle forces acting across the joint. These joint moments by themselves provide useful information about movement. Even more so than the human, the horse, with its four multi-jointed limbs frequently acting as closed-chain mechanisms, may redistribute its joint moments without visual gait changes. For instance, a visually identical hindlimb extension in late stance may be accomplished by only hip extensor muscles, only knee extensor muscles, or any combination of these. Inverse dynamic analysis allows us to 'see' these differences in muscle coordination. One further useful step in inverse dynamic analysis is the quantification of joint power profiles. This allows investigation of the sources of mechanical power for movement. We will show in this chapter how joint moment and joint power can be used to estimate force and power output in musculotendinous structures.

It must be stressed that results of inverse dynamic analysis are sensitive to the protocol for data collection and the methods for data analysis. Since the horse is not a set of perfect rigid body segments, and kinematic data are contaminated by measurement errors and soft tissue deformation, results can only be an approximation. This is acceptable, as long as the methodology is well understood and used consistently so that results can be compared between studies.

An indication of the potential applications of inverse dynamic analysis can be obtained from examples in the human literature. A well-known finding is that knee extensor moments during gait are significantly reduced after anterior cruciate ligament injury. Inverse dynamic analysis provides a tool to monitor the patient's progress during rehabilitation and decide when surgical treatment is required (Andriacchi & Birac, 1993). Using out-of-sagittal plane joint moments, it has been shown that a certain bracing method reduces the medial compartment loads in the knee joint (Lindenfeld et al., 1997). Especially noteworthy is the success of gait analysis, including inverse dynamic and joint power analysis, in surgical decision making for children with cerebral palsy (Rose et al., 1993). In research, useful information for understanding of injury mechanisms and design of joint replacements is obtained from inverse dynamic analysis of muscle and joint forces during various activities (Paul, 1971; van den Bogert et al., 1999). Similar clinical applications can be found for horses when using inverse dynamics to analyze equine gait. It has, for example, been used successfully to analyze the influence of heel wedges in horses with tendinitis (Clayton et al., 2000).

Before such applications are possible, it is imperative that valid test protocols are established and normative data are collected (Ounpuu et al., 1991). Movements of horses are remarkably planar and the function of most muscles, especially those in the distal limbs, is limited to flexion and extension in the sagittal plane. Therefore, two-dimensional analysis is sufficient for most purposes. This chapter presents in detail the procedure for inverse dynamic analysis for sagittal plane movement, with specific reference to development of protocols for equine applications. Some applications require a full three-dimensional analysis. A short introduction of this more complex analysis therefore concludes this chapter.

INVERSE DYNAMIC ANALYSIS

Linked segment model

For the inverse dynamic calculations a simplified model of the horse is used. This model is called a linked-segment model since it consists of rigid segments, which are linked to each other. The segments can rotate in the joints that link the segments. In a two-dimensional model, these joints are assumed to be ideal hinge joints: there is no friction, there is no translation possible and the only movement is a pure rotation around a fixed point, the center of rotation. Since the segment is assumed to be rigid, its length, or the distance between the joints, is constant. Furthermore the inertial properties, mass (*m*), location of the center of mass and moment of inertia (*I*), of the segments are constant (Winter, 1990). In mechanical terms the moment of inertia is the rotational equivalent to the mass. While the mass determines the resistance to linear accelerations, the moment of inertia determines the resistance to angular accelerations. The force needed for a certain (linear) acceleration equals the mass times the acceleration ($F = m \cdot a$). In a similar way the moment needed for a certain angular acceleration

equals the moment of inertia times the angular acceleration ($M = I \cdot \alpha$). This moment of inertia is determined by the spatial distribution of the mass within the segment. The mass of the segment equals the total mass between the joints; it represents not only the bone but also the soft tissue surrounding it. The mass of all segments together is therefore equal to the body mass of the horse. Figure 13.2 gives a graphical representation of a linked-segment model.

The action of the muscles is represented by the moment they generate around the joint. This moment generating function is explained in Figure 13.3. If a muscle is activated it generates a tensile force at the bones. Due to this force the bones are compressed at the joint. This causes a bone-to-bone force from both bones onto each other. So, because of the muscular activity there are two forces acting on each bone: one from the muscle at the attachment site and one from the other bone at the joint. Since these two forces are equal in magnitude and opposite in direction they form a couple. The moment associated with this couple equals the force times the distance between the two forces. Since the two forces are equal in magnitude and opposite in direction they cancel each other out and the muscle action can be represented by the moment (Elftman,

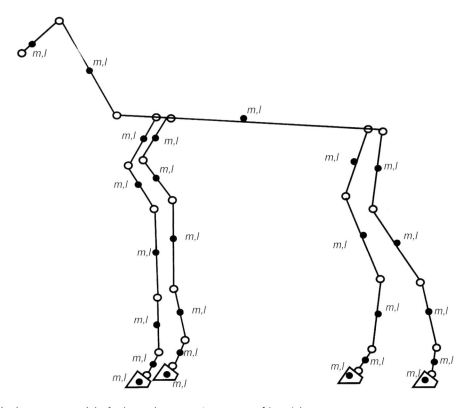

Fig. 13.2 Linked-segment model of a horse (*m*: mass; *I*: moment of inertia).

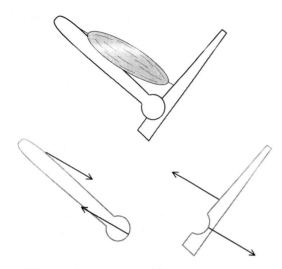

Fig. 13.3 Muscle activity causes a bone-to-bone force at the joint. The muscle action can thus be represented by a moment.

1939). In a similar way the forces exerted by ligaments can also be represented by moments. It should be noted that the bone-to-bone force of Figure 13.3 does not represent the complete joint contact force, it is only the part of this force that is caused by the activity of the muscle.

Inverse dynamic calculations

In inverse dynamic calculations the movement of the linked segment model is used to calculate the underlying forces (Elftman, 1939; Winter, 1990). The calculations are based on the principles of Newton's laws of motion. In order to apply these principles the linked segment model is split into separate segments. The interaction between the segments is summarized in a net joint force and a net joint moment. The net joint force is the resultant of all forces between the two segments. The net joint moment is the sum of the moments of all muscles and ligaments crossing the joint. All moments and forces acting on each segment are depicted in a free body diagram. The moments are the net joint moments at both joints. The forces are the gravitational force, the net joint forces at both joints and, sometimes, an external force. The most important external force is the ground reaction force (GRF) acting on the hoof segment during stance. Other external forces can be the weight of a rider or the force needed to pull a load. All those external forces are measured. Furthermore, the linear and angular accelerations are calculated from the (measured) movements of the segments. The inverse dynamic calculations can then start by analyzing either the most proximal or the most distal segment.

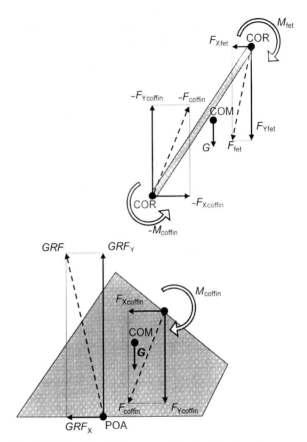

Fig. 13.4 Free body diagrams of the hoof and pastern segments (POA: point of application of the *GRF*; COM: segmental center of mass; COR: joint center of rotation).

The free body diagram of the most distal segment, the hoof segment, is drawn in Figure 13.4. The amplitude and direction of the coffin joint moment and force are not yet known. They are therefore drawn in an arbitrary direction. After the calculations the real direction and magnitude will be known. According to Newton's Second Law the sum of all forces on the segment must equal its mass times acceleration:

$$\sum F_{\mathrm{X}} = m_{\mathrm{hoof}} \cdot a_{\mathrm{Xhoof}} \qquad (1)$$

where the subscript $_{\mathrm{X}}$ denotes the horizontal components of the force (see Fig. 13.4), m_{hoof} is the mass of the hoof segment and a_{Xhoof} is the horizontal acceleration of the center of mass of the hoof. Using this equation the horizontal components of the net joint force can be calculated from measurements, as is illustrated in Example I. Complete formulas can be found in the Appendix. A similar equation can be written for the vertical direction to calculate the vertical component of the net joint force at the coffin joint:

Example 1: *Calculation of the net coffin joint moment and force*

A horse lands on a force plate after clearing a fence. At midstance, the ground reaction force vector (GRF) is directed forward and up, as depicted in the free body diagram (Fig. E1). The inertial properties and accelerations are listed in Table E1. From the given data the net coffin joint force can be calculated:

$$\sum F_X = m_{hoof} \cdot a_{Xhoof}$$
$$F_{Xcoffin} = m_{hoof} \cdot a_{Xhoof} - GRF_X$$
$$= 1.08 \cdot (-0.2) + 1750$$
$$= 1750 \text{ N}$$

$$\sum F_Y = m_{hoof} \cdot a_{Yhoof}$$
$$F_{Ycoffin} = m_{hoof} \cdot a_{Yhoof} - GRF_Y - m_{hoof} \cdot g$$
$$= 1.08 \cdot 0.6 - 8000 + 1.08 \cdot 9.81$$
$$= -7989 \text{ N}$$

Note that the horizontal GRF and the gravitational force are negative, $-GRF_X$ therefore equals $+1750$. Furthermore $F_{Xcoffin}$ turns out to be positive and points right. $F_{Ycoffin}$ is negative, and points downward. Now the net joint force is known the net joint moment can be calculated from equation 3:

$$\sum M = I_{hoof} \cdot \alpha_{hoof}$$
$$M_{coff} = I_{hoof} \cdot \alpha_{hoof} - GRF_X \cdot (y_{hoof} - y_{GRF}) - GRF_Y \cdot$$
$$(x_{GRF} - x_{hoof}) - F_{Xcoff} \cdot (y_{hoof} - y_{coff}) - F_{Ycoff} \cdot$$
$$(x_{coff} - x_{hoof})$$
$$= 0.0015 \cdot 14 + 1750 \cdot 0.045 - 8000 \cdot (-0.008)$$
$$- 1750 \cdot (-0.03) + 7989 \cdot 0.002$$
$$= 211 \text{ Nm}$$

Note that the distances are in meters, whereas the distances in the Fig. EI are in cm. The coffin joint moment is positive, acting counterclockwise on the hoof: a flexing moment generated by the flexor muscles.

Table E1 Inertial properties and accelerations.

	Hoof
m (kg)	1.08
I (kg m^2)	0.0015
a_X (m/s^2)	−0.2
a_Y (m/s^2)	0.6
α (rad/s^2)	14

Note that the horizontal GRF and the gravitational force are negative, $-GRF_X$ therefore equals $+1750$. Furthermore $F_{Xcoffin}$ turns out to be positive and points right. $F_{Ycoffin}$ is negative, and points downward. Now the net

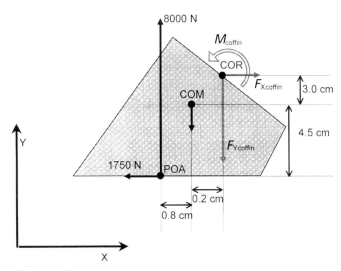

Fig. E I Free body diagram of the hoof segment.

$$\sum F_Y = m_{hoof} \cdot a_{Yhoof} \qquad (2)$$

where the subscript $_Y$ denotes the vertical components of the force and acceleration. Of course, the gravitational force (G) should now be taken into account.

All forces, except the gravitational force, generate a moment relative to the center of mass. The magnitude of the moment is determined by the amplitude of the force and its perpendicular distance from the center of mass. Moments that tend to rotate the segment counterclockwise are defined

Example II: *Calculation of the net fetlock joint moment and force*

The free body diagram of the hoof from Example I is redrawn with all forces and moments in the correct direction. Furthermore, the free body diagram of the pastern segments in added (Fig. EII). The force and moment from the hoof on the pastern are known since they are the opposite of F_{coffin} and M_{coffin}. They are drawn in their actual direction. The fetlock joint force can be calculated:

$$\sum F_X = m_{past} \cdot a_{Xpast}$$
$$F_{Xfet} - F_{Xcoffin} = m_{past} \cdot a_{Xpast}$$
$$F_{Xfet} - 1750 = 0.73 \cdot (-6.0)$$
$$F_{Xfet} = 1746 \text{ N}$$

$$\sum F_Y = m_{past} \cdot a_{Ypast}$$
$$F_{Yfet} - F_{Ycoffin} + G_{past} = m_{past} \cdot a_{Ypast}$$
$$F_{Yfet} + 7989 - 0.73 \cdot 9.81 = 0.73 \cdot 13.4$$
$$F_{Yfet} = -7972 \text{ N}$$

Finally, the net fetlock joint moment can be calculated:

$$\sum M = I_{past} \cdot \alpha_{past}$$
$$M_{fet} - M_{coff} + F_{Xfet} \cdot (y_{past} - y_{fet}) + F_{Yfet} \cdot (x_{fet} - x_{past})$$
$$- F_{Xcoff} \cdot (y_{past} - y_{coff}) - F_{Ycoff} \cdot (x_{coff} - x_{past}) = I_{past} \cdot \alpha_{past}$$
$$M_{fet} - 211 + 1746 \cdot (-0.05) - 7972 \cdot 0.04 - 1750 \cdot 0.06$$
$$+ 7989 \cdot (-0.07) = 0.0012 \cdot 170$$
$$M_{fet} = 1282 \text{ Nm}$$

The fetlock joint moment is positive, this flexor moment is generated by the flexor muscles of the fetlock joint.

Table E II Inertial properties and accelerations.

	Pastern
m (kg)	0.73
I (kg m^2)	0.0012
a_X (m/s^2)	−6.0
a_Y (m/s^2)	13.4
α (rad/s^2)	170

positive whereas moments that tend to rotate clockwise are defined negative. For the hoof of Figure 13.4 this means that positive moments tend to flex the coffin joint. Note that this association between flexion or extension and the sign of the moment is dependent on the way the free body diagram is drawn since it is reversed for mirrored images. The sum of the net coffin joint moment and the moments of all forces must equal the moment of inertia times the angular acceleration of the hoof segment (α_{hoof}):

$$\sum M = I_{hoof} \cdot \alpha_{hoof} \qquad (3)$$

From this equation the net joint moment can be calculated. Now all forces and moments acting on the hoof segment are known and the analysis of this segment is complete. The calculations can be continued by analyzing the next segment, the pastern segment. The movement of the pastern joint is often neglected and the remaining part of the digit is represented by one segment.

The free body diagram of the pastern segment (Fig. 13.4, upper part) contains the moment and force acting from the hoof on the pastern. According to Newton's Third Law (action equals minus reaction) the force from the hoof on the pastern is the exact opposite of the force from the pastern on the hoof. Similarly, the moment from the hoof on the pastern is the opposite of the coffin joint moment. The net joint force at the fetlock joint can now be calculated in a similar way as was previously done for

the coffin joint. The horizontal acceleration is used to calculate the horizontal component of the net joint force and the vertical acceleration is used to calculate the vertical component (see Example II):

$$\sum F_X = m_{past} \cdot a_{Xpast} \qquad (4)$$

$$\sum F_Y = m_{past} \cdot a_{Ypast} \qquad (5)$$

Finally, the angular acceleration is used to calculate the net joint moment:

$$\sum M = I_{past} \cdot \alpha_{past} \qquad (6)$$

After the pastern segment, the metacarpal segment can be analyzed in the same manner, again using the principle of action and reaction. This can be continued, segment after segment, until the most proximal segment, most often the head segment. The only forces on this segment are the gravitational force and the net joint force at the distal side. The only moment is the distal net joint moment. In theory these forces and this moment should balance the linear and angular accelerations of the final segment. However, most often a residual force and moment are found. This is caused by measurement errors and non-rigidity of the segments. Although errors are present in all calculated joint forces and moments, they are largest for the final joint since they accumulate during the calculations. In order to prevent this accumulation of errors, and to remove the residual moment

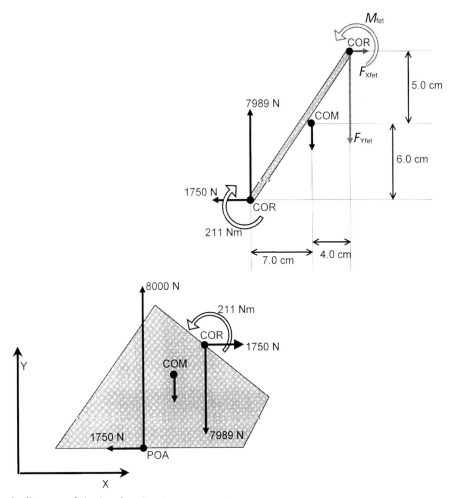

Fig. EII Free body diagram of the hoof and pastern segment.

and force at the final segment, an alternative method has been developed (Kuo, 1998). This method solves the equations for all segments simultaneously. Because there are more equations than there are unknown forces and moments, they cannot be solved exactly. However an approximate solution can be calculated using a least squares method. In this way the errors are distributed evenly over all joints. The errors of the final joint are therefore smaller than in the segment-after-segment approach, however, the errors of the distal joints will be larger. Furthermore, the simultaneous least squares method is only useful if the whole horse is analyzed. If only part of the horse is analyzed, e.g. only one limb, both methods will give the same result.

Measurement of input variables

In order to perform inverse dynamic calculations several input variables are needed. These variables can be sub-

divided into three categories: inertial properties, movement data and external force data. The inertial properties are mass, moment of inertia and location of the center of mass for all segments. These properties have been measured in cadaver segments and are represented as regression equations (van den Bogert *et al.*, 1989; Buchner *et al.*, 1997). This allows scaling to horses of different size by using individual body mass and/or segment lengths. The position of the center of mass is represented in a segment-based coordinate system. The origin of this coordinate system is located at the proximal joint center of rotation, the *x*-axis runs through the distal joint center of rotation and the *y*-axis is perpendicular to the *x*-axis and points cranially or dorsally (Fig. 13.5).

The inertial data of ponies and Dutch Warmblood horses are presented in Tables 13.1 and 13.2. Using the regression equations it is possible to interpolate the data to live horses. However, some care should be taken with these interpolations. They only hold for horses with a similar body

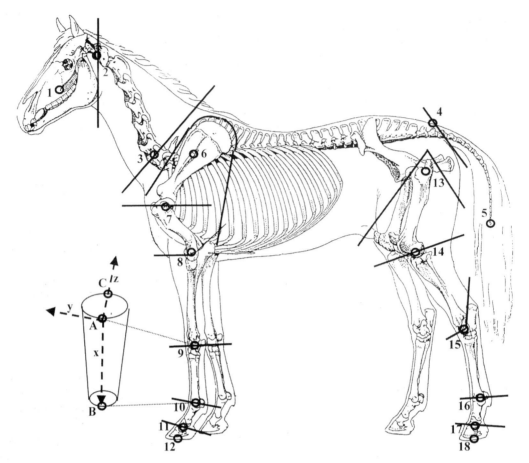

Fig. 13.5 Definition of the segments and their coordinate systems. Thick lines represent the segment boundaries. The schematic enlargement shows the coordinate system. The z-axis is used only in three-dimensional analyses. (Reprinted from Buchner, H.H.F. Savelberg, H.H.C.M. Schamhardt, H.C. and Barneveld, A. (1997) Inertial properties of Dutch Warmblood horses. *J. Biomech.* **30**: 653–658, with permission from Elsevier Science.)

composition and body weight as the cadaver specimens. Extrapolation of Tables 13.1 and 13.2 outside the measured range (165–240 kg for the ponies and 470–620 kg for the warmblood horses), or for horses with another conformation, may give erroneous results.

The movement data consist of the position of the joints and the angular and linear acceleration of all segments. The measurement of position data is discussed in chapter 3. However, for inverse dynamic calculations not only the joint angles but also the position of the joints should be known. The easiest way to measure these positions is by putting the markers on the joint centers of rotation (Leach & Dyson, 1988). Joint moments are sensitive to joint center location, so it is important to know the inaccuracies introduced by this procedure. Alternatively, two markers are applied to each segment and the position of the joint center of rotation relative to these markers is determined in a

separate measurement with additional markers on the joints. For some joints this procedure can limit the skin movement artifacts because the markers can be applied on places with minimal skin movement (van Weeren *et al.*, 1992a). Further discussion of the skin movement problem in equine movement analysis may be found in chapter 3 of this volume. After the movements are measured they must be differentiated twice to obtain the accelerations. This can be done with a spline function, as described in chapter 3, or with a finite difference method (see Appendix). When using the finite difference method excessive noise must first be removed from the data (see chapter 3, Fig 3.6). This can be done by filtering or by averaging several trials.

The external force data consist of the amplitude, direction and point of application of the external forces, most often the GRF. The GRF can be measured with a force plate, force shoe or instrumented treadmill as described in chapter 3. For

Table 13.1 Inertial properties of ponies.

Segment	Mass (kg)	x-position (m)	y-position (m)	Moment of inertia (kg m²)
Trunk[*]	$0.613M - 19.5$	0.289	−0.140	$0.0825mL^2 + 0.186$
Head	8.8	$0.403L$	0.015	0.125
Neck	$0.0404M + 4.94$	$0.429L$	−0.029	$0.0736mL^2 + 0.0802$
Scapula	4.3	−0.135	$0.00032L$	0.054
Brachium	$0.0177M+0.0337$	0.089	−0.016	$0.341mL^2 - 0.0223$
Antebrachium	2.11	0.1092	−0.0079	$0.185mL^2 - 0.0159$
Metacarpus	0.588	$0.469L$	−0.002	0.0034
Fore pastern	$3.17L - 0.111$	0.050	−0.010	$0.00783mL^2 - 0.000612$
Fore hoof	$0.00350M - 0.162$	0.032	−0.013	$0.169mL^2 - 0.000400$
Thigh	$0.0357M + 4.763$	0.138	−0.034	0.16
Crus	$-10.8L + 5.9$	$0.482L$	−0.010	0.0183
Metatarsus	0.98	$0.355L$	−0.0161	$0.378mL^2 - 0.0146$
Hind pastern	0.22	$0.478L$	−0.0067	0.00020
Hind hoof	$0.00221M - 0.110$	0.048	−0.0146	$-0.0142L + 0.00174$

For the boundaries between the segments see Fig. 13.5. Position of the center of mass (x, y) is expressed in a segment-based coordinate system (see text). M: body mass (in kg); m: segmental mass (in kg); L: segmental length (in m); *: including tail. (Adapted from van den Bogert *et al.*, 1989).

Table 13.2 Inertial properties of Dutch Warmblood horses.

Segment	Mass (kg)	x-position (m)	y-position (m)	Moment of inertia (kg m²)
Trunk[*]	$0.912M - 139$	0.732	$-0.861L + 1.181$	$0.0774mL^2 - 0.399$
Head	23.1	$0.825L - 0.030$	−0.027	0.71
Neck	26.8	0.248	0.059	0.94
Scapula	$41.83L + 0.047$	$0.714L - 0.121$	−0.033	$0.191L - 0.10783$
Brachium	$0.248M - 4.751$	$0.462L + 0.012$	−0.013	$0.103L + 0.0552$
Antebrachium	$17.76L - 1.017$	$0.423L - 0.032$	−0.0091	$0.05128mL^2 + 0.063668$
Metacarpus	1.59	$0.499L - 0.018$	−0.0029	$0.0913mL^2 + 0.00265$
Fore pastern	$4.283L + 0.152$	$0.510L - 0.007$	−0.015	$0.157mL^2 - 0.00088$
Fore hoof	$15.95L - 0.510$	$0.383L - 0.010$	$-0.326L + 0.012$	$0.143mL^2 - 0.00005$
Thigh	18.6	$0.685L - 0.033$	−0.043	0.34
Crus	$18.53L + 0.242$	0.164	−0.036	$0.078mL^2 + 0.02260$
Metatarsus	$5.753L + 0.812$	$0.593L - 0.095$	−0.024	$0.0246mL^2 + 0.00285$
Hind pastern	0.89	0.061	−0.018	0.00194
Hind hoof	$15.00L - 0.538$	$0.456L - 0.0143$	−0.022	$0.1149mL^2 + 0.00005$

For the boundaries between the segments see Fig. 13.5. Position of the center of mass (x, y) is expressed in a segment-based coordinate system (see text). M: body mass (in kg); m: segmental mass (in kg); L: segmental length (in m); * excluding tail, mass of the tail: $10.646L - 3.824$. (Adapted from Buchner *et al.*, 1997).

inverse dynamic calculations not only the magnitude and direction of the GRF must be measured but also the point of application. Force plates, although very accurate with respect to the force amplitude, often have systematic errors in the point of application (Bobbert & Schamhardt, 1990). These errors can be corrected with a calibration procedure in which static loads are applied at known positions. Instrumented treadmills or force shoes give the opportunity to measure consecutive strides. However, the accuracy of these systems should be evaluated carefully.

The movement and GRF data must be aligned and synchronized. Some motion analysis systems can capture the force data directly and do not need additional synchronization. For other systems synchronization pulses from the video camera can be sampled simultaneously with the force data to synchronize the force data. Alternatively, a counter operated by the force sampling equipment and visible in the camera image can be used to synchronize the motion data. The coordinate systems of the force plate and motion analysis systems can be aligned by putting markers on the edges of the force plate and measuring them with the motion analysis system. This can be performed in a separate session to prevent interference with the normal data collection.

Net joint moment and muscle force

The net joint moment is generated by the muscles. The polarity of the moment indicates whether flexors or extensors are active, whereas the amplitude is a measure of the amount of activity. Based on the net joint moments the activity of muscle groups (flexors and extensors of the different joints) can be analyzed. However, sometimes it is desirable to estimate forces of individual muscles. Depending on the number of muscles crossing the joint, the muscle forces can either be calculated or estimated from the net joint moment (Fig. 13.6).

In some joints there is only one muscle that can flex the joint. The deep digital flexor muscle (DDF), for instance, is the only muscle that can flex the coffin joint. (The navicular ligaments can generate a flexor moment but only if the joint is (hyper) extended.) In a flexed joint the moment generated by DDF will equal the net coffin joint moment:

$$M_{coffin} = F_{DDF} \cdot d_{DDF} \qquad (7)$$

where d_{DDF} is the moment arm of the deep digital flexor – the perpendicular distance between the joint center of rotation and the line of action of the muscle (Fig. 13.6A, Example III). This

moment arm can be measured from radiographs (Jansen *et al.*, 1993) or from longitudinal sections of an *in vitro* limb. For some muscles the moment arm depends on the joint angle. A model containing the origin, insertion and possible curvatures of the muscle can then be used to calculate the moment arm from the joint angles (van den Bogert & Sauren, 1989). When calculating F_{DDF} from M_{coffin} using equation 7 it is assumed that there is no other active muscle or force generating ligament at the coffin joint. The antagonistic muscles – the digital extensors – are assumed to be inactive. If these muscles, contrary to the assumption, are active they will generate an extensor moment, which should be compensated by the DDF. The actual F_{DDF} will then be higher than the calculated force. The calculated force is therefore the lower limit of the actual muscle force. This type of analysis has shown that desmotomy of the distal accessory ligament causes a decrease in the DDF force that does not disappear within 6 months (Buchner *et al.*, 1996; Becker *et al.*, 1998).

For joints with only one muscle at each side, the calculation of muscle force is simple. However, most joints, e.g. the hip joint of Figure 13.6B, are crossed by more than one muscle. In order to calculate muscle forces from the net moments at these joints, assumptions must be made about the distribution of the moment among the available muscles. To estimate muscle forces the moments are most often distributed in such a way that a certain criterion or cost function is minimized. Computer algorithms are available to solve the distribution problem by minimizing a given cost function. This procedure is called optimization. Some commonly used cost functions are the sum of all muscle forces, the sum of the squared or cubed muscle forces and the highest muscle force. In order to correct for size differences between the muscles the force is sometimes replaced by stress: muscle force divided by physiological cross-sectional area. Other cost functions might include measures for muscle fatigue, energy costs or joint contact forces (Crowninshield & Brand, 1981; Dul *et al.*, 1984; Glitsch & Baumann, 1997).

A major problem in optimization is that it is difficult to validate the cost function. The real muscle forces can only be

---

Example III: *Calculation of the deep digital flexor force*

The net coffin joint moment of Example I is positive. It is a flexor moment that is generated by the flexor muscle of the coffin joint: the deep digital flexor (DDF). The moment arm of the DDF is approximately 3.3 cm (or 0.033 m). The force of the DDF can therefore be calculated as:

$$M_{coffin} = F_{DDF} \cdot d_{DDF}$$
$$211 = F_{DDF} \cdot 0.033$$
$$F_{DDF} = 6394 \text{ N}$$

For a horse with a body mass of 570 kg this tendon force exceeds the body weight (570 · 9.81 = 5592 N) of the horse.

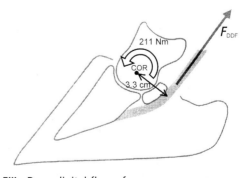

Fig. EIII Deep digital flexor force.

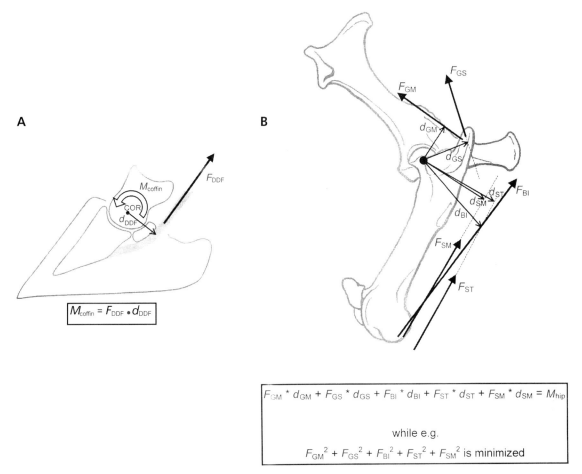

$$M_{coffin} = F_{DDF} \cdot d_{DDF}$$

$$F_{GM} * d_{GM} + F_{GS} * d_{GS} + F_{BI} * d_{BI} + F_{ST} * d_{ST} + F_{SM} * d_{SM} = M_{hip}$$

while e.g.

$$F_{GM}{}^2 + F_{GS}{}^2 + F_{BI}{}^2 + F_{ST}{}^2 + F_{SM}{}^2 \text{ is minimized}$$

Fig. 13.6 Different ways to estimate muscle forces (*F*) from net joint moments (*M*) and muscular moment arms (*d*). **A** With only one muscle the force can be calculated from the moment (COR: coffin joint center of rotation; DDF: deep digital flexor). **B** With several muscles, optimizations are needed to distribute the moment (GM: gluteus medius; GS: gluteus superficialis; BI: biceps femoris; ST: semitendinosus; SM: semimembranosis).

found when the cost function represents the principles by which the nervous system solves the distribution problem. These principles, however, are not known. Another problem is that realistic boundary conditions must be included in the optimizations. For each muscle, the force it can generate is limited to a certain maximum. This maximum is influenced by the momentary length and the contraction velocity of the muscle fibers. Predicted forces should of course not exceed this maximum force. Furthermore, muscle force can only increase and decrease gradually, muscles cannot be either 'on' or 'off' momentarily. Dynamic models of muscle in which these properties are incorporated can be used in optimization based on inverse dynamics (Thunnissen, 1993).

These more sophisticated *dynamic optimization* models, as opposed to *static optimizations* that do not consider muscle properties (both based on inverse dynamic analysis of

movement!), have not been used other than in research, presumably because more complicated calculations are required. However, they will result in more realistic estimates of muscle force. In rare cases, results from optimizations have been compared to direct measurements using invasive methods. In cats, the load sharing among synergistic muscle was not correctly predicted by *static* optimization (Herzog & Leonard, 1991) when compared to tendon force transducer data.

Most muscles can be represented by moment generators. This is possible because the bones are connected by joints that can be modeled as hinge or ball joints and can generate the bone-to-bone force at a known joint center. However in the shoulder synsarcosis there is no joint (Dyce *et al.*, 1987). Therefore the muscles of the shoulder synsarcosis are not moment generators. Furthermore, the movement of the scapula

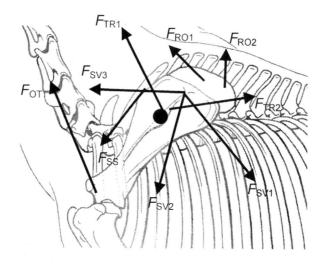

$$\Sigma F_{X,TRi} + \Sigma F_{X,ROi} + \Sigma F_{X,SVi} + F_{X,OT} + F_{X,SS} = F_{Xscapula}$$

$$\Sigma F_{Y,TRi} + \Sigma F_{Y,ROi} + \Sigma F_{Y,SVi} + F_{Y,OT} + F_{Y,SS} = F_{Yscapula}$$

and

$$\Sigma(F_{TRi} * d_{TRi}) + \Sigma(F_{ROi} * d_{ROi}) + \Sigma(F_{SVi} * d_{SVi}) + F_{OT} * d_{OT} + F_{SS} * d_{SS} = M_{scapula}$$

while e.g.

$$\Sigma(F_{TRi}^2) + \Sigma(F_{ROi}^2) + \Sigma(F_{SVi}^2) + F_{OT}^2 + F_{SS}^2 \text{ is minimized}$$

Fig 13.6 (Contd) C The muscles of the shoulder synsarcosis generate both the net moment *and the net forces* ($F_{Xscapula}$, $F_{Yscapula}$) (TR: trapezius; RO: rhomboideus; SV: serratus ventralis; OT: omotransversarius; SS: subscapularis. Muscles with large origins are represented by several (numbered) force vectors; in the formulas the influence of these vectors are summed. $_X$ and $_Y$ subscripts denote the horizontal and vertical components of the forces).

relative to the trunk is not limited to rotation around a fixed point. Due to the absence of a joint, substantial translations are also possible. The linked-segment model will become more realistic if the hinge joint between scapula and trunk is replaced by a free movement and the muscles are represented by force generators. The net moment and net force can still be calculated relative to a fixed point on the scapula – this can be any point, for instance the center of mass. However, the point of application of the net force on the trunk is not fixed any more. The forces of the muscles can still be calculated exactly if there are three active muscles in the model (since there are three equations of motion for a body segment), or using optimization methods if there are more than three. The only difference in the equations is that the muscles should not only generate the net moment between scapula and trunk but also the net force. Therefore the position of the muscle should not be represented by the moment arm but by their actual line of action between trunk and scapula (Fig. 13.6C).

Net joint force and joint contact force

The net joint force, calculated from the equations of motion, represents the sum of all forces between the two segments. It should not be confused with the joint contact force, which can be measured between the bones in the joint. The joint contact force is only one of the forces between the segments; other forces are the muscle and ligament forces. The real contact force therefore equals the difference between net joint force and the summed muscle (and ligament) forces (see Example IV):

$$F_{contact} = F_{net} - \sum F_{muscle} \qquad (8)$$

When calculating the joint contact force, the forces of all active muscles should be taken into account. In calculating muscle forces from the net joint moment it is often assumed that there are no antagonistic co-contractions. This is implied by most of the static optimization methods. These co-contractions will cancel each other out with respect to the joint moment and are therefore 'invisible' to a mechanical analysis. However both muscles add a bone-to-bone force and increase the joint contact force. Ignoring antagonistic co-contractions therefore results in an underestimation of the joint contact force. Similarly, the joint contact force will be influenced by the way the net joint moment is distributed over muscles with different moment arms. Muscles with a larger moment arm need a smaller force to generate a similar moment than muscles with a smaller moment arm. The joint contact force will therefore be smaller if the contribution of muscles with a larger moment arm is higher. In humans, the contact force in the hip joint was estimated by static optimization of muscle forces and compared to measurements from an instrumented prosthesis (Brand *et al.*, 1994). It was found that the model calculations overestimated the joint contact force, mainly due to incorrect moment arms in the model.

Continued calculations: power

The muscles are the motors of the body. The moments and forces generated by the muscles have been analyzed in the previous paragraphs. However, a motor does not only generate moments or forces; it also produces or converts mechanical energy. The muscles obtain their energy from the oxidation of foods and convert it to mechanical energy. The energy is distributed over the segments and is used internally, to accelerate or elevate the segments, or externally, e.g. to

overcome air resistance or to pull a load. Energy production, distribution and use can be analyzed with calculations based on inverse dynamic results. If a force acts on a moving object, energy is produced or absorbed. The amount of energy equals the force times displacement of the point of application in the direction of the force. Power is the time derivative; it equals energy production divided by time, which is equal to force times velocity of the point of application:

$$P = F_X \cdot v_X + F_Y \cdot v_Y \qquad (9)$$

For rotational movements the power equals moment times angular velocity ($P = M \cdot \omega$). Note that power will be calculated in Watts if the moment is expressed in Newton-meters and the angular velocity in radians per second. In power analyses of linked-segment models, the powers associated with all forces and moments on the segments are calculated. The sum of these powers equals the rate of change of the kinetic and potential energy of the entire system. This power balance follows from Newton's laws of motion and may be used to determine the contributions of each joint to the movement of the entire system (van Ingen Schenau & Cavanagh, 1990).

For most forces and moments the power calculation is straightforward. However, the GRF needs special attention. The point of application of the GRF shifts forward during stance. It is tempting to multiply the velocity of this shift with the GRF to obtain the power. However this is not the power flow associated with the GRF (van Ingen Schenau & Cavanagh, 1990). On a hard, non-deformable surface the GRF does not perform work. The ground reaction force is a distributed force, which is summarized to one resultant force with a certain point of application. In Figure 13.7 the GRF is represented as five smaller forces acting on different positions of the hoof surface. During stance the amplitude of these five partial forces changes, whereas their position stays constant. This causes the point of application of the resultant GRF to shift forward. However, none of the partial forces generates power since their velocity is zero. The resultant force, which is simply the summation of all partial forces, does not generate power. In reality there are, of course, more

---

Example IV: *Calculation of the joint contact force*

The net coffin joint force of Example I was 1750 N in the horizontal and −7989 N in the vertical direction. It is important to remember that these forces were calculated from the equations of motion for the hoof segment, so it is a force acting on the hoof segment, a vector pointing down and right. From this the force of the DDF tendon must be subtracted, a vector pointing up and right. The DDF was assumed to be the only active muscle. The force in this muscle, as calculated in Example III, was 6394 N. Let us assume that the DDF makes an angle of 45° with the horizontal. The joint contact force vector, acting on the coffin bone, is then:

$$F_{Xcontact} - F_{XDDF} = 1750 - 6394 \cdot \cos(45°) = -2771 N$$
$$F_{Ycontact} = F_{Ynet} - F_{YDDF} = -7989 - 6394 \cdot \sin(45°)$$
$$= -12510 N$$

This contact force is substantially larger than the GRF. Furthermore, it is over twice the body weight of the horse. An equal and opposite force acts on the pastern bone.

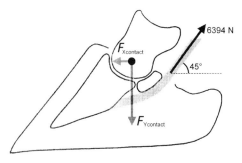

Fig. EIV Joint contact force.

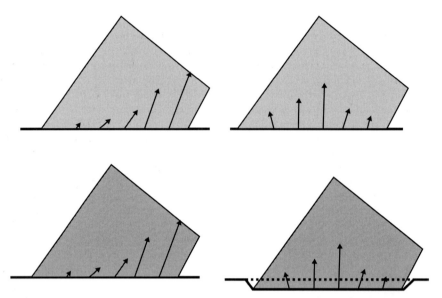

Fig. 13.7 Shifts and movements of the point of application of the ground reaction force. (See text for details.)

than five partial forces, but the same reasoning applies. On a deformable surface, like sand, the situation is different. When the hoof penetrates the surface the point of application not only shifts due to amplitude changes but also moves due to hoof movements. The position of the five partial forces changes and they generate power (see Fig. 13.7). Therefore, on deformable surfaces, power can be associated with the GRF. This power is related to the movement of the surface; it equals the velocity of the hoof surface times the amplitude of the GRF. This power is used to deform the surface. This example illustrates that valid power results are only obtained if a force is multiplied by the velocity of a point on a physical body to which the force is applied. The velocity of a point that is not rigidly attached to a mass is not suitable.

When analyzing the powers of the linked-segment model two different approaches are used: a segment oriented approach (Elftman, 1939; Winter & Robertson, 1978; Robertson & Winter, 1980) and a joint-oriented approach (van Ingen Schenau & Cavanagh, 1990). The segment-oriented approach is used to analyze *internal* use and the *distribution* of energy, or power flow, whereas the joint-oriented approach is used to analyze power *production* and *external* use. In the segment-oriented approach two power flows are distinguished at both the proximal and distal end of the segment: the power flow associated with the net joint force and the power flow associated with the net joint moment. The power flow associated with the net joint force is a passive power flow from the adjacent segment, or, if negative, a passive power flow into the adjacent segment. At the joint, the passive power flow into the proximal segment equals the passive power flow out of the distal segment

(or reversed). This is caused by the fact that the net joint forces on the distal and proximal segments are each other's opposites while the velocities at the point of application, the center of rotation, are equal. The power flow associated with the net joint moment is an active power flow generated by the muscles. At the joint, the angular velocities of the two segments are normally different and therefore the power flow associated with the net joint moment is different for the two segments. This difference is generated (or absorbed) by the muscles.

All four power flows, passive and active proximal and distal flow, can either be positive or negative. Most often some of them are positive whereas others are negative and power flows from one segment to the other. However the sum of the four flows is not always zero. If the sum is positive the energy of the segment increases. This energy is converted into potential or kinetic energy as the height or the velocity of the segment increases. Similarly, a negative power flow is converted from potential and/or kinetic energy when the height and/or velocity decreases.

Using this kind of analysis the power flow within the limb can be analyzed. This has been done for the distal front limb during walk (Colborne *et al.*, 1997). During the major part of the stance phase the power flow of the metacarpal and pastern segments was distal to proximal. This probably reflects the propulsion of the proximal part of the body. During final stance the power flowed in at both ends of the segments and was probably used to accelerate and elevate the segments for the swing phase. Care must be taken with this kind of analysis because results are dependent on the velocity of the coordinate system in which the movements are represented. This will influence the results when measuring on a treadmill. We recommend that the analysis be performed only in a coordinate system attached to the ground, which implies a moving coordinate system for treadmill analysis.

In the joint-oriented approach of power analyses the power flows of all segments are summed (van Ingen Schenau & Cavanagh, 1990). The power associated with the net joint force is opposite for two adjacent segments. When adding the powers of the different segments the powers associated with the net joint forces cancel each other out. The only power, therefore, is the power associated with the net joint moment. At each joint the powers for the two segments are summed to one joint power. This power equals the net joint moment multiplied by the difference in angular velocity between the segments:

$$P_{\text{joint}} = M_{\text{joint}} \cdot \left(\omega_{\text{prox}} - \omega_{\text{dist}} \right) \qquad (10)$$

This power is generated by the muscles crossing the joint and is therefore a measure of the activity of the muscles. The joint powers of all joints can be summed to obtain the total power production. This power is used for external power production (e.g. pulling a load, air resistance) and kinetic and potential energy changes of the segments. Power production at the joints can therefore be compared with external power losses due to air resistance, friction, etc. In human research this approach has been applied successfully in movements where most of the power is used externally and where internal loss of power is minimal. Examples can be found for bicycling, swimming and speed skating (van Ingen Schenau & Cavanagh, 1990). In walking and running the external power production is very small; most power is used to accelerate and decelerate the limbs and to provide a shock-absorbing support against gravity. Apart from the high-speed gallop, where air resistance might become substantial, the same holds for the gaits of a horse. Although it is not useful to apply this approach to the equine walk and trot, it can be used when the external power output is substantial, e.g. in pulling a load, during accelerating and in jumping.

Apart from the external power production the joint-oriented analyses might give insight into muscle function during movement (de Koning et al., 1991; Devita & Skelly, 1992). Positive joint power indicates power production that might originate from concentric activity of the muscles crossing the joint. Large positive power production peaks indicate important propulsive muscles whereas timing of the different peaks indicates the coordination of the movement. Furthermore, negative joint power indicates power absorption which might be related to eccentric muscle contraction. These contractions are assumed to be a major cause of muscle soreness and a risk for muscle injuries (Jones & Round, 1990). Power analyses can therefore be used to find muscles that are at high risk for injuries. This type of analysis has been used for the equine forelimb during walk (Colborne et al., 1998).

Moment peaks of the carpal and fetlock joints were of similar magnitude whereas the coffin joint moment was much smaller. The carpal joint power was almost zero due to the small movements of this joint. The fetlock joint had alternating periods of power absorption and production whereas the coffin joint predominantly absorbed power.

The two approaches, segment-oriented and joint-oriented power analyses, are closely related. They emphasize different aspects of the power balance. The joint-oriented approach emphasizes the external power production and the places where this power is produced whereas the segment-oriented approach emphasizes the power flow within the body and the internal use (see Example V). In both approaches power production and absorption have simply been related to concentric and eccentric contraction of muscles at the joint. However the biological reality is a bit more complex for two reasons: elastic structures can temporarily store energy and most muscles cross more than one joint (van Ingen Schenau & Cavanagh, 1990).

Elastic structures, like tendons and ligaments, store energy when elongated. This energy is released when they return to their normal length. The long and stiff tendons in the distal limbs of horses are able to store substantial amounts of elastic energy (Alexander & Bennet-Clark, 1977). Furthermore, the deep palmar ligament of the carpus might also absorb a substantial amount of energy during hyperextension of the carpus. Power absorption is therefore not always associated with eccentric muscle contraction but can also be caused by elastic energy storage in tendons and ligaments. The subsequent power production can originate from the release of elastic energy instead of concentric muscle contraction. If elastic properties of tendons are known, and tendon force is estimated from inverse dynamic analysis, the amount of energy storage can be estimated separately.

Power production and absorption are usually analyzed at a joint level but many muscles span more than one joint. These muscles can therefore absorb power at one joint and simultaneously produce power at another joint. This has, for instance, been described for the gastrocnemius muscle in human vertical jumping: at the end of push-off, the muscle generates positive power at the ankle and negative power at the knee. This function of biarticular muscles is referred to as power transport between joints (Gregoire et al., 1984). It is assumed to be a major function of these muscles. Power transport can take place during isometric contraction without power production by the transporting muscle. Therefore, no muscle fibers are needed to transport power and tendons can also transport power. In the lower limbs of horses there are several more or less tendinous bi- or polyarticular muscles. It has been hypothesized that the proximal muscles generate the power and that this power is transported to the distal joints by the tendinous biarticular muscles (van Ingen Schenau, 1994). The major advantage of this system is that the lower limbs are very lightweight while the joints can still be actively moved and can contribute to the propulsion.

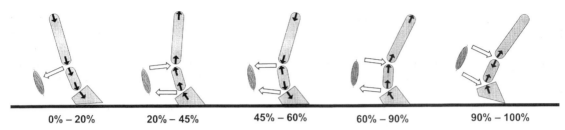

0% – 20%   20% – 45%   45% – 60%   60% – 90%   90% – 100%

Fig. EV   Five parts of stance phase.

The lower limbs undergo large accelerations during gait; if they are lightweight the accelerations will cost less energy and can be performed more rapidly, enabling a faster and more economical gait.

Example V: *Power analysis during walk*

The results of joint power analysis (Colborne *et al.*, 1998) and power flow analysis (Colborne *et al.*, 1997) for the equine walk can be combined to obtain a more complete description of the power production, absorption and transport in the distal limb during the stance phase. Because the data are obtained from different horses, they might contain small inconsistencies and there are unknown changes in the mechanical energy of the segments. Nevertheless, the stance phase can be described in five parts:

- In the first 20% of the stance phase, the power flows in proximally and is absorbed by the flexors of the fetlock joint.
- From 20% till 45%, the power flow is reversed: the fetlock muscle produces power, which is transported proximally, probably to propel the trunk. Simultaneously, the coffin flexors absorb some power from the hoof.
- From 45% to 60%, the power flows in proximally and is absorbed by the fetlock and coffin joint flexors.
- From 60% till 90%, the fetlock flexors again produce power which is transported proximally. Simultaneously, the coffin flexors absorb power from the pastern and hoof.
- In the final 10% of the stance phase, both the fetlock and coffin flexors produce power which is used to increase the mechanical energy of the distal segments.

The fetlock flexors have alternating periods of power absorption and power production. Part of this power might be stored as elastic energy in the long tendons of these muscles.

To prevent the problems with biarticular power transport, power production can also be analyzed at the level of the muscles, using the muscle force estimation methods described previously. The estimated muscle force is multiplied by the contraction velocity of the muscle. The contraction velocity can be obtained from kinematic data (Riemersma *et al.*, 1988; van den Bogert *et al.*, 1988) or by multiplying the joint angular velocity by the moment arm of the muscle. For human cycling, energy expenditure predictions obtained from power analysis at the muscle level differed greatly from predictions using power analysis at the joint level (Neptune & van den Bogert, 1998). This is due to the fact that joint power does not consider power transport by biarticular muscles nor antagonistic co-contraction. Estimates of energy expenditure should therefore not be obtained from analyses at the joint level but from analyses at the muscle level. Power analysis at the joint level can still be used to describe and analyze the control of movement.

Apart from the segment-oriented and joint-oriented approaches there is a third power analysis approach, which is used in gaits without substantial external power production. This approach does not use the joint moments and forces but focuses on mechanical energy changes. During a stride cycle both the potential and the kinetic energy of the segments change constantly. Based on comparison of patterns of these energy changes gaits have been classified as either inverted pendulum or bouncing gaits (Cavagna & Kaneko, 1977). In inverted pendulum gaits like walk, the limbs act as rigid struts over which the body vaults – the kinetic energy and potential energy changes are each other's opposites. In the bouncing gaits like trot, the limbs act as springs and the body center of mass moves like a bouncing ball – the kinetic and potential energy increase and decrease simultaneously. Equine gallop might have both bouncing and pendulum aspects (Minetti *et al.*, 1999). Apart from this classification of gaits, attempts have been made to relate the changes in mechanical energy to metabolic energy consumption (Cavagna & Kaneko, 1977; Minetti *et al.*, 1999). The major problem is that when moving at a constant speed the mechanical energy at the end of the stride equals the mechanical energy at the beginning of the stride and no net work is performed. Nevertheless, to enable analysis, negative and positive changes of energy of the segments are treated differently. Either all positive changes are added, ignoring negative powers, or different efficiencies are used to add positive and negative power production. However the efficiencies of positive and negative muscular work are speculative. Furthermore, energy can be stored temporarily in elastic structures or it can be transferred between segments and probably also between limbs. The relative importance of these processes is not known. Results of internal power analyses, therefore, are largely dependent on the assumptions of internal power transport, energy storage and efficiency. This necessitates careful validation of the mechanical energy analysis, and estimation of error bounds due to assumptions regarding power transfer, efficiency and elastic storage (Thys *et al.*, 1996).

Accuracy of inverse dynamic calculations

All direct and indirect measurements of biological variables are influenced by certain sources of errors and, therefore, have a limited accuracy. Inverse dynamic calculations are no exception to this rule. The errors influencing the accuracy of inverse dynamic calculations can be subdivided in two categories: errors in the measurement of input variables and errors originating from model assumptions. The most important measurement errors are caused by estimation of the inertial properties from *in vitro* data, misalignment of markers with the joint rotation center, skin displacement relative to the underlying bones, the use of noisy data to calculate accelerations, inaccuracies in the measurement of the point of application of the ground reaction force and misalignment of force and movement data. Further details on some of these inaccuracies may be found in chapter 3. The major assumptions influencing the accuracy of the calculations are the rigidity of the segments and the fixed rotation point. If muscle forces are calculated, two major assumptions are often added: the absence of antagonistic co-contractions and the cost function used to distribute the moment among the available muscles. The influence of all these errors and assumptions on the final accuracy depends, of course, on the magnitude of the errors. This magnitude is determined by the equipment used and the conditions of the actual measurements. However, some general considerations can be made on the order of the errors and their influence on the final results.

The assumptions of a fixed rotation center can be questioned for the stifle and carpal joints, whereas the alignment of the markers with the rotation center is difficult in the coffin joint and the proximal joints. Even relatively small errors in the coffin joint marker placement can seriously influence the results for this joint because of the small moment arms in the hoof segment. Radiographs should therefore be used to validate and, if necessary, correct this marker position. Due to similar small moment arms, measurement errors in the point of application of the GRF relative to the hoof will also seriously influence the coffin joint results (Bartel *et al.*, 1978). These errors can arise from systematic errors in the point of application or from misalignment of the coordinate systems of the force and movement data. The systematic errors in the point of application should be corrected (Bobbert & Schamhardt, 1990) and the two coordinate systems should be aligned carefully. Although the errors in the point of application, in the alignment and in the marker placement will influence the accuracy for other joints, the relative influence is much smaller due to the larger moment arms.

The accuracy of the inertial properties differs for the proximal and distal segments (Buchner *et al.*, 1997). In general the proximal segments have a large mass, are not quite rigid and it is difficult to separate them from each other. The distal limb segments, in contrast, have a small mass, are quite rigid and the boundary between these segments is clear. Therefore, the inertial data for the distal segments is quite accurate and does not seriously influence the accuracy of the results. Furthermore, the accelerations of the distal segments are very small, at least during stance, and errors in the inertial data or the accelerations hardly influence the results for these segments. Similarly, the total ignorance of the accelerations, as is done in a quasi-static analysis, seems to be acceptable for these segments. During the swing phase, however, the results are determined completely by the accelerations. Errors in these accelerations or the inertial data seriously influence the accuracy. Skin displacements for the distal joints are small and will not influence the accuracy. However, for the proximal joints they are very large, influence the accuracy and should be corrected, using the available correction algorithms (van Weeren *et al.*, 1992b).

The effect of random errors on the final results can be determined with Monte Carlo simulation (van den Bogert *et al.*, 1994). In this simulation the analysis is performed multiple times, with multiple copies of the input data that are modified by adding random errors according to known probability distributions. The standard deviation of these multiple results provides an estimate of the error in the final result. Systematic errors, such as skin movement, are not random and should be modeled as a hypothetical function of time or joint angle in such an error analysis.

Three-dimensional analysis

The methodology presented above applies to a two-dimensional analysis, usually in the sagittal plane. Movement of horses seems remarkably planar, but for some applications the small mediolateral movements may also be important. In Trotters, these out of plane movements were reproducible, highly individual, and presumably related to performance (van Weeren *et al.*, 1993). It is therefore conceivable that analysis of the sources of those movements is useful. Furthermore, the magnitude of out-of-plane moments is presently unknown.

In human walking, it has been shown that a two-dimensional analysis underestimates the average joint power at the hip by 23% because the hip abductor moment is ignored (Eng & Winter, 1995). Similar underestimations might be obtained in horses and a full 3D analysis should be undertaken to determine for which movements and which applications the out-of plane moments can be neglected. Finally, out-of-plane moments might provide useful information about joint loading. In humans adductor–abductor moments reflect load distribution between the medial and lateral compartments of the knee (Lindenfeld et al., 1997).

Extension of inverse dynamic analysis to three dimensions is mathematically straightforward (Vaughan et al., 1992; van den Bogert, 1994). The equation of motion for force (equation 1 and 2) is the same, with the only difference that force is now a vector with three, rather than two components. The equation of motion for moments (equation 3) has an extra term in three dimensions, and uses a matrix **I** for the moment of inertia rather than a single scalar value:

$$\sum M = \mathbf{I} \cdot \alpha + \omega \times (\mathbf{I} \cdot \omega) \qquad (11)$$

Joint moments M are vectors in 3D, as are angular velocities ω and angular accelerations α. In the force equation, vectors are usually expressed in a global, ground-based coordinate system. In the moment equation, however, all vectors and matrices must be expressed relative to a segment-fixed coordinate system. The final term is proportional to the square of the magnitude of the angular velocity and accounts for centrifugal effects when the axis of rotation is not aligned with an axis of symmetry (principal axis) of the body segment. Note the cross product symbol '×', which makes this moment perpendicular to the axis of rotation. The inertia matrix **I** is a 3×3 matrix which is diagonal (only three elements are non-zero) when the axes of the segment coordinate system are aligned with the principal axes; otherwise **I** has 9 non-zero elements that reflect the non-symmetrical distribution of the mass. Three-dimensional inertial properties for equine segments have been measured with respect to anatomically defined coordinate systems (Buchner et al. 1997). When expressed in a suitable segment-fixed coordinate system, the three components of the moment vector M can be interpreted as flexion–extension, abduction–adduction and internal–external rotation moment, respectively. The angular velocity vector ω must be decomposed along the same three axes in order to obtain the joint power by taking the dot product of moment and angular velocity.

Instrumentation for collecting three-dimensional movement and GRF data is now standard equipment in biomechanical laboratories. However, problems arise from modeling assumptions and the standardization of the experimental protocol. These problems may lead to inaccuracies that are, in some cases, larger than the magnitude of the results of the calculations. In those cases, a three-dimensional

analysis does not provide useful additional information compared to a sagittal plane analysis.

In the experimental protocol, three markers must be attached to each segment in order to obtain all six degrees of freedom – three translations and three rotations – for each segment. It is no longer possible to have markers coincide with the joint center in 3D, since the joint center is inside the body. Markers must therefore be attached to standardized anatomical landmarks, relative to which the location of the joint center is known. Suitable protocols have been developed for human analysis (Bell et al., 1990; Vaughan et al., 1992), and first attempts have been made for equine analysis (Nicodemus et al., 1999).

Soft tissue movement may be more of a problem in 3D because of the indirect method for locating joint centers. Joint moments are known to be sensitive to errors in the joint center location (Burdett, 1982). Also, three markers may not be representative of the motion of the entire body segment when the segment undergoes complex soft tissue movements during impacts. This may lead to errors in the inertial terms of the equations of motion, the terms which are proportional to masses and moments of inertia. On segments such as the thigh, using more than three markers should be considered. Least-squares techniques can then provide the best estimate of 3D rigid segment movement that is consistent with data from all markers (Soderkvist & Wedin, 1993). Note that there are two conflicting requirements for a marker placement protocol: for location of joint centers, markers should closely follow the bone movement; for accurate estimation of inertial forces, markers should follow the 'average' of the mass distribution, of which the muscles can be an important component. Different marker sets for these two calculations should be considered.

Accelerations for certain out-of-plane movements in the horse may be small relative to the errors associated with differentiation of noisy movement data (see chapter 3). It is therefore important to have good estimates of these errors, so that the accelerations that are smaller than the noise can simply be neglected, rather than introduce extra noise into the results.

In modeling, the body is typically represented as rigid segments linked by ball joints. For estimation of muscle forces, three moment arms must be known for each muscle, one for rotation about each axis of the segment coordinate system. Three-dimensional models of the muscle path from origin to insertion (e.g. Brand et al., 1982) are typically used to determine the instantaneous moment arms, as well as the orientation of muscle force vectors during movement. Interactive software tools are now available to develop such models of the 3D musculoskeletal anatomy (Delp & Loan, 1995).

Many joints in horses and humans are hinge joints where rotations other than flexion and extension are prevented by the articular surfaces and ligaments. Such joints have an axis of rotation rather than a center of rotation. The 'joint center' used for the inverse dynamic analysis lies on this axis; typically, the midpoint of the part of the axis within the bone is used. The moment components associated with internal–external rotation and abduction–adduction components do not represent muscle function. Interpreting these moments as muscle moments may lead to severe overestimation of muscle forces and joint loading (Burdett, 1982; Glitsch & Baumann, 1997). Instead, these moments can indicate load distributions in articular contact and ligaments (Lindenfeld *et al.*, 1997).

REFERENCES

Alexander, R.McN. and Bennet-Clark, H.C. (1977) Storage of elastic strain energy in muscle and other tissues. *Nature* **265**: 114–117.

Andriacchi, T.P. (1993) Functional analysis of pre and post-knee surgery: total knee arthroplasty and ACL reconstruction. *J. Biomech. Eng.* **115**: 575–581.

Andriacchi, T.P. and Birac, D. (1993) Functional testing in the anterior cruciate ligament-deficient knee. *Clin. Orthop.* 40–47.

Back, W., Barneveld, A., van Weeren, P.R. and van den Bogert, A.J. (1993) Kinematic gait analysis in equine carpal lameness. *Acta Anat. (Basel)* **146**: 86–89.

Back, W., Schamhardt, H.C., Hartman, W., Bruin, G. and Barneveld, A. (1995) Predictive value of foal kinematics for the locomotor performance of adult horses. *Res. Vet. Sci.* **59**: 64–69.

Bartel, D.L., Schryver, H.F., Lowe, J.E. and Parker, R.A. (1978) Locomotion in the horse: a procedure for computing the internal forces in the digit. *Am. J. Vet. Res.* **39**: 1721–1727.

Becker, C.K., Savelberg, H.H., Buchner, H.H. and Barneveld, A. (1998) Long-term consequences of experimental desmotomy of the accessory ligament of the deep digital flexor tendon in adult horses. *Am. J. Vet. Res.* **59**: 347–351.

Bell, A.L., Pedersen, D.R. and Brand, R.A. (1990) A comparison of the accuracy of several hip center location prediction methods. *J. Biomech.* **23**: 617–621.

Biewener, A.A., Thomason, J.J. and Lanyon, L.E. (1988) Mechanics of locomotion and jumping in the horse (*Equus*): in vivo stress in the tibia and metatarsus. *J. Zool.* **214**: 547–565.

Bobbert, M.F. and Schamhardt, H.C. (1990) Accuracy of determining the point of force application with piezoelectric force plates. *J. Biomech.* **23**: 705–710.

Brand, R.A., Crowninshield, R.D., Wittstock, C.E., Pedersen, D.R., Clark, C.R. and van Krieken, F.M. (1982) A model of lower extremity muscular anatomy. *J. Biomech. Eng.* **104**: 304–310.

Brand, R.A., Pedersen, D.R., Davy, D.T., Kotzar, G.M., Heiple, K.G. and Goldberg, V.M. (1994) Comparison of hip force calculations and measurements in the same patient. *J. Arthroplasty* **9**: 45–51.

Buchner, H.H.F., Savelberg, H.H.C.M., Schamhardt, H.C. and Barneveld, A. (1997) Inertial properties of Dutch Warmblood horses. *J. Biomech.* **30**: 653–658.

Buchner, H.H.F., Savelberg, H.H.C.M., and Becker, C.K. (1996) Load redistribution after desmotomy of the accessory ligament of the deep digital flexor tendon in adult horses. *Vet. Quart.* **18**: S70–74.

Burdett, R.G. (1982) Forces predicted at the ankle during running. *Med. Sci. Sports Exerc.* **14**: 308–316.

Cavagna, G.A. and Kaneko, M. (1977) Mechanical work and efficiency in level walking and running. *J. Physiol. (Lond.)* **268**: 647–681.

Clayton, H.M. (1996) Instrumentation and techniques in locomotion and lameness. *Vet. Clin. North Am.: Equine Pract.* **12**: 337–350.

Clayton, H.M., Lanovaz, J.L., Schamhardt, H.C., Willemen, M.A. and Colborne, G.R. (1998) Net joint moments and powers in the equine forelimb during the stance phase of the trot. *Equine Vet. J.* **30**: 384–389.

Clayton, H.M., Willemen, M.A., Lanovaz, J.L. and Schamhardt, H.C. (2000) Effects of a heel wedge in horses with superficial digital flexor tendinitis. *Vet. Comp. Orthop. Traum.* **13**: 1–8.

Colborne, G.R., Lanovaz, J.L., Sprigings, E.J., Schamhardt, H.C. and Clayton, H.M. (1997) Power flow in the equine forelimb. *Equine Vet. J.* (Suppl **23**): 37–40.

Colborne, G.R., Lanovaz, J.L., Sprigings, E.J., Schamhardt, H.C. and Clayton, H.M. (1998) Forelimb joint moments and power in the walking stance phase of horses. *Am. J. Vet. Res.* **59**: 609–614.

Crowninshield, R.D. and Brand, R.A. (1981) A physiologically based criterion of muscle force prediction in locomotion. *J. Biomech.* **14**: 793–801.

de Koning, J.J., de Groot, G. and van Ingen Schenau, G.J. (1991) Coordination of leg muscles during speed skating. *J. Biomech.* **24**: 137–146.

Delp, S.L. and Loan, J.P. (1995) A graphics-based software system to develop and analyze models of musculoskeletal structures. *Comput. Biol. Med.* **25**: 21–34.

Deuel, N.R. and Park, J. (1993) Gallop kinematics of Olympic three-day event horses. *Acta Anat. (Basel)* **146**: 168–174.

Devita, P. and Skelly, W.A. (1992) Effect of landing stiffness on joint kinetics and energetics in the lower extremity. *Med. Sci. Sports Exerc.* **24**: 108–115.

Dow, S.M., Leendertz, J.A., Silver, I.A. and Goodship, A.E. (1991) Identification of subclinical tendon injury from ground reaction force analysis. *Equine Vet. J.* **23**: 266–272.

Dul, J., Townsend, M.A., Shiavi, R. and Johnson, G.E. (1984) Muscular synergism – I. On criteria for load sharing between synergistic muscles. *J. Biomech.* **17**: 663–673.

Dyce, K.M., Sack, W.O. and Wensing, C.J.G. (1987) Textbook of veterinary anatomy. Saunders company, Philadelphia.

Elftman, H. (1939) Forces and energy changes in the leg during walking. *Am. J. Physiol.* **125**: 339–356.

Eng, J.J. and Winter, D.A. (1995) Kinetic analysis of the lower limbs during walking: what information can be gained from a three-dimensional model? *J. Biomech.* **28**: 753–758.

Glitsch, U. and Baumann, W. (1997) The three-dimensional determination of internal loads in the lower extremity. *J. Biomech.* **30**: 1123–1131.

Gregoire, L., Veeger, H.E., Huijing, P.A. and van Ingen Schenau, G.J. (1984) Role of mono- and biarticular muscles in explosive movements. *Int. J. Sports Med.* **5**: 301–305.

Hartman, W., Schamhardt, H.C., Lammertink, J.L. and Badoux, D.M. (1984) Bone strain in the equine tibia: an in vivo strain gauge analysis. *Am. J. Vet. Res.* **45**: 880–884.

Herzog, W. and Leonard, T.R. (1991) Validation of optimization models that estimate the forces exerted by synergistic muscles. *J. Biomech.* **24**: 31–39.

Jansen, M.O., van den Bogert, A.J., Riemersma, D.J. and Schamhardt, H.C. (1993) In vivo tendon forces in the forelimb of ponies at the walk, validated by ground reaction force measurements. *Acta Anat. (Basel)* **146**: 162–167.

Jones, D.A. and Round, J.M. (1990) Skeletal muscle in health and disease. Manchester University Press, Manchester.

Kuo, A.D. (1998) A least-squares estimation approach to improving the precision of inverse dynamics computations. *J. Biomech. Eng.* **120**: 148–159.

Leach, D.H. and Dyson, S. (1988) Instant centres of rotation of equine limb joints and their relationship to standard skin marker locations. *Equine Vet. J.* (Suppl **6**): 113–119.

Lindenfeld, T.N., Hewett, T.E. and Andriacchi, T.P. (1997) Joint loading with valgus bracing in patients with varus gonarthrosis. *Clin. Orthop.* **344**: 290–297.

Merkens, H.W. and Schamhardt, H.C. (1988) Evaluation of equine locomotion during different degrees of experimentally induced lameness. II: Distribution of ground reaction force patterns of the concurrently loaded limbs. *Equine Vet. J.* (Suppl. **6**): 107–112.

Minetti, A.E., Ardig, O.L., Reinach, E. and Saibene, F. (1999) The relationship between mechanical work and energy expenditure of locomotion in horses. *J. Exp. Biol.* **202**: 2329–2338.

Neptune, R.R. and van den Bogert, A.J. (1998) Standard mechanical energy analyses do not correlate with muscle work in cycling. *J. Biomech.* **31**: 239–245.

Nicodemus, M.C., Lanovaz, J.L., Corn, C. and Clayton, H.M. (1999) The application of virtual markers to a joint coordinate system for equine three-dimensional motions. *Proc. 16th Equine Nutr. Physiol. Symp.*, pp. 24–25.

Ounpuu, S., Gage, J.R. and Davis, R.B. (1991) Three-dimensional lower extremity joint kinetics in normal pediatric gait. *J. Pediatr. Orthop.* **11**: 341–349.

Paul, J.P. (1971) Load actions on the human femur in walking and some resultant stresses. *Exp. Mech.* **11**: 121–125.

Pratt, G.W. Jr. and O'Connor, J.T. Jr. (1976) Force plate studies of equine biomechanics. *Am. J. Vet. Res.* **37**: 1251–1255.

Riemersma, D.J., van den Bogert, A.J., Jansen, M.O. and Schamhardt, H.C. (1996) Tendon strain in the forelimbs as a function of gait and ground characteristics and in vitro limb loading in ponies. *Equine Vet. J.* **28**: 133–138.

Riemersma, D.J., van den Bogert, A.J., Schamhardt, H.C. and Hartman, W. (1988) Kinetics and kinematics of the equine hind limb: in vivo tendon strain and joint kinematics. *Am. J. Vet. Res.* **49**: 1353–1359.

Robertson, D.G. and Winter, D.A. (1980) Mechanical energy generation, absorption and transfer amongst segments during walking. *J. Biomech.* **13**: 845–854.

Rose, S.A., DeLuca, P.A., Davis, R.B.d., Ounpuu, S. and Gage, J.R. (1993) Kinematic and kinetic evaluation of the ankle after lengthening of the gastrocnemius fascia in children with cerebral palsy. *J. Pediatr. Orthop.* **13**: 727–732.

Schryver, H.F., Bartel, D.L., Langrana, N. and Lowe, J.E. (1978) Locomotion in the horse: kinematics and external and internal forces in the normal equine digit in the walk and trot. *Am. J. Vet. Res.* **39**: 1728–1733.

Soderkvist, I. and Wedin, P.A. (1993) Determining the movements of the skeleton using well-configured markers. *J. Biomech.* **26**: 1473–1477.

Thunnissen, J. (1993) Muscle force prediction during human gait. *PhD thesis, University of Twente.*

Thys, H., Willems, P.A. and Saels, P. (1996) Energy cost, mechanical work and muscular efficiency in swing-through gait with elbow crutches. *J. Biomech.* **29**: 1473–1482.

van den Bogert, A.J. (1994) Analysis and simulation of mechanical loads on the human musculoskeletal system: a methodological overview. *Exerc. Sport Sci. Rev.* **22**: 23–51.

van den Bogert, A.J. and Sauren, A.A.H.J. (1989) Implementation of curves musculotendinous structures in rigid body dynamics. In: van den Bogert, A.J. Computer simulation of locomotion in the horse. *PhD thesis, University of Utrecht*, pp. 37–55.

van den Bogert, A.J., Schamhardt, H.C. and Hartman, W. (1988) Relationship between simultaneously measured muscle activation, length, force and power in the horse. In: *Proc. 6th Congr. Europ. Soc. Biomech.* p C 32

van den Bogert, A.J., Hartman, W. and Sauren, A.A.H.J. (1989) Measurement and computation of inertial parameters in the horse. In: van den Bogert, A.J. Computer simulation of locomotion in the horse. *PhD thesis, University of Utrecht*, pp. 67–89.

van den Bogert, A.J., Smith, G.D. and Nigg, B.M. (1994) In vivo determination of the anatomical axes of the ankle joint complex: an optimization approach. *J. Biomech.* **27**: 1477–1488.

van den Bogert, A.J., Read, L. and Nigg, B.M. (1999) An analysis of hip joint loading during walking, running, and skiing. *Med. Sci. Sports Exerc.* **31**: 131–142.

van Ingen Schenau, G.J. (1994) Proposed actions of bi-articular muscles and the design of hindlimbs of bi- and quadrupeds. *Hum. Movem. Sci.* **13**: 665–681.

van Ingen Schenau, G.J. and Cavanagh, P.R. (1990) Power equations in endurance sports. *J. Biomech.* **23**: 865–881.

van Weeren, P.R., Jansen, M.O., van den Bogert, A.J. and Barneveld, A. (1992a) A kinematic and strain gauge study of the reciprocal apparatus in the equine hind limb. *J. Biomech.* **25**: 1291–1301.

van Weeren, P.R., van den Bogert, A.J., Back, W., Bruin, G. and Barneveld, A. (1992b) Correction models for skin displacement in equine kinematic gait analysis. *J. Equine Vet. Sci.* **12**: 178–192.

van Weeren, P.R., van den Bogert, A.J., Back, W., Bruin, G. and Barneveld, A. (1993) Kinematics of the standardbred trotter measured at 6, 7, 8 and 9 m/s on a treadmill, before and after 5 months of prerace training. *Acta Anat. (Basel)* **146**: 154–161.

Vaughan, C.L. (1984) Computer simulation of human motion in sports biomechanics. *Exerc. Sport Sci. Rev.* **12**: 373–416.

Vaughan, C., Davis, B. and O'Connor, J. (1992) Dynamics of Human gait. 1st edition Human Kinetics Publishers, Champaign, Illinois.

Winter, D.A. and Eng, P. (1995) Kinetics: our window into the goals and strategies of the central nervous system. *Behav. Brain Res.* **67**: 111–120.

Winter, D.A. and Robertson, D.G. (1978) Joint torque and energy patterns in normal gait. *Biol. Cybern.* **29**: 137–142.

Winter, D. (1990) Biomechanics and motor control of human movement. 2nd edn. Wiley, New York.

Yeadon, M.R. and Challis, J.H. (1994) The future of performance-related sports biomechanics research. *J. Sports Sci.* **12**: 3–32.

APPENDIX: FORMULAS FOR INVERSE DYNAMIC CALCULATIONS

Hoof segment

The sum of all forces on the segment must equal its mass times acceleration. In the horizontal direction this gives the following equation:

$$\sum F_X = m_{hoof} \cdot a_{Xhoof} \Leftrightarrow GRF_X + F_{Xcoffin} = m_{hoof} \cdot a_{Xhoof}$$

or:

$$F_{Xcoffin} = m_{hoof} \cdot a_{Xhoof} - GRF_X$$

For symbols see Figure A1 and the symbol list below.

For the vertical direction the gravitational force (G) should be taken into account:

$$\sum F_Y = m_{hoof} \cdot a_{Yhoof} \Leftrightarrow GRF_Y + F_{Ycoff} + G_{hoof} = m_{hoof} \cdot a_{Yhoof}$$

or

$$F_{Ycoffin} = m_{hoof} \cdot a_{Yhoof} - GRF_Y - m_{hoof} \cdot g$$

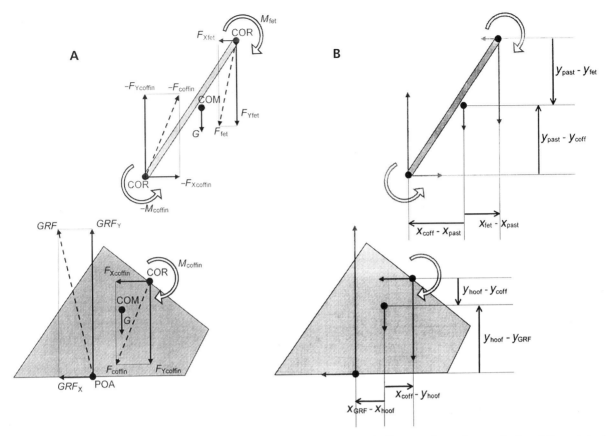

Fig. A1 Free body diagrams of the hoof and pastern segments. **A** Free body diagrams; **B** x and y coordinates of the points of application of the forces.

The sum of the net coffin joint moment and the moments of all forces must equal the moment of inertia times the angular acceleration of the hoof segment:

$$\sum M = I_{\text{hoof}} \cdot \alpha_{\text{hoof}}$$

or

$$M_{\text{coffin}} + GRF_{\text{X}} \cdot (y_{\text{hoof}} - y_{\text{GRF}}) + GRF_{\text{Y}} \cdot (x_{\text{GRF}} - x_{\text{hoof}})$$
$$+ F_{\text{Xcoffin}} \cdot (y_{\text{hoof}} - y_{\text{coff}}) + F_{\text{Ycoffin}} \cdot (x_{\text{coff}} - x_{\text{hoof}})$$
$$= I_{\text{hoof}} \cdot \alpha_{\text{hoof}}$$

or:

$$M_{\text{coffin}} = I_{\text{hoof}} \cdot \alpha_{\text{hoof}} - GRF_{\text{X}} \cdot (y_{\text{hoof}} - y_{\text{GRF}}) - GRF_{\text{Y}} \cdot$$
$$(x_{\text{GRF}} - x_{\text{hoof}}) - F_{\text{Xcoffin}} \cdot (y_{\text{hoof}} - y_{\text{coff}}) - F_{\text{Ycoffin}} \cdot$$
$$(x_{\text{coff}} - x_{\text{hoof}})$$

Note the different subtraction of the x and y coordinates: the x coordinate of the joint center of rotation is subtracted from the x coordinate of the point of application of the force whereas the y coordinate of the point of application is subtracted from the y coordinate of the center of rotation. In this way moments produced by the forces will automatically get a

correct sign: positive for counterclockwise and negative for clockwise moments.

Pastern segment

Horizontal and vertical forces:

$$\sum F_{\text{X}} = m_{\text{past}} \cdot a_{\text{Xpast}} \Leftrightarrow F_{\text{Xfet}} - F_{\text{Xcoffin}} = m_{\text{past}} \cdot a_{\text{Xpast}}$$

$$\sum F_{\text{Y}} = m_{\text{past}} \cdot a_{\text{Ypast}} \Leftrightarrow F_{\text{Yfet}} - F_{\text{Ycoffin}} + G_{\text{past}} = m_{\text{past}} \cdot a_{\text{Ypast}}$$

Note that the net coffin joint force (the force from the pastern of the hoof) is inverted to obtain the force from the hoof on the pastern.

Moments:

$$\sum M = I_{\text{past}} \cdot \alpha_{\text{past}}$$

or

$$M_{\text{fet}} - M_{\text{coffin}} + F_{\text{Xfet}} \cdot (y_{\text{past}} - y_{\text{fet}}) + F_{\text{Yfet}} \cdot (x_{\text{fet}} - x_{\text{past}})$$
$$- F_{\text{Xcoffin}} \cdot (y_{\text{past}} - y_{\text{coff}}) - F_{\text{Ycoffin}} \cdot (x_{\text{coff}} - x_{\text{past}})$$
$$= I_{\text{past}} \cdot \alpha_{\text{past}}$$

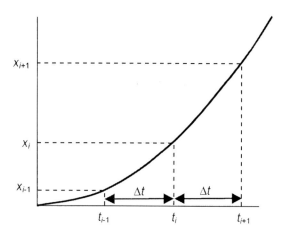

Fig. A2 Finite differences can be used to calculate velocity and acceleration.

Velocity and accelerations

Velocity and acceleration can be calculated using a finite difference method. The difference in position between frame number i and $i+1$ is divided by the time difference to obtain an approximation of the velocity at frame $i+1/2$ (see Fig. A2):

$$v_{i+1/2} = \frac{\Delta x}{\Delta t} = \frac{x_{i+1} - x_i}{t_{i+1} - t_i}$$

Subsequently the difference in velocity between $i+1/2$ and $i-1/2$ is used to calculate the acceleration:

$$a_i = \frac{\Delta v}{\Delta t} = \frac{v_{i+1/2} - v_{i-1/2}}{\Delta t} = \frac{x_{i+1} - x_i - (x_i - x_{i-1})}{\Delta t \cdot \Delta t}$$
$$= \frac{x_{i+1} - 2x_i + x_{i-1}}{(\Delta t)^2}$$

For power calculations the velocity at i instead of $i+1/2$ must be known; this velocity can be calculated from the difference in position at frame $i-1$ and $i+1$:

$$v_i = \frac{\Delta x}{\Delta t} = \frac{x_{i+1} - x_{i-1}}{t_{i+1} - t_{i-1}} = \frac{x_{i+1} - x_{i-1}}{2\Delta t}$$

Symbols

α	angular acceleration of the segment
a	linear acceleration of the segment
F	force
F_{coffin}	net coffin (coff) joint force
F_{fetlock}	net fetlock (fet) joint force
GRF	ground reaction force
g	gravitational acceleration: 9.81 m/s^2
I	moment of inertia
m	segmental mass
M	moment
M_{coffin}	net coffin (coff) joint moment
M_{fetlock}	net fetlock (fet) joint moment
t	time
v	velocity
x	horizontal coordinate of point of application or center of mass
X	horizontal component of force or acceleration (subscript)
y	vertical coordinate of point of application or center of mass
Y	vertical component of force or acceleration (subscript).

14
Metabolic Energetics of Locomotion

Mathew P. Gerard and David R. Hodgson

INTRODUCTION

Vertebrate locomotion requires the controlled integration of numerous physiological and metabolic pathways. These then impact on the musculoskeletal system thereby providing the organism with mobility. Perhaps the most important pathways are those concerned with the production of energy, for without energy muscles cannot contract and mobility is not achieved. The horse represents one of the more efficient species in terms of locomotion, designed to move a relatively large mass with great speed and endurance. One of the major survival mechanisms for the wild equid is swift retreat from threatening circumstances.

Muscular movement requires the transformation of chemical energy stored in metabolic fuels to the kinetic energy of muscular contraction. All pathways integral to

energy supply are concerned with the ultimate production of adenosine triphosphate (ATP), the final carrier of energy 'packages' utilized by muscle for contraction. For muscles to contract there is a coupling of thin actin and thick myosin filaments to form cross-bridges and then these filaments slide relative to each other by a change in orientation of the cross-bridges (Guyton, 1986). Energy is necessary for the change in orientation of the cross-bridges to occur. Cleavage of a high-energy phosphate bond from ATP results in adenosine diphosphate (ADP), free phosphate, a proton and the release of energy. This hydrolysis reaction of ATP occurs at the head of each myosin filament and is catalyzed by the enzyme myosin ATPase (Fig. 14.1). The energy released is utilized by the working muscle (Cain & Davies, 1962).

In addition, ATP is the source of energy required to restore the contracted muscle to a relaxed or resting

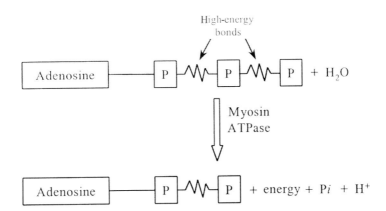

Fig. 14.1 Hydrolysis of ATP to ADP by the enzyme myosin ATPase, with the release of energy for use by working muscle. P: Phosphate; P*i*: orthophosphate. (Modified from Clayton, 1991.)

state via the distribution of calcium ions (Åstrand & Rodahl, 1986). Under normal conditions there is a finite store of ATP within muscle, sufficient to maintain muscular activity for only a few seconds (Lindholm, 1979; Åstrand & Rodahl, 1986). Therefore to perform continuous muscular exertion it is necessary to resynthesize ATP and this is done by the pathways of aerobic (oxidative) and anaerobic phosphorylation.

PRODUCTION OF ENERGY

Aerobic phosphorylation

Production of ATP via aerobic pathways occurs within the inner membrane of mitochondria in a series of single oxidation reactions known as the *electron transport* or *respiratory chain*. *Oxidation* is the donation or loss of electrons (often in the form of hydrogen) from an atom or molecule, while *reduction* is the acceptance of electrons (hydrogen) by an atom or molecule. When electrons are donated, considerable chemical energy is liberated and a portion of this energy is captured for the rephosphorylation of ADP to ATP, with the remainder being lost as heat energy (Guyton, 1986). Nicotinamide adenine dinucleotide (NAD) and flavin adenine dinucleotide (FAD) act as hydrogen carriers (acceptors) during glycolysis, beta oxidation and the tricarboxylic acid (TCA) cycle and therefore are reduced to NADH and $FADH_2$. These coenzymes are essential for aerobic and anaerobic phosphorylation but their concentrations within the muscle are low. Therefore, NADH and $FADH_2$ must be reoxidized to NAD^+ and FAD via the electron transport chain. Specific mitochondrial enzymes incorporated in the electron transport chain catalyze the oxidation through a process of dehydrogenation. The donated hydrogen atoms provide the electrons that are transported from one enzyme complex to another by electron carriers, e.g. *cytochrome c*. The importance of oxygen (O_2) in this whole process is that it acts as the final hydrogen acceptor to form water. The energy released by the step-by-step transfer of electrons from NADH or $FADH_2$ to O_2 via the electron carriers is used to pump protons from the inner matrix of the mitochondrion into the outer chamber between the inner and outer mitochondrial membranes. This creates a strong transmembrane electric potential. Energy for the phosphorylation of ADP to ATP is obtained as the protons flow back through an inner membrane enzyme complex called *ATP synthetase* (Guyton, 1986; Stryer, 1988).

The availability of O_2 to the exercising muscle is the rate-limiting step for oxidative phosphorylation. Oxygen immediately available to the muscle at the onset of exercise, from myoglobin within the muscle (MbO_2),

hemoglobin within the circulatory system (HbO_2) or O_2 dissolved in the body fluids, is in sufficient quantities for only a few seconds of exercise. Therefore the delivery of O_2 to the exercising muscles via the cardiorespiratory system is crucial for the capacity to continuously produce energy via aerobic means.

The two major electron donor substrates for aerobic phosphorylation are carbohydrates (CHO) and fatty acids. Glucose is the main CHO and if it is not used for immediate energy production, it is stored as glycogen, mostly in skeletal muscle and to a lesser extent in the liver (Lindholm, 1979; Hodgson *et al.*, 1983, 1984). Adipose tissue constitutes the largest store of fatty acids (FA) (Robb *et al.*, 1972; Stryer, 1988). Adipocytes store fat within their cytoplasm as triglycerides. Triglyceride storage also occurs to a much lesser extent in muscle (Lindholm, 1979).

Aerobic glycolysis

The importance of CHO as a substrate for energy production increases as exercise intensity increases (Hodgson, 1985; Lawrence, 1990). Glucose diffuses into the muscle cell cytoplasm from the circulation and is phosphorylated to glucose-6-phosphate (G-6-P) in a reaction catalyzed by the enzyme *hexokinase* (HK) and requiring one ATP molecule. Glucose-6-phosphate is then transferred into the glycolytic pathway for immediate energy production or reversibly converted to glucose-1-phosphate (G-1-P) and then glycogen for storage. Glycogen stores provide most of the glucose required for energy production during exercise. In the glycolytic pathway, G-6-P is phosphorylated to fructose-6-phosphate (F-6-P). Fructose-6-phosphate is then phosphorylated to fructose-1,6-bisphosphate (F-1,6-BP) in a reaction catalyzed by *phosphofructokinase* (PFK) and at the expense of one ATP molecule. Fructose-1,6-bisphosphate is subsequently split into the triose phosphate isomers, glyceraldehyde-3-phosphate (Gl-3-P) and dihydroxyacetone-phosphate (DiH-P). Dihydroxyacetone-phosphate is readily converted into Gl-3-P by *triose phosphate isomerase* (TPI). So one molecule of glucose or glycogen gives 2 molecules of Gl-3-P. Glyceraldehyde-3-phosphate then proceeds through a series of reactions with the end result being the production of pyruvate, ATP, NADH, water and hydrogen ions. The net reaction for the glycolytic pathway utilizing glucose is:

$$\text{Glucose} + 2Pi + 2ADP + 2\,NAD^+ \rightarrow 2\,\text{Pyruvate} + 2\,\text{ATP} + 2\,\text{NADH} + 2H^+ + 2H_2O$$

Under aerobic conditions the hydrogen atoms are transferred to the electron transport chain and pyruvate is transported into the mitochondrial matrix as a substrate for acetyl coenzyme A (acetyl CoA). Acetyl CoA then enters the TCA cycle by combining with oxaloacetate to form citrate. The normal function of the TCA cycle requires 3 NAD^+ and 1 FAD to accept hydrogen atoms during the oxidative conversion of citrate back to oxaloacetate. When O_2 is available, the NADH and $FADH_2$ are then reoxidized back to NAD^+ and FAD in the electron transport chain, thus replenishing the adenine dinucleotide stores and producing ATP (Fig. 14.2). The complete aerobic utilization of one mole of glucose generates 36–38 ATP. When O_2 is not available, pyruvate is converted to lactate as described later.

Fatty acid utilization

Following lipolysis, non-esterified fatty acids (NEFAs) are released into the circulation and are subsequently available as hydrogen donors for energy production in skeletal muscle. NEFAs likely diffuse into muscle cells down a concentration gradient (Hodgson, 1985) as well as being actively transported across the cell membrane. At the cytoplasmic surface of the outer mitochondrial membrane, the NEFAs are esterified (activated) enzymatically forming long-chain acyl CoA molecules. The acyl CoA molecules are then linked to carnitine and shuttled across to the matrix side of the inner mitochondrial membrane. In the mitochondria the acyl CoA molecules undergo a series of four reactions known as *beta oxidation*. With each cycle of beta oxidation two-carbon (C_2) units are sequentially removed from the acyl CoA molecule and acetyl CoA, NADH and $FADH_2$ are produced (see Fig. 14.2). NADH and $FADH_2$ subsequently donate their electrons in the electron transport chain generating ATP and being reoxidized to NAD^+ and FAD in the process. Acetyl CoA is utilized in the TCA cycle as previously described. The splitting of C_2 units from the parent acyl CoA molecule is repeated until the whole chain has been cleaved into the acetyl CoA molecules. The number of carbon atoms in the parent FA chain will determine the net energy yield from beta oxidation. Complete oxidation of one palmitic acid molecule produces 129 molecules of ATP.

Anaerobic phosphorylation

The pathways of anaerobic phosphorylation occur solely in the muscle cell cytoplasm, with no reactions in the mitochondria as there are for aerobic phosphorylation. With the initiation of exercise there is a lag period before oxidative energy production becomes an important source of ATP. During this time rapid supplies of ATP must still be available if muscular contraction is to continue. Stores of ATP in skeletal muscle are limited (4–6 mmol/kg wet muscle) and contribute little to the total energy supply (Lindholm & Piehl, 1974; McMiken,

1983). Until aerobic phosphorylation makes a substantial contribution to energy supply, rapid regeneration of ATP must occur in the absence of O_2. The anaerobic phosphorylation of ADP is achieved by three pathways: the phosphocreatine reaction, the myokinase reaction and anaerobic glycolysis. The former two pathways may be described as anaerobic alactic reactions because no lactate is produced as it is in the latter process (Clayton, 1991).

Phosphocreatine reaction

In this pathway the enzyme *creatine kinase* catalyzes a reversible reaction where creatine phosphate (CP or phosphocreatine) donates its high-energy phosphate to ADP producing ATP:

$$CP + ADP \xrightleftharpoons[]{\text{creatine kinase}} Creatine + ATP$$

In the gluteus medius muscle of Standardbreds, the size of the CP pool is estimated to be 15–20 mmol/kg wet muscle (Lindholm & Piehl, 1974; Lindholm, 1979). This source of ATP replenishment would support maximum intensity exercise for no more than a few seconds (Åstrand & Rodahl, 1986; Clayton, 1991).

Myokinase reaction

The *myokinase* enzyme catalyzes the synthesis of ATP and adenosine monophosphate (AMP) from two ADP molecules:

$$ADP + ADP \xrightleftharpoons[]{\text{myokinase}} ATP + AMP$$

At rest, this reaction proceeds at an approximately equal rate in both directions with little net ATP being produced. In working muscle, *AMP-deaminase* reduces AMP concentration by converting it to ionosine monophosphate (IMP) and ammonia. This provides the driving force for the myokinase reaction towards the production of ATP (McMiken, 1983). Again this pathway only has the capabilities of providing small amounts of ATP.

Anaerobic glycolysis

The anaerobic production of 2 molecules of pyruvate from 1 molecule of glucose or glycogen is identical to that described for aerobic glycolysis. In the absence of available O_2, pyruvate accepts hydrogen atoms from NADH and is converted to lactate, rather than being converted to acetyl CoA and entering the TCA cycle. The reaction is catalyzed by *lactate dehydrogenase* and the regeneration of NAD^+ during the reduction of pyruvate to lactate sustains glycolysis under anaerobic conditions (Fig.14.2). The net result of anaerobic gly-colysis is the production of 3 molecules of ATP from 1 molecule of glycogen or 2 molecules of ATP from 1 molecule of glucose. This form of energy production is relatively rapid compared to aerobic glycolysis but yields a significantly lower amount of ATP and sub-strates are limited.

Regulation of aerobic and anaerobic pathways

At all exercise levels both systems of energy supply are active; however, one will predominate, depending in par-ticular on the intensity and duration of the activity. A complex method of metabolic regulation controls the input of each pathway. Substrate and enzyme availability, end product concentrations and various feedback mecha-nisms contribute to pathway dynamics.

Oxygen supply to muscle and the ratio of ATP:ADP are the most significant regulators of the energy produc-ing pathways. While there is adequate O_2 available aero-bic phosphorylation persists, providing a driving force for substrate to enter the TCA cycle and produce high concentrations of citrate. Citrate retards the activity of PFK, the enzyme responsible for the irreversible conver-sion of F-6-P to F-1,6-BP in the glycolytic pathway. This has the effect of inhibiting glucose and glycogen metab-olism. Accumulation of glycolytic intermediates before the PFK step, including G-6-P, inhibits the activities of HK and phosphorylase, thus also dampening the gly-colytic pathway. High cellular concentrations of ATP (i.e. a high ATP:ADP ratio) also inhibits PFK activity. *Pyruvate kinase*, the third control site in glycolysis, is inhibited by ATP and activated by F-1,6-BP. When the relatively slow production of energy by oxidative phosphorylation is unable to meet the demands for ATP, the ATP:ADP ratio swings in favor of ADP and this in turn stimulates PFK and enhances glycolysis and the utilization of glucose and glycogen stores. The pyruvate produced is metabo-lized to lactate and this allows the reoxidization of NADH to NAD$^+$ for continued electron acceptance in the glycolytic pathway.

Control of the TCA cycle starts with regulation of the irreversible oxidative decarboxylation of pyruvate to acetyl CoA by *pyruvate dehydrogenase* (PDH). Acetyl CoA, NADH and ATP inhibit PDH activity. Once acetyl CoA is formed, its combination with oxaloacetate to produce citrate is inhibited by high concentrations of ATP. At least two other sites in the TCA cycle have regulatory mechanisms that respond to the cellular concentrations of ATP. Overall the rate of the TCA cycle is reduced when abundant ATP is present but it should also be remembered the TCA cycle operates only under aero-bic conditions because of the constant need for NAD$^+$ and FAD.

The rate of oxidative phosphorylation is regulated by the cellular ADP concentration. This is known as *respiratory control*. For electrons to flow through the elec-tron transport chain to O_2 the simultaneous phosphory-lation of ADP to ATP is usually required. When ATP is utilized ADP concentrations increase and therefore the rate of oxidative phosphorylation increases, assuming an adequate O_2 supply is available. So oxidative phosphory-lation is coupled to ATP utilization via the relative ADP concentration.

Enzymes in the beta oxidation pathway are inhibited by NADH and acetyl CoA; however, the rate of FA oxida-tion is determined greatly by substrate availability.

Energy pathway contributions in the exercising horse

The duration and intensity of exercise determine the metabolic requirements of muscle. At any given time the most effective combination of the various energy-pro-ducing pathways will occur and, again, it should be emphasized that no form of exercise by the horse is entirely aerobic or anaerobic in nature.

At the initiation of exercise, the immediate source of energy is locally available ATP (McMiken, 1983). As pre-viously noted, this supply of ATP is limited and rapidly depleted, so for exercise to continue ATP must be replenished by other processes. Creatine phosphate and the phosphocreatine pathway provide the next rapidly available ATP source; however, this energy supply is also of limited capacity. The myokinase reaction provides a further means of regenerating ATP but it is restricted to certain muscle fiber types and is used in anaerobic exer-cise only when these fibers are recruited (Meyer, *et al.*, 1980). The myokinase reaction is believed to have a minor role in energy production overall.

The glycolytic pathway with the production of pyruvate and lactate provides the main ongoing ATP source and reaches peak metabolism within about 30 seconds of the onset of exercise (McMiken, 1983). The delay in maximal glycolytic output is possibly due to the multiple and complex reactions required (McMiken, 1983). The large stores of glycogen in equine muscle (Lindholm & Piehl, 1974; Lindholm, *et al.*, 1974; Lindholm, 1979; Nimmo & Snow, 1983; Hodgson *et al.*, 1984) allow this pathway to provide an early consistent source of energy, but still there is a finite limit to this substrate.

Aerobic mechanisms for ATP replenishment repre-sent the most efficient means of substrate production. However, it is the slowest pathway to respond to exercise demands, owing to the cardiovascular lag in supplying O_2 to the cells and the intricacy of the reactions. Oxidative processes are in full production approximately 1 minute after the onset of exercise and then muscular

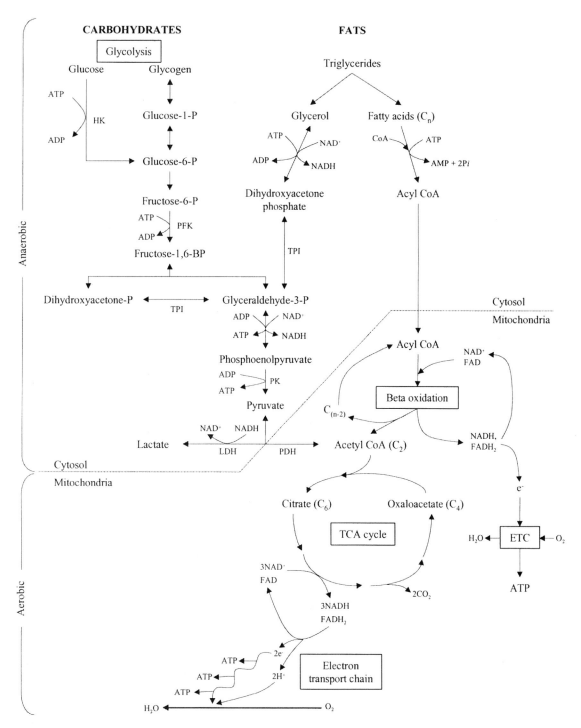

Fig. 14.2 Schematic representation of the principal components of glycolysis, fatty acid oxidation, the tricarboxylic acid (TCA) cycle and the electron transport chain (ETC) in a muscle cell. ATP: Adenosine triphosphate; ADP: adenosine diphosphate; P: phosphate; BP: bisphosphate; C: carbon; HK: hexokinase; PFK: phosphofructokinase; TPI: triose phosphate isomerase; PK: pyruvate kinase; LDH: lactate dehydrogenase; PDH: pyruvate dehydrogenase; CS: citrate synthase; NAD+, NADH: nicotinamide adenine dinucleotide; FAD, FADH₂: flavin adenine dinucleotide.

Table 14.1 Rates of glycogen utilization in horses performing various types of athletic activities. (Adapted from Hodgson, 1985.)

Type of exercise	Average speed (m/min)	Glycogen utilization*
Endurance ride		
40 km	187	1.47
110 km	173	0.41
160 km	180–135	0.69
Three-day event		
cross-country	293	4.08
phase (23.1 km)	(range 220–690)	
Trotting		
4 hr	300	0.50†(2.0)
1 hr	500	0.175†(7.0)
5 min	750	15.0†(60)
Racing		
506 m	870	149.4
800 m	920	191.9
1025 m	846	129.3
1200 m	960	126.5
1600 m	756	66.5
3620 m	684	18.8

Note: At speeds greater than 500 to 600 m/min, intensity of exercise is such that aerobic phosphorylation is unable to meet all the energy needs of the working muscle; therefore anaerobic glycolysis plays a major role in the supply of energy. As a result, glycogen utilization at these speeds and greater increases dramatically.
* Millimoles glucose units per kg muscle per min (dry weight); †Millimoles glucose units per kg muscle per min (wet weight). Approximate figures for dry weight values are presented in parentheses.

Table 14.2 Mean plasma non-esterified fatty acid concentration in horses performing various athletic activities. (Adapted from Hodgson, 1985.)

Type of exercise	Mean plasma NEFA concentration (µmol/L)
80 km endurance ride	
Pre-exercise	47
Post-exercise	1254
Three-day event (cross-country phase)	
Pre-exercise	156
After steeplechase and roads and tracks section	586
After cross-country section	324
Galloping (1.2 km)	
Pre-exercise	246
Post-exercise	279

(see Table 14.1). Galloping and bursts of intense exercise, such as during polo and jumping, rely heavily on anaerobic energy supply. The self-limiting nature of anaerobic power output (substrate exhaustion) means the horse can only maintain maximal speed for about 600 to 800 meters. After this distance, energy supply falls back to the slower aerobic pathways, necessitating a reduction in speed of exercise (McMiken, 1983; Hodgson, 1985).

ENERGY SUBSTRATES

Scientific data on the relationship between nutrition and equine performance has occupied the attention of many researchers in recent years; however, it is difficult to design controlled experiments that only isolate nutritional influences on performance. Subtle, yet important effects of nutritional alterations may go undetected partly because the power of statistical studies is limited by the small numbers of horses often used in experiments (Hintz, 1994). The relationship between energy and exercise is complex and inseparable. The amount of energy required depends on the type and duration of activity and the horse's body weight. Maintenance digestible energy (DE) requirements are linearly related to body weight (Pagan & Hintz, 1986a). During submaximal exercise energy expenditure is exponentially related to speed and proportional to the body weight of the riderless horse or the combined weight of the horse plus rider (Pagan & Hintz, 1986b). The method used by Pagan and Hintz (1986b) for calculating energy requirements was based only on the amount of work performed and may not account for any follow-on demands for energy in recovery that the work bout stimulates (Lawrence, 1990).

energy is more likely to be dependent on the rate of oxygen transport to the cells rather than substrate availability (McMiken, 1983).

At rest and during low-intensity exercise (walking and trotting), aerobic pathways provide most energy requirements after the initial lag period (Åstrand & Rodahl, 1986). At this exercise intensity the ratio of ATP to ADP will be high; PFK will therefore be inhibited and beta oxidation of fatty acids will provide the main method for ATP regeneration (Hodgson, 1985; Lawrence, 1990). Such is the case during endurance rides where it is well recorded that blood concentrations of NEFA increase and the glycogen utilization rate is low (Lucke & Hall, 1980; Snow et al., 1982; Hodgson, et al., 1983; Hodgson, 1985) (Tables 14.1 and 14.2).

As exercise intensity increases, ADP accumulates and this stimulates anaerobic glycolytic energy production with a dramatic increase in the use of CHO substrates

The stores of major fuels in the horse for muscular contraction are outlined in Table 14.3 as calculated by McMiken (1983). It is clear that 'fast' energy stores (i.e. ATP, creatine phosphate and glycogen) are limited despite the high capacity for glycogen storage in equine muscle. The primary dietary sources of energy stores for the horse are soluble and fiber CHOs and fats. Protein is considered to play a minor role as an energy source.

Carbohydrates

Absorbed CHO is immediately available as an energy source in the form of blood glucose. Muscle and liver provide the reservoirs for excess CHO where it is stored as glycogen. Numerous studies have documented the depletion of muscle glycogen stores that occurs with exercise in the horse (Lindholm, *et al.*, 1974; Lindholm, 1979; Hodgson, *et al.*, 1983; Nimmo & Snow, 1983, 1984). The rate of, and percentage, depletion that results is a function of the intensity and duration of exercise. Muscle glycogen utilization/minute is greatest at the faster speeds over shorter distances (Nimmo & Snow, 1983; Hodgson *et al.*, 1984) (Table 14.1) but the total percentage of glycogen depletion increases with increasing duration of exercise (Snow, *et al.*, 1981; 1982; Hodgson, *et al.*, 1983). Liver glycogen stores are also depleted significantly during exercise (Lindholm, *et al.*, 1974; Lindholm, 1979).

Fat

Assimilated fats are stored as triglycerides (uncharged esters of glycerol) in adipose tissue and muscle. Quantitatively, adipose tissue constitutes the largest energy store in the body (see Table 14.3). Triglyceride concentrations in muscle are considerably less than in fat (Lindholm, 1979). The triglycerides are highly concentrated stores of energy because they are reduced and anhydrous (Stryer, 1988). The initial event in the utilization of triglycerides as an energy substrate is their hydrolysis by lipases to glycerol and free fatty acids (FFA). Lipolysis is stimulated by epinephrine, norepinephrine, glucagon and adrenocorticotrophic hormone and inhibited by insulin. Glycerol is converted in a number of steps to Gl-3-P, which is an intermediate in both the glycolytic and gluconeogenic pathways. The FFAs undergo beta oxidation and enter the TCA cycle as previously described. Oleic, palmitic and linoleic acids represent the major FAs in the equine species (Robb *et al.*, 1972).

Fat has been shown to be the major energy substrate during low-intensity exercise. This is best evidenced by a decrease in the respiratory exchange ratio (R) (McMiken, 1983; Pagan *et al.*, 1987; Rose, *et al.*, 1991) and an increase in plasma NEFA concentrations (Lindholm, 1979; Rose *et al.*, 1980; Essen-Gustavsson *et al.*, 1991) that occurs with prolonged submaximal exercise. R is calculated by dividing the volume of carbon dioxide (CO_2) expired by the volume of O_2 consumed during exercise. R values around 0.7 indicate fat utilization whereas for CHO utilization the value is 1.0. Values within this range reflect various mixtures of FA and CHO metabolism. When anaerobic metabolism predominates R values will exceed 1.0 because lactate production is high, thereby adding to the CO_2 load to be eliminated.

Protein

Digested protein is absorbed from the small intestine as amino acids and small peptides. When amino acids are available in excess of the animal's requirements they may be broken down to provide energy. Degradation by deamination or transamination reactions occurs mostly in the liver, with the final product being acetyl CoA for utilization in the TCA cycle. Leucine, a branched-chain amino acid, may undergo oxidation directly in muscle (Lawrence, 1990). The contribution of amino acids to energy production during exercise is minor compared to that of CHO and FA (Åstrand & Rodahl, 1986), perhaps in the range of 1% to 15% (Lawrence, 1990). High protein diets (up to 16%) were once thought necessary to sustain the performance of mature equine athletes but now it is considered that approximately 10% protein in the diet is adequate (Snow, 1994).

Effects of dietary alterations on energy substrate utilization

Many published reports have described the effect that altering components of the normal diet has on substrate utilization and performance in the horse. The

Fuel	Energy	
	kJ	kcal
ATP	38	9
Creatine phosphate	188	45
Glycogen	75 300	17 988
Fat	640 000	152 889

Table 14.3 Energy stores. (Adapted from McMiken, 1983. ©EVJ Ltd.)

Note: These values are estimations for a 500 kg horse with a muscle mass of 206 kg (approximately 55 kg being locomotor muscles), adipose tissue of 25 kg and a liver of 6.5 kg.

consumption of large amounts of digestible CHO within a few hours of strenuous activity may depress the performance of that exercise (Åstrand & Rodahl, 1986). This is possible because insulin-stimulated uptake of blood glucose results in hypoglycemia and a greater dependence on muscle glycogen and therefore earlier onset of fatigue. Free FA mobilization is also inhibited by insulin. Frape (1988) summarized the effects of consumption of CHO or fat before or during exercise on metabolism, as depicted in Figure 14.3.

On the other hand, a lack of available CHO during submaximal exercise can also limit performance and there is strong evidence supporting the use of high CHO diets by humans for endurance exercise (Lawrence, 1990). In humans, muscle glycogen loading was achieved by performing intense exercise and then consuming a CHO-rich diet (Lindholm, 1979). Current practice is to combine a program of decreased activity with increased CHO consumption a few days before competition to achieve a glycogen load. Glycogen loading in horses has been accomplished but no obvious improvement in work performance has been demonstrated (Topliff *et al.*, 1983, 1985; Frape, 1988; Lawrence, 1990; Snow, 1994). Intravenous, but not oral, glucose supplementation has increased glycogen repletion rates after exercise (Snow *et al.*, 1987; Davie *et al.*, 1994, 1995; Snow, 1994). Although glycogen loading is not recommended in the horse adequate CHO intake must still be ensured (Hintz, 1994). A low CHO diet and regular exercise leads to glycogen depletion and decreased performance in horses (Topliff *et al.*, 1983, 1985). In a study where fit Standardbreds were exercised strenuously for 3 consecutive days to achieve a 55% depletion of the muscle glycogen store, anaerobic, but not aerobic, capacity was impaired (Lacombe *et al.*, 1999). However the association between glycogen depletion and impaired anaerobic metabolism is not conclusive as confounding effects of other exercise-induced changes on performance could not be eliminated (Lacombe *et al.*, 1999). When muscle glycogen was depleted by 22% there was no significant effect on performance of Thoroughbreds exercising at high intensities (Davie *et al.*, 1996).

A CHO supplement taken an hour or two before exercise does not seem to benefit endurance performance but intake of glucose during exercise may supplement waning plasma concentrations and delay onset of fatigue (Lawrence, 1990) (see Fig. 14.3).

The beneficial effects of feeding high-fat diets to horses remains shrouded in controversy. Differences in the condition of the horses, type of exercise, the length of the adaptation period to the diets, the type of fat used as the supplement, and the level of fat supplemented, particularly in relation to CHO, make comparing the published results difficult (Lawrence, 1990; Hintz, 1994). Many variations in study designs influence results obtained. Feeding an increased level of fat is suggested to cause metabolic adaptations that permits horses to preferentially utilize fat and spare glycogen during exercise but the evidence to support such a proposal is inconclusive (Lawrence, 1990; Hintz, 1994; Snow, 1994).

Interest in amino acid requirements of the performance horse is growing and there is a suggestion that improvements in oxidative capacity can be brought about by certain amino acid supplements (Lawrence, 1990; Hintz, 1994). Higher than necessary protein diets are often fed to performance horses but studies to indicate that this practice enhances exercise capabilities are lacking (Lawrence, 1990). On CHO-rich and fat-rich diets, plasma concentrations of glucose, ammonia, lactate, alanine and the muscle concentrations of G-6-P and lactate were higher at the end of exercise compared to normal diets (Essén-Gustavsson *et al.*, 1991). Higher pre-exercise muscle glycogen concentrations and FFA concentrations were present in the horses fed a CHO-rich diet when compared to the fat-rich and normal-diet fed periods. No significant difference in performance during trotting at submaximal intensity on a horizontal treadmill was detected between the three diets (Essén-Gustavsson *et al.*, 1991) with the average time to fatigue being 51 to 56 minutes. Whether or not the diets would alter performance in shorter or longer exercise periods remains unanswered. The effects on protein metabolism need to be further investigated as both the CHO-rich and the fat-rich diets were associated with significant increases in branched-chain amino acids in the plasma during and at the end of exercise compared to the normal diet (Essén-Gustavsson *et al.*, 1991). The resting plasma concentration of the branched-chain amino

---

Starch/glucose → ↑ insulin → ↓ catecholamines → ↓ lipolysis → ↑ glycogenolysis → ↓ endurance and speed?

Fats → ↑ citrate → ↓ phosphofructokinase → ↓ glycogenolysis

Glucose during exercise → ↑ glycemia, extends endurance time?

Fig. 14.3 Effect of consumption of carbohydrate or fat immediately before or during exercise on energy metabolism (Frape, 1988).

acids was increased 26% on the fat-rich diet but only 8% on the CHO-rich diet.

A 9% (control) or 18.5% (high) crude protein diet had no effect on hepatic or muscular glycogen utilization and did not affect exercise performance in Quarterhorses exercising at submaximal intensities (Miller-Graber *et al.*, 1991). Performance of Arabian endurance horses was not augmented by excessive protein in their diet (Hintz, 1983). In contrast, Standardbreds fed a high protein diet (20%) or high fat diet (15% soybean oil) showed greater muscle and liver glycogen utilization during prolonged exercise compared to when fed a control diet of 12% crude protein (Pagan *et al.*, 1987). During higher-intensity, shorter-duration exercise, glycogen utilization was less when horses were fed the high-protein or high-fat diets.

The timing of feeding and what to feed before exercise has considerable influence on the metabolic and physiological responses to exercise (Lawrence *et al.*, 1995; Harris & Graham-Thiers, 1999). In one study, it was concluded that feeding only hay shortly before exercise would not adversely affect performance but feeding grain would, and that therefore grain should be withheld (Pagan & Harris, 1999).

Of course, many other nutritional components not discussed in this chapter may play roles in equine performance. These include water, electrolytes, acid–base balance, minerals and vitamins.

ENERGY EXPENDITURE

Aerobic power

Oxygen uptake

The oxygen consumed by the body at a given time is a measure of the body's total aerobic metabolic rate and is termed the oxygen uptake ($\dot{V}O_2$). Units of measurement are usually milliliters of oxygen per kilogram of body weight per minute (ml/kg/min) or liters per minute (L/min), therefore representing a rate of consumption and not a finite capacity. The maximum rate of oxygen uptake is called the $\dot{V}O_{2max}$. Oxygen consumption by the body is principally a function of the cardiorespiratory system to supply oxygen and the capacity of end organs to utilize oxygen. The sequence of events is described as the *oxygen transport chain* (Fig. 14.4). It is influenced by the O_2 concentration in the air, ventilation of the lungs, diffusion of O_2 through the alveolar wall, circulatory perfusion of the lungs and affinity of hemoglobin (Hb) for O_2, distribution of O_2 to the periphery by the circulation, extraction by the end organ (muscle) and, finally, O_2 utilization by the mitochondria. A large number of physiological variables contribute to the capacity of the oxygen transport chain.

Oxygen uptake at rest and during submaximal exercise

At rest, $\dot{V}O_2$ is in the order of 3 to 5 ml/kg/min or 1.5 to 2.5 L/min for a 500 kg horse (Thornton *et al.*, 1983; Eaton, 1994). It can be difficult to accurately obtain a basal $\dot{V}O_2$ prior to exercise as often horses are excited in anticipation of impending activity. Therefore a resting $\dot{V}O_2$ level of 2 ml/kg/min may be more realistic (Eaton, 1994).

During submaximal exercise a number of factors will influence the level of $\dot{V}O_2$, including speed of exercise, load being carried, degree of incline on which exercise is being performed, duration of exercise, thermoregulation and track surface.

There is a well-established linear relationship between $\dot{V}O_2$ and the speed of exercise at submaximal intensities in horses (Hoyt & Taylor, 1981; Hörnicke, *et al.*, 1983; Evans & Rose, 1987, 1988a; Rose, *et al.*, 1990a; Eaton, 1994) and humans (Åstrand & Rodahl, 1986). When speed increases such that $\dot{V}O_{2max}$ is approached, this linear relationship is lost as $\dot{V}O_2$ plateaus and anaerobic sources of energy production become significant. In addition, if horses exercise at unnatural (extended or restricted) gaits the linear relationship will be lost due to a loss in economy of locomotion (Hoyt & Taylor, 1981; Eaton, 1994) (see later discussion).

Few equine sports are performed without the horse carrying an extra load in the form of a rider or driver. Oxygen consumption (or energy expenditure) increases in proportion to the load carried (Taylor *et al.*, 1980; Pagan & Hintz, 1986b; Thornton, *et al.*, 1987; Gottlieb-Vedi, *et al.*, 1991). Taylor and colleagues (1980) reported that when a 10% load was added to the horse when trotting, $\dot{V}O_2$ increased approximately 10% and this direct proportionality was consistent for loads between 7% and 27% of the horse's body mass. A direct proportionality between load and $\dot{V}O_2$ was also demonstrated for trotting rats, trotting and galloping dogs and running humans (Taylor *et al.*, 1980). As a consequence, small animals use more oxygen and expend more energy to carry each gram of a load a given distance than do large animals, be it their own body mass or an additional load carried. Pagan and Hintz (1986b) demonstrated that a 450 kg horse with a 50 kg rider would expend the same amount of energy as a 500 kg horse. Thornton and colleagues (1987) found no significant difference in the oxygen cost per kilogram per meter traveled between loaded and unloaded horses. The increase in $\dot{V}O_2$ due to load is achieved largely by an increase in ventilation until maximum tidal volume is approached (Thornton, *et al.*, 1987) and this is readily explained by the close and linear relationship between $\dot{V}O_2$ and pulmonary ventilation (Hörnicke *et al.*, 1983; Gottlieb-Vedi, *et al.*, 1991).

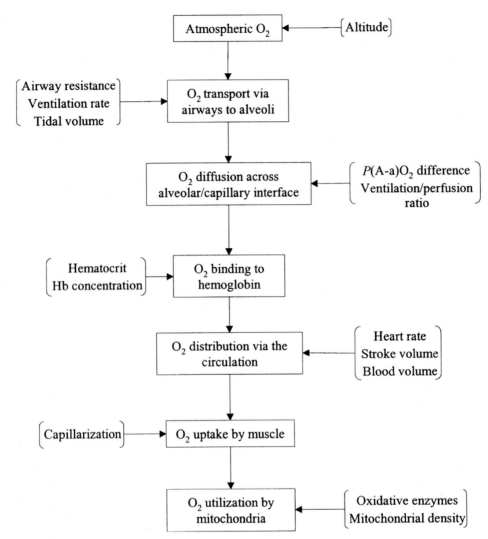

Fig. 14.4 The oxygen transport chain, indicating the steps in the transfer of oxygen from the inspired air to the final utilization by the mitochondria. Physiological variables that will influence the capacity of the oxygen transport chain are listed beside each step they affect. P (A–a) O_2: Alveolar – arterial oxygen pressure; Hb: hemoglobin

The implications for racing performance should be considered. A horse of less mass will expend proportionally less total energy to move the same distance when compared to a heavier horse.

The degree of incline on which exercise is being performed has a significant impact on $\dot{V}O_2$. For Standardbreds, trotting on a 6.25% inclined treadmill at an average speed of 5.2 m/s, $\dot{V}O_2$ increased from a mean of 17.7 L/min on the flat to 31.1 L/min on the slope (mean change of 13.4 L/min (76%, $p < 0.001$) (Thornton, *et al.*, 1987). The addition of a load when doing the inclined exercise did not significantly add to the oxygen cost of the exercise. Thoroughbreds exer-

cising on a treadmill at speeds of 1 to 13 m/s also showed a substantial increase in $\dot{V}O_2$ when the treadmill slope was elevated from 0% to 5% and 10% (Eaton *et al.*, 1995a). Exercising on a 10% slope can double the energy expenditure at some speeds. The terrain of endurance rides and cross-country tracks in three-day events ensure that much work up and down gradients will be performed and this will play a large role in determining energy expenditure. Little investigation has been done regarding the effect of a downhill gradient on energy expenditure in horses but in humans the energy cost of moving down a slope decreases up to a certain steepness and then becomes more expensive compared to level exercise (Åstrand & Rodahl, 1986). A similar response is likely for the horse.

The effect that duration of exercise has on $\dot{V}O_2$ has not been frequently investigated. Rose and Evans (1986) monitored cardiorespiratory and metabolic alterations during 90 minutes of submaximal exercise in Standardbreds. The horses trotted on a slope of 2% at 3 m/s. Many respiratory variables measured, including $\dot{V}O_2$, reached a steady state within 5 minutes of the start of exercise and remained stable for the duration of the exercise period. Oxygen consumption from 5 minutes onwards did not alter significantly until a slight decrease was identified at 90 minutes. It was proposed that fluid and electrolyte losses in the sweat, contributing to thermoregulatory and circulatory problems, would be key factors in the horse's ability to perform endurance activity (Rose & Evans, 1986). Naturally, the intensity of exercise will be a determinant of the duration of any activity.

The effect of temperature on $\dot{V}O_2$ will be a consequence of any impedence that altered thermoregulation may have on energy demands. Redistribution of cardiac output to skin for heat dissipation, fluid shifts and metabolic disturbances may all contribute to a less-efficient oxygen transport chain and therefore diminished performance. The optimum temperature range for oxygen utilization has yet to be established.

Track surfaces may affect the economy of locomotion due to altered stride patterns (change in frequency and length of stride) in slippery, uneven or 'heavy' conditions. Quantifying track effects on energy expenditure is difficult but Thoroughbreds and endurance horses have longer race times in heavy conditions (Eaton, 1994).

Maximum aerobic power

When $\dot{V}O_2$ no longer increases despite an increase in workload, the horse is defined as having reached $\dot{V}O_{2\ max}$. This value represents the 'gold standard' measure for maximum or peak aerobic power. Thoroughbred horses have mean $\dot{V}O_{2max}$ values around 150 to 170 ml/kg/min (Evans & Rose, 1987; Rose, *et al.*, 1990), easily twice the values for elite human athletes (69 to 85 ml/kg/min), 1.5 times those of greyhounds (100 ml/kg/min) and 3 times those of racing camels (51 ml/kg/min) (Derman & Noakes, 1994). Oxygen consumption can be calculated by the following equation:

$$\dot{V}O_2 = CO \times (a\text{-}v)O_2$$

where CO = cardiac output (heart rate × stroke volume) and $(a\text{-}v)O_2$ is the arterio-mixed venous oxygen difference.

The horse's tremendous ability to achieve a higher $\dot{V}O_{2max}$ than other athletic species is related to its massive heart rate response and ability to substantially augment its circulating red blood cell mass, and therefore oxygen-carrying capacity, during exercise (Thomas & Fregin, 1981). Trends indicate that top human athletes (for example, runners, cyclists and cross-country skiers) will generally have higher $\dot{V}O_{2max}$ values; however, there is considerable variation between athletes of similar ability (Derman & Noakes, 1994). In horses, a positive correlation between running speed and $\dot{V}O_{2max}$ has been described and this correlation became stronger as the distance ran increased (Harkins *et al.*, 1993). It was suggested that faster horses utilize more oxygen during maximal exercise intensity.

Anaerobic power

Anaerobic energy supply becomes significant when exercise intensity is at a level beyond that which aerobic pathways can accommodate alone. The faster glycolytic pathways may be recruited under two conditions: when energy demand increases so rapidly that the slower aerobic systems cannot match the supply rate required; or when the total energy demand exceeds what the aerobic pathways are capable of supplying at peak capacity. Workloads at intensities beyond that provided for by $\dot{V}O_{2max}$ have been referred to as *supramaximal* intensities. This level of energy utilization is experienced by racing Thoroughbreds, Standardbreds and Quarterhorses during competition. Shorter duration races, e.g. Quarterhorse 400 m sprints, rely predominately on the rapid supply of energy by anaerobic means (Eaton, 1994). Anaerobic power is considered a finite capacity and not a rate because the supply of substrates for anaerobic phosphorylation is limited. Factors that influence anaerobic capacity are depicted in Figure 14.5.

Theorizing that anaerobic capacity is a function of the area of type II fibers in the locomotor muscles, McMiken (1983) stated that to measure maximal anaerobic capacity one should calculate the type II fiber area and the activities of anaerobic pathway enzymes in the muscle. More recently, *maximum accumulated oxygen deficit* (MAOD) has been investigated as a measure of anaerobic capacity in horses (Eaton *et al.*, 1992, 1995b; Eaton, 1994) following preliminary studies indicating its usefulness in humans (Mebø *et al.*, 1988; Scott *et al.*, 1991).

Oxygen deficit refers to the deficiency in $\dot{V}O_2$ that occurs at the commencement of exercise until the responding cardiorespiratory system meets the oxygen demand of the tissues (Åstrand & Rodahl, 1986). The total oxygen deficit that accumulates during exercise at supramaximal intensities is the MAOD and this is the difference between the oxygen demand and the actual

$\dot{V}O_2$ achieved. The O_2 demand is calculated by extrapolating from the linear relationship between $\dot{V}O_2$ and speed at submaximal intensities (Fig. 14.6). To determine MAOD, horses on a treadmill are rapidly accelerated to speeds equivalent to supramaximal intensities (defined as a percentage of $\dot{V}O_{2max}$ measured in a pre-vious exercise test and extrapolated from the $\dot{V}O_2$ versus speed plot) (Rose *et al.*, 1988; Eaton *et al.*, 1995b). The $\dot{V}O_2$ is measured at frequent intervals until the horse fatigues. The area between the O_2 demand and the $\dot{V}O_2$ curve is the MAOD (Eaton *et al.*, 1995b) (Fig. 14.6).

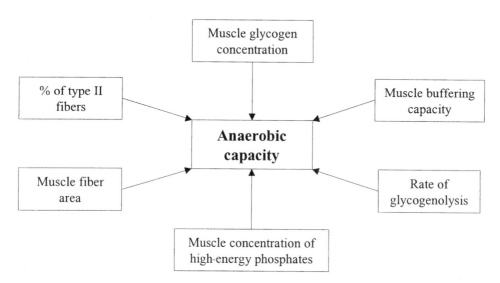

Fig. 14.5 Major factors contributing to anaerobic capacity.

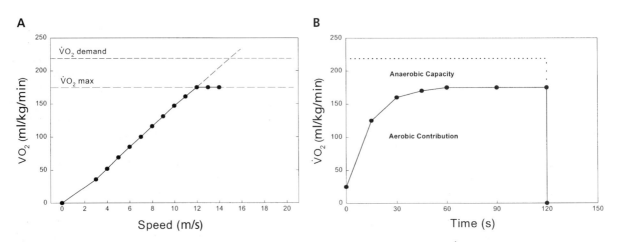

Fig. 14.6 Determination of maximum accumulated oxygen deficit (MAOD). **A** Initially, the $\dot{V}O_2$ versus speed plot is generated by performing a standardized incremental exercise test on an inclined treadmill. The $\dot{V}O_{2max}$ is 175 ml/kg/min, and for this horse to exercise at an intensity of 125% of $\dot{V}O_{2max}$, by extrapolation it can be seen that the $\dot{V}O_2$ demand would be 219 ml/kg/min. To exercise at this supramaximal intensity the horse would need to run at 15 m/s. **B** This figure demonstrates the relationship between $\dot{V}O_2$ and time for the horse exercising at 125% of $\dot{V}O_{2max}$. The previously calculated O_2 demand is drawn in as the dotted line at 219 ml/kg/min. At the onset of the exercise there is a lag in $\dot{V}O_2$ but it quickly reaches $\dot{V}O_{2max}$. The exercise ceases when the horse can no longer keep pace with the treadmill. The difference in the O_2 demand and the actual oxygen uptake is defined as the MAOD and is a measure of the anaerobic capacity. (Adapted from Eaton, 1994.)

For exercise intensities requiring 105% to 125% $\dot{V}O_{2max}$ the MAOD was similar at 31 ml O_2 equivalents per kg of bodyweight but the proportion of energy supplied by anaerobic processes increased from 14% to 30% (Eaton *et al.*, 1995b). $\dot{V}O_{2max}$ was not correlated to MAOD, suggesting that anaerobic capacity is unlikely to be dependent on the rate of oxygen uptake. Eaton and colleagues (1995b) proposed from their results that anaerobic energy supply would contribute less than 30% of the total energy input in Thoroughbred and Standardbred races, which is considerably lower than previously suggested (Bayly, 1985). Using peak blood or plasma lactate concentrations as an indicator of anaerobic capacity appears limited because of the many variables that affect lactate concentrations including rates of flux between fluid compartments.

In humans, the power vs. time-to-fatigue (P:TTF) relationship has been used as an accepted method for assessing anaerobic work capacity and this relationship has now been investigated in horses (Lauderdale & Hinchcliff, 1999). In humans, the relationship is best described by the hyperbolic equation:

$$t = W' / (P - \varnothing_{PA})$$

where t is the time to fatigue (s); P is power (watts); $\varnothing_{PA}$ is power asymptote, or critical power, which represents the maximum sustainable power output or anaerobic threshold, and W' is a constant representing anaerobic capacity or the finite amount of work that can be performed above $\varnothing_{PA}$ (Fig. 14.7). Similarly to humans, the P:TTF relationship in Standardbreds is best represented by a hyperbolic function; however, the technique needs to be validated against the more traditional MAOD measure of anaerobic capacity before its usefulness in horses as a predictor of fitness and anaerobic capacity can be investigated (Lauderdale & Hinchcliff, 1999). The P:TTF does not require collection of respiratory gases or blood for its calculation and this may be an advantage over the more intensive effort required to measure blood lactate concentrations or determine MAOD. However, currently a high-speed treadmill and multiple high-intensity exercise tests are still a prerequisite, as the ability to calculate the P:TTF relationship in field trials is yet to be determined.

For any measure of anaerobic capacity in the horse, it remains to be examined what relationship exists between performance and anaerobic capacity.

Anaerobic threshold

Anaerobic threshold is defined as the level of work or $\dot{V}O_2$ consumption just below that at which metabolic acidosis and the associated changes in pulmonary gas exchange

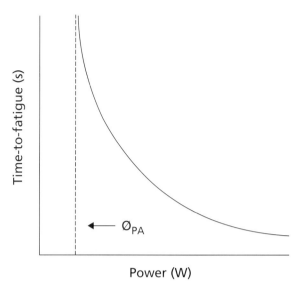

Fig. 14.7 Schematic of the hyperbolic relationship between power (*P*) and time-to-fatigue (*t*) represented by the equation $t = W'/(P - \varnothing_{PA})$. W': anaerobic capacity; $\varnothing_{PA}$: critical power; power units = watts (W).

occur (Wasserman *et al.*, 1973). It represents the transition when anaerobic means of energy supply becomes important during exercise. In humans, this level of work has been correlated with a blood lactate concentration of 4 mmol/L (Åstrand & Rodahl, 1986). As exercise intensity increases, lactate accumulation in the circulation rises in an exponential manner. Hence the anaerobic threshold has also been described as the *onset of blood lactate accumulation (OBLA)*. The velocity or intensity of work at which a blood lactate concentration of 4 mmol/L (V_{LA4}) is reached has been used to assess the relative fitness of horses and humans and their response to training (Persson, 1983; Thornton *et al.*, 1983; Rose *et al.*, 1990a; Auvinet, 1996). The V_{LA4} increases with training (Thornton *et al.*, 1983; Eaton *et al.*, 1999) and in general, the higher the V_{LA4} the fitter the horse (Rose & Hodgson, 1994a).

Anaerobic threshold and OBLA are determined during an incremental exercise test. Anaerobic threshold is identified by the point of non-linear increase in respiratory variables such as minute ventilation and carbon dioxide production (Wasserman *et al.*, 1973). It is assumed that this point is highly correlated with the OBLA but this may not be the case (Åstrand & Rodahl, 1986).

Postexercise oxygen consumption

At the cessation of exercise, O_2 continues to be consumed above basal rates as it declines in an exponential manner to resting levels. This is referred to as *excess post-exercise oxygen consumption* (EPOC) or *oxygen debt*. The EPOC may only account for a small fraction of the net total oxygen cost (NTOC) of exercise. In humans exercising at 30 to 70% of $\dot{V}O_{2max}$ for up to 80 minutes the EPOC was only 1.0 to 8.9% of the NTOC of the exercise (Gore & Withers, 1990). In the only comprehensive study to date in horses, Rose and colleagues (1988) measured oxygen debt as the area under the O_2 recovery curve following a bout of exhaustive exercise at an intensity equivalent to 120% of $\dot{V}O_{2max}$. Oxygen debt represented nearly 52% of the NTOC, which is dramatically higher than that in the previously quoted study of humans. This can be attributed in part to the very different exercise intensities performed in the two studies and the relative fitness of the subjects.

EPOC is considered to have an initial fast phase and then a slower phase. In the horse these phases were complete by 1.4 and 18.3 minutes, respectively, after supramaximal exercise (Rose *et al.*, 1988). The fast phase is associated with the resaturation of myoglobin and hemoglobin and the replenishment of the high-energy phosphagen pool (CP and ATP). Perhaps less than 1.5% of the EPOC was required to restore the muscle CP pool in the horse and this occurred at a slower pace than may have been expected (Rose *et al.*, 1988). Post-exercise tachycardia and tachypnea would also contribute small components to the EPOC because of increased consumption of O_2 by the myocardium and respiratory muscles until resting levels are reached. The slow phase is associated with the oxidation of lactate that accumulates during exercise. However, not all the lactate that is metabolized is accounted for by the EPOC and some is utilized in gluconeogensis and amino acid synthesis. A poor relationship existed between the restoration of muscle metabolites to pre-exercise levels and the recovery of $\dot{V}O_2$. Muscle and plasma lactate concentrations remained elevated after 60 minutes of recovery whereas $\dot{V}O_2$ had returned to near pre-exercise levels (Rose *et al.*, 1988).

A number of other factors considered associated with EPOC, including exercise-induced hyperthermia, have not been quantified in the horse.

Economy of locomotion

The *economy of locomotion* refers to the net energy cost in milliliters of O_2 per kilogram of body weight per meter traveled (ml O_2/kg/m). It is independent of speed and load (or body weight) (Eaton, 1994). There are conflicting reports on the values for economies of locomotion but the importance of gait in these studies needs to be recognized (Eaton, 1994). Horses on treadmills may be forced to work at defined speeds, and in doing so, utilize extended or restricted gaits that might alter the true cost

of locomotion they would otherwise naturally incur if allowed to control their own pace. Thorton and colleagues (1987) have reported values of 0.122 ml O_2/kg/m for speeds of 4.5 to 6.25 m/s and 0.124 ml O_2/kg/m for speeds of 6.5 to 8.14 m/s obtained on a horizontal plane. These results are similar to the 0.133 ml O_2/kg/m that can be derived from the results of Taylor and coworkers (1980) for a 119 kg pony working at 3.11 m/s. Eaton and colleagues (1995a) recorded a range of 0.10 to 0.16 ml O_2/kg/m at speeds of 5 to 13 m/s on a horizontal treadmill. Exercising on a positively inclined treadmill will increase the oxygen cost of work about 2 to 2.5 times that measured on a flat plane, depending on the steepness of the slope (Thornton, *et al.*, 1987; Eaton *et al.*, 1995a). When averaging a range of speeds for each gait, Hönicke and colleagues (1983) reported higher values for the walk (0.21 ml O_2/kg/m) and for the trot and gallop (0.19 ml O_2/kg/m) for horses exercising on the track. By averaging the economies of a number of speeds, a higher oxygen cost can be expected as values will include less-efficient gait velocities than that at which the horses may be required to exercise. (Hörnicke *et al.*, 1983).

It is well documented that horses will choose a gait at any speed that results in the least possible expenditure of energy (Hoyt & Taylor, 1981). Ponies (110–170 kg) were trained to walk, trot and gallop, and to extend their gait on command on a treadmill. Rates of oxygen consumption increased curvilinearly with speed for walking and trotting. The maximum speed of the treadmill prevented sufficient data from being obtained for galloping velocities. Gait transition occurred at speeds when the oxygen consumption was similar for the two gaits, but when the ponies were forced to exercise at an extended gait beyond the normal range of speeds, oxygen consumption was higher (Hoyt & Taylor, 1981). Thus, there was a speed for each gait where the energy cost of locomotion was minimal and this cost was similar for the walk, trot and gallop (Hoyt & Taylor, 1981) (Fig. 14.8). So, at the optimal speed of each gait, the amount of energy consumed to move a given distance is much the same. When a horse was allowed to move at its natural pace freely, it did so by selecting speeds within each gait around the most energy efficient speed (Hoyt & Taylor, 1981). The optimal value for economy was similar to the 0.122 to 0.133 ml O_2/kg/m values derived elsewhere for flat treadmill exercise (Taylor *et al.*, 1980; Thornton, *et al.*, 1987).

The effect of the training and athletic activities horses are subjected to needs to be considered with regard to the economy of locomotion. Endurance horses forced to use extended gaits for prolonged periods may fatigue more rapidly than if they were to move at their natural speed for each gait. Clearly, it becomes a matter of

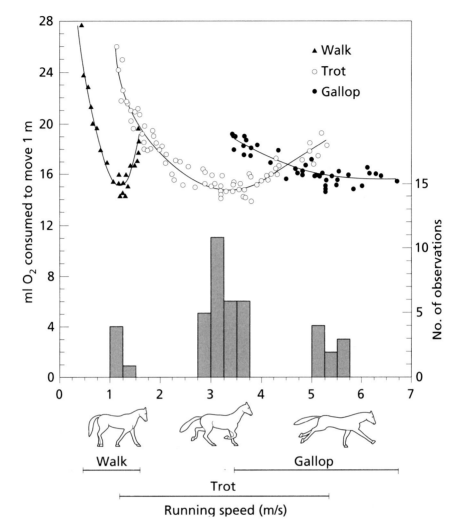

Fig. 14.8 Economy of locomotion. The oxygen cost to move a unit distance (rate of oxygen consumption divided by speed) declined to a minimum and then increased with increasing speed in a walk and trot. It also declined to a minimum in a gallop but the treadmill did not go fast enough to observe any increase at higher galloping speeds. The minimum oxygen cost to move a unit distance was almost the same in all three gaits. The histogram shows gaits when a horse was allowed to select its own speed while running on the ground. The three speeds chosen coincided with the energetically optimal speed for each gait. (From Hoyt & Taylor, 1981. Reprinted with permission from *Nature*; ©Macmillan Magazines.)

achieving the right balance of speed and energy consumed to complete the distances and be successful in such events.

Standardbred trotters and pacers may be able to work at a wide range of speeds using a single gait without any loss of economy (Thornton, *et al.*, 1987; Eaton, 1994).

Fatigue

Fatigue is a complex and intricate physiological response to exercise, leading to the inability to sustain further activity at the current intensity. Fatigue can be categorized as structural, acute or chronic. Structural fatigue refers to biomechanical failure of tissues, for example tendons, ligaments and bone, that inadequately adapt to the stresses placed upon them. Chronic fatigue is a function of prolonged conditions such as chronic anemia and starvation. Acute fatigue is directly related to energy production in the muscle and occurs in events requiring maximal work effort for short periods, e.g. Thoroughbred or Standardbred racing. It has been labeled *anaerobic fatigue* (McMiken, 1983) and has different causal factors to those that limit aerobic performance in endurance type events. Fatigue appears to involve central (psychologic/neurologic) and peripheral (muscular) contributions (Hodgson & Rose, 1994a). Overtrained horses can become listless and 'sour' and decline in performance and this may be partly a manifestation of psychological fatigue. Peripheral causes of fatigue have been studied more widely as they are easier to define.

Fatigue in response to high-intensity exercise is likely due to a combination of factors including depletion of the phosphagen pool (ATP and CP), decreased intracellular pH, and possibly accumulation of lactate (McMiken, 1983; Hodgson, 1985; Hodgson & Rose, 1994a; Essén-Gustavsson et al., 1999). The main event appears to be a reduction in the concentration of ATP. Acidity can impair the respiratory capacity of muscle and have a direct effect on the contractile apparatus. In addition, acidosis and increased muscle temperature could be associated with impaired sarcoplasmic reticulum function. Finally, altered electrolyte gradients (potassium and calcium) will add to the overall deleterious effects on muscle metabolism.

During prolonged, submaximal exercise, hyperthermia, altered fluid and electrolyte balance, and fuel depletion have all been considered as contributors to fatigue during this type of exercise (Lucke & Hall, 1980; Snow et al., 1982; Hodgson, 1985; Hodgson & Rose, 1994a). Performance capacity or onset of fatigue in horses and humans has been correlated with a depletion in glycogen stores in working muscle (Snow et al., 1981, 1982; McMiken, 1983; Åstrand & Rodahl, 1986). A decline in extracellular glucose concentrations may also be important. However, fatigue or reduced muscle power occurs before the complete depletion of any substrate and it is the rate of ATP production that appears crucial. Neural fatigue in short events is considered very unlikely but may be important in endurance events (McMiken, 1983). However, in supramaximal exercise lasting only a few seconds, fatigue may be related to an inability of the neuromuscular junction to maintain the propagation of excitatory action potentials into the muscle fibers.

TRAINING PROGRAMS

The implications of the various energy supply pathways are far-reaching in terms of specific training programs for horses competing in different athletic events. An understanding of the patterns of energy substrate supply and utilization in different althetic events allows tailored training strategies to be adopted to maximize the adaptations in various body systems. Although no activity is exclusively aerobic or anaerobic in nature, aerobic energy production is vital in all cases. Hence an emphasis on establishing a good 'aerobic foundation' is considered paramount in any training program.

Even today, there is probably more desire to use training methods that have 'stood the test of time' over many years and have been passed on from generation to generation, than to develop a training program based on current scientific knowledge. Naturally, the successful training of any athlete relies on far more than simple physiologic adaptations to exercise. The maintenance of motivation, the skill of predicting a horse's tolerance levels and the fostering of that psychogenic factor, 'the will to win,' are vitally important and unquantifiable. The ability to train a horse to its limits without causing it to 'break down' is necessary. These 'human factor' components of any training program separate the elite trainers from their average peers.

Training may be of a continuous or intermittent nature. Continuous training, also known as endurance training, refers to exercise performed in a single bout that can vary in intensity and duration. Intermittent or interval training implies a series of intense work sessions interspersed with rest periods of varying duration. The intensity and duration of training are two variables that must be considered in any training program. It seems that the shorter the race the more consideration should be given to the intensity of training and the longer the race the more important endurance training becomes (Bayly, 1985). A basic model of training incorporates three phases (Derman & Noakes, 1994; Evans, 1994);

1. a foundation phase
2. a cardiovascular or aerobic phase
3. an anaerobic interval phase.

The foundation phase is considered continuous or endurance-type training and is vital for the cardiovascular and musculoskeletal systems to make early adaptations to the stresses placed upon them. With each next phase more intense, shorter runs are included in the program.

Improvement in $\dot{V}O_{2\,max}$ is independent of submaximal training intensity when horses are exercised for the same distance (Knight, et al., 1991; Eaton et al., 1999) and as little as 10 to 14 days of training is all that is required to achieve an increase in aerobic capacity (Knight, et al., 1991; Geor, et al., 1999). Geor and colleagues (1999) reported an 8.9% increase in $\dot{V}O_{2max}$ after 10 days of moderate-intensity training at 55% $\dot{V}O_{2max}$ for 60 min each day. Concurrent metabolic studies revealed a decrease in muscle glycogenolysis and anaerobic metabolism but no concomitant increase in muscle oxidative enzyme activities. So, although there was improvement in the aerobic capacity of the horses the mechanisms underlying it were not clear (Geor, et al., 1999). Guy and Snow (1977) reported an increase in muscle glycogen content and an increase in aerobic and anaerobic enzymes in response to training.

Various conditioning programs studied by Gansen and colleagues (1999) revealed significant increases in muscle glycogen storage in Haflinger stallions after low-intensity, long-duration exercise but not after higher-intensity, shorter-duration exercise. This adaptation in the middle gluteal muscle fibers was only noted at 6 cm depth and not at 2 cm depth, demonstrating the variable response of different regions of muscle fibers to training.

Scientific studies comparing conventional and interval training techniques for Thoroughbreds have been infrequently reported. In one study it was concluded that interval training led to higher lactate production and increased plasma lactate clearance during a 1000 m sprint compared to conventionally trained horses and this was equated with greater anaerobic capacity (Harkins et al., 1990). An earlier study failed to identify significant differences in the response to conventional and interval training techniques but the total slow- and fast-work distances undertaken were the same in both training schedules (Gabel et al., 1983).

The various physiologic adaptations that occur in response to training in the horse have been extensively reviewed elsewhere (Hodgson & Rose, 1994b).

MEASURING ENERGY EXPENDITURE

Until the 1980s, some veterinarians and horse trainers relied on the complete blood count and the plasma or serum biochemistry panel in an attempt to assess clinical and subclinical disease in performance horses. Evaluation of resting and/or post-exercise hematology and biochemistry to assess fitness capacity or response to training is of limited use.

A range of equipment to determine various performance indices has now been available and extensively used for the last decade and a half, including treadmills, heart rate meters and rapid lactate analyzers.

Treadmills

The first use of a high-speed equine treadmill for experimental purposes was in 1960 in Stockholm, Sweden (Sloet van Oldruitenborgh-Oosterbaan & Clayton, 1999). Early studies focused on metabolic variables with locomotor studies becoming more common in later years. During the last 15 years, equine treadmills have been installed in many university veterinary colleges and equine research centers for ongoing studies of exercise physiology and for the diagnosis of poor performance conditions, in particular dynamic upper airway obstructions. In addition, treadmills are now commonly used in training stables as a complementary training tool and, by stud farms, to walk and trot yearlings for conditioning prior to sale.

Most current knowledge concerning the physiologic response of the horse to exercise has come from numerous treadmill-based studies. Cardiovascular, respiratory, metabolic, hematologic, thermoregulatory, hormonal, musculoskeletal and locomotory changes in the horse, exercising over various intensities and durations, have been thoroughly examined. The vast accumulation of literature appears to be almost exponential as evidenced by the recent publication of papers from the 5th International Conference on Equine Exercise Physiology (Equine Veterinary Journal, Supplement 30, 1999).

Treadmill exercise is not equivalent to track exercise (Sloet van Oldruitenborgh-Oosterbaan & Clayton, 1999). The effects of air movement, track surface and rider impact are not duplicated on the treadmill and horses have no forward momentum on the treadmill because the moving belt provides the driving force (Rose & Hodgson, 1994b). So the amount of work performed by a horse on the treadmill is quantitatively different from work on the track. For a track exercise test, horses require only a short habituation period and can be worked in their standard manner, often with the usual rider or driver (Sloet van Oldruitenborgh-Oosterbaan & Clayton, 1999). Nevertheless, there are clear advantages to studying responses to exercise on the treadmill. A consistent exercise surface, controlled environmental conditions, precise control over intensity of exercise and ease of measuring physiologic variables to monitor fitness are all strong indications to pursue treadmill-based studies (Rose & Hodgson, 1994b; Sloet van Oldruitenborgh-Oosterbaan & Clayton, 1999). By positively inclining the treadmill, a horse can be exercised at its maximum power output at a relatively slower speed than if it were on a flat plane (Sexton & Erickson, 1990). This potentially reduces the risk of musculoskeletal injury because speeds above 12 to 13 m/s are unnecessary, but the steeper the slope the more an adverse impact is likely on normal biomechanical function. It is suggested that muscles may be recruited differently when the horse is exercised on a slope versus the flat (Sloet van Oldruitenborgh-Oosterbaan & Barneveld, 1995). A slope of 10% (5.71°) is recommended for treadmill testing as most horses will reach their maximum oxygen uptake at speeds of 10 to 12 m/s compared with 14 to 15 m/s on the flat (Rose & Hodgson, 1994b). It is desirable to standardize the incline that exercise tests are performed on, to allow better comparison between studies from different institutions (Sloet van Oldruitenborgh-Oosterbaan & Clayton, 1999).

Significant differences in locomotor and metabolic variables have been reported in studies comparing track versus treadmill exercise (Sloet van Oldruitenborgh-Oosterbaan & Clayton, 1999) and future research may continue to elucidate the etiology of these differences. Currently, treadmill tests are preferable for most research purposes but track tests may be of greater importance when examining locomotor variables and fitness of sport horses (Sloet van Oldruitenborgh-Oosterbaan & Clayton, 1999).

Oxygen consumption

The measurement of $\dot{V}O_2$ by the exercising body is the single most important step in the evaluation of exercise capacity. In the horse, various mask systems have been investigated and an open-flow mask without valves is the currently accepted apparatus. Bayly and colleagues (1987) compared flow-through mask systems with valved masks and found a funnel-shaped, valveless flow-through system to have the least impedence on airway function at flow rates of 6300 L/min. Evans and Rose (1988b) investigated a valved mask system and showed a negative influence on arterial blood gases, namely an exacerbation of the exercise-induced hypercapnea and hypoxemia. Respiratory frequency was lower when the mask was worn but arterial acid–base tensions and heart rate were minimally affected. The respiratory effects were attributed to alveolar hypoventilation (Evans & Rose, 1988b). The most appropriate exercise test to determine $\dot{V}O_{2max}$ is a standardized rapid incremental test on a 10% treadmill incline (Rose et al., 1990b) and the repeatability of results is good (Evans & Rose, 1988a; Seeherman & Morris, 1990). Oxygen uptake can improve quickly with the onset of training but relative training intensity, when kept constant and submaximal, does not appear to effect the rate of change of $\dot{V}O_{2\,max}$ (Knight, et al., 1991).

Lactate analysis

Response to training and the relative intensity of an exercise session can be assessed by the simple measurement of blood or plasma lactate, during or after exercise (Milne et al., 1977). Lactate increases at an exponential rate with increasing workload, and fitter horses show a slower accumulation during submaximal exercise. The V_{LA4} is often calculated to compare fitness between horses and response to training. Classically, the V_{LA4} has been considered to approximate the anaerobic threshold, mirroring the metabolic transition from predominantly aerobic to anaerobic energy sources, and this calculated value increases with improved fitness (Hodgson & Rose, 1994b). Plasma lactate values are 30 to 50% higher than whole blood lactate (Rose & Hodgson, 1994b). However, because of great inter-individual variation in lactate distribution between plasma and red blood cells (RBCs) after exercise and in the rate of lactate influx into RBCs, there is no consistent relationship between the two lact-

ate reservoirs (Pösö et al., 1995; Vaihkonen & Poso, 1998). Recent evidence suggests that whole blood lactate concentrations should be measured when estimating the accumulation of lactate from exercising muscle, to minimize variation due to factors that influence transport of lactate from plasma into RBCs (Väihkönen, et al., 1999). If whole blood is to be used, the sample should be immediately deproteinized to halt post-collection production of lactate within the RBC (Ferrante, 1995); however, storage at 0°C for up to an hour before deproteinization does not effect the lactate concentration (Ferrante & Kronfeld, 1994).

Whether plasma or whole blood lactate is assessed one method should be adhered to by the laboratory or investigator, to reduce variability in measurements. Post-exercise blood and plasma lactate concentrations were significantly correlated with race performance for Thoroughbreds undergoing a submaximal treadmill exercise test (Evans, et al., 1993). Harkins and colleagues (1993) found the V_{LA4} to be one of the best correlates of running speed for Thoroughbreds. This was a negative correlation, indicating that faster horses attained a plasma lactate of 4 mmol/L at a lower velocity than did slower horses. The faster horses also had the highest peak lactate concentrations, implying that plasma lactate concentrations of faster horses rise more rapidly and to higher levels than do those of slower horses. However, no correlation was found between performance and post-exercise blood or plasma lactate concentrations taken after maximal activity during a field trial (Evans, et al., 1993).

Heart rate

Heart rate is measured to monitor exercise intensity on the basis that there is a linear relationship between heart rate and work performed in the range of 120 to 210 beats per minute (bpm) (Persson, 1983). The velocity at a heart rate of 200 bpm (V_{200}) has been used to assess fitness and response to training but care should be taken when evaluating this variable (Rose & Hodgson, 1994a). Conflicting reports on the correlation between V_{200} and $\dot{V}O_{2max}$ have been published (Evans & Rose, 1987; Rose et al., 1990a) but this is attributed to the dissimilar numbers of horses tested in each study and it is accepted that the two variables are significantly positively correlated. The usefulness of V_{200} to assess response to training in the field using Thoroughbreds has been confirmed (Kobayashi, et al., 1999). A number of heart rate meters are available with generally good accuracy (Evans & Rose, 1986; Rose & Hodgson, 1994b; Holopherne, et al., 1999). Telemetry electrocardiography is the favored technique in treadmill laboratories. To achieve accurate heart rate values good electrode contact with the skin is required, and this can be difficult to maintain in the galloping horse. Electrode gels can enhance contact and glue adhesives can hold electrode casings firmly on the skin (Hill *et al.*, 1977; Rose & Hodgson, 1994b).

Blood gases

Respiratory disorders that may interfere with the transport of oxygen from the atmosphere to the pulmonary vasculature can be assessed for their significance by measuring arterial blood gas tensions. Arterial blood samples are normally collected from a catheterized transverse facial artery during a treadmill exercise test. Values should be corrected for central venous blood temperature. Hypoxemia and hypercapnea are recognized responses to high-intensity exercise (Bayly *et al.*, 1983; 1987) and the severity of hypoxemia increases with training (Christley *et al.*, 1997). There is a strong negative correlation between minimum arterial oxygen content and VO_{2max} in trained horses, indicating the importance of assessing both variables before interpreting blood gas data (Christley *et al.*, 1997). Horses with functional airway obstructions may have a greater degree of hypoxemia or hypercapnea when approaching, and at, maximal exercise intensities compared to normal horses (Rose & Hodgson, 1994a). The degree of hypoxemia in normal Thoroughbreds performing a standardized treadmill exercise test was not correlated with their running speed on an 800 m track (Harkins, *et al.*, 1993).

Blood volume

The Evans blue dye technique of measuring the plasma volume (PV) in horses was first described by Persson in 1967. It is a simple and highly reproducible technique with a coefficient of variation of 3–4%. To ensure an accurate assessment of the plasma volume, the splenic erythrocyte pool must be mobilized either by intense exercise or an epinephrine injection. A post-exercise hematocrit is preferred and is typically measured for blood volume calculations. A major determinant of the oxygen-carrying capacity of the horse is the red cell volume (RCV) which can be calculated from the hematocrit and PV. Evaluation of the hematocrit alone as an indicator of RCV can be misleading due to variations in PV. Plasma volume increases in response to training in all species studied (Oscai, *et al.*, 1968; Persson, 1968; McKeever *et al.*, 1985, 1987). Total blood volume (TBV) has been positively correlated with fitness level and may be a useful measure of such as long as variations due to body size, age, sex and breed of horse are taken into account (Persson, 1968). A significant positive correlation has also been found between TBV and racing performance in Standardbred trotters (Persson, 1968). During a single high-intensity exercise bout TBV increases substantially in the horse mainly due to the release of red cells from the splenic reservoir. It remains to be elucidated whether PV or RCV can be used to predict performance in horses.

Muscle biopsy

Needle biopsy of skeletal muscle was first described in the horse 25 years ago by Lindholm and Piehl (1974). The middle gluteal muscle was used as the preferred site of sampling and continues to be favored today although other muscles, e.g. the semitendinosis and biceps femoris, have been examined. Examination of muscle tissue has allowed fiber typing and evaluation of responses to exercise and training, particularly alterations in substrate utilization and the oxidative capacity of muscle. One concern with the use of muscle biopsies is the degree of variation in samples from very similar sites. A standardized approach to the muscle biopsy procedure in French trotters has been described, incorporating anatomical landmarks, age, sex and hip width of the horses (Valette *et al.*, 1999). Interestingly, muscle fiber composition has been correlated with locomotor patterns in horses (stride frequency and stride length) (Rivero & Clayton, 1996) and therefore may indirectly influence the economy of locomotion.

CONCLUSION

It is imperative that anyone with an interest in the equine as an athlete should understand energy production and utilization in the horse. Both aerobic and anaerobic pathways of energy supply are necessary for all forms of exercise. In recent years evidence suggests that the aerobic system has a much greater role to play than previously thought, in short-duration, supramaximal exercise bouts. The effect of nutrition on performance has been heavily investigated but continues to be an area of considerable controversy. Comparison between studies is difficult and at this time meaningful conclusions cannot be drawn. Well thought-out training programs tailored to the horse's particular activity are important for preparing the horse for athletic endeavors. Every program should have an initial low-intensity foundation phase to allow body tissues to adapt to the stresses placed upon them. The economy of locomotion refers to the optimal gait at a given speed of exercise at which the energy cost is least and this gait is naturally chosen by freely moving horses. The measurement of VO_{2max} remains the single most important assessor of a horse's relative fitness.

Fundamental differences between track and treadmill exercise tests make both methods of performance evaluation attractive; however, because of more controllable conditions treadmill exercise tests continue to be favored. The emphasis is on further development and evaluation of procedures that can be readily and reliably applied to the field situation.

REFERENCES

Åstrand, P.-O. and Rodahl, K. (1986) *Textbook of Work Physiology: Physiological Bases of Exercise*, 3rd edn. New York: McGraw-Hill Book Company.

Auvinet, B. (1996) Performance testing and improvement in human athletes. *Pferdeheilkunde* **12**(4): 455–456.

Bayly, W.M. (1985) Training programs. *Vet. Clin. N. Amer.: Equine Pract.* **1**(3): 597–610.

Bayly, W.M., Grant, B.D., Breeze, R.G. and Kramer, J.W. (1983) The effects of maximal exercise on acid-base balance and arterial blood gas tension in Thoroughbred horses. In: Snow, D.H., Persson, S.G.B. and Rose, R.J. (eds) *Equine Exercise Physiology* . Cambridge UK: Granta Editions, pp. 400–407.

Bayly, W.M., Schulz, D.A., Hodgson, D.R. and Gollnick, P.D. (1987) Ventilatory responses of the horse to exercise: effect of gas collection systems. *J. Appl. Physiol.* **63**(3): 1210–1217.

Cain, D.F. and Davies, R.E. (1962) Breakdown of adenosine triphosphate during a single contraction of working muscle. *Biochem. Biophys. Res. Comm.* **8**(5): 361–366.

Christley, R.M., Hodgson, D.R., Evans, D.L. and Rose, R.J. (1997) Effects of training on the development of exercise-induced arterial hypoxemia in horses. *Am. J. Vet. Res.* **58**(6): 653–657.

Clayton, H.M. (1991) Energy production. In: Clayton, H.M. (ed.) *Conditioning Sport Horses.* Saskatoon: Sport Horse Publications, pp. 31–43.

Davie, A.J., Evans, D.L., Hodgson, D.R. and Rose, R.J. (1994) The effects of an oral glucose polymer on muscle glycogen resynthesis in standardbred horses. *J. Nutr.* **124**: 2740S–2741S.

Davie, A.J., Evans, D.L., Hodgson, D.R. and Rose, R.J. (1995) Effects of intravenous dextrose infusion on muscle glycogen resynthesis after intense exercise. *Equine Vet. J.*, **18**(Suppl.): 195–198.

Davie, A.J., Evans, D.L., Hodgson, D.R. and Rose, R.J. (1996) Effects of glycogen depletion on high intensity exercise performance and glycogen utilization rates. *Pferdeheilkunde* **12**(4): 482–484.

Derman, K.D. and Noakes, T.D. (1994) Comparative aspects of exercise physiology. In: Hodgson, D.R. and Rose, R.J. (eds) *The Athletic Horse: Principles and Practice of Equine Sports Medicine.* Philadelphia: WB Saunders, pp. 13–25.

Eaton, M.D. (1994) Energetics and performance. In: Hodgson, D.R. and Rose, R.J. (eds) *The Athletic Horse: Principles and Practice of Equine Sports Medicine.* Philadelphia: WB Saunders, pp. 49–61.

Eaton, M.D., Rose, R.J., Evans, D.L. and Hodgson, D.R. (1992) The assessment of anaerobic capacity of Thoroughbred horses using maximal accumulated oxygen deficit. *Aust. Equine Vet.* **10**(2): 86.

Eaton, M.D., Evans, D.L., Hodgson, D.R. and Rose, R.J. (1995a) Effect of treadmill incline and speed on metabolic rate during exercise in Thoroughbred horses. *J. Appl. Physiol.* **79**(3): 951–957.

Eaton, M.D., Evans, D.L., Hodgson, D.R. and Rose, R.J. (1995b) Maximum accumulated oxygen deficit in Thoroughbred horses. *J. Appl. Physiol.* **78**(4): 1564–1568.

Eaton, M.D., Hodgson, D.R., Evans, D.L. and Rose, R.J. (1999) Effects of low- and moderate-intensity training on metabolic responses to exercise in Thoroughbreds. *Equine Vet. J.* **30**(Suppl.): 521–527.

Equine Exercise Physiology 5 (1999) *Equine Veterinary Journal Supplement 30.* Newmarket: Equine Veterinary Journal Limited.

Essén-Gustavsson, B., Blomstrand, E., Karlstrom, K., Lindholm, A. and Persson, S.G.B. (1991) Influence of diet on substrate metabolism during exercise. In: Persson, S.G.B., Lindholm, A. and Jeffcott, L.B. (eds) *Equine Exercise Physiology 3.* Davis, California: ICEEP Publications, pp. 288–298.

Essén-Gustavsson, B., Gottlieb-Vedi, M. and Lindholm, A. (1999) Muscle adenine nucleotide degradation during submaximal treadmill exercise to fatigue. *Equine Vet. J.* **30**(Suppl.): 298–302.

Evans, D.L. (1994) Training Thoroughbred racehorses. In: Hodgson, D.R. and Rose, R.J. (eds) *The Athletic Horse: Principles and Practice of Equine Sports Medicine.* Philadelphia: WB Saunders, pp. 393–397.

Evans, D.L. and Rose, R.J. (1986) Method of investigation of the accuracy of four digitally-displaying heart rate meters suitable for use in the exercising horse. *Equine Vet. J.* **18**(2): 129–132.

Evans, D.L. and Rose, R.J. (1987) Maximum oxygen uptake in racehorses: changes with training state and prediction from submaximal cardiorespiratory measurements. In: Gillespie, J.R. and Robinson, N.E. (eds) *Equine Exercise Physiology 2* Davis, California: ICEEP Publications, pp. 52–67.

Evans, D.L. and Rose, R.J. (1988a) Determination and repeatability of maximum oxygen uptake and other cardiorespiratory measurements in the exercising horse. *Equine Vet. J.* **20**(2): 94–98.

Evans, D.L. and Rose, R.J. (1988b) Effect of a respiratory gas collection mask on some measurements of cardiovascular and respiratory function in horses exercising on a treadmill. *Res. Vet. Sci.* **44**(2): 220–225.

Evans, D.L., Harris, R.C. and Snow, D.H. (1993) Correlation of racing performance with blood lactate and heart rate after exercise in Thoroughbred horses. *Equine Vet. J.* **25**(5): 441–445.

Ferrante, P.L. (1995) Lactate measurement and interpretation: blood vs. plasma. *Equine Vet. J.* **18**(Suppl.): 478–479.

Ferrante, P.L. and Kronfeld, D.S. (1994) Effect of sample handling on measurement of plasma glucose and blood lactate concentrations in horses before and after exercise. *Am. J. Vet. Res.* **55**(11): 1497–1500.

Frape, D.L. (1988) Dietary requirements and athletic performance of horses. *Equine Vet. J.* **20**(3): 163–172.

Gabel, A.A., Milne, D.W., Muir, W.W., Skarda, R.T. and Weingold, M.F. (1983) Some physiological responses of Standardbred horses to a submaximal exercise test following conventional and interval training. In: Snow, D.H., Persson, S.G.B. and Rose, R.J. (eds) *Equine Exercise Physiology.* Cambridge UK: Granta Editions, pp. 497–504.

Gansen, S., Lindner, A., Marx, S., Mosen, H. and Sallmann, H-P (1999) Effects of conditioning horses with lactate-guided exercise on muscle glycogen content. *Equine Vet. J.* **30**(Suppl.): 329–331.

Geor, R.J., McCutcheon, L.J. and Shen, H. (1999) Muscular and metabolic responses to moderate-intensity short-term training. *Equine Vet. J.* **30**(Suppl.): 311–317.

Gore, C.J. and Withers, R.T. (1990) Effect of exercise intensity and duration on postexercise metabolism. *J. Appl. Physiol.* **68**(6): 2362–2368.

Gottlieb-Vedi, M, Essén-Gustavsson, B. and Persson, S.G.B. (1991) Draught load and speed compared by submaximal tests on a treadmill. In: Persson, S.G.B., Lindholm, A. and Jeffcott, L.B. (eds) *Equine Exercise Physiology 3*. Davis, California: ICEEP Publications, pp. 92–96.

Guy, P.S. and Snow, D.H. (1977) The effect of training and detraining on muscle composition in the horse. *J. Physiol.* **269**: 33–51.

Guyton, A.C. (1986) *Textbook of Medical Physiology*, 7th edn. Philadelphia: WB Saunders.

Harkins, J.D., Kamerling, S.G., Bagwell, C.A. and Karns, P.A. (1990) A comparative study of interval and conventional training in Thoroughbred racehorses. *Equine Vet. J.* **9**(Suppl.): 14–19.

Harkins, J.D., Beadle, R.E. and Kamerling, S.G. (1993) The correlation of running ability and physiological variables in Thoroughbred racehorses. *Equine Vet. J.* **25**(1): 53–60.

Harris, P. and Graham-Thiers, P.M. (1999) To evaluate the influence that 'feeding state' may exert on metabolic and physiological responses to exercise. *Equine Vet. J.* **30** (Suppl.): 633–635.

Hill, G., Atkins, R., Littlejohn, A., Kruger, J.M. and Bowles, F. (1977) Exercise studies in horses: 1. A simple telemetry system for recording exercise ECGs in horses. *Equine Vet. J.* **9**(2): 72–74.

Hintz, H.F. (1983) Nutritional requirements of the exercising horse – a review. In: Snow, D.H., Persson, S.G.B., and Rose, R.J. (eds) *Equine Exercise Physiology*. Cambridge, UK: Granta Editions, pp. 275–290.

Hintz, H.F. (1994) Nutrition and equine performance. *J. Nutr.* **124**: 2723S–2729S.

Hodgson, D.R. (1985) Energy considerations during exercise. *Vet. Clin. N. Am.: Equine Pract.* **1**(3): 447–460.

Hodgson, D.R. and Rose, R.J. (1994a) Evaluation of performance potential. In: Hodgson, D.R. and Rose, R.J. (eds) *The Athletic Horse: Principles and Practice of Equine Sports Medicine.* Philadelphia: WB Saunders, pp. 231–243.

Hodgson, D.R. and Rose, R.J. (1994b) Training regimens: physiologic adaptations to training. In: Hodgson, D.R. and Rose, R.J. (eds) *The Athletic Horse: Principles and Practice of Equine Sports Medicine*. Philadelphia: WB Saunders, pp. 379–385.

Hodgson, D.R., Rose, R.J. and Allen, J.R. (1983) Muscle glycogen depletion and repletion patterns in horses performing various distances of endurance exercise. In: Snow, D.H., Persson, S.G.B. and Rose, R.J. (eds) *Equine Exercise Physiology*. Cambridge, UK: Granta Editions, pp. 229–236.

Hodgson, D.R., Rose, R.J., Allen, J.R. and Dimauro, J. (1984) Glycogen depletion patterns in horses performing maximal exercise. *Res. Vet. Sci.* **36**: 169–173.

Holopherne, D.L.M., Hodgson, D.R., and Rose, R.J. (1999) Investigation of the accuracy of a new heart rate meter for use in exercising horses. *J. Equine Vet. Sci.* **19**(9): 552.

Hörnicke, H., Meixner, R. and Pollmann, U. (1983) Respiration in exercising horses. In: Snow, D.H., Persson, S.G.B., and Rose, R.J. (eds) *Equine Exercise Physiology*. Cambridge, UK: Granta Editions, pp. 7–16.

Hoyt, D.F. and Taylor, C.R. (1981) Gait and the energetics of locomotion in horses. *Nature* **292**: 239–240.

Knight, P.K., Sinha, A.K. and Rose, R.J. (1991) Effects of training intensity on maximum oxygen uptake. In: Persson,

S.G.B., Lindholm, A. and Jeffcott, L.B. (eds) *Equine Exercise Physiology 3*. Davis, California: ICEEP Publications, pp. 77–82.

Kobayashi, M., Kuribara, K. and Amada, A. (1999) Application of V200 values for evaluation of training effects in the young Thoroughbred under field conditions. *Equine Vet. J.* **30**(Suppl.): 159–162.

Lacombe, V., Hinchcliff, K.W., Geor, R.J. and Lauderdale, M.A. (1999) Exercise that induces substantial muscle glycogen depletion impairs subsequent anaerobic capacity. *Equine Vet. J.* **30**(Suppl.): 293–297.

Lauderdale, M.A. and Hinchcliff, K.W. (1999) Hyperbolic relationship between time-to-fatigue and workload. *Equine Vet. J.* **30**(Suppl.): 586–590.

Lawrence, L.M. (1990) Nutrition and fuel utilization in the athletic horse. *Vet. Clin. N. Am.: Equine Pract.* **6**(2): 393–418.

Lawrence, L.M., Hintz, H.F., Soderholm, L.V., Williams, J. and Roberts, A.M. (1995) Effect of time of feeding on metabolic response to exercise. *Equine Vet. J.* **18**(Suppl.): 392–395.

Lindholm, A. (1979) Substrate utilization and muscle fiber types in Standardbred trotters during exercise. *Proc. Am. Assoc. Equine Pract*. **25**: 329–336.

Lindholm, A. and Piehl, K. (1974) Fibre composition, enzyme activity and concentrations of metabolites and electrolytes in muscles of Standardbred horses. *Acta Vet. Scand.* **15**: 287–309.

Lindholm, A., Bjerneld, H. and Saltin, B. (1974) Glycogen depletion pattern in muscle fibres of trotting horses. *Acta Physiol. Scand.* **90**: 475–484.

Lucke, J.N. and Hall, G.N. (1980) Further studies on the metabolic effects of long distance riding: Golden Horseshoe Ride 1979. *Equine Vet. J.* **12**(4): 189–192.

McKeever, K.H., Schurg, W.A. and Convertino, V.A. (1985) Exercise training-induced hypervolemia in greyhounds: role of water intake and renal mechanisms. *Am. J. Physiol. (Regulatory, Integrative and Comparative Physiology)* **248**(17): R422–R425.

McKeever, K.H., Schurg, W.A., Jarrett, S.H. and Convertino, V.A. (1987) Exercise training-induced hypervolemia in the horse. *Med. Sci. Sports Exerc.* **19**(1): 21–27.

McMiken, D.F. (1983) An energetic basis of equine performance. *Equine Vet. J.* **15**(2): 123–133.

Medbø, J.I., Mohn, A-C., Tabata, I., Bahr, R., Vaage, O. and Sejersted, O.M. (1988) Anaerobic capacity determined by maximum accumulated O_2 deficit. *J. Appl. Physiol.* **64**(1): 50–60.

Meyer, R.A., Dudley, G.A. and Terjung, R.L. (1980) Ammonia and IMP in different skeletal muscle fibers after exercise in rats. *J. Appl. Physiol. (Respiration, Environment and Exercise Physiology)* **49**(6): 1037–1041.

Miller-Graber, P.A., Lawrence, L.M., Foreman, J.H., Bump, K.D., Fisher, M.G. and Kurcz, E.V. (1991) Dietary protein level and energy metabolism during treadmill exercise in horses. *J. Nutr.* **121**(9): 1462–1469.

Milne, D.W., Gabel, A.A., Muir, W.W. and Skarda, R.T. (1977) Effects of training on heart rate, cardiac output, and lactic acid in Standardbred horses, using a standardized exercise test. *J. Equine Med. Surg.* **1**(4): 131–135.

Nimmo, M.A. and Snow, D.H. (1983) Changes in muscle glycogen, lactate and pyruvate concentrations in the thoroughbred horse following maximal exercise. In: Snow, D.H., Persson, S.G.B. and Rose, R.J. (eds) *Equine Exercise Physiology*. Cambridge, UK: Granta Editions, pp. 237–244.

Oscai, L.B., Williams, B.T. and Hertig, B.A. (1968) Effect of exercise on blood volume. *J. Appl. Physiol.* **24**(5): 622–624.

Pagan, J.D. and Harris, P.A. (1999) The effects of timing and amount of forage and grain on exercise response in Thoroughbred horses. *Equine Vet. J.* **30**(Suppl.): 451–457.

Pagan, J.D. and Hintz, H.F. (1986a) Equine energetics. 1. Relationship between body weight and energy requirements in horses. *J. Anim. Sci.* **63**(3): 815–821.

Pagan, J.D. and Hintz, H.F. (1986b) Equine energetics. 2. Energy expenditure in horses during submaximal exercise. *J. Anim. Sci.* **63**(3): 822–830.

Pagan, J.D., Essén-Gustavsson, B., Lindholm, A. and Thornton, J. (1987) The effect of dietary energy source on exercise performance in Standardbred horses. In: Gillespie, J.R. and Robinson, N.E. (eds) *Equine Exercise Physiology 2*. Davis, California: ICEEP Publications, pp. 686–700.

Persson, S.G.B. (1967) On blood volume and working capacity. *Acta. Vet. Scand.* **19**(Suppl.): 1–189.

Persson, S.G.B. (1968) Blood volume, state of training and working capacity of race horses. *Equine Vet. J.* **1**: 52–58.

Persson, S.G.B. (1983) Evaluation of exercise tolerance and fitness in the performance horse. In: Snow, D.H., Persson, S.G.B. and Rose, R.J. (eds) *Equine Exercise Physiology*. Cambridge, UK: Granta Editions, pp. 441–457.

Pösö, A.R., Lampinen, K.J. and Räsänen, L.A. (1995) Distribution of lactate between red blood cells and plasma after exercise. *Equine Vet. J.* **18**(Suppl.): 231–234.

Rivero, J-L.L. and Clayton, H.M. (1996) The potential role of the muscle in kinematic characteristics. *Pferdeheilkunde* **12**(4): 635–640.

Robb, J., Harper, R.B., Hintz, H.F. *et al.* (1972) Chemical composition and energy value of the body, fatty acid composition of adipose tissue, and liver and kidney size in the horse. *Anim. Prod.* **14**: 25–34.

Rose, R.J. and Evans, D.L. (1986) Metabolic and respiratory responses to prolonged submaximal exercise in the horse. In: Saltin, B. (ed.) *Biochemistry of Exercise VI*. Champaign, Illinois: Human Kinetics Publishers, pp. 459–466.

Rose, R.J. and Hodgson, D.R. (1994a) Clinical exercise testing. In: Hodgson, D.R. and Rose, R.J. (eds) *The Athletic Horse: Principles and Practice of Equine Sports Medicine*. Philadelphia: WB Saunders, pp. 245–257.

Rose, R.J. and Hodgson, D.R. (1994b) An overview of performance and sports medicine. In: Hodgson, D.R. and Rose, R.J. (eds) *The Athletic Horse: Principles and Practice of Equine Sports Medicine*. Philadelphia: WB Saunders, pp. 3–11.

Rose, R.J., Ilkiw, J.E., Arnold, K.S., Backhouse, J.W. and Sampson, D. (1980) Plasma biochemistry in the horse during 3-day event competition. *Equine Vet. J.* **12**(3): 132–136.

Rose, R.J., Hodgson, D.R., Kelso, T.B. *et al.* (1988) Maximum O_2 uptake, O_2 debt and deficit, and muscle metabolites in Thoroughbred horses. *J. Appl. Physiol.* **64**(2): 781–788.

Rose, R.J., Hendrickson, D.K. and Knight, P.K. (1990a) Clinical exercise testing in the normal Thoroughbred racehorse. *Aust. Vet. J.* **67**(10): 345–348.

Rose, R.J., Hodgson, D.R., Bayly, W.M., and Gollnick, P.D. (1990b) Kinetics of VO_2 and VCO_2 in the horse and comparison of five methods for determination of maximum oxygen uptake. *Equine Vet. J.* **9**(Suppl.): 39–42.

Rose, R.J., Knight, P.K. and Bryden, W.L. (1991) Energy use and cardiorespiratory responses to prolonged submaximal exercise. In: Persson, S.G.B., Lindholm, A. and Jeffcott, L.B. (eds) *Equine Exercise Physiology 3*. Davis, California: ICEEP Publications, pp. 281–287.

Scott, C.B., Roby, F.B., Lohman, T.G. and Bunt, J.C. (1991) The maximally accumulated oxygen deficit as an indicator of anaerobic capacity. *Med. Sci. Sports Exerc.* **23**(5): 618–624.

Seeherman, H.J. and Morris, E.A. (1990) Methodology and repeatability of a standardised treadmill exercise test for clinical evaluation of fitness in horses. *Equine Vet. J.* **9**(Suppl.): 20–25.

Sexton, W.L. and Erickson, H.H. (1990) Effects of treadmill elevation on heart rate, blood lactate concentration and packed cell volume during graded submaximal exercise in ponies. *Equine Vet. J.* **9**(Suppl.): 57–60.

Sloet van Oldruitenborgh-Oosterbaan, M.M. and Barneveld, A. (1995) Comparison of the workload of Dutch warmblood horses ridden normally and on a treadmill. *Vet. Rec.* **137**: 136–139.

Sloet van Oldruitenborgh-Oosterbaan, M.M. and Clayton, H.M. (1999) Advantages and disadvantages of track vs. treadmill tests. *Equine Vet. J.* **30**(Suppl.): 645–647.

Snow, D.H. (1994) Ergogenic aids to performance in the race horse: nutrients or drugs. *J. Nutr.* **124**: 2730S–2735S.

Snow, D.H., Baxter, P. and Rose, R.J. (1981) Muscle fibre composition and glycogen depletion in horses competing in an endurance ride. *Vet. Rec.* **108**: 374–378.

Snow, D.H., Kerr, M.G., Nimmo, M.A. and Abbott, E.M. (1982) Alterations in blood, sweat, urine and muscle composition during prolonged exercise in the horse. *Vet. Rec.* **110**: 377–384.

Snow, D.H., Harris, R.C., Harman, J.C. and Marlin, D.J. (1987) Glycogen repletion following different diets. In: Gillespie, J.R. and Robinson, N.E. (eds) *Equine Exercise Physiology 2* Davis, California: ICEEP Publications, pp. 701–710.

Stryer, L. (1988) *Biochemistry*, 3rd edn. New York: WH Freeman and Company.

Taylor, C.R., Heglund, N.C., McMahon, T.A. and Looney, T.R. (1980) Energetic cost of generating muscular force during running: a comparison of large and small animals. *J. Exp. Biol.* **86**: 9–18.

Thomas, D.P. and Fregin, G.F. (1981) Cardiorespiratory and metabolic responses to treadmill exercise in the horse. *J. Appl. Physiol. (Respiratory, Environmental and Exercise Physiology)* **50**(4): 864–868.

Thornton, J., Essén-Gustavsson, B., Lindholm, A., McMiken, D. and Persson, S. (1983) Effects of training and detraining an oxygen uptake, cardiac output, blood gas tensions, pH and lactate concentrations during and after exercise in the horse. In: Snow D.H., Persson, S.G.B. and Rose, R.J. (eds) *Equine Exercise Physiology*. Cambridge, UK: Granta Editions, pp. 470–486.

Thornton, J., Pagan, J. and Persson, S.G.B. (1987) The oxygen cost of weight loading and inclined treadmill exercise in the horse. In: Gillespie, J.R. and Robinson, N.E. (eds) *Equine Exercise Physiology 2*. Davis, California: ICEEP Publications, pp. 206–215.

Topliff, D.R., Potter, G.D., Dutson, T.R., Kreider, J.L. and Jessup, G.T. (1983) Diet manipulation and muscle glycogen in the equine. In: *Proc. 8th Equine Nutr. Physiol. Symp.* Lexington, Kentucky, pp. 119–124.

Topliff, D.R., Potter, G.D., Kreider, J.L., Dutson, T.R. and Jessup, G.T. (1985) Diet manipulation, muscle glycogen metabolism and anaerobic work performance in the equine. In: *Proc. 9th Equine Nutr. Physiol. Symp.* East Lansig, Michigan, pp. 224–229.

Väihkönen, L.K. and Pösö, A.R. (1998) Interindividual variation in total and carrier-mediated lactate influx into red blood cells. *Am. J. Physiol. (Regulatory, Intergrative and Comparative Physiology)* **274**(43): R1025–R1030.

Väihkönen, L.K., Hyyppä, S. and Pösö, A.R. (1999) Factors affecting accumulation of lactate in red blood cells. *Equine Vet. J.* **30**(Suppl.): 443–447.

Valette, J.P., Barrey, E., Jouglin, M., Courouce, A., Auvinet, B. and Flaux, B. (1999) Standardisation of muscular biopsy of gluteus medius in French trotters. *Equine Vet. J.* **30** (Suppl.): 342–344.

Wasserman, K., Whipp, B.J., Koyal, S.N. and Beaver, W.L. (1973) Anaerobic threshold and respiratory gas exchange during exercise. *J. Appl. Physiol.* **35**(2): 236–243.

15

Scaled Energetics of Locomotion

At L. Hof

INTRODUCTION

Horses come in quite different sizes (Fig. 15.1), raising the question as to how the performance of a small and large horse should be compared. In Figure 15.1 the two breeds of horses shown are about the biggest (British Shire) and smallest (Argentinean Fallabella) that exist. Imagine a situation in which the Shire (height 1.91 m, weight 1000 kg) moves alongside the Fallabella (height 0.80 m, weight 60 kg). The Fallabella will be trotting, maybe even galloping, while the Shire is still walking. Obviously, the speeds of both horses should be scaled to their size, but how should this be achieved? Is it proportional to weight? This is not likely, since in that case the Shire would move 1000/60 = 17 times as fast as the Fallabella. Is it, then, proportional to height? This seems more plausible, but it will be shown that it is not correct either. Questions of this type will be examined in this chapter. It will be seen that the outcome depends not only on the question asked – a common situation – but also on the assumptions made. Recognizing assumptions is a trickier problem.

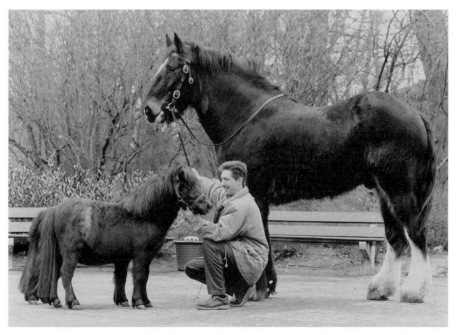

Fig. 15.1 The smallest and biggest breeds of horse: the Fallabella, height 0.80 m, mass 60 kg, with foal (weight at birth 8 kg); and the Shire, height 1.91 m, mass *ca.* 1000 kg. (Photograph courtesy of Noorder Zoo, Emmen, The Netherlands.)

There is a vast amount of literature in the field of scaling. It has been produced by generations of biologists and a few engineers, who have always been fascinated by questions like why an ant can carry 20 times its own weight, and why a horse evidently cannot. There are several books on this subject (Alexander & Goldspink, 1977; McMahon & Bonner, 1983; McMahon, 1984; Schmidt-Nielsen, 1984; Pennycuick, 1992), all of which make fascinating reading as their authors are talented writers.

GEOMETRIC SCALING

Problem

The first problem to be handled is the most elementary. Assume that animal B is in all aspects twice as large as animal A. A consequence is that B can take steps that are twice as long as A. Can it also run twice as fast? And what stride frequency will it use?

In a first approximation it will be assumed that the bigger animal is just an enlarged version of the smaller one, that all linear measures (leg length, leg diameter, trunk circumference, etc.) are proportional to a single length measure. An example is given in Figure 15.2. The big horse has been obtained by enlarging the small one on a photocopier. For the reference length, the height at the withers will be taken and denoted as l. A second assumption to be made relates to the consideration of which two categories of forces are the most important to our problem? For overground locomotion,

the answer is acceleration forces ($= ma$) and gravitational forces ($= mg$) (Hof, 1996).

Having made this assumption, our scaling should now be made such that for animals of different sizes ma and mg should scale in proportion. One reason is that forces are vector quantities, they have both a magnitude and a direction, and the direction of the forces should be the same irrespective of the size. The constant of gravity g is practically the same (9.81 m/s^2) anywhere on earth, and as long as our horses don't walk on the moon, where $g = 2$m/s^2, it may be assumed to be constant. Acceleration is calculated as distance divided by time squared (unit: m/s^2). When distance increases, the time scale should thus be made longer as well. When one animal has height l_1 and the other height l_2, all temporal variables, stance time, stride time, etc., should be scaled in the proportion t_1/t_2. The argument goes as follows:

$$\frac{ma_1}{mg} = \frac{ma_2}{mg} \Rightarrow \frac{a_1}{g} = \frac{a_2}{g} \Rightarrow \frac{l_1}{gt_1^2} = \frac{l_2}{gt_2^2} \tag{1}$$

This leads to:

$$\frac{t_1}{t_2} = \sqrt{\frac{l_1}{l_2}} \tag{2}$$

Time and temporal variables should thus be scaled as the square root of height. A consequence is that speed and velocity should be scaled inversely with the square root of height:

$$\frac{v_1}{v_2} = \frac{l_1/t_1}{l_2/t_2} = \frac{l_1}{l_2}\sqrt{\frac{l_2}{l_1}} = \sqrt{\frac{l_1}{l_2}} \tag{3}$$

A method to account for this scaling with size is to use so-called dimensionless numbers, the definition of which is given in Table 15.1.

It can easily be verified that these numbers are indeed dimensionless by noting that the factors in the denominator have the same units as the quantity in the numerator. The dimensionless number for speed (or sometimes the square of it, which can be confusing) is known as the 'Froude number.' Examples of the possibilities of these dimensionless numbers are given in Figures 15.3 and 15.4, both from Alexander (1977). Figure 15.4 gives dimensionless stride length (the distance traveled in a complete walking stride) as a function of dimensionless speed for a number of very diverse animals.

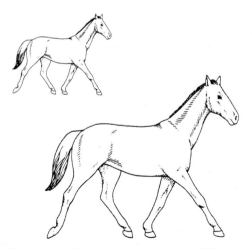

Fig. 15.2 Geometric scaling. Two horses of different size, but with the same proportions.

Table 15.1 Dimensionless numbers for length, time, speed/ velocity and acceleration.			
Length	Time	Velocity	Acceleration
$\hat{l} = \dfrac{l}{l_0}$	$\hat{t} = \dfrac{t}{\sqrt{l_0/g}}$	$\hat{v} = \dfrac{v}{\sqrt{l_0 g}}$	$\hat{a} = \dfrac{a}{g}$

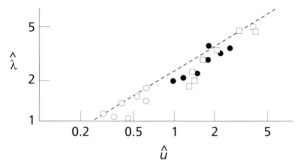

Fig. 15.3 Relationship between stride length and speed. Dimensionless stride length $\hat{\lambda} = \lambda/l_0$ plotted against dimensionless speed $\hat{u} = \nu/\sqrt{l_0 g}$ in logarithmic coordinates. The dashed line gives the regression $\hat{\lambda} = 2.3\hat{u}^{0.6}$. Data are from Muybridge (1887) on horses, mostly with riders. (From Alexander & Goldspink, 1977.)

Answer

If animal B is twice as big as animal A, it will make strides twice as long. Animal A, on the other hand, can make faster steps. Unjust as it is, it turns out that A does not make the steps with twice the frequency of B, but at a rate proportional to the square root of 2, i.e. about 1.4 times as quickly. As a consequence, a corresponding speed of B, e.g. the speed at which the horse changes from walk to trot or from trot to gallop, is 1.4 times as fast as in A. If horses of unequal size are to be compared, speeds and temporal variables should thus be corrected by a factor equal to the square root of the ratio of the respective heights at the withers.

It can be seen that by using dimensionless numbers, i.e. by accounting for geometric scaling, the differences due to size are eliminated. The data for all animals could be expressed in a single formula:

$$\hat{\lambda} = 2.3\hat{v}^{0.6} \qquad (4)$$

Figure 15.4 shows a diagram with the gaits adopted as a function of speed. It can be seen that all animals change from walking to trotting or running at a dimensionless speed of around 0.8. They change from trot to gallop somewhere between 1.3 and 2.0.

An example might be helpful. Imagine the Shire going along with the Fallabella at a speed of 2.5 m/s (9 km/h). Dimensionless speed for Shire is $2.5/\sqrt{1.91 \times 9.81} = 0.58$, a walking speed. Dimensionless speed for Fallabella, on the

other hand, is $2.5/\sqrt{0.80 \times 9.81} = 0.89$, and it will be trotting. A small dog, with a height of 30 cm, may gallop at this speed, as its dimensionless speed is $2.5/\sqrt{0.3 \times 9.81} = 1.46$. The mouse (height 5 cm), which is chased by the dog, has $\hat{v} = 2.2/\sqrt{0.05 \times 9.81} = 3.1$, and is galloping at top speed. Stride length λ of the big horse can be estimated from equation 4 as $\lambda = 1.91 \times \hat{\lambda} = 1.91 \times 2.3 \times (0.58)^{0.6} = 1.91 \times 1.65 = 3.16$ m. Stride frequency is thus $2.5/3.16 = 0.79$ strides/s. The mouse, at the other extreme, will have a stride length of only 23 cm, but a stride frequency of 11 strides/s.

A practical application was given by Back et al. (1995) in a study in which kinematic variables were employed in 4-month-old foals in order to predict the same variables in adult (26-month-old) horses.

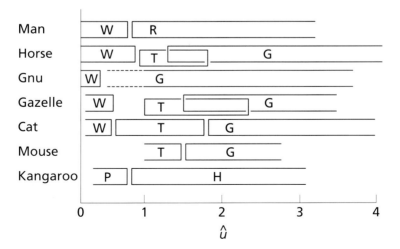

Fig. 15.4 Diagram showing the ranges of speed, expressed as the dimensionless number $\hat{u}$, at which mammals commonly use their various gaits. W: walk; R: run; T: trot; G: gallop or canter; H: hop; P: pentapedal gait (slow gait, typical for kangaroos). (From Alexander & Goldspink, 1977.)

DIFFERENCES IN PROPORTION

Problem

Horses of different breeds are not just bigger or smaller copies of each other, there are substantial differences in morphology. This section will explore what difference it makes whether a horse is compact or slender. Which type can carry heavier loads?

Table 15.2 Some properties of power functions, as used in this chapter.

$$ax^b \cdot cx^d = acx^{b+d}$$

$$\frac{x^a}{x^b} = x^{a-b}$$

$$\sqrt[n]{\sqrt{x^b}} = x^{b/n}$$

$$(x^a)^b = x^{ab}$$

$$x^0 = 1$$

In the preceding section the scaling was purely geometric: every measure was multiplied by the same scaling factor. When looking at a picture of various horse breeds, it is obvious that this is only an approximate picture. Even a layman can see differences in the proportions of Shetland ponies and Thoroughbreds, and the expert can distinguish many dozens of breeds. In a purely geometric scaling, as used in the previous section, it will hold that mass (m) is

specific mass times volume, while volume is proportional to l_0 to the third power. The overall relation can be written as $m \propto l_0^3$.

In the subsequent parts of this chapter some mathematics cannot be avoided. Many of the scaling relations that follow will be expressed in the so-called allometric form, as functions of the form $y = ax^b$. As a reminder, some properties of functions with exponents have been given in Table 15.2.

One factor that distinguishes between breeds is whether they are of slender or compact build. This might be expressed in a ratio d/l_0, in which d is a characteristic width measure, e.g. the thickness of the midshaft of a forelimb or the circumference of the trunk, and l_0 is a characteristic length measure, such as the height at the withers, as used in the first section. If the form of our horses may be approximated with a stack of cylinders (Fig. 15.5), this leads to the following proportionalities for volume or body mass and surface area, respectively:

$$\text{Body mass}: \quad m \propto d^2 l_0 \qquad (5)$$

$$\text{Surface area}: \quad S \propto d l_0 \qquad (6)$$

An important item to be scaled is muscle force. It is generally known from physiology that the force of a muscle is proportional to its physiological cross-section, around $20\,\text{N/cm}^2$. Determining the physiological cross-sectional area of a muscle is not an easy task, as most muscles have quite a complex architecture. It is plausible, however, to assume that it is proportional to the cross-section of the limb, thus with d^2:

$$\text{Muscle force}: \quad F_m \propto d^2 \qquad (7)$$

The moment that is exerted by the muscle is the product of force and moment arm. The moment arm can be assumed proportional to d, so that:

$$\text{Moment}: \quad M \propto d^3 \qquad (8)$$

When a bent limb has to support a force F_s (Fig. 15.6), the muscle has to supply a moment equal to $F_s x$, in which x is the perpendicular distance between the joint that is spanned by the muscle and the line between the joints proximal and

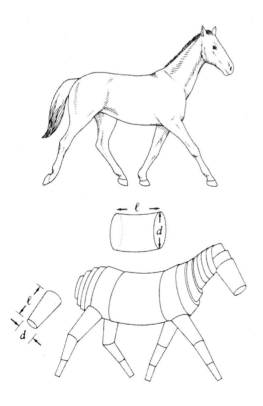

Fig. 15.5 Approximation of the form of a horse by a stack of cylinders. Surface area is proportional to dl and volume to $d^2 l$. (McMahon & Bonner, 1983.)

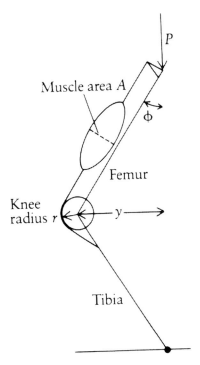

Fig. 15.6 Relation between muscle force, moment and support force (see text). (From McMahon & Bonner, 1983.)

distal of it. When the angle of the limb is not related to size, it can be assumed that x is proportional to l, and thus

$$\text{Supported force :} \quad F_s \propto d^3/l_0 \quad (9)$$

Here we are confronted with a problem. In standing, walking or running the supported force will be equal to 1 to $2 \times$ body weight, respectively. According to equation 5, body mass, and thus body weight, is proportional to $d^2 l_0$. Thus, supported weight and body weight depend in different ways on d and l_0:

$$\frac{F_s}{mg} \propto \frac{d^3/l_0}{d^2 l_0} = \frac{d}{l_0^2} \quad (10)$$

This means that bigger animals need higher stresses in their muscles to support their weight. At some point it becomes too much, and that may explain why whales are too big to walk. Horses are far from the largest species, fortunately, and even elephants are able to walk. There are some effects, nevertheless. Small animals walk and run with strongly angulated limbs and stand in a rather crouched position, while large animals keep their legs much straighter. A lying dog or cat can quickly jump into a standing position, but a horse (or an elephant for that matter) needs considerably more time and effort to assume a standing posture.

A possible 'solution' to this problem would be to make width d proportional to l_0^2, 'constant stress scaling' as it is called, in contrast to true geometric scaling in which all sizes scale in the same proportion: $d \propto l_0$. A third alternative is 'elastic similarity scaling' (McMahon & Bonner, 1983; McMahon, 1984) which leads to a proportionality $d^2 \propto l_0^3$. It can indeed be observed that large animals (elephants) have in general proportionally thicker legs than small ones (mice), and the general trend suggests that elastic similarity scaling is followed. Within the horse family, however, the differences in d/l_0 ratio between breeds are more interesting than a general trend over the widest possible range of animal sizes.

A second application for equation 10 is to assess maximum acceleration or sprinting power. According to Newton's Second Law $a = F/m$, and thus maximum acceleration should scale according to equation 10.

While data on the height l_0 and the mass are commonly available, a problem is to find data on a measure related to thickness d. A way to circumvent this problem is to use equation 5 and replace d in equations 7–10 by $m^{1/2} l_0^{-1/2}$. This results in the alternative forms:

$$\text{Supported force :} \quad F_s \propto m^{3/2} l_0^{-5/2} \quad \text{force factor} \quad (9a)$$

$$\text{and} \quad \frac{F_s}{m} \propto m^{1/2} l_0^{-5/2} \quad \text{force/weight} \quad (10a)$$

In Table 15.3 'force factor' F_s (/1000) and (force/weight) factor F_s/m have been calculated for a number of common breeds. It can be seen that an ordering according to the force factor is in agreement with common sense. It increases with body mass, and thus with muscle mass, and is highest for heavy horses with relatively short limbs. The Belgian horse is the champion in force. The Shire, which has about the same weight, is second in force, due to its longer legs. The force/weight factor is highest in the ponies, with their small mass and short legs. The Quarter horse also stands out for its high acceleration. The data also indicate that the Mustang holds some promise in this respect. Thoroughbreds, on the other hand, have low force/weight factors; they are selected for speed at longer distances. Standardbreds have factors in between these extremes.

The biggest land animal, the African elephant, is the strongest, but not per kg of body weight. In this respect it is far surpassed by the ant (mass 2 mg, leg length 3 mm), which sports an F_s/m of almost 3000, and indeed is able to carry loads many times its body weight.

Table 15.4 gives F_s and F_s/m for a growing warmblood foal. As it seems, foals are born with excessively long limbs, compared to their weight. When the force/weight ratio is calculated, however, it appears to remain quite constant during the growth process, from 57 kg at birth to an almost full-grown 534 kg.

The proportionalities (9a) and (10a) also indicate that although large horses can draw or carry heavier loads than

Table 15.3 Size data of some breeds of horses. Most data on height of the withers and mass were obtained from Sambraus (1989). Data from the horses of Figure 15.1 are marked with an * (personal communication Dr Kooi, Noorder Zoo). Calculated values are the force factor (eqn 9a), the force/weight ratio (eqn 10a), predicted maximum speed unloaded (eqn 19a) and loaded with 50 kg (eqn 19b), and predicted maximum climbing speed (eqn 20).

Breed	Mass (kg)	Height (m)	F_s / 1000	F_s/m	v_{max} (m/s)	v_{max} (km/h)	With rider (m/s)	50 kg (km/h)	v_{climb} (m/s)
Ponies									
Fallabella*	60	0.800	0.81	13.53	14.61	52.61			0.95
Shetland	150	0.980	1.93	12.88	13.48	48.51			0.79
Icelandic	350	1.300	3.40	9.71	13.75	49.49	12.03	43.30	0.66
Fjord	350	1.350	3.09	8.83	14.28	51.39	12.49	44.97	0.66
Coldblood									
Shire*	1000	1.910	6.27	6.27	14.59	52.51	13.89	50.01	0.53
Belgian	1100	1.720	9.40	8.55	12.75	45.91	12.20	43.91	0.52
Warmblood									
Arabian	450	1.550	3.19	7.09	15.16	54.58	13.65	49.12	0.62
Mustang	450	1.450	3.77	8.38	14.18	51.06	12.77	45.95	0.62
Thoroughbred	500	1.700	2.97	5.93	16.09	57.94	14.63	52.67	0.61
Standardbred	600	1.630	4.33	7.22	14.58	52.50	13.46	48.46	0.59
Quarterhorse	680	1.560	5.83	8.58	13.43	48.34	12.51	45.02	0.57
Various									
Donkey, small	150	0.900	2.39	15.94	12.38	44.55	9.28	33.41	0.79
Donkey, middle	300	1.300	2.70	8.99	14.42	51.91	12.36	44.49	0.68
African elephant	5700	3.200	23.49	4.12	14.25	51.29	14.12	50.85	0.37

Table 15.4 Sizes and calculated force and speed for a growing Dutch warmblood foal. Data on height and weight from Smolders (1989). Calculations as in Table 15.3.

Age (months)	Mass (kg)	Height (m)	F_s/1000	F_s/m	v_{max} (m/s)	v_{max} (km/h)
0	57	1.013	0.42	7.31	18.80	67.69
1	101	1.109	0.78	7.76	17.24	62.06
3	178	1.239	1.39	7.81	16.16	58.16
6	262	1.352	2.00	7.62	15.64	56.30
9	331	1.428	2.47	7.47	15.36	55.31
12	395	1.492	2.89	7.31	15.20	54.71
15	452	1.532	3.31	7.32	14.97	53.87
18	494	1.565	3.58	7.25	14.87	53.54
21	510	1.584	3.65	7.15	14.90	53.66
24	519	1.606	3.62	6.97	15.03	54.11
27	534	1.624	3.67	6.88	15.06	54.23

small ones (high force factor), small ones are stronger per kg of body weight. This may explain why donkeys and mules are favored as pack animals over larger horses. On the other hand, for drawing a heavy cart or plowing, large horses with thick legs are best. Even without the help of biomechanics, equine experts have known this for ages. The Shire horse in Figure 15.1, for example, is said to descend from the horses that carried the knights in their heavy armour in the Middle Ages. It stands out more as a riding than a pulling horse, in contrast to the Belgian.

Answer

In this section the consequences of the fact that animals can have different proportions of thickness and length were considered. Muscle force is proportional to cross-sectional area of the muscle. When this effect is accounted for, it turns out that:

1. large animals are stronger than small ones, but that this increase is less than proportional to body weight, therefore—
2. large animals can carry less load per kg of body weight.

These two effects are expressed in, respectively, a force factor F_s and the force divided by body mass F_s/m. The latter factor explains why an ant can carry many times its body weight, while a horse cannot. Table 15.3 gives both factors for a number of horse breeds, Table 15.4 for a growing warmblood foal.

ENERGY COST OF LOCOMOTION

A running horse consumes energy; this is obvious to the observer and to the horse. The laws of mechanics do not provide an easy answer, however, to the question how much energy is needed per meter of progression. According to Newton's First Law, in an ideal frictionless world the cost of locomotion on the level should be nil. Only uphill locomotion would require an energy equal to $mg\Delta h$, body weight (mg) times rise (Δh). Going upward with a speed of rise v_{rise} would thus require a power:

$$P_{rise} = mgv_{rise} \qquad (11)$$

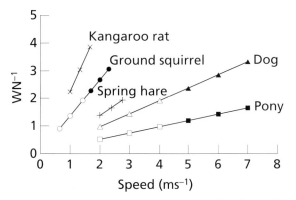

Fig. 15.7 Energy consumption per newton of body weight, P^*_{trans}/mg, as a function of speed for (in order of size) a kangaroo rat, a ground squirrel, a spring hare, a dog and a pony. (Kram & Taylor, 1990. Reprinted with permission from *Nature*; ©Macmillan Magazines.)

For level walking, theory is of no help, and we should rely on measurement. A convenient way to measure energy consumption is to measure oxygen consumption and recalculate this to the power of transport P^*_{trans} in watts. In the following an asterisk (*) will be used to denote work and energy values derived from oxygen consumption. Figure 15.7 gives data on running for animals of different sizes, in which power has already been divided by body weight (in newtons, N). Two things are apparent from this figure: first, P^*_{trans} increases linearly with speed in running, without intercept of the vertical axis. This means that P^*_{trans} divided by speed v, i.e. the energy per meter traversed, E^*_{trans}, is independent of speed. The second aspect is that E^*_{trans} depends on size; after dividing by body mass m it is smaller for big animals (see Fig. 15.8A). With m in kg and E^*_{trans} in J, the relation can be expressed as:

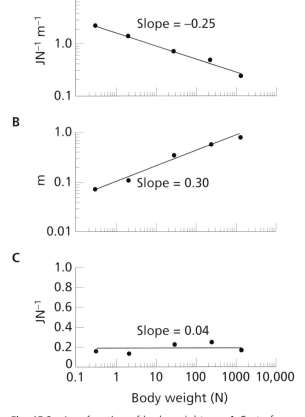

Fig. 15.8 As a function of body weight mg: **A** Cost of transport per unit of body weight, E^*_{trans}/mg, in running; **B** step length l_c, defined as the distance the body moves forward in a single foot contact; **C** the product of both, $E^*_{trans}l_c/mg$, is constant and equal to 0.183 ± 0.045 J/N. Same animals as shown in Fig. 15.7. (Kram & Taylor, 1990. Reprinted with permission from *Nature*; ©Macmillan Magazines.)

$$E^*_{\text{trans}}/m = 8.8m^{-0.25} \qquad (12a)$$

Another way to express the same relationship is:

$$\frac{P^*_{\text{trans}}}{v} = E^*_{\text{trans}} = 8.8m^{0.75} \qquad (12b)$$

When Kram and Taylor (1990) first published this figure, the phenomenon had already been known for a considerable time. (Kram and Taylor used body weight mg instead of body mass m, which is more correct, but makes their formulae somewhat more difficult to compare with those of others.) It is to their merit that they provided an interpretation, by observing that while E^*_{trans}/mg decreases, step length l_c increases by about the same factor (Fig. 15.8B). The latter will not come as a great surprise to the attentive reader, as step length l_c will be proportional to leg length or height l_0, and in geometric scaling it would hold that $l_0 \propto m^{1/3}$. In fact the exponent is slightly less, 0.30. This may be because of the fact that small animals run with more angulated legs, while big animals keep their legs straighter. The overall consequence is that the product $(E^*_{\text{trans}} \, l_c)/mg$ is constant (Fig. 15.8C), and is equal to 0.183 ± 0.045 J/N or m. This means that for all animals the energy cost per newton of body weight is the same per step: for each step an energy is needed equal to what is required to make an upward movement of about 20 cm (0.183 ± 0.045 m):

$$\frac{P^*_{\text{trans}}}{v} = 0.183 \cdot \frac{mg}{l_c} \qquad (12c)$$

This is a comprehensive summary of a great amount of data. It nicely sums up why large animals need less energy to cover a certain distance; it is simply because they can make bigger steps. It further suggests that animals with long legs have an advantage, a fact that breeders of whippets and racing horses will readily admit. To give an explanation for these simple facts, on the other hand, is not so easy. In the following section some considerations will be given.

One reservation should be made at this point. Kram and Taylor (1990) found their experimental relationship from experiments on widely different animals (see Fig. 15.7). The decrease of energy consumption per unit mass and distance and the increase of step length with body size (Fig. 15.8) are

> There is not a simple mechanical reasoning to predict how much energy is needed for horizontal overground locomotion. It can be measured experimentally in a reasonably simple way, however, by assessment of oxygen consumption. It turns out that big animals consume less energy (or oxygen) per kilogram of body mass and per meter traveled. This can be expressed in a remarkably simple way: the (gross) energy needed to make a single step is equal to body weight times 20 cm, irrespective of size.

undoubtedly valid for the range of animals studied. The question, however, is whether these two effects have a causal relationship. To answer this question it would have been more convincing if animals had been studied with different step lengths but similar weight, e.g. dachshunds vs. whippets or Shetland ponies vs. warmblood foals.

MUSCLE WORK AND POWER

> This section attempts to provide some arguments for the decrease in energy consumption per meter and per kg, as presented in the previous one. This will require quite a complicated reasoning that may be omitted on first reading.

Muscles can exert force, and when they are allowed to shorten, they can do work: force times shortening. The unit of work is the joule (J). The rate at which the work is done is called power, measured in watts (W) or joule/s. The relations between force, work and velocity in muscle are depicted in Figure 15.9. When a muscle shortens at a certain speed, the force it develops decreases according to the so-called Hill relation (Hill, 1938), (Fig. 15.9A). As long as there is no lengthening or shortening, the muscle develops its 'isometric' force F_0. With increasing shortening speed muscle force becomes less, until at a speed v_0 force has decreased to zero. In lengthening (negative speed in the figure), force can increase somewhat above isometric, maybe 20–40%. This relation has often been observed in all kinds of muscle. It explains the common observation that a light load can be moved faster than a heavy one.

Mechanical power is force times shortening speed: $P = Fv$. It can be calculated for muscle from the Hill relation (Fig. 15.9B). Power is zero at two points, when speed is zero, i.e. when the muscle is isometric, and at (and above) the maximum speed, when force is zero. The maximum power is developed at an intermediate speed, around $0.3v_0$. At that point force has declined to $0.3F_0$. Power is thus (with some rounding-off) equal to about $0.1F_0v_0$, with a fairly flat maximum. An active muscle not only can do mechanical work but it can generate heat as well, a kind of unavoidable waste, not different from any other motor. Two components of heat development can be discerned: a constant part and one that increases with shortening speed (Fig. 15.9C). In Figure 15.9C the mechanical power of Figure 15.9B has also been drawn, reminding the reader that both mechanical work and heat are forms of energy. From this figure can be seen that the ratio (mechanical power)/(total energy delivered) is not constant for all speeds. It is, of course, zero for $v = 0$ and $v = v_0$ and it has again a maximum in between, but now at a

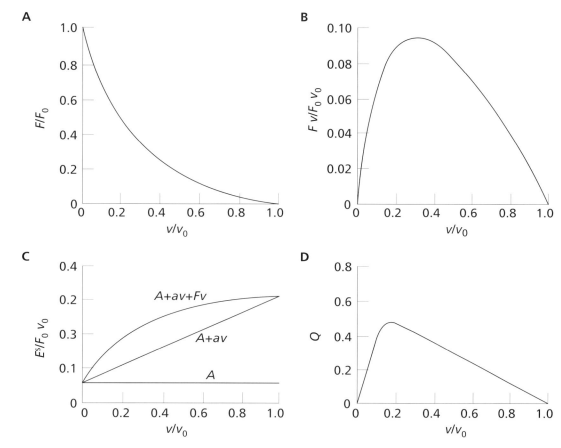

Fig. 15.9 Force, velocity and power in muscle. **A** Muscle force F as a function of shortening speed v. F is shown relative to F_0, the force in an isometric contraction. Shortening speed v expressed relative to the muscle's maximum shortening speed v_0. **B** Mechanical power Fv (work per unit time), unit $F_0 v_0$. **C** Energy production in the form of activation heat A, shortening heat av, and mechanical power Fv, as in panel **B**. **D** Efficiency of work production $Fv/(A + av + Fv)$. Only the efficiency of muscle force production is shown, from ATP to Fv, the processes leading to ATP production reduce the maximal efficiency to about 25%.

speed around $0.2v_0$. At this optimum speed, mechanical work is generated at an efficiency of about 25%. In this respect a horse does better than a motor car, which has an efficiency no greater than 15%. Note that energy and power here are net values, to be differentiated from the gross values with an asterisk in the preceding paragraph.

In equation 7 it has already been noted that maximum isometric muscle force F_0 is proportional to muscle physiological cross section, about $20\,N/cm^2$. In a single contraction, muscle can shorten to about 50% of its initial fiber length, but if this is to be done at a reasonably efficient speed, force is no higher than $0.3F_0$. As energy is force times shortening, 1 cm^3 of muscle (length $0.01\,m$) can thus produce $20\,N \times 0.3 \times 0.005\,m = 0.03\,J$. With a specific mass of muscle fibers around $1\,g/cm^3$, this gives an energy output of $30\,J/kg$ of muscle for a single contraction. In a real muscle, part of the

mass may be due to connective and fat tissue, which may make an estimate of $20\,J/kg$ more realistic. Maximum energy output of a muscle is thus directly proportional to its mass.

Remembering that the work needed to raise the center of gravity by an amount Δh in a jump is $mg\Delta h$, this explains why animals of any size, from fleas to horses, can jump about the same height, from 0.5 to 1.0 m. For a 80 kg human, the legs have mass of about 30 kg. Assuming that muscle mass is 20 kg, one would predict an energy output of $20 \times 20 = 400\,J$ and a jumping height of $400/(80.10) = 0.50\,m$. This is exactly the height well-trained volleyball players can jump in a standing jump. Horses seem to perform better; they are reported to jump up to 2.00 m. Taking into account the height of the trunk in standing, *ca.* 1 m, a rise of 1 m is still performed. Such jumps will be made only after a run, however, and with a run and a fiberglass jumping pole

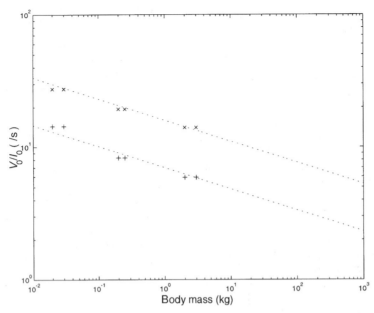

Fig. 15.10 Maximal shortening speed divided by muscle fiber length, v_0/l_0, of slow (soleus) and fast (extensor digitorum longus) muscles of mouse, rat and cat. (Data from Close, 1972.) Bigger animals have slower muscles per unit muscle length. The lines are drawn according to equation 13. No liability is accepted for extrapolations of these data to the size of horses.

humans can reach almost 6 m. (With a final running speed of 10 m/s, the human athlete has gained a kinetic energy of $\frac{1}{2}mv^2 = 4000$ J. This corresponds to a rise in center of gravity of 5.0 m.)

Maximum shortening speed v_0 is proportional to muscle length: a longer muscle contains more sarcomeres in series. In physiology it is therefore usual to give relative muscle speed in muscle lengths per second: v/l_0. In Figure 15.10 a number of data on the maximum muscle shortening speed v_0/l_0 have been given for animals of different sizes, and for a fast muscle (extensor digitorum longus) and a slow muscle (soleus). It can be seen that maximum shortening speed consistently decreases with size of the animal:

$$v_0/l_0 = c_v m^{-0.16} \tag{13}$$

with $c_v = 6$ muscle lengths/s for slow muscles like soleus and $c_v = 14$ for fast muscles and body mass in kg. For horses between 200 and 1000 kg one might thus expect v_0/l_0 to be 2–2.6/s for slow, and 4.6–6.0/s for fast muscles.

We will turn our attention at first to the exponent of m. The data of Figure 15.10 reflect activities at the cellular level: myosin ATP-ase activity. On the other hand, it is very practical. Remember, from Table 15.1 that in geometric scaling all speeds should be scaled as $l_0^{1/2}$, and next that $m \propto l^3$. Taken together, this means that v/l_0 should scale as $m^{-1/6} = m^{-0.167}$, which is in very good agreement with the measured data of Figure 15.9. It seems that muscle intrinsic speeds, related to enzyme activities, are closely adapted to the

speeds that can be expected in an animal of the given size. These size-related differences are probably genetically determined, as they are already present in newborn animals and are rather insensitive to training. It is not known whether this size dependency occurs not only between species of widely different size but also within species, e.g. horses.

In a similar reasoning as for the work, the maximum mechanical power that can be generated by 1 cm³ tissue, area 1 cm² and length 1 cm can now be calculated:

$$P(1\text{cm}^3) = 0.1 F_0 v_0 = 0.1 \cdot 20 \cdot 0.01 \cdot c_v m^{-0.16}$$
$$= 0.02 \cdot c_v m^{-0.16} \tag{14a}$$

Calculated for a muscle mass of m kg, this leads to:

$$P_{\text{muscle, peak}} = 20 c_v m^{0.84} \tag{14b}$$

For horses between 200 and 1000 kg, this results in $P_{\text{muscle, peak}} = 40$–50 W/kg for slow and 90–120 W/kg for fast muscle. These are peak power values. In a series of cyclic contractions, averages of $\frac{1}{3}$ of the above will be the maximum.

Even when it just generates force, without shortening, muscle generates heat and consumes energy. Data on this heat production/resting energy consumption are very scarce, but there are good reasons to assume that it is proportional to the maximal work production according to equation 13. Thus:

$$P^*_{\text{iso}} \propto F_0 c_v m^{-0.16} \tag{15a}$$

In Table 15.1 it was seen that time should be scaled by $\sqrt{l_0}$, and as in geometric scaling $\sqrt{l_0} \propto m^{1/3}$, by temporal factors, like step time t_c should be proportional to $m^{1/6}$. Kram and Taylor's (1990) argument was that:

$$P^*_{\text{iso}} \propto \frac{F_0 c_v}{t_c} \qquad (15b)$$

To arrive at running cost of locomotion, they assumed that (a) the average weight to be supported by muscles is equal to body weight, and (b) muscle contraction in running is nearly isometric. The latter seems rather improbable, but there are good arguments for it, related to the role of muscle elasticity in locomotion. Even if it is not completely true, if there is indeed muscle work done, it should be considered that this work would still be proportional to F_0 and to intrinsic muscle speed v_0. The simple expressions (equations 12abc) thus require a complex explanation, related to intramuscular enzyme activities.

> The simple experimental fact that energy consumption in locomotion per meter and per kg body weight decreases with increasing body size, has probably to do with the fact that the muscles of large animals are slower than those of small ones. This is an innate property and related to specific enzyme activities. It is quite functional, as the large limbs of big animals move more slowly.

MAXIMUM AEROBIC CAPACITY

The power that can be sustained for more than a few minutes is determined by the aerobic capacity, the maximum oxygen consumption. Taylor *et al.* (1981) have determined a general equation for aerobic capacity as a function of body mass. Recalculated in W, and with body mass m in kg, they found:

$$P^*_{\text{max}} = 39m^{0.79} \text{ (all animals)} \qquad (16a)$$

Remarkably, horses (and dogs) are in an exceptional position, as their maximum aerobic capacity is substantially above the average line. For horses the following seems to hold:

$$P^*_{\text{max}} = 90m^{0.79} \text{(horses)} \qquad (16b)$$

This equation contains some extrapolation. It relies on measurements of a single 100 kg pony. It is not really known whether the data for horses really scale according to the 0.79 power of body mass, as they do in the whole range of animals.

> The maximal aerobic power production, the power that can be generated for longer than a few minutes, can be measured as the maximal oxygen consumption. It increases with body weight, not in proportion but as mass to the power 0.79. This means that an animal twice as heavy as a smaller one has not twice the aerobic power, but only 1.73 times as much.

MAXIMUM SPEED

In the above an expression for the aerobic capacity (equation 16b) and on page 358 for the cost of locomotion (equation 12c) were found. Combining these two an estimate can be given of the maximum aerobic speed, i.e. the maximum speed a horse can sustain for more than a few minutes

$$v_{\text{max}} = \frac{P^*_{\text{max}}}{P^*_{\text{trans}}/v} = \frac{90m^{0.79}}{0.184mg/l_c} = 50m^{-0.21}l_c \qquad (17)$$

Here we run into a problem. Data on l_c as defined by Kram and Taylor (1990), the distance the horse goes forward while one limb is on the ground, are hard to get. McMahon (1975) has given data on some average animals: mouse, rat, dog and horse. He found that the angular excursion of the legs decreased with $m^{-0.10}$. This leads to an estimate:

$$l_c \approx 1.3m^{-0.10}l_0 \qquad (18)$$

Combining equations 17 and 18 gives an estimated top aerobic speed:

$$v_{\text{max}} = 65m^{-0.31}l_0 \qquad (19a)$$

Equation (19a) is valid for unloaded horses. For horses, body mass m_b, loaded on the back with a rider or a pack with mass m_l, P^*_{trans} increases proportionally with total mass $(m_b + m_l)$, but aerobic capacity (equation 14b) and step length (equation 18) are still related to m_b only. Taking this into account, it will hold that:

$$v_{\text{max}} = 65 \frac{m_b^{0.69}}{m_b + m_l} l_0 \quad \text{(with back load } m_l) \qquad (19b)$$

Calculated values have been given in Tables 15.3 and 15.4. In Table 15.3 values for a rider of 50 kg have been given in addition. The record on the three-mile race (McWhirter, 1984) stands at 5 min 15 s, corresponding to an average speed of 15.32 m/s or 55.18 km/h. The predicted value of 14.63 m/s is a surprisingly good estimation, considering the rough assumptions made in the derivation, and the fact that champion horses are by definition exceptional. In addition, exact values of masses for horse and jockey, and of horse height, were not available. More importantly, differences between breeds correspond roughly with experience.

Looking more closely at equation 19a, it is striking that in geometrically similar animals about the same maximum speed is predicted. In that case l_0 scales in proportion to $m^{1/3}$, and thus v_{max} is almost independent of size. This may explain why fox, hounds and hunting horses are quite closely matched in speed. The proportions make the difference: fast animals should have long legs for their mass. This effect is also shown when maximum speed according to equation 19a is calculated for the foal of Table 15.4. The calculated values are already at their top immediately after birth. This is not realistic, of course; newborn foals will not have a similar aerobic capacity to adult horses and their running technique leaves room for improvement. Their seemingly odd proportions – excessive long legs for their mass – are thus very functional: it allows them to keep up with the herd within a short time after birth.

Three factors contribute to the estimated speed: maximum aerobic capacity, cost of locomotion and step length. Individual differences in any of these three factors will affect the final result. Aerobic capacity is different between individuals. Muscle fiber composition and technique affect the cost of transport. A running technique with longer steps is advantageous. Several other aspects may also influence speed, which could not be included in the present simple model.

The model presented here is restricted to aerobic speed: maximum speed over times longer than 2 minutes or distances over 2000 m. Horses, and racing horses in particular, have an excessively high aerobic capacity compared to other species. This is reflected in the high speed at longer distances (Fig. 15.11), about 15 m/s. In man long-distance speed is a relatively poor 6 m/s (Fig. 15.11), corresponding to a lower aerobic capacity and a less suitable build for running. A good model to predict speed over short distances, including the

acceleration phase, will be much more complicated than the simple reasoning presented above and is not available at present. The same holds for trotting; this requires data on oxygen consumption for horses drawing a load and on the force needed to draw a sulky on a track, data that are not available. Speed with a sulky seems not to be much lower than with a rider (see Fig. 15.11).

Similarly, no data are available on the energy cost for uphill locomotion. A simple guess is to consider pure upward movement, quite unlikely for horses, which are not suited for climbing up ladders. Combining the expressions for maximum aerobic capacity (equation 16b) and for mechanical power in upward movement (equation 11), and assuming that muscle power is generated at an efficiency of 25%, results in:

$$v_{\text{rise, max}} = \frac{0.25 \cdot 90 \cdot m^{0.79}}{mg} = 2.25 \cdot m^{-0.21} \quad (20)$$

This formula gives unrealistically high speeds of rise (Table 15.3, rightmost column); no animal seems to climb at maximum speed. It does show that climbing speed is inversely related to body mass: small animals, like mice or squirrels, climb easily, while for bigger animals it requires considerable effort. It is well known that inhabitants of mountain areas prefer smaller breeds of horse, or alternatively donkeys or mules. One should wonder at the perseverance of Hannibal in marching elephants over the Alps.

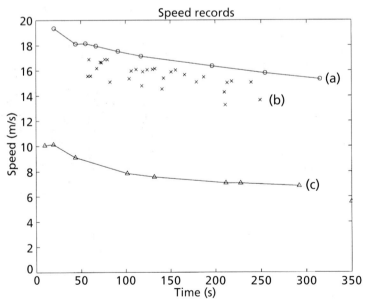

Fig. 15.11 Speed records for horse and man. **(a)** World records of horse racing, 0.25 mile up to 3 miles; **(b)** course records of the trotting course Duindigt, The Netherlands, distances from 900 m to 3600 m; **(c)** world records for men running in 1983, distances 100 m to 2000 m and 30 km (shown at far right). (Data from McWhirter, 1984.)

Expressions are given (equations 19, 19a) for the maximum speed of horses, unloaded and loaded with a rider, respectively. The outcome is that maximum speed decreases with mass and increases with leg length, in such a way that animals of similar shape but different size will run equally fast, but that animals with proportionally longer legs have an advantage.

Concluding remarks

After this brief journey around the outposts of biology and engineering, it is hoped that the reader has been as much entertained by the reading as the author has with the writing. Hesitatingly, the question of practical applicability of the above might be brought forward. In our opinion such applicability is small, but not completely futile. Scaling theories give a frame of reference for the problems discussed: the order of magnitude of the effect is taken into account, based on very elementary considerations, and often rough approximations. For details one should go further into the problem. To give an example, page 352 gives the theory of geometric scaling. According to this theory stride time and step time in animals of different sizes should be scaled to the square root of a characteristic length. Sound physical arguments are given for this. This theory explains some relevant findings, e.g. why your Dachshund is galloping while you are still walking. Other findings are not explained, e.g. why Standardbreds trot and Thoroughbreds gallop. Scaling theory should certainly be used when one tries to relate findings on locomotion patterns in rats to the situation in horses. Without doubt, there will remain major differences between rats and horses, but the agreements will emerge more clearly. Pages 361 and 362, on the other hand, bring together some experimental findings on metabolic capacity and cost of transport, and try to find some of the consequences. The outcome of these exercises gives an idea what can be expected on the basis of very simple assumptions. Any predictions from it will be inferior to the insights from experts, but the charming thing is that even simple models can produce realistic predictions.

Acknowledgements

I thank Dr. Agaath Kooi from the Noorder Zoo at Emmen, for data on and photographs of the Fallabella and Shire horses (Fig. 15.1) and Dr Roger Kram for providing the original data for Figures 15.7 and 15.8.

REFERENCES

Alexander, R.McN. and Goldspink, G. (1977) Mechanics and energetics of animal locomotion. London: Chapman and Hall.

Back, W., Schamhardt, H. C., Hartman, W., Bruin, G. and Barneveld, A. (1995) Predictive value of foal kinematics for the locomotor performances of adult horses. *Res. Vet. Sci.* **59**: 64–69.

Close, R.I. (1972) Dynamic properties of mammalian skeletal muscles. *Physiol. Rev.* **52**: 129–197.

Hill, A.V. (1938) The heat of shortening and the dynamic constants of muscle. *Proc. Royal Soc. Series B.* **126**: 136–195.

Hof, A.L. (1996) Scaling gait data to body size. *Gait and Posture* **4**: 222–223.

Kram, R. and Taylor, C.R. (1990) Energetics of running: a new perspective. *Nature* **346**: 265–267.

McMahon, T.A. (1975) Using body size to understand the structural design of animals: quadripedal locomotion. *J. Appl. Physiol.* **39**: 619–627.

McMahon, T.A. (1984) *Muscles, Reflexes and Locomotion.* Princeton: Princeton University Press.

McMahon, T.A. and Bonner, J.T. (1983) *On Size and Life.* New York: WH Freeman & Co.

McWhirter, N. (1984) *The Guiness Book of Records*, Dutch edn. Utrecht: Luitingh. [In more recent editions, data on horse racing are absent.]

Muybridge, E. (1887) *Animals in Motion*, modern reprint 1979. New York: Dover.

Pennycuick, C.J. (1992) *Newton Rules Biology. A Physical Approach to Biological Problems.* Oxford: Oxford University Press.

Sambraus, H.H. (1989) *Atlas van Huidierrassen.* (Atlas of Domestic Animals.) Zutphen: Terra.

Smolders, G. (1989) Groei en ontwikkeling van rijpaarden. (Growth and development of riding horses.) *PR Praktijkonderzoek* **2**: 26–28.

Schmidt-Nielsen, K. (1984) *Scaling: Why is Animal Size so Important?* Cambridge: Cambridge University Press.

Taylor, C.R., Maloiy, G.M.O., Weibel, E.R. *et al.* (1981) Design of the mammalian respiratory system. III Scaling maximum aerobic capacity to body mass: wild and domestic mammals. *Resp. Physiol.* **44**: 25–37.

16

Modeling of Locomotion

Adam K. Arabian and Hilary M. Clayton

INTRODUCTION

Computer modeling is generally defined as the process of creating a representation of an object or system within the computer. The origins lie in tools developed by engineers to assist them in the industrial design process. These models allowed the engineer to create each component of a product, assemble them 'virtually' in the computer, and ensure a good fit before manufacturing. Using computer mathematical analysis tools, it is also possible to predict the forces that the component will see and make certain that it will not fail under that loading.

For biological systems, computer models are useful for many of the same reasons. Instead of having to perform *in vivo* studies, a computer representation of an anatomical structure can be created and examined in ways that would be prohibitively difficult in a live animal. The advantages are obvious; if the model is reliable, it can be used to examine many biomechanical systems including the motion of a complex joint, such as the tarsus, the loading and motion in regions that are not visible to the human eye such as within the hoof capsule, or the loading that causes a bone to fracture. These can be studied by modeling, which does not require the use of live subjects.

History of computer modeling

The origins of computer modeling can be traced back to a program developed in 1963 at the Massachusetts Institute of Technology (Encarnacao *et al.*, 1990). Its capabilities were limited to what would be called a simple drawing program in modern terms, but many of the fundamental drawing subroutines and standards were established by this work. Although developments were made in subsequent years, it wasn't until the late 1970s that computer-based design moved from the realm of

academic theory into mainstream science. As the increasing power of computers allowed for more advanced applications, a new technique was developed in the 1980s called 'solid modeling.' In this process a three-dimensional representation of a structure is created within a computer, rather than the older method of simply having a number of two-dimensional projections (Fig. 16.1).

Using this new technology, designers could view parts of a system and their interactions without the cost and time involved in creating a prototype. Assemblies of independent components, structural supports, or even entire complex mechanisms such as automotive engines could be examined for fit and accuracy before any real monetary investment was made by the company.

COMPUTER MODELING AND BIOMECHANICS

Even before solid modeling became an industry standard, anatomists and biomechanists had recognized the opportunities it represented. One of the earliest uses of computers to model a musculoskeletal system represented an approximation of the human body as a series of rigid links with simple hinge or pin joints (Chaffin, 1969). Although this was useful in visualization of human motion, it was not a tool for examining specific bones or joints. It was not until medical imaging devices such as computed tomography (CT) and magnetic resonance imaging (MRI) scanners were used as the basis for the geometry that truly representative anatomy could be created in a computerized model.

After the techniques of modeling had been proven in human studies, the veterinary community began to use

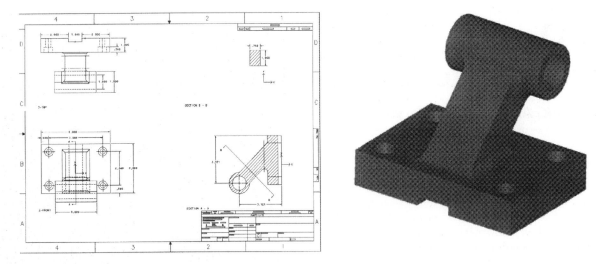

Fig. 16.1 A comparison of two-dimensional versus three-dimensional modeling methods.

the same methods to explore the complexities of motion in animals. An early equine study using the fundamentals of joint motion developed for human protocols modeled the entire forelimb distal to the metacarpophalangeal joint (Cheung & Thompson, 1993), but subsequent research has typically focused on a single joint, such as the carpus (Les *et al.*, 1997) or fetlock (Thompson & Cheung, 1993).

Applications of computer models

There are four typical applications of computer models in biomechanics: visualization, kinetics, dynamics and finite element analysis.

Visualization

The potential of computer models in visualization represents one of the great emerging applications of this technology. A well-known example is the use of CT or MRI data by a veterinarian or physician to produce a three-dimensional recreation of a bone or joint, rather than looking at it as a series of two-dimensional projections. This functionality is included in a number of commercial medical imaging products. The operator uses specific areas as 'edges' of structures and the computer rebuilds a visualization of the bone, soft tissue or any other object of interest. This type of modeling is useful for viewing different structures and the relationships between them in live subjects, but some of its most promising practical applications arise from the ability to produce physical objects by the processes of rapid prototyping and machining.

Rapid prototyping is a method by which a sample part is made from a soft plastic (typically nylon or epoxy) that can be held and examined, not just viewed on a computer screen. The process consists of creating a solid model in the computer, then sending the information to a rapid prototyping machine, which recreates it as a series of layers of plastic. In industry, entire prototype engines have been constructed this way to demonstrate new technology and concepts that would be difficult to otherwise describe. Similarly, anatomical structures can be recreated and examined in the same way as a dissected specimen. This has been explored in humans as a method of preparing surgeons to perform operations, including neurological and orthopedic procedures (McGurk *et al.*, 1997).

Machining is a process by which a product is manufactured from a permanent material. For orthopedic procedures, this allows preliminary evaluation of surgeries and the manufacturing of custom implants. Using CT data obtained preoperatively, the joint can be recreated precisely in the computer and a surgeon can have an exact fit for the orthopedic implant prepared prior to surgery or even constructed during the procedure (Mulier *et al.*, 1989).

One of the most exciting areas into which visualization techniques are expanding is the field of virtual reality. The concept of virtual reality has become something of a buzzword of the media in recent years due to proliferation of home computers, increased distance interaction on the internet, and incredible advances in computer graphics. The true concept of virtual reality is that, by recreating a situation in the processor of a computer and by using highly realistic graphics, the human brain can be fooled into believing that the computer-generated images are real. Although technological limitations still prevent complete immersion in a virtual reality environment, some early and very impressive demonstrations of its medical applications have been performed, such as the National Library of Medicine's Visible Human Project. This is an ambitious program to develop a complete database of human anatomy based on cryosections and CT scans of male and female cadaver specimens. The results of this research have already been used to develop educational and research tools for audiences ranging from school-age children to medical professionals.

Another focus for the development for visualization tools in medicine is in preoperative planning. An entire surgery can be simulated and performed any number of times to rehearse the mechanics of the procedure prior to a single incision being made on a live patient. However, the use of a purely anatomical model cannot completely prepare the student for all situations and complications that may arise during a procedure and that necessitate a rapid and accurate response by the surgeon. However, in the same way that pilots can practice emergency maneuvers and landings in jet simulators, critical conditions could be simulated to prepare a student for surgical emergencies.

The application of virtual reality in the field of equine biomechanics is surprisingly advanced. One of the most remarkable examples is 'Persival,' a mechanical horse simulator (Fig. 16.2) developed by Patrick Galloux of the Ecole Nationale d'Equitation in Saumur, France (Galloux *et al.*, 1994). His group has constructed a mechanical simulator that recreates the movements of a horse at a walk, trot and canter, as well as during jumping. Virtual reality is used to allow the rider to follow a show jumping course by watching a screen in front of the simulator or by wearing virtual reality glasses. The rider sees the obstacles, and sensors are used to detect and react to the rider's aids. It has been found that by using this simulator, the time required to train a rider was shorter than when using a real horse, and the novice rider was able to learn safely and without the need for 'lesson' horses.

Kinematics

Kinematics is defined as the observation of motion in a mechanical system. It encompasses a spectrum that ranges from the rotation of a horse's limbs as it gallops across a polo field, to the movements of a player's arm and mallet as a shot is made, to the way the polo ball arcs through the air after it has been hit. Kinematic studies have described the horse's movement at various gaits and during jumping. This information can be used to create an accurate simulation of the motion of a par-

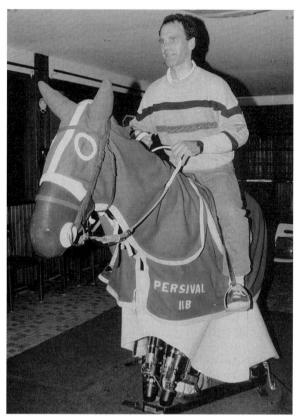

Fig. 16.2 Persival, the Ecole Nationale d'Equitation's mechanical horse simulator.

ticular joint that shows how the various components interact and allows the user to visualize the effects of disease, lameness or surgeries. Other types of computer simulations might show deformation of the structures within the hoof during weight bearing, or the actions of the rider in giving a horse the aids for different movements.

It is important to recognize that kinematics is limited to the process of observation; it does not have the ability to make inferences. For example, kinematics can be used to study how a bone, joint, limb or animal moves based on a set of data describing that movement, but it cannot predict the results of a perturbation of the system, such as an injury or lameness. Using computer models as kinematic simulations is, to a great extent, a specific application of the previously discussed visualization tools. However, it goes beyond simple visualization because the kinematic information represents a bridge between visualization, a purely external observation, and dynamics, an understanding of the forces that are responsible for creating the movement and the forces that arise as a consequence of the movement.

Dynamics

As stated above, kinematics is a passive observation of how a system moves. Dynamics uses kinematic data, combined with additional information, to evaluate the forces within the system. Having calculated the dynamics, much more complex simulations can be performed. Two methods are primarily used for the development of dynamic results: inverse dynamics, and forward or direct dynamics. In general, inverse dynamics is a technique by which internal forces are estimated using data from external observations, while forward dynamics predicts external forces and motions by prescribing internal forces.

An application of computer modeling using inverse dynamics involves the calculation of net joint moments and joint powers from knowledge of the kinematics, ground reaction forces (GRFs) and morphological data using a link-segment model. In this type of model, the complex structure of the limbs is simplified by representing the limb segments as rigid bodies linked by hinge joints (e.g. Schryver *et al.*, 1978; Hjertén & Drevemo, 1987; Clayton *et al.*, 1998; Colborne *et al.*, 1998; Lanovaz *et al.*, 1999) (Fig. 16.3).

The musculature that drives the limb has a complex geometry and many mechanical and material properties that are difficult to quantify. In order to study the effect of muscle action without defining all of the specific parameters of the system, the net muscular action within the limb is represented in the model as net torques or net joint moments acting at each of the joints. Realistic inertial parameters such as mass and moment of inertia are assigned to each segment of the computer model. Kinematic data and GRFs are measured and used as inputs to the model. An inverse dynamics solution is used to calculate the torques required to cause the observed motion and forces. This 'net effect' of muscle action derived from the model can be applied in both clinical and research settings to study the function and dysfunction of the limb at the different joints (Buchner *et al.*, 1996; Clayton *et al.*, 1999). Additional information can be added to the model to increase the level of sophistication. For example, knowledge of the orientation of anatomic structures such as the line of action of tendons can allow for a more detailed estimation of internal muscle and tendon forces (Riemersma *et al.*, 1988; Jansen *et al.*, 1993).

Forward or direct dynamics utilizes data describing muscle activation patterns and the force of muscular contraction to determine the position of each segment of the limb. Although this method is theoretically ideal, as it is the most accurate representation of what is actually occurring in the system, it is practically difficult to measure these inputs with the accuracy needed to produce a model that represents the internal forces and interac-

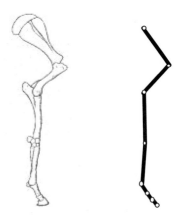

Fig. 16.3 Link-segment model of the equine forelimb.

tions. A variation on this type of dynamic analysis was performed for an entire horse in 1987 using a mechanical mechanism analysis package (Bogert, 1989). The horse was represented by a series of rigid bodies connected by springs, dampers and torque producers representing tendons and ligaments. The innovative aspect of this simulation was that, instead of simply prescribing the motion of a segment by kinematic data, an intelligent model was created that prescribed the limitations of joints, the reaction forces created by the tension in ligaments and muscle activations. The model was analyzed and validated through both kinematic and ground reaction force data. However, in order to simulate the entire horse, a number of assumptions had to be made due to the complexity of the project and the limitations in computer power at the time. The entire system was assumed to be purely two dimensional with the segments of the horse moving in the sagittal plane. Complex joints, such as the carpus and tarsus, were approximated as simple hinges, and it was necessary to completely ignore certain joints, such as the coffin joint and the articulation of the spine. In spite of these assumptions, the simulation was found to accurately recreate the ground reaction force patterns measured in research studies.

The availability of a complete and accurate model of even a single joint opens up incredible opportunities. Should a specific treatment be recommended, such as a tenectomy, the outcome can be predicted by incorporating into the model the loss of the forces transmitted by that tendon. The model could then be used to predict the effectiveness of the treatment, allowing for a more educated and confident recommendation of the likely benefits. This application was validated by a study in which the human lower leg was recreated in a computer to evaluate orthopedic surgical procedures. It was found that the model accurately predicted the effects of tendon transfers and lengthening procedures (Delp *et al.*,

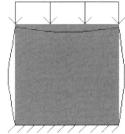

Fig. 16.4 Typical deformation of objects under various load conditions.

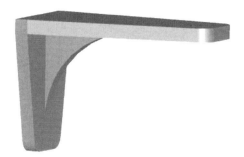
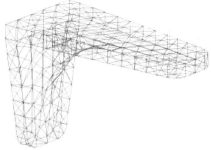

Fig. 16.5 A simple finite element model.

1990). It is within the realm of possibility that a sufficiently complex model of the equine limb could be created that it would be capable of assessing the effects of orthopedic shoeing, changes in the physical properties of the footing, muscular atrophy, or surgical procedures such as tenectomy or arthrodesis.

Finite element analysis

The stress on a structure can be measured through a dynamic analysis as described above or it can be computed through application of mechanical measurement techniques such as strain gauges. Having determined the stress on a structure, it is of great interest to know what effect this might have on the structure in terms of causing deformation (strain) or stimulating biological adaptation. For example, hoof deformation at impact could be used to evaluate how energy is dampened or dissipated. Observation of the habitual patterns of stress in a bone can be related to the way in which that bone adapts to its environment and reconstructs itself. The complexity of these types of calculations makes it almost impossible to accurately determine or calculate by hand the way in which forces will be distributed across a particular structure.

In the field of engineering, this problem has been solved by the development of the process called finite element analysis (FEA) or finite element modeling (FEM).

To understand the process of FEA, consider a very simple piece of geometry, a cube. It is relatively easy to predict the way a cube deforms based on the forces applied (Fig. 16.4) and the properties of the material from which the cube is made. A steel cube deforms in a specific way, which is different from an aluminum or wood cube.

Most objects are more complicated than simple cubes. They are made up of very complex surfaces and curves, which make it difficult, if not impossible, to predict how the structure will deform under stress. The process of FEA consists of breaking up a piece of complex geometry into a series of simple shapes, such as cubes or pyramids (Fig. 16.5). These subdivisions, called elements, react to stress in a mathematically predictable way. The entire structure is represented by numerous elements, which are each described in terms of the motion of their corners, or in more complex models, the motions of the midpoints between the corners as well. When the model is analyzed, the deformation of one element defines the force on the next element, and subsequently its force on the next, and so on. The minimal requirement is to analyze each corner of each element in three directions (up/down, left/right and forward/backwards). When we take into account the fact that a finite element model can consist of thousands of these elements, it becomes evident that a powerful computer is an essential tool in performing this type of analysis.

Biological structures are even more complex than most products manufactured in industry, making finite element analysis invaluable for predicting their behavior under various loading conditions. For example, by creating a computer model of a particular bone and applying forces to the bone from data known *a priori*, the type and location of fractures in that bone may be predicted.

A number of equine studies have been performed using finite element analysis. One of the earliest was an analysis of the structure of the hoof. The intent of the project was to examine the role of mechanical factors in lameness and degenerative diseases within the hoof capsule (Hogan *et al.*, 1991). A two-dimensional finite element analysis was performed, and the deformation results were examined to determine motions that were not visible through direct observation. The results indicated that during weight-bearing the coffin bone moved downward toward the sole, and rotated away from the dorsal hoof wall (Fig. 16.6). Additionally, approximations of the stresses induced in the laminar tissue during loading were determined. The stress values within the hoof derived from this and similar studies have given a much more comprehensive understanding of the behavior of the hoof. The results were of particular interest because, at that time, there was little direct information describing the motion of the coffin bone with respect to the hoof wall during loading.

A more recent analysis looked at stresses in the equine metacarpus (Les *et al.*, 1997) (Fig. 16.7). Due to improvements in computing capabilities and finite element programs, this analysis was a more comprehensive three-dimensional model than that of Hogan *et al.* (1991). Using CT data, an accurate model of the metacarpus was created in the computer, and it was then subdivided into a series of quadrilateral elements. This model was compared to *ex vivo* loading results, and the accuracy of the FEA was validated. This study was an excellent example of the opportunities opened up by FEM. Once a particular model has been validated, many different loading conditions can be simulated and analyzed within the computer and an accurate representation of the stress

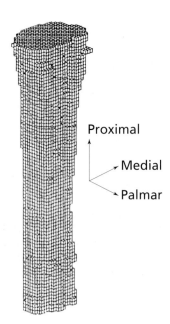

Fig. 16.7   Finite element model of the equine metacarpus. (Reprinted from Les *et al.* (1997) *J. Biomech.* **30**: 737–742.)

response can be determined without the need to use additional live subjects.

DEVELOPMENT OF A COMPUTER MODEL

Although the end result of computer models can vary greatly between applications, the steps involved in the process are quite similar. Visualization requires the greatest accuracy in the overall form and appearance of structures. When attempting to simulate a surgical procedure, it is critical that the anatomy appear as realistic as possible. The model must accurately predict what the surgeon sees during the procedure if it is to have any practical value. In order to reproduce anatomical structures accurately, it is necessary to use very advanced medical imaging techniques. When studying skeletal structures, CT scans can be used to build a representation of structures with high X-ray absorbance. Soft tissue structures are typically visualized more clearly using MRI images. Regardless of the source of data, the process of recreating the region in question is the same. The resulting images are stored as a series of pictures that are then analyzed to locate the edge of the structure of interest. These interface locations are stored in the computer and are used to define the edges. Graphics tools are subsequently used to rebuild the edges into a solid

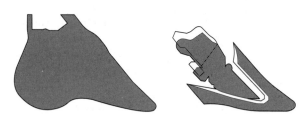

Fig. 16.6   Finite element model of the hoof and coffin bone. (Reprinted from Hogan *et al.* (1991) *Proc. 10th Ann. Mtg. Assoc. Equine Sports Med.*, p. 43.)

structure. By this method, almost any complex anatomical structure can be recreated for a visual examination.

These techniques are also useful in kinematic and dynamic modeling. Regardless of how it may appear, joint motion is never as simple as a two-dimensional rotation. Using the techniques specified above, a more comprehensive representation can be constructed which will allow for a much more accurate study of the dynamics of joint motion, and hence a better understanding of pathologies.

Finite element models perhaps require the most comprehensive and accurate descriptions of skeletal and accessory structures and their properties. The accuracy of the analysis is directly dependent upon how closely the model approximates the original geometry. Although this analysis technique is inherently an approximation due to its very nature of subdividing curved surfaces into linear segments, without an accurate framework on which to build the structure of the finite element model, the analysis will be inherently flawed. The model itself is only as good as the information from which it was created, and without a great deal of precision in the original model, the results will be useless.

If a kinematic or dynamic model is being developed, another major step is necessary to the completion of the simulation. External data, such as kinematic information describing the motion of the horse and GRFs, are necessary for a comprehensive model. There are, however, two ways in which these data can be used. The first is to apply the information as the perturbation input to the model. By specifying the kinematic and force input, data such as joint torques, moments and temporal responses may be analyzed. The second method is to use the external data to verify a solution arrived at by other means. In the full body equine simulation of Bogert (1989), an intelligent system was used to describe the motion of the segments of the horse. A standard muscular model controlled some joints with activation timing based on the percent of stride, while others were controlled by constraints based on approximate joint angles. Since the force data were indepedent of the solution, they could be used to confirm the veracity of the solution.

Needless to say, computer modeling will never fully replace the use of live subjects in all cases. However, its clinical and diagnostic capabilities are likely to be exploited to an even greater extent in the future.

REFERENCES

Bogert, A.J. van den (1989) Computer simulation of locomotion in the horse. *PhD thesis, University of Utrecht.*

Buchner, H.H.F., Savelberg, H.H.C.M. and Becker, C.K. (1996) Load redistribution after desmotomy of the accessory ligament of the deep digital flexor tendon in adult horses. *Vet. Quart,* **18**, (Suppl. 2): 570–574.

Chaffin, D.B. (1969) A computerized biomechanical model development and used in studying gross body actions. *J. Biomech.* **2**: 429–441.

Cheung, T.K. and Thompson, K.N. (1993) Development of a three dimensional electronic solids model of the lower forelimb of the horse. *Vet. Radiol. Ultrasound* **34**: 331–333.

Clayton, H.M., Lanovaz, J.L., Schamhardt, H.C., Willemen, M.A. and Colborne, G.L. (1998) Net joint moments and powers in the equine forelimb in the stance phase of the trot. *Equine Vet. J.* **30**: 384–389.

Colborne, G.R., Lanovaz, J.L., Sprigings, E.J., Schamhardt, H.C. and Clayton, H.M. (1998). Forelimb joint moments and power during the walking stance phase of horses. *Am. J. Vet. Res.* **59**: 609–614.

Delp, S.L., Loan, J.P., Hoy, M.G., Zajac, F.E., Topp, E.L. and Rosen, J.M. (1990) An interactive graphics-based model of the lower extremity to study orthopaedic surgical procedures. *IEEE Trans. Biomed. Engin.* **37**: 757–767.

Encarnacao, J.L., Linder, R. and Schlechtendahl, E.G. (1990) *Computer-Aided Design. Fundamentals and System Architectures,* 2nd edn. Springer-Verlag, Berlin.

Galloux, P., Richard, N., Dronka, T. *et al.* (1994) Analysis of equine gait using three dimensional accelerometers fixed on the saddle. *Equine Vet. J.* **17**(Suppl.): 44–47.

Hjertén, G. and Drevemo, S. (1987) A method to analyse forces and moments in the extremities of the horse during the stance phase at the trot. In: *Equine Exercise Physiology 2* N.E. Robinson and J.R. Gillespie eds., Davis, California: ICEEP Publications, pp. 587–598.

Hogan, H.A., Wichtmann, A.D. and Hood, D.M. (1991) Finite element analysis of the internal deformation and stresses in the equine distal digit. *Proc. 10th Ann. Mtg. Assoc. Equine Sports Med.,* p. 43.

Jansen, M.O., Bogert, A.J., van den, Riemersma, D.J. and Schamhardt, H.C. (1993) In vivo tendon forces in the forelimb of ponies at the walk, validated by ground reaction force measurements. *Acta. Anat.* **146**: 162–167.

Lanovaz, J.L., Clayton, H.M., Colborne, G.R. and Schamhardt, H.C. (1999) Forelimb kinematics and net joint moments during the swing phase of the trot. *Equine Vet. J.,* **30**(Suppl.): 235–239.

Les, C.M., Keyak, J.H., Stover, S.M. and Taylor, K.T. (1997) Development and validation of three dimensional finite element models of the equine metacarpus. *J. Biomech.* **30**: 737–742.

McGurk, M., Amis, A.A., Potamianos, P. and Goodger, N.M. (1997) Rapid prototyping techniques for anatomical modeling in medicine. *Annals Royal Coll. Surg. England* **79**: 169–174.

Mulier, J.C., Mulier, M., Brady, L.P. *et al.* (1989) A new system to produce intraoperatively custom femoral prosthesis from measurements taken during the surgical procedure. *Clin. Orthop. Related Res.* **249**: 97–112.

Riemersma, D.J., Schamhardt, H.C., Hartman, W. and Lammertink, J.L.M.A. (1988). Kinetics and kinematics of the equine hind limb: In vivo tendon loads and force plate measurements in ponies. *Am. J. Vet. Res.* **49**: 1344–1352.

Schryver, H.F., Bartel, D.L., Langrana, N. and Lowe, J.E. (1978) Locomotion in the horse: kinematics and external and internal forces in the normal equine digit in the walk and trot. *Am. J. Vet. Res.* **39**: 1728–1733.

Thompson, K.N. and Cheung, T.K. (1993) A finite element model of the proximal sesamoid bones of the horse under different loading conditions. *Vet. Comp. Orthop. Traumatol.* **7**: 35–39.

Index

Note: page numbers in *italics* refer to figures and tables